Handbook of
Clinical Behavior
Therapy with Adults

Handbook of Clinical Behavior Therapy with Adults

Edited by

MICHEL HERSEN
Western Psychiatric Institute and Clinic
University of Pittsburgh School of Medicine
Pittsburgh, Pennsylvania

and

ALAN S. BELLACK
Medical College of Pensylvania at EPPI
Philadelphia, Pennsylvania

Plenum Press • New York and London

Library of Congress Cataloging in Publication Data

Main entry under title:

Handbook of clinical behavior therapy with adults.

Includes bibliographies and index.
1. Behavior therapy. I. Hersen, Michel. II. Bellack, Alan S. [DNLM: 1. Behavior
Therapy—in adulthood—handbooks. 2. Mental Disorders—therapy—handbooks.
WM 34 H236]
RC489.B4H375   1985   616.89′142   85-9503
ISBN 0-306-41875-4

©1985 Plenum Press, New York
A Division of Plenum Publishing Corporation
233 Spring Street, New York, N.Y. 10013

Printed in the United States of America

To
Our
Parents

Contributors

MARGRET A. APPEL, *Department of Psychology, Porter Hall, Ohio University, Athens, Ohio*

JACK S. ANNON, *The Royal Queen Emma, Suite 604, 222 South Vineyard Street, Honolulu, Hawaii*

BERNARD J. BALLEWEG, *Department of Psychology, University of Montana, Missoula, Montana*

ROBERT E. BECKER, *Behavior Therapy Unit, Department of Psychiatry, Medical College of Pennsylvania at EPPI, 3200 Henry Avenue, Philadelphia, Pennsylvania*

ALAN S. BELLACK, *The Medical College of Pennsylvania at EPPI, 3200 Henry Avenue, Philadelphia, Pennsylvania*

MARY JANE BLACK, *Department of Psychiatry, St. Luke's Hospital, Cleveland, Ohio*

PHILIP H. BORNSTEIN, *Department of Psychology, University of Montana, Missoula, Montana*

HENRY M. BOUDIN, *Center for Psychological Services, Suite 310, Chin Hills Building, 3915 Talbot Road South, Renton, Washington*

DIANNE L. CHAMBLESS, *Department of Psychology, The American University, Washington, District of Columbia*

CAROL E. CORNELL, *J. Hillis Miller Health Center, Department of Basic Dental Sciences, University of Florida, Box J-424, Gainesville, Florida*

LINDA WILCOXON CRAIGHEAD, *Division of Counseling and Educational Psychology, The Pennsylvania State University, University Park, Pennsylvania*

JAMES P. CURRAN, *Veterans Administration Medical Center, Brown University Medical School, Providence, Rhode Island*

C. J. DAVIS, *Department of Psychology, Louisiana State University, Baton Rouge, Louisiana*

STEPHEN V. FARAONE, *Veterans Administration Medical Center, Brown University Medical School, Providence, Rhode Island*

VIVIAN FERNANDEZ, *Department of Psychology, University of Southern California, Seeley G. Mudd Building, University Park, Los Angeles, California*

SUZANNE M. FISCHER, *Department of Psychology, Memphis State University, Memphis, Tennessee*

EDNA B. FOA, *Department of Psychiatry, Behavior Therapy Section, Eastern EPPI, 3300 Henry Avenue, Philadelphia, Pennsylvania*

K. GUNNAR GÖTESTAM, *Department of Psychiatry and Behavioural Medicine, University of Trondheim, Trondheim, Norway*

JONATHAN B. GRAYSON, *Department of Psychiatry, Behavior Therapy Section, Eastern EPPI, 3300 Henry Avenue, Philadelphia, Pennsylvania*

SIMONE GUENETTE, *Veterans Administration Medical Center, Davis Park, Providence, Rhode Island*

FRANCIS C. HARRIS, *Western Psychiatric Institute and Clinic, University of Pittsburgh School of Medicine, Pittsburgh, Pennsylvania*

RICHARD G. HEIMBERG, *Center for Stress and Anxiety Disorders, State University of New York at Albany, 1535 Western Avenue, Albany, New York*

MICHEL HERSEN, *Western Psychiatric Institute and Clinic, University of Pittsburgh School of Medicine, Pittsburgh, Pennsylvania*

STEVEN D. HOLLON, *Department of Psychology, University of Minnesota and St. Paul-Ramsey Medical Center, Minneapolis, Minnesota*

KENNETH A. HOLROYD, *Department of Psychology, Porter Hall, Ohio University, Athens, Ohio*

VIRGINIA JACOBSON, *Ramsey County Adult Mental Health Center, St. Paul, Minnesota*

JEFFREY A. KELLY, *Department of Psychiatry, University of Mississippi Medical Center, 2500 North State Street, Jackson, Mississippi*

DANUTA M. LAMPARSKI, *Department of Psychiatry, University of Mississippi Medical Center, 2500 North State Street, Jackson, Mississippi*

DAVID M. LAWSON, *Division of Psychology, Shaughnessy Hospital, 4500 Oak Street, Vancouver, British Columbia and Department of Psychology, University of British Columbia, 2136 West Mall, Vancouver, British Columbia, Canada*

PAUL M. LEHRER, *Department of Psychology, Rutgers Medical School, University of Medicine and Dentistry of New Jersey, Piscataway, New Jersey*

KENNETH L. LICHSTEIN, *Department of Psychology, Memphis State University, Memphis, Tennessee*

STEVEN J. LINTON, *Department of Occupational Medicine, Örebro Medical Centre Hospital, Örebro, Sweden*

GAYLA MARGOLIN, *Department of Psychology, University of Southern California, Seeley G. Mudd Building, University Park, Los Angeles, California*

NATHANIEL McCONAGHY, *Psychiatry Unit, Prince of Wales Hospital, Randwick, New South Wales, Australia*

F. DUDLEY McGLYNN, *J. Hillis Miller Health Center, Department of Basic Dental Sciences, University of Florida, Box J-424, Gainesville, Florida*

JAMES R. MOON, *Department of Aging Programs, Florida Mental Health Institute, The University of South Florida, Tampa, Florida*

ROGER L. PATTERSON, *Director, Geriatric Rehabilitation Project (116B), Veterans Administration Medical Center, Tuskegee, Alabama*

CAROLYN F. PHELPS, *Department of Psychology, University of Pittsburgh, Pittsburgh, Pennsylvania*

PATRICIA A. RESICK, *Department of Psychology, University of Missouri–St. Louis, St. Louis, Missouri*

C. STEVEN RICHARDS, *Department of Psychology, College of Arts and Sciences, Syracuse University, Syracuse, New York*

CRAIG H. ROBINSON, *The Royal Queen Emma, Suite 604, 222 South Vineyard Street, Honolulu, Hawaii*

LAURIE RUGGIERO, *Department of Psychology, Louisiana State University, Baton Rouge, Louisiana*

PATRICE G. SAAB, *Department of Psychiatry, University of Pittsburgh, Pittsburgh, Pennsylvania*

HAROLD E. SCHROEDER, *Department of Psychology, Kent State University, Kent, Ohio*

GAIL STEKETEE, *Department of Psychiatry, Temple University, Philadelphia, Pennsylvania*

ROBERT G. SUTTON, *Veterans Administration Medical Center, Davis Park, Providence, Rhode Island*

SUSAN R. WALEN, *Baltimore Center for Cognitive Therapy, 6303 Greenspring Avenue, Baltimore, Maryland*

CHARLES E. WEISSER, *Department of Psychology, University of Montana, Missoula, Montana*

DONALD A. WILLIAMSON, *Department of Psychology, Louisiana State University, Baton Rouge, Louisiana*

ROBERT L. WOOLFOLK, *Department of Psychology, Busch Campus, Rutgers University, New Brunswick, New Jersey*

Preface

Despite the occasional outcries to the contrary, the field of behavior therapy is still growing, and the asymptote has not been reached yet. The umbrella of behavior therapy continues to enlarge and still is able to encompass new theories, new concepts, new research, new data, and new clinical techniques. Although the number of new behavioral journals now has stabilized, we still see a proliferation of books on the subject.

In the past few years, however, we have seen considerable specialization within behavior therapy. No longer is it possible to be a generalist and remain fully abreast of all the relevant developments. Thus, we see behavior therapists who deal with adults, those who deal with children, those whose specialty is hospital psychiatry, and those who see themselves as practitioners of behavioral medicine. Even within a subarea such as behavioral medicine, specialization runs supreme to the extent that there are experts in the specific addictions, adult medical problems, and child medical problems.

Given the extent of specialization, there are numerous ways "to skin" the proverbial "cat." We therefore have chosen to look at the contemporary work in behavior therapy that is being carried out with adults, in part, of course, because of our long-standing interest in this area as teachers, researchers, and clinicians. In so doing, we have chosen to highlight the clinical aspects of the endeavor but not at the expense of the rich research heritage for each of the specific adult disorders.

The thrust of this handbook is more clinical than competing works because we find that many of our students and some colleagues with differing theoretical persuasions still consider what behavior therapists do in their clinical encounters to be somewhat of a mystery. Thus, for pedagogic reasons, we have asked each of our contributors to follow, to the extent feasible, a general outline for the discussion of the specific disorders: (a) introduction and description; (b) assessment; (c) range of treatment techniques available; (d) limitations and problems with the techniques; (e) illustrative case study, with actual therapist–patient dialogue when available; and (f) problems encountered during the course of treatment. But all of the aforementioned does appear within the context of extant clinical-research findings.

The book is divided into six parts. Following Part I (Introduction) we have five chapters dealing with the Anxiety Disorders (Part II). Part III (Depression) includes two different treatment approaches currently being carried out for the depressive disorders, whereas Part IV (Behavioral Medicine) includes seven chapters dealing with medical problems. Two approaches (inpatient and outpatient) are devoted to the treatment of Schizophrenia in Part V. Finally, in Part VI we have eight chapters on a variety of issues that fall under the general rubric of Special Problems.

Many people have devoted time and effort to the development and production of this handbook. First and foremost are our contributors who agreed to share their expertise with us. To them, we express our heartfelt thanks. Second are our secretaries and technicians (Susan Capozzoli, Florence Levito, Mary Newell, and Janet Twomey) without whom we could not have carried out a project of this magnitude. Finally, we thank the good people at Plenum Press for their excellent workmanship, and particularly Eliot Werner, our editor, who agreed as to the timeliness of this project in the first place.

MICHEL HERSEN
ALAN S. BELLACK

Contents

Introduction

I

General Considerations

ALAN S. BELLACK AND MICHEL HERSEN

Introduction

Selecting a title for a book is a deceptively difficult task. First and foremost, the title should reflect the content and purpose of the volume. It must also be brief and distinct from other books on the same or similar topics. This poses a special challenge with a book on such a heavily published topic as *behavior therapy*. These restrictions place a premium on each and every word in the title. There really is no room for any extra words or words that are subject to misinterpretation. This brief discourse underscores our very careful and pointed use of the word *clinical* to modify *behavior therapy* in the title of this book. At first glance, the word might seem redundant. After all, behavior therapy is an applied discipline. Surely, there is no such thing as nonclinical behavior therapy. Yet, in some respects there are two behavior therapies.

One is the behavior therapy described in textbooks and the method sections of countless journal articles. In this behavior therapy, client/subjects come for help with single, narrowly defined problems, the nature of which is seemingly so obvious that it must be tatooed on their foreheads. There are no treatment decisions to be made, and therapists are able to conduct all treatments exactly as specified. Client/subjects dutifully report for all sessions and are cooperative throughout. They never raise questions about such prosaic issues as inability to pay fees or the fact that treatment does not seem to be getting at their real problems. Nor do they ever disclose facts in the middle of treatment that change the diagnosis and direction of treatment. Client/subjects do not all improve in this behavior therapy, but treat-

ALAN S. BELLACK • The Medical College of Pennsylvania at EPPI, 3200 Henry Avenue, Philadelphia, Pennsylvania 19129. MICHEL HERSEN • Western Psychiatric Institute and Clinic, University of Pittsburgh School of Medicine, Pittsburgh, Pennsylvania 15213.

ment rarely requires more than 8 or 10 sessions, regardless of outcome or individual variability.

The second behavior therapy is the one practiced in clinics, hospitals, and consulting offices. It rarely appears to be as simple and straightforward as the former type. Client/patients present with multiple problems that are most difficult to separate and categorize. Moreover, they frequently have the annoying habit of disrupting treatment plans by divulging new information as they become more comfortable with the therapist or by having crises that require immediate attention. They do not always attend weekly sessions, follow instructions, or cooperate. For their part, therapists in this behavior therapy feel a need to be responsive to these vagaries on the part of their client/patients. They also frequently enjoy talking to them more than conducting repetitive, highly structured tasks. Consequently, the treatment for each client is individualized and difficult to describe in the objective fashion preferred in the first type of behavior therapy. Needless to say, this type of behavior therapy typically requires many more than 8 to 10 sessions.

The word *clinical* in our title refers to this second type of behavior therapy. The purpose of the book is to present what experienced clinicians actually do with their patients. Later in this chapter we will amplify on some of the differences between research and practice alluded to before. The remaining chapters will then discuss the clinical enterprise as it occurs with diverse adult disorders. However, we first will consider how behavior therapy evolved into this bifurcated discipline despite the intentions of most behavior therapists to develop an integrated clinical science.

Evolution of Behavior Therapy

The history of behavior therapy has been well documented (Kazdin, 1978). Many core "behavioral" techniques, such as exposure for reducing fears, shaping in the development of new skills, and positive reinforcement have been used throughout history, albeit without the specific labels and conceptualization provided by behavior therapy. They make intuitive sense and have simply been an ongoing part of man's attempt to control and improve the behavior of others. Beginning in the 20th century, such procedures have been systematized and tied more closely with scientific advances and theories about behavior. Two lines of study were especially critical in this regard. First, the Russian physiologists Sechenov, Pavlov, and Bechterev began their studies of reflexes, which led to the development of classical conditioning. At the same time, the American psychologist John B. Watson stimulated the movement away from mentalism and introspection by the development of behaviorism. Together, these two lines of work emphasized the critical effect of the environment on behavior and the value of studying behavior objectively (rather than subjectively, as by introspection).

The period between 1920 and 1950 saw marked progress in understanding of conditioning and learning. There were scattered demonstrations of how these new principles could be applied to human psychopathology. However, behavior therapy as a nascent discipline did not really begin until the late 1950s and early 1960s. During that period, the seminal work of B. F. Skinner, Joseph Wolpe, and Hans J. Eysenck combined to provide a beginning set of procedures, a theoretical framework, and a raison d'être for the behavioral revolution. The procedures were, of course, systematic desensitization and operant conditioning strategies (e.g., positive reinforcement, shaping). The theoretical framework was learning theory, or more specifically, the principles of classical and operant conditioning.

Reflecting on our experiences as graduate students during the 1960s, our sense is that the raison d'être may well have been the most critical ingredient of the three. To be sure, desensitization and operant conditioning were not the first exciting new treatment procedures to be developed since psychoanalysis was first introduced. For example, the client-centered therapy of Carl Rogers was equally revolutionary and had a major impact on clinical psychology, but it did not have the lasting effect of behavior therapy. The application of learning theory to psychopathology was also not unique to the new behavioral movement. Dollard and Miller had provided a lucid reinterpretation of psychoanalytic concepts in terms of learning theory as early as 1950. The catalyst that helped launch behavior therapy seems to have been a reaction to the failings of alternative approaches as much as the positive features of the initial behavioral procedures and model.

Two sources of dissatisfaction were especially paramount. First, there was a sense that traditional verbal psychotherapies (notably psychoanalytic therapies) were not effective. This sense was crystallized by Eysenck's landmark papers that purportedly documented that psychotherapy was no more effective than no treatment (Eysenck, 1952, 1960). Regardless of the scientific merits of his case, these arguments were based on data rather than on belief *per se*. Hence, they had added impact because they underscored the second major area of dissatisfaction with the psychoanalytic establishment: the failure to employ sound empirical methods to evaluate either theory or therapy practice.

The development of behavior therapy has been intimately tied to the development of clinical psychology after World War II. Trained in a research-oriented discipline, the burgeoning number of psychologists brought a strong empirical orientation to the clinical arena. They were adamant that progress in understanding and alleviating maladaptive behavior would only come through sound research. Conversely, psychoanalytic concepts and procedures were explicitly not amenable to systematic empirical evaluation. They were poorly defined and impossible to measure objectively. Perhaps most importantly, they were not subject to verification or disproof, in essence placing them "above" science. This was a source of great philosophical dissatisfaction above and beyond questions about effectiveness and validity.

In contrast, the new behavioral orientation was distinctly empirical. It initially eshewed obtuse intervening variables. Procedures and concepts were easy to define and measure objectively and were thus amenable to research evaluation. Moreover, they were based on the core learning principles that were taught in graduate seminars, providing a strong scientific patina. At times, the behavioral-analytic conflict seemed to be a struggle between science and philosophy as much as a debate between alternative views about the nature of human behavior.

We have emphasized our belief that behavior therapy developed, at least in part, as a reaction against traditional practices because that accounts for some of its current limitations as well as its strengths. In some respects, behavior therapy threw the proverbial baby out with the bathwater. Despite the many problems with psychoanalysis, many of its practitioners were brilliant clinicians. Their observations about a good number of clinical phenomena, including the importance of the therapeutic relationship and the fact that many problems are much more complex than is apparent in the client's initial presentation, were highly accurate. Yet, in an effort to establish its own position, behavior therapy rejected anything that smacked of an analytic, nonempirical approach (London, 1972).

In keeping with the rigidly empirical orientation, an undue premium was placed on conceptual and tactical simplicity. Subjective phenomena and complex procedures were discouraged, in part, because they were not amenable to easy investigation. This resulted in theories and techniques that, with 20/20 hindsight, seem naive. The use of simple aversive conditioning paradigms to treat alcoholism and punishment procedures to suppress schizophrenic hallucinations are two cases in point.

We are by no means arguing that all early behavioral interventions were naive or that subjectivity and complexity are inherently desirable. Procedures such as the token economy and systematic desensitization are elegant in their parsimony and are dramatically effective. But the excessive emphasis on simplicity and operationalism has significant limitations, many of which have become apparent as the field has accrued research and clinical experience. The recent development of cognitive behavior therapy is, perhaps, the most notable example (Mahoney, 1974; Meichenbaum, 1977).

Early efforts to explain all aspects of behavior by nonmediational, operant parameters (and to base all interventions accordingly) were simply not adequate. Cognitive phenomena are now widely incorporated in behavioral interventions, either as components of broad-based interventions or as the primary vehicle for change. Beck's cognitive therapy for depression (Beck, Rush, Shaw, & Emery, 1979) is a prime example of a new treatment based primarily on a cognitive-behavioral orientation. Depression is seen as a result of unrealistic and irrational beliefs about oneself, the world, and the future. Treatment entails teaching the patient new, more reasonable ways to think.

The evolution of early, narrowly conceived operant treatments toward a more multifaceted, integrated perspective is well illustrated by recent advances in behavioral marital therapy (Weiss & Weider, 1982). Early behavioral approaches to improving marital relationships focused almost exclusively on the spouses' exchange of reinforcers. "Love" was interpreted, essentially, as the direct consequence of the exchange of positive reinforcers and punishments in the relationship. Therapy, therefore, was viewed as a procedure to increase the ratio of positive reinforcers. More recently, behavioral marital therapists have emphasized communication training and the attributions spouses make about one another's behavior. In fact, the quid pro quo contracts formerly employed are now viewed as insufficient at best and harmful at worst because spouses appraise the motives underlying behavior (i.e., make attributions) rather than simply tallying the valences received.

As behavior therapy has increased in popularity, the field has broadened as well as having become more sophisticated. New interventions were developed for a broad range of problems. As indicated previously, other problems have been reconceptualized, and dramatically different types of interventions have been applied. Many of these new approaches fall under the *behavioral* umbrella more because their developers identify themselves as behavior therapists than because the techniques and theoretical underpinnings are specifically *behavioral*. Although they often are loosely tied to conditioning principles, these new procedures frequently defy easy categorization or operational definition. They owe their development more to clinical experience than to carefully controlled research programs.

The limited role accorded to research in the recent evolution of behavior therapy is in no small way due to the research strategies employed. It is extremely difficult to conduct well-controlled research in *real clinical settings*. The costs involved, ethical constraints, and limited numbers of matched patients available at any one time have precluded some types of research and made it virtually impossible for many behavior therapists to conduct even simple studies. As a result, the field has relied extensively on *analog* research. This term refers loosely to research employing subclinical populations (e.g., snake-phobic college students) and analogs of real clinical techniques (e.g., four sessions of group desensitization) in lieu of actual clinical patients and full-scale clinical interventions. Until recently, analog studies had been widely accepted as directly comparable to full-scale clinical trials. In fact, the research base of the field lies substantially on such research. However, it is now generally agreed that such research often is not a valid model of the clinical arena (Barlow, 1980; Hersen, 1981; Kazdin, 1979). College student volunteers with subclinical fears or depression are not fully equivalent to middle-aged patients spontaneously requesting treatment. Such mild problems often can be eliminated with minimal interventions, including education and persuasive placebos. Consequently, many of the principles and procedures developed in studies with these subjects are neither valid nor powerful enough for the clinical arena. Bibliotherapy and automated desensitization are prime examples. Clinicians have long complained about the limitations of analog research and the associated claims of quick and easy cures. Behavioral researchers have now also reached this conclusion as large-scale clinical research trials have supported the clinicians' observations.

Research and Clinical Distinctions

During the course of the last two decades we have been most privileged to have seen the tremendous developments in behavior therapy from a number of vantage points. In short, we have worn "different hats" at different times. Thus, we have evaluated the process of behavioral assessment (Hersen & Bellack, 1976, 1981), conducted single-case and controlled group outcome research (e.g., Bellack, Hersen, & Turner, 1976; Hersen, Bellack, Himmelhoch, & Thase, 1984; Turner, Hersen, Bellack, & Wells, 1979), taught behavioral principles to graduate students and psychiatric residents (e.g., Bellack & Hersen, 1977; Hersen & Bellack, 1978a), provided consultation to others (e.g., Bellack & Franks, 1975; Hersen & Bellack, 1978b), and have practiced clinically (e.g., Hersen, 1970, 1983). By wearing so many "hats," we have been in a position to observe the differences between the theory and research of behavior therapy and its clinical applications.

Although differences between textbook descriptions of clinical research projects and what practicing clinicians actually do in the consulting room are fewer in behavior therapy than the other theoretical approaches, *they do exist.* The purpose of this portion of our chapter is to document and discuss the vital differences. Of course, use of the single-case strategy (Hersen & Barlow, 1976) and its application by the empirically minded clinician (Barlow, Hayes, & Nelson, 1984) are attempts to diminish the research/clinical gap. But the very nature of the clinical endeavor makes it most difficult to carry out. Let us therefore consider why this may be the case.

Where Have All the Good Behavioral Cases Gone?

Some of the earlier behavior therapists may have done us an inadvertent disservice by repeatedly publishing their successful and rapid clinical treatments of monosymptomatic phobics. We take this position for several basic reasons. *First,* despite being on the decrease, in many circles (psychoanalytic, psychiatric) the prevailing notion remains that behavior therapy is limited to the application of very specific strategies with only highly defined problems. *Second,* as previously noted, there is the erroneous notion that treatment will be successful in 8 to 10 sessions or less (see Hersen, 1979, 1981, for further discussion of this issue) for the majority of cases referred. *Third,* there also is a misunderstanding that application of behavior therapy is inconsistent with the concurrent use of some other strategy, such as pharmacotherapy.

In our supervision of psychiatric residents in particular and to a somewhat lesser extent with graduate students and psychology interns, we have noted the resulting naive approaches to patient care due to the aforementioned misconceptions. We frequently hear the complaint that a given case "is not appropriate" for behavior therapy because there are no focal symptoms or because the patient is suffering from an "existential" problem or is "borderline." However, the student obviously has missed the point. Any case can be conceptualized as *behavioral, psychoanalytic,* or *Rogerian.* It is the specific task of the therapist to ferret out the relevant information that will make the case behavioral. That is, the specific circumstances and controlling variables maintaining inappropriate behavior or cognitions need to be determined. Generally, this will require a more protracted behavioral analysis than when the patient presents with phobia, obsessiveness, ritualistic behavior, sexual dysfunction, sexual deviation, or some other focal problem. We still are looking for the perfect textbook case but have not yet found it. Indeed, the ones that have appeared in the literature undoubtedly are the reconstruction of the therapist, not how the patient appeared at the first interview session.

There Are No Simple Cases

We (Hersen, 1981; Hersen & Bellack, 1977) and others (e.g., Wolpe, 1976) have tried to impress our readers with the fact that the behavioral enterprise is considerably more complicated than the outsider (i.e., nonbehavioral practitioner) peering in would imagine. And this is especially so when contrasting experimental behavioral treatment dictated by protocol to the more "freewheeling" and flexible approach carried out at the clinical level. That is not to say that clinicians treating patients in an approved research protocol are unaware of the intracacies and complexities of a particular case. However, when one closely follows a therapeutic protocol in, say, a grant, "secondary" features of the case will be directed less attention and perhaps neglected altogether. This should not be interpreted as a direct indictment of clinicians hired to provide clinical services on that grant. To the contrary, they are fulfilling the requirements of the protocol to ensure experimental precision. Thus, if the behavioral treatment is for an individual approach to depression, the therapist will not, in midcourse, switch to a conjoint marital therapy if the patient's sagging marriage is implicated as etiological. In short, the luxury of rapidly switching therapeutic gears is not readily available in the therapy research protocol unless a "doctor's choice" approach to treatment is being followed. Unfortunately, however, many tainted views of what behavior therapists do with complex cases are based on the experimental limitations imposed on protocol therapists.

Let us now turn to the clinical complexities that are presented to us by most of our patients. Even in the very few instances where a well-defined problem appears, exigencies in the patient's life experience undoubtedly will alter the therapist's game plan. Let us assume that we are treating a 26-year-old female phobic patient with standard systematic desensitization. Let us also assume that good progress has been attained after going up the hierarchy of items by the 9th treatment session. At the 10th session the patient appears for treatment one-half hour earlier than scheduled and visibly upset. She begins the session by recanting how she and her boyfriend just had a major quarrel over what she perceives to be his inattentiveness and neglect of her. During the course of the quarrel both partners have said things they now regret. Our patient, in particular, has alluded to the possibility of "breaking up." But, of course, this was said in the heat of the argument, and now she is fearful that he, too, feels rejected and that he may initiate separation in retaliation.

As for presentation of the aforementioned material, our patient does so under apparent distress and anxiety and with much affectual display. Several times during her presentation she breaks into tears. Faced with such a presentation, even the least sensitive of therapists would be cognizant of his or her patient's distress and know that some attention to the interpersonal crisis would be warranted (see Eisler

& Hersen, 1973). Only the most naive of student therapists would consider going on with the desensitization strategy planned for session 10. The sensitive therapist clearly understands the patient's need for catharsis, reassurance, and some attention to the interpersonal problem. Furthermore, the astute clinician begins to wonder how the particular phobia and the interpersonal stress relate to one another. Is there some causal connection? Was the initial behavioral analysis of her problem correct? Does systematic desensitization need to be supplemented or even supplanted by a strategy that remediates the interpersonal problem? Or will some counseling on boyfriend–girlfriend relations and expectations suffice? Of course, there is no protocol at this point that dictates how the clinician should operate, other than that he or she should be exquisitely sensitive to the nuances of the case as it unfolds over time. As a general rule of thumb, we have advised our students that when emergencies occur in otherwise straightforward cases, it behooves them to carefully evaluate the crisis, and to deal with it therapeutically but with the background of initial treatment in mind. In some such instances, the therapist is well advised to separate treatment sessions into (a) what's going on in your life now; and (b) implementation of original treatment plan and homework exercises. How much of each, of course, depends on the clinical presentation. But generally the sensitive clinician will be able to carry out a two-pronged approach to treatment.

Fishman and Lubetkin (1983), in their excellent chapter, "Office Practice of Behavior Therapy," also have commented on the complexity of clinical cases seen by behavior therapists. They point out that

> As patients' problems have become less circumscribed and multifaceted (this distinction may be more apparent than real—the change may be due to the way problems are currently assessed) over the decade of our practice, our own emphasis has shifted from a problem-centered, technique-oriented approach to strategies that provide our patients with more general coping capabilities. . . . Our goals for therapy are to provide the patient with skills for exercising greater control over their presenting problems and further, to provide them with the means for both assessing and remediating problems that may arise in their future functioning. This shift in emphasis in our own treatment planning is reflected in the fact that our mean number of sessions from intake to termination has increased from approximately 22 sessions, 10 years ago, to about 50 sessions per patient currently. (p. 23)

Are There Two Kinds of Behavioral Assessments?

In our experience, it is quite apparent that there is a considerable discrepancy between how behavioral assessment is applied during the course of group-controlled and single-case research and in clinical practice. Such discrepancies, of course, are due to financial, equipment, practical, and personnel limitations inherent in the clinical situation. Indeed, there can be no doubt that the evaluation a patient will receive in a research protocol will be significantly more comprehensive than the comparable one received clinically. This is highlighted by the fact that extensive motoric and physiological assessments of patients in the consulting room setting often are not possible, perhaps with the exception of those practitioners specializing in behavioral medicine and biofeedback. That is, most clinical behavioral practitioners do not have extensive electronic monitoring devices required for making precise physiological determinations. Nor do they have at their disposal the needed trained judges for making observations of actual motoric behavior in the natural environment.

To illustrate the aforementioned points, let us first consider the extensive diagnostic assessment afforded our female unipolar depressed patients seen in a controlled clinical trial pitting psychotherapy, social skills training, and amitriptyline against one another (see Bellack, Hersen, & Himmelhoch, 1981; Hersen, Bellack, Himmelhoch, & Thase, 1984). Prior to the study, all patients were withdrawn from psychotropic medication (if any), given a complete physical, EKG, and EEG, and other relevant laboratory tests. Then, during the extensive assessment phase, the self-report, observer rating, behavioral, and significant-other measures listed in Table 1 were administered. In this elaborate evaluation, the only category of assessment omitted was the physiological.

Let us now consider the type of behavioral assessment that might be conducted in the single-case experimental design study (e.g., Hersen & Bellack, 1976; Hersen, Turner, Edelstein, & Pinkston, 1975; Turner *et al.*, 1979). In one study (Hersen & Bellack, 1976), involving the social skills training of chronic schizophrenics, behavioral assessment consisted of eliciting role played responses to eight

Table 1. Measures Used in Bellack, Hersen, and Himmelhoch (1981) and Hersen, Bellack, Himmelhoch, and Thase (1984)

Type	Description
Self-Report	Beck Depression Inventory (Beck, Ward, Mendelson, Mock, & Erbaugh, 1961)
	Lubin Depression Adjective Check L (Lubin, 1965)
	Hopkins Symptom Checklist (Derogatis, Lipman, Rickles, Uhlenhath, & Covi, 1974)
	Wolpe–Lazarus Assertiveness Scale (Wolpe & Lazarus, 1966)
	Eysenck Personality Inventory (Eysenck & Eysenck, 1968)
Observer Ratings	Raskin Eligibility Depression Scale (Raskin, Schulterbrandt, Reatig, & Rice, 1967; Raskin, Schulterbrandt, Reatig, & McKeon, 1969)
	Hamilton's Rating Scale for Depression (Hamilton, 1960)
	Paykel *et al.*'s Assessment of Social Adjustment (Paykel, Weissman, Prusoff, & Tonks, 1971)
Behavioral	Behavioral Assertiveness Test-Revised (Eisler, Hersen, Miller, & Blanchard, 1975)
Significant Other	Katz Adjustment Scale-Relative (Katz & Lyerly, 1963)

scenarios requiring assertive responding. As noted in the method section of the article, the following was required to carry out the assessment:

> The behavioral assessment of subjects' responses to role-played interactions was conducted in a videotape studio arranged in a comfortable living room setting. Female and male role models sat next to the subject on a small two-seat sofa and provided prompts to facilitate responses. An adjoining control room separated by a one-way mirror contained videotape recording equipment and several videotape monitors. Role-played scenes were narrated by a research assistant (therapist) over the intercom from the control room. (Hersen & Bellack, 1976, p. 240)

All videotapes were subsequently rated by two independent judges on the following target behaviors: ratio of eye contact to speech duration, speech duration, number of requests, number of compliances, ratio of speech durations to words spoken, number of appropriate smiles, appropriate effect, and overall assertiveness.

In a second single-case experimental analysis (Turner *et al.*, 1979), ritualistic behavior (checking and washing) of a 66-year-old female compulsive was observed three times daily for 1-hour periods by a BA-level research technician. This was accomplished by observing the patient in her hospital room, using a 30 seconds on–30 second off method of recording data. A second BA-level research technician made independent judgments for one-third of the observation intervals for purposes of obtaining a reliability check. Behaviors recorded were as follows: hand-washing, possession washing, folding, arm rubbing, possession touching, possession marking, and placing/checking.

We might note that yet more elaborate behavioral assessment schemes have been followed to evaluate therapeutic progress during the course of single-case and group comparison analyses. Without belaboring the point, then, what can the behavioral clinician do in the way of assessment, given the limitations of the consulting room practice? In tackling this issue, Fishman and Lubetkin (1983) have articulated some broad goals with respect to the conceptualization of problems.

> Problem conception and subsequent treatment planning are not as straightforward as some therapists would like to believe. A multitude of factors must be taken into consideration during the assessment period: factors that ultimately affect treatment planning and eventual outcomes. From our perspective, the goals of behavioral assessment are multifold: (1) to cull out the parameters of the manifest problem, that is, the overt and covert or mediational determinants; (2) to identify trouble spots or dysfunctional thinking and behavior in all spheres of clients' functioning (e.g., familial, social, sexual, academic, and vocational) from an historical perspective to their current functioning; (3) to determine how each of the clients' problems is differentially weighted and interrelated, particularly with regard to the manifest problem; (4) to assess for the more subtle factors such as "secondary gain" and other such maintenance factors, which are discussed below; and (5) to prioritize treatment focus. These elements, along with keeping a watchful eye on the so-called unspecified variables, then become building blocks for the conceptual framework from which treatment planning follows. (p. 26)

In pursuing these broad objectives the clinician may (a) use structured interviews; (b) obtain ancillary information from family and friends; (c) have the patient self-monitor targeted behaviors; (d) observe behavior during the course of the therapeutic hour; (e) actually accompany the patient in some naturalistic settings and record behaviors (as in the case of agoraphobia; and (f) use records and permanent products of behavior (e.g., school grades, promotions at work, reconciliation with estranged wife) as evidence of therapeutic progress.

In some of the preceding strategies, however, there is a great reliance on the veracity of the patient's self-report (see Hersen, 1978), earlier eschewed by the pioneering behavior therapists. In fact, we are most amused by this course of events because behaviorists seem to have made a 180-degree turn on this issue, once so hotly debated as anathema to the principles of behaviorism. Indeed, the marked influence of cognitive therapists (e.g., Meichenbaum, 1976) undoubtedly appears to have taken hold, in that the self-report has been relegitimized by the behavioral practitioners. Thus, very much as in traditional dynamic psychotherapy, the patient's self-report seems to be one of the main vehicles for obtaining relevant information and gauging therapeutic progress. But how it is used is, of course, so vastly different in the two theoretical approaches.

In contrast to the clinical situation, in most single-case research studies the favored criterion is the patient's recorded motoric or physiological behavior (Hersen & Barlow, 1976). And in controlled group outcome studies, both motoric and self-report measures seem to have been accorded equal criterion status. To recapitulate, then, there are some major differences in how behavioral assessments are carried out, depending on whether they are in a clinical or research setting. This is both in terms of mode of the assessment and its complexity and comprehensiveness. To answer our original question, then, "Yes, there are two kinds of behavioral assessments!" Indeed, there may be three, especially if differences in assessment between single-case and group comparison research also are considered.

How Important Is the Therapist–Patient Relationship?

In responding to the question that is raised in this section, the answer, of course, is a resounding *extremely!* In fact, here again we are left with the legacy of earlier behavior therapists who, in attempts to underscore the unique features of their approach, highlighted technical aspects of treatment at the expense of the therapeutic relationship. Along these lines, in the late 1960s, Lang (1969) and Krapfl and Nawas (1969) reported the successful use of automated procedures, i.e., the Device for Automated Desensitization (DAD) for ameliorating minor fears (e.g., test anxiety, public speaking) experienced by college students. The DAD was a programmed apparatus that contained relaxation instructions and a tape-recorded hierarchy. In addition, subjects' physiological responses to item presentation were automatically recorded. Items presented on the hierarchy were controlled according to predetermined criteria (number of the subjects' nonanxious repetitions).

Although these were highly specific applications of systematic desensitization that certainly did not represent the norm of actual clinical practice, they did set the stage for presenting behavior therapy in a cold and mechanistic light. Other accounts of the therapist as a "social reinforcement machine" (Krasner, 1962) similarly did little to portray the behavior therapist as he or she really is (i.e., a warm, empathetic, understanding, and caring professional).

Perhaps it is the classic Sloane, Staples, Cristol, Yorkston, and Whipple (1975) controlled clinical trial contrasting behavior therapy and psychotherapy that did the most to dispel the myth of the "cold, calculating behavior therapist." Indeed, in an empirical evaluation of Truax therapist variables, Sloane *et al.* (1975) documented that

> behavior therapists showed a significantly higher level of interpersonal contact than did psychotherapists. In addition, behavior therapists showed a significant higher level of Accurate Empathy and of Therapist Self-Congruence than did psychotherapists. Both showed an equal degree of warmth or unconditional positive regard towards the patient. (pp. 147–148)

In a similar evaluation in one of our own clinical trials (Greenwald, Kornblith, Hersen, Bellack, & Himmelhoch, 1981), behavior therapists showed more initiative, seemed more supportive, and made more directive and nondirective statements than their psychotherapist counterparts.

Of all of the extant therapeutic schools, it is in behavior therapy that the therapeutic alliance with the patient is most critical (cf. DeVoge & Beck, 1978; Fishman & Lubetkin, 1983; Hersen, 1983; Martin & Worthington, 1982). Fishman and Lubetkin (1983), strictly from a clinical perspective, make it crystal clear why this is the case.

> First, generally, behavior therapy is a directive psychotherapeutic approach and presupposes both the cooperation and the active participation of the client in the therapy process. Without the establishment of a constructive therapeutic relationship, it is doubtful whether the client will carry out the between-session home practice that is necessary for behavior therapy to be maximally efficacious. . . . Second, a high percentage of patients' presenting problems fall in the interpersonal-social sphere. Role-playing and behavior rehearsal which involve the therapist and the client "playing out" a number of the situations in which the client is experiencing difficulties comprise a significant part of treatment. By means of this process, the therapist can supply constructive and corrective feedback to the client about the verbal and nonverbal behavior that seems to be interfering with his or her optimal functioning. The socially reticent client, unless the therapeutic relationship is sound, will be reluctant to participate in the role-playing process and, in all likelihood, will be unresponsive to the therapist's feedback. . . . Third, . . . many of the methods and techniques in behavior therapy involve skill acquisition, which requires a continuity of between-session practice on the part of the client. Additionally, in keeping with the "canon of gradualness," the client is typically asked to progress by approximations; such progress is predicated on the assumption that the behavior therapist can keep the client sufficiently motivated to continue with his or her independent practice. . . . Finally, frequently used techniques, participant modeling and "in vivo" desensitization, require the therapist to accompany the client into their [*sic*] fear-producing situations and to model "nonfearful behavior." In such instances the therapist must provide a sense of support and encouragement and,

more importantly, impart a sense of security to the client. Unless such relationship factors are operative, it is highly doubtful that behavior therapy would have much value in the treatment of a clinical population. (pp. 25–26)

Behavior Therapy and Pharmacotherapy

Although behavior therapy is still carried out primarily by nonmedical practitioners, there have been some judicious attempts to combine it with pharmacotherapy by those clinical psychologists who work in psychiatric in- and outpatient settings (cf. Hersen *et al.*, 1975; Turner, Hersen, & Alford, 1974; Wells, Turner, Bellack, & Hersen, 1978). As noted elsewhere, integration of pharmacological and behavioral approaches has been carried out basically under four circumstances: (a) experimental analyses of pharmacological treatment; (b) behavioral strategies to motivate drug compliance; (c) drugs applied to facilitate behavioral treatment (and the reverse as well); and (d) the comparative assessment of drugs and behavioral treatment. The marriage of these two empirical approaches can only be conceptualized as natural and needed, despite the parallel paths they have taken until relatively recently. We say this because pharmacotherapy and behavior therapy are the two most empirical and data-based therapeutic approaches seen in the last two decades. Indeed, many calls for the rapprochement of the two strategies have been noted in the recent literature (Alford & Williams, 1980; Stern, 1978).

The use of pharmacotherapy in behavior therapy with adult patients is of particular importance. Let us consider a few illustrative examples. *First,* when dealing with day-hospital schizophrenics, use of neuroleptics is essential to bring psychotic features under control in order to facilitate social skills strategies (see Hersen & Bellack, 1976). Put more simply, the actively psychotic schizophrenic patient will not be able to attend sufficiently to benefit from a skills program until primary symptomatology is suppressed pharmacologically. Second, in some instances, the management of anxiety is enhanced by use of anxiolytics on a short-term basis (Turner *et al.*, 1974). In still other instances (Roth, Bielski, Jones, Parker, & Osborne, 1982; Thase, Hersen, Bellack, & Himmelhoch, 1984; Wilson, 1982), a combination of behavior therapy and pharmacotherapy will yield significantly more rapid initial symptomatic relief, although ultimately over 6 to 12 weeks the result will be the same as if behavior therapy were administered alone. However, this is a most critical issue for the patient who is unable to tolerate any delay in symptomatic relief. For the depressed patient in particular, this is important with regard to compliance in therapy, the ability to perform the activities of daily living, and with respect to suicide potential. Given these three factors, for selected depressed patients who are at greater risk for suicide and a prolonged episode of depression, use of drugs along with behavior therapy or preceding it definitely is indicated.

We are convinced that the combined approach to treatment is the wave of the future. Indeed, we expect to see an increased number of innovative clinical papers in the literature that highlight the synergistic effects of pharmacotherapy and behavior therapy with disturbed adult patients.

In the preceding sections, we have highlighted several limitations of contemporary behavior therapy, especially as related to the clinical arena. It seems apparent that the field is entering a new era. It is facing two critical questions, the answers to which will determine its future course and existence. The first question concerns the effectiveness of behavioral procedures in real clinical settings. The second involves determining what behavior therapy is. In this final section, we will briefly address these questions and consider some possible solutions.

We have already addressed the first question at some length. In summary, the core of research supporting the efficacy of behavioral treatments lies in analog studies, whose generality is questionable. To be sure, this research has contributed significantly in advancing the field. For example, the tripartite composition of fears was uncovered through analog studies (Bellack, 1980) as was the fact that both exposure and response prevention are necessary in the treatment of obsessive compulsive disorder (Rachman, 1982). Yet it is essential that the pendulum now shift to more clinically relevant studies. A recent issue of the journal *Behavioral Assessment* (Summer/Fall, 1981) was devoted specifically to this problem. In his lead editorial upon assuming the editorship of *Behavior Therapy*, David Barlow (1983) called for the publication of clinical replication series in order to document the clinical validity of our procedures. This issue has also been a significant theme in most recent presidential addresses at the annual meetings of the Association for Advancement of Behavior Therapy.

Numerous recommendations have been made to encourage this change. These include such diverse proposals as changing tenure requirements in academic settings so as to discourage quick and easy publications, changing journal review and acceptance criteria, stimulating the research interests of clinicians so as increase their roles in generating research, and placing increased emphasis on single-case research so as to foster the intensive study of individual cases (Hayes & Nelson, 1981). Increasing the clinical relevance of analog studies, as by employing more rigid subject selection criteria and *in vivo* measures of change, has also been recommended (Kazdin, 1979). Our own feeling is that these specific suggestions all have merit but that the critical factor is to alter the orientation and values of the field. We simply must become more sensitive to the generality of our research. Clinical relevance must attain equal status with methodological purity in the planning and evaluation of research. If we can maintain this dual focus, no other specific changes will be necessary. If we do not, other changes will be insufficient.

The second major problem facing the field concerns its very identity: What is behavior therapy? Early definitions emphasized its base in learning theory as well as a commitment to behavioral principles (e.g., operationism) and research. It is now clear that the relationship of behavior therapy techniques to learning theory is remote at best (Kazdin & Wilson, 1978). Conditioning principles, broadly conceived, have served as a model and stimulus for our thinking. However, few techniques employ the precise stimulus-response sequencing associated with laboratory conditioning paradigms. Most employ a loose mélange of cognitive inputs and a variable pattern of stimulus-response pairing. Moreover, few techniques actually evolved directly from the laboratory or conditioning principles. Many of our most effective procedures, including the bell-and-pad method for enuresis, overcorrection, response prevention, and exposure, owe their development more to clinical insight than to any experimental or theortical pedigree.

As the field has shaken off its supposed ties to learning theory and narrowly conceived research models, it has become more and more difficult to arrive at a definition that is sufficiently broad to encompass its diverse aspects, while at the same time reflecting some characteristics that set it apart from other orientations (Franks & Barbrack, 1983). The most widely accepted current definition is the one endorsed by the Association for Advancement of Behavior Therapy (Franks & Barbrack, 1983). The two key elements of that definition are that behavior therapy techniques are based on principles derived from research in experimental and social psychology (not specifically learning principles) and that it emphasizes empirical evaluation of effectiveness. These are certainly noteworthy principles, and they are, regrettably, not inherent aspects of all other approaches. However, they are certainly not unique to behavior therapy, and they do not delimit the field. Essentially, any empirical approach, including pharmacotherapy and psychosurgery, could qualify. We are not presumptuous enough to set limits on what should or should not be categorized as a behavior therapy technique, but we do strongly believe that the field does need a more specific identity. As indicated before, many current "behavioral" techniques are behavioral primarily because of the professional identity of the developer rather than because of anything inherent to the procedure. Often, these individuals developed their professional identities in the earlier days of the field and have simply continued their allegiance. If this trend continues, there will be decreasing rationale for current and future students to become behavior therapists, as opposed to empirical eclectics. Given the dramatic and significant contributions made by behavior therapy up to this point, it would be tragic for the field to disappear by default. Our highest priority must be to forge an identity that is broad enough to facilitate further growth in diverse areas but that at the same time is specific enough to set us apart and highlight our contributions to the mental health and educational arenas.

References

Alford, G. S., & Williams, J. G. (1980). The role and uses of psychopharmacological aspects in behavior therapy. In M. Hersen, R. M. Eisler, & P. M. Miller (Eds.), *Progress in behavior modification* (Vol. 20). New York: Academic Press.

Barlow, D. H. (1980). Behavior therapy: The next decade. *Behavior Therapy, 11,* 315–328.

Barlow, D. H. (1983). Announcement. *Behavior Therapy, 14,* i–ii.

Barlow, D. H., Hayes, S. C., & Nelson, R. O. (1984). *The scientist practitioner: Research accountability in clinical and educational settings.* New York: Pergamon Press.

Beck, A. T., Ward, C. H., Mendelson, M., Mock, J., & Erbaugh, J. (1961). An inventory for measuring depression. *Archives of General Psychiatry, 4,* 561–571.

Beck, A. T., Rush, A. J., Shaw, B. F., & Emery, G. (1979). *Cognitive therapy of depression.* New York: Guilford Press.

Bellack, A. S. (1980). Anxiety and neurotic disorders. In A. E. Kazdin, A. S. Bellack, & M. Hersen (Eds.), *New perspectives in abnormal psychology*. New York: Oxford University Press.

Bellack, A. S., & Franks, C. M. (1975). Behavioral consultation in the community mental health center. *Behavior Therapy, 6,* 388–391.

Bellack, A. S., & Hersen, M. (1977). *Behavior modification: An introductory textbook*. New York: Oxford University Press.

Bellack, A. S., Hersen, M., & Himmelhoch, J. (1981). Social skills training compared with pharmacotherapy and psychotherapy in the treatment of unipolar depression. *American Journal of Psychiatry, 12,* 1562–1567.

Bellack, A. S., Hersen, M., & Turner, S. M. (1976). Generalization effects of social skills training in chronic schizophrenics: An experimental analysis. *Behaviour Research and Therapy, 14,* 391–398.

Derogatis, L. R., Lipman, R. S., Rickles, K., Uhlenhuth, E. H., & Covi, L. (1974). The Hopkins Symptom Checklist (HSCL): A self-report symptom inventory. *Behavioral Science, 19,* 1–15.

DeVoge, J. T., & Beck, S. (1978). The therapist–client relationship in behavior therapy. In M. Hersen, R. M. Eisler, & P. M. Miller (Eds.), *Progress in behavior modification* (Vol. 6). New York: Academic Press.

Eisler, R. M., & Hersen, M. (1973). Behavioral techniques in family-oriented crisis intervention. *Archives of General Psychiatry, 28,* 111–116.

Eysenck, H. J. (1952). The effects of psychotherapy: An evaluation. *Journal of Consulting Psychology, 16,* 319–324.

Eysenck, H. J. (1960). The effects of psychotherapy. In H. J. Eysenck (Ed.), *Handbook of abnormal psychology: An experimental approach*. London: Pittman Press.

Eysenck, H., & Eysenck, S. (1968). *The Eysenck Personality Inventory*. San Diego: Educational and Industrial Testing Service.

Fishman, S. T., & Lubetkin, B. S. (1983). Office practice of behavior therapy. In M. Hersen (Ed.), *Outpatient behavior therapy: A clinical guide*. New York: Grune & Stratton.

Franks, C. M., & Barbrack, C. R. (1983). Behavior therapy with adults: An integrative perspective. In M. Hersen, A. E. Kazdin, & A. S. Bellack (Eds.), *The clinical psychology handbook*. New York: Pergamon Press.

Greenwald, D. P., Kornblith, S. J., Hersen, M., Bellack, A. S., & Himmelhoch, J. M. (1981). Differences between social skills therapists and psychotherapists in treating depression. *Journal of Consulting and Clinical Psychology, 49,* 757–759.

Hayes, S. C., & Nelson, R. O. (1981). Clinically relevant research: Requirements, problems, and solutions. *Behavioral Assessment, 3,* 209–216.

Hamilton, M. (1960). A rating scale for depression. *Journal of Neurology, Neurosurgery, and Psychiatry, 23,* 56–61.

Hayes, S. C., & Nelson, R. O. (1981). Clinically relevant research: Requirements, problems, and solutions. *Behavioral Assessment, 3,* 209–216.

Hersen, M. (1970). The use of behavior modification techniques within a traditional psychotherapeutic context. *American Journal of Psychotherapy, 25,* 308–313.

Hersen, M. (1978). Do behavior therapists use self-reports as major criteria? *Behavioural Analysis and Modification, 2,* 328–334.

Hersen, M. (1979). Limitations and problems with clinical application of behavioral techniques in psychiatric settings. *Behavior Therapy, 10,* 65–80.

Hersen, M. (1981). Complex problems require complex solutions. *Behavior Therapy, 12,* 15–29.

Hersen, M. (Ed.). (1983). *Outpatient behavior therapy: A clinical guide*. New York: Grune & Stratton.

Hersen, M., & Barlow, D. H. (1976). *Single case experimental designs: Strategies for studying behavior change*. New York: Pergamon Press.

Hersen, M., & Bellack, A. S. (1976). Multiple-baseline analysis of social-skills training in chronic schizophrenics. *Journal of Applied Behavior Analysis, 9,* 239–245.

Hersen, M., & Bellack, A. S. (1977). Behavior modification: Sophisticated or naive? *Behavior Modification, 1,* 3–6.

Hersen, M., & Bellack, A. S. (1978). *Behavior therapy in the psychiatric setting*. Baltimore: Williams & Wilkins.

Hersen, M., & Bellack, A. S. (1978). Staff training and consulation. In M. Hersen & A. S. Bellack (Eds.), *Behavior therapy in the psychiatric setting*. Baltimore: Williams & Wilkins.

Hersen, M., & Bellack, A. S. (Eds.). (1981). *Behavioral assessment: A practical handbook*. New York: Pergamon Press.

Hersen, M., Bellack, A. S., Himmelhoch, J. M., & Thase, M. E. (1984). Effects of social skills training, amitriptyline, and psychotherapy in unipolar depressed women. *Behavior Therapy, 15,* 21–40.

Hersen, M., Turner, S. M., Edelstein, B. A., & Pinkston, S. G. (1975). Effects of phenothiazines and social skills training in a withdrawn schizophrenic. *Journal of Clinical Psychology, 31,* 588–594.

Katz, M. M., & Lyerly, S. B. (1963). Methods for measuring adjustment and social behavior in the community: Vol. 1. Rationale, description, discriminative validity and scale development. *Psychological Reports, 13,* 503–535.

Kazdin, A. E. (1979). Fictions, factions, and functions of behavior therapy. *Behavior Therapy, 10,* 629–654.

Kazdin, A. E., & Wilson, G. T. (1978). *Evaluation of behavior therapy: Issues, evidence, and research strategies.* Cambridge, MA: Ballinger.

Krapfl, J. E., & Nawas, M. M. (1969). Client-therapist relationship factors in systematic desensitization. *Journal of Consulting and Clinical Psychology, 33,* 435–439.

Krasner, L. (1962). The therapist as a social reinforcement machine. In H. H. Strupp & L. Luborsky (Eds.), *Research in Psychotherapy* (Vol. 2). Washington, DC: American Psychological Association.

Lang, P. J. (1969). The mechanics of desensitization and the laboratory study of human fear. In C. M. Franks (Ed.), *Behavior therapy: Appraisal and status.* New York: McGraw-Hill.

London, P. (1972). The end of ideology in behavior modification. *American Psychologist, 27,* 913–920.

Lubin, B. (1965). Adjective checklists for the measurement of depression. *Archives of General Psychiatry, 12,* 57–62.

Mahoney, M. J. (1974). *Cognition and behavior modification.* Cambridge, MA: Ballinger.

Martin, G. A., & Worthington, E. L. (1982). Behavioral homework. In M. Hersen, R. M. Eisler, & P. M. Miller (Eds.), *Progress in behavior modification* (Vol. 13). New York: Academic Press.

Meichenbaum, D. (1976). A cognitive-behavior modification approach to assessment. In M. Hersen & A. S. Bellack (Eds.), *Behavioral assessment: A practical handbook.* New York: Pergamon Press.

Meichenbaum, D. H. (1977). *Cognitive behavior modification.* New York: Plenum Press.

Paykel, E. S., Weissman, M., Prusoff, B. A., & Tonks, C. M. (1971). Dimensions of social adjustment in depressed women. *Journal of Nervous and Mental Disease, 152,* 158–172.

Rachman, S. J. (1982). Obsessive-compulsive disorders. In A. S. Bellack, M. Hersen, & A. E. Kazdin (Eds.), *International handbook of behavior modification and therapy.* New York: Plenum Press.

Raskin, A., Schulterbrandt, J., Reatig, N., & Rice, C. (1967). Factors of psychopathology in interview, ward behavior and self-report ratings of hospitalized depressions. *Journal of Consulting Psychology, 31,* 270–278.

Raskin, A., Schultenbrandt, J., Reatig, N., & McKeon, J. J. (1969). Replication of factors of psychopathology in interview, ward behavior and self-report ratings of hospitalized depressions. *Journal of Nervous and Mental Disease, 148,* 87–98.

Roth, D., Bielski, R., Jones, M., Parker, W., & Osborne, G. (1982). A comparison of self-control therapy and combined self-control therapy and antidepressant medication in the treatment of depression. *Behavior Therapy, 13,* 133–144.

Sloane, R. B., Staples, F. R., Cristol, A. H., Yorkston, N. J., & Whipple, K. (1975). *Psychotherapy versus behavior therapy.* Cambridge: Harvard University Press.

Stern, R. (1978). Behavior therapy and psychotropic medication. In M. Hersen & A. S. Bellack (Eds.), *Behavior therapy in the psychiatric setting.* Baltimore: Williams & Wilkins.

Thase, M., Hersen, M., Bellack, A. S., & Himmelhoch, J. M. (1984). *Combining cognitive-behavioral and pharmacological treatments for depression: A review and some new data.* Unpublished manuscript.

Turner, S. M., Hersen, M., & Alford, H. (1974). Effects of massed practiced and meprobamate on spasmodic torticollis: An experimental analysis. *Behaviour Research and Therapy, 12,* 259–260.

Turner, S. M., Hersen, M., Bellack, A. S., & Wells, K. C. (1979). Behavioral treatment of obsessive-compulsive neurosis. *Behaviour Research and Therapy, 17,* 95–106.

Weiss, R. L., & Weider, G. B. (1982). Marital distress. In A. S. Bellack, M. Hersen, & A. E. Kazdin (Eds.), *International handbook of behavior modification and therapy.* New York: Plenum Press.

Wells, K. C., Turner, S. M., Bellack, A. S., & Hersen, M. (1978). Effects of cue-controlled relaxation on psychomotor seizures: An experimental analysis. *Behaviour Research and Therapy, 16,* 51–53.

Wilson, P. H. (1982). Combined pharmacological and behavioural treatment of depression. *Behaviour Research and Therapy, 20,* 173–184.

Wolpe, J. (1976). *Theme and variations: A behavior therapy casebook.* New York: Pergamon Press.

Wolpe, J., & Lazarus, A. A. (1966). *Behavior therapy techniques.* New York: Pergamon Press.

Anxiety Disorders

II

Simple Phobia

F. DUDLEY MCGLYNN AND CAROL E. CORNELL

Introduction

The term *simple phobia* refers to a large but clinically rare class of specific anxiety disorders characterized by uncommon fear/avoidance of tangible objects and/or situations. Using the rules of the third edition of the *Diagnostic and Statistical Manual of Mental Disorders* (DSM-III) (American Psychiatric Association, 1980), the most common clinically seen simple phobias are fears of heights (acrophobia), fears of confinement (claustrophobia), and fears of animals (zoophobia). If the rules of DSM-III are relaxed, then fairly widespread fears such as motoring, flying, medical, and weather-related phobias are among the most common. In principle, however, virtually any object or situation can become a functional cue for phobic fear/avoidance. Mental health professionals of past generations equipped themselves with very long lists of simple-phobia "diagnoses": for example, parthenophobia (fear of virgins), and necrophobia (fear of corpses).

DSM-III prompts the diagnosis of simple phobia for those anxiety disorders characterized by "a persistent, irrational fear of, and compelling desire to avoid an object or situation." Various qualifications also are provided, that is, care should be taken to differentially diagnose social phobia, agoraphobia, delusion-related avoidance, and obsessive-compulsive disorder. However, the DSM-III narrative will not suffice to guide behavioral assessment and treatment of the problem.

Behavioral Models of the Problem

At a gross level the problem of simple phobia lends itself readily to an analysis in S-R terms. On the stimulus side of the general S-R equation we usually have

F. DUDLEY McGLYNN and CAROL E. CORNELL • J. Hillis Miller Health Center, Department of Basic Dental Sciences, University of Florida, Box J-424, Gainesville, Florida 32610.

tangible or real-world antecedents to deal with, antecedents such as "a dog up the street and another one two blocks over," "that little dog chasing the covered wagon on television," or "the furry collar on Aunt Minnie's Sunday coat." On the response side of the general equation we have measurable responses to use, such as "following a circuitous route to the market," or "keeping records of times when dogs appear in television commercials," or "cardiac acceleration while riding to church with Aunt Minnie." Beyond a crude S-R connectionism, however, behavioral analysis of the problem of simple phobia is less straightforward.

Early mental health professionals learned the psychodynamic theory of phobia etiology, a theory in terms of which phobic avoidance mirrors displaced projection of hostile and/or erotic unconscious impulses (cf. Cameron, 1963). Not surprisingly, therefore, professionals' treatments for the phobic neuroses focused on "problems" seemingly far removed from the phobic behavior itself.

Early behavior therapists learned a conditioned emotionality theory of phobic *anxiety.* In the orthodox Pavlovian account, an unconditional stimulus (UCS) that evokes anxiety as an unconditional response (UCR) repeatedly follows in close temporal contiguity some conditional stimulus (CS) that did not initially elicit any anxiety. Later behavior therapists noted clear empirical shortcomings in the orthodox Pavlovian model. Some responded by offering revised or expanded "conditioning" formulations of the problem (Eysenck, 1976; Rachman, 1976). Others filled the gaps in a Pavlovian account with cognitive (e.g., expectancy) models of fear ontogeny (Carr, 1979; Reiss, 1980).

Early behavior therapists also learned the dual process fear-mediation theory of phobic *avoidance.* According to this view (Dollard & Miller, 1950; Mowrer, 1947), anxiety is first acquired by the aversive Pavlovian mechanism just described,

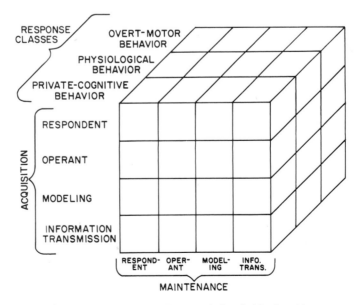

Figure 1. A multifaceted framework for phobic disorders.

and subsequently it serves as an aversive drive state whose contingent removal (or reduction) negatively reinforces instrumental escape/avoidance of the cues that produce it. Again, the light of history has revealed significant empirical weaknesses in the early account (cf. Bolles, 1970; Herrnstein, 1969). And, again, subsequent writers have offered alternative views of the avoidance problem (Bandura, 1977; Seligman & Johnston, 1973).

Delprato and McGlynn (1984) have offered a "multifaceted framework for anxiety disorders" that seems to distill contemporary behavior therapists' thinking about the ontogeny of simple phobias. A variant of the framework is shown in Figure 1. The model incorporates the three-systems view of fear (Lang, 1978; Rachman, 1977, 1978) in terms of which physiological behavior, overt motor behavior, and private/cognitive behavior are three substantially independent fear response classes. It proposes that fear behaviors within *any* of these response classes can be acquired via any one of four ontogenetic mechanisms; that is, by respondent conditioning, by operant contingencies, by modeling processes, and by the transmission of information. It also suggests that maintenance of fear behaviors within any response class is similarly, though independently, organized. To the clinician, the principal implication of the "multifaceted framework" is that simple phobias are not so simple after all—they entail uniquely interrelated physiological and/or motoric and/or private/cognitive fear behaviors, each with its own partially independent ontogeny.

General Approaches to Behavior Therapy

There seem to be three general orientations to the conduct of behavior therapy for phobias. One is an "orthodox behavior therapy" orientation (e.g., Wolpe, 1973), in terms of which controlled assessments of autonomic, motoric, and private/cognitive fear targets are used to guide selection of desensitization, fearless modeling, or flooding as the treatment mode. A second is a "monolithic exposure" orientation (e.g., Marks, 1975), in terms of which naturalistic assessments within the three classes of fear targets are used to guide exposure therapy—doing whatever it takes to expose the patient to feared stimulation. A third is a "cognitive behavior therapy" orientation (e.g., Bandura, 1977), in terms of which inferentially constructed performance-outcome expectations and/or generalized self-efficacy expectations are used to guide therapy tactics like self-directed mastery trials and rational restructuring.

For this chapter the cognitive behavior therapy approaches are omitted from the assessment section but are characterized in the treatment narrative. Our crystal ball tells us that monolithic exposure approaches will be the most popular treatments of phobias (including simple phobias) for the foreseeable future. At the same time we think it would be a mistake for behavior therapists to forget about orthodox behavior therapy methods. Hence, even though we agree with Marks (1975) that exposure is a fundamental ingredient common to successful fear reduction methods, we treat exposure *technology* here as a subset of classical behavioral methods.

Assessment

CHAPTER 2

Importance of Assessment

The general task of behavior therapy for simple phobia is threefold: (a) to pinpoint the precise stimuli that occasion the fear/avoidance; (b) to identify the exact nature and instrumental functions of the fear/avoidance (i.e., its physiological, behavioral, and private/cognitive manifestations); and (c) to implement, in a supportive but directive context, a therapy regimen that will replace anxious behaviors with nonanxious conduct in the presence of phobic stimuli. The first two of these are assessment activities, and they are important to reliable therapeutic success. Indeed, when behavior therapy for simple phobia does fail, defective or incomplete assessment probably is at fault.

The Goals of Assessment

As noted, the specific goals and techniques of assessment differ according to three general orientations. One general goal of orthodox behavioral assessment in cases of simple phobia is that of pinpointing the "type" of stimulus control that is involved with those fear/avoidance behaviors that prompted the patient to seek help. One or both of two types of stimulus control will be discovered. In the *first,* the patients' anxious behaviors are more or less automatically cued by encountering an actual phobic stimulus. This is seen, for example, in the cockroach-phobic patient who telephones the therapist while perched atop a kitchen chair where she finds she has just sought refuge from the roach in the laundry. In the *second* type of stimulus control, the patient encounters an environmental event that is not aversive in and of itself but that does serve reliably as a cue for fear-related activities. This is seen, for example, in the dog-phobic patient who begins ruminating about the dog up the street or who begins privately rehearsing a "safe" route to the market in response to viewing a dog on television. In any given patient, his or her help seeking might have been prompted by fear behaviors regulated in either or both of the preceding ways.

A second general goal of orthodox behavioral assessment in cases of simple phobia is that of specifying the "content" of the controlling stimulus involved with the targeted fear behaviors. This involves specifying exhaustively the exact stimuli (e.g., specific rooms, stairways, hallways, elevators, vehicles, animals, etc.) that pose adaptive hazards. Sometimes it is helpful also to understand the dimensions of the feared stimuli in terms of which fear intensity is regulated. For example, rooms and hallways vary in size, in lighting, and in ease of escape; stairways vary in narrowness, in length, and in where they lead to; elevators vary in size, in cleanliness, in quality of ventilation, and so forth.

A third general goal of behavioral assessment is that of determining the specific forms and instrumental properties of the patient's phobic behaviors. Three sets of separate determinations are involved: (a) To what extent does the patient speak of suffering *subjectively* from fear, terror, dread, apprehension, and the like? (b) In what way does the patient *behaviorally* escape or avoid feared stimuli or otherwise allow his or her behavior in the world to be impacted by the phobia? and (c) To what degree does the patient respond *physiologically* during encounters with phobic stimuli?

In addition to the goals stated, assessment in simple phobia has the objective of allowing a realistic prognosis. Hence the following questions typically are answered: (a) How long has the phobia persisted? (b) By what tactics and with how much perseverance has the patient attempted to overcome the phobia on his or her own? (c) What previous experiences with chemotherapy, psychotherapy, and behavior therapy has the patient had? (d) Does the patient expect that therapy will succeed? and (e) Does the patient have roughly accurate expectations regarding how therapy will proceed? A realistic prognosis is also sometimes related to important background information concerning familial, social, and sexual interaction patterns. Routine gathering of such information will serve to minimize therapy failures caused by factual blind spots; for example, the spouse who sabotages treatment.

Sources of Assessment Data

Ideally, clinical assessment of physiologic, motoric, and private/cognitive phobic activities will take place during adaptively significant interactions with problematic subsets of the patients' natural environment. More and more professional therapists seem to be working toward this ideal. Even so the most economical and still very common tools of assessment are indirect and retrospective measures of the patients' problematic naturalistic functioning.

The Behavioral Interview

The face-to-face interview is a very important clinical assessment procedure. The purpose of behavioral interviewing is to seek broad-band (Cronbach, 1970) answers to the assessment questions discussed previously, answers that serve to guide preliminary treatment planning and subsequent assessment work. Some authorities (e.g., Goldfried & Davison, 1976) hold that during behavioral interviews therapists should strive to warmly but firmly address themselves to seeking information about their patients' anxiety behaviors and to providing information about behavior therapy. Other well-known therapists (e.g., Lazarus, 1971) have historically argued for a "softer," relatively more nondirective behavioral interview style. In general, behavior therapists should undertake systematic behavioral interviewing very early in therapy but should, at the same time, be prepared to forego this activity and to respond to clearly evidenced needs for interest, hope, reassurance, and the like.

For patients who report a history of psychotherapy for their phobia(s) or other problems, it is important that the therapist take time during the initial interview to describe a behavioral model of simple phobia and to describe some of the forms that behavior therapy might take. For patients who appear dubious regarding the power of behavior therapy, the therapist might benefit from setting aside some time early on for a "therapy preview" (e.g., brief muscular relaxation training). For all patients, it is important to spell out clearly who is responsible for the success of therapy. In general, behavior therapy is based on an explicit partnership in which the patient and therapist have complementary responsibilities. Ideally, these joint responsibilities should be mutually endorsed in an early interview.

As noted, a major purpose of behavioral interviewing is to provide broad-band assessment of the phobic stimuli and related fear behaviors that prompted the patient to seek help. The purpose of further assessment is to provide more detailed and more accurate views of the problem.

General and Specific Fear Questionnaires

Questionnaire measures have an uncertain history within the academic wing of the behavior therapy movement. Yet, few clinicians would deny the occasional value of such instruments. Self-reports can be acquired concerning physiological and motoric behaviors as well as concerning subjective anxiety. That is, self-reports do *not* represent windows to consciousness as much as they represent a response domain within which diverse assessment information can be sought.

General fear surveys, like the Fear Survey Schedule-II (Geer, 1965), are readily available and should be used routinely in assessing phobic patients, as the omnibus questionnaires occasionally point to areas of difficulty overlooked during interviewing. Clinicians should remember, however, that general fear surveys were not designed to assess fear in specific situations.

Measures of specific fears, such as fear of snakes, fear of spiders, fear of mutilation, fear of public speaking, and fear of testing taking also are available. Ordinarily, such instruments are used more for research than for clinical diagnosis because, by and large, they are insufficiently idiographic for the latter purpose. Nonetheless, several of these measures do have demonstrable reliability and discriminant validity, and occasional well-timed use can point toward fine-grain therapy targets. For example, Kleinknecht, Klepac, and Alexander (1973) have provided a specific questionnaire about fear of dentistry (odontophobia) that can be scored so as to quantify separate factors involving reports about dental avoidance, reports about autonomic behavior in the presence of dentists, and reports about "fear" of dental stimuli (see Kleinknecht, McGlynn, Thorndike, & Harkavy, 1984). For clinicians who view motoric, physiological, and private/cognitive behaviors as more or less separate fear-response systems, self-reports on the Dental Fear Survey can guide further assessment and early treatment planning for a patient with dental phobia. Similarly conceived and usable questionnaires exist for other problems.

Self-Reports of Fear Intensity

In both omnibus and specific fear inventories the actual stimuli for self-report responses are language descriptions of objects and situations that are not present at the time of assessment. Of course, it is preferable to use real objects or situations to occasion self-reports about fear intensity, hopefully objects or situations closely akin to clinically focal ones.

A well-known situation-specific self-report format used to measure subjective distress is Walk's (1956) Fear Thermometer. This is a 10-point rating scale ("completely calm" to "absolute terror") that the patient uses to rate degrees of subjective distress during encounters with phobic stimuli. It is completely portable and is easily used at various points during assessment of motor and physiologic behavior. For example, in the assessment of acrophobia, the therapist might ask for Fear Thermometer ratings of anxiety at various points during a naturalistic and/or clinic height approach task (e.g., Ritter, 1969). A well-known research example is the use of Fear Thermometer ratings during behavioral approach tasks in the early snake-fear desensitization experiments. Other approaches have also been used to measure naturalistically regulated subjective fear. Anxiety differential ratings (Husek & Alexander, 1963) and ratings on the State-Trait Anxiety Inventory A-State Scale (Spielberger, Gorsuch, & Lushene, 1970) are common examples.

Sometimes it is not feasible to acquire reports of fear intensity during actual contact with phobic stimuli. In such cases, therapists can provide instructions for imagery that are pertinent to the phobia and can evaluate the patient's subjective fear intensity during the imagery trials. Wolpe's (1973) use of SUDs (subjective units of discomfort) scaling exemplifies this approach. Using anchor points of 0 (absolute calmness) and 100 (maximum fear), the patient assigns numerical SUDs values to phobic stimuli "presented in imagination."

Contrived Behavioral Approach Tests

Three major contrived situations are used by behavior therapists to assess anxiety at the level of overt motor behavior: the behavioral approach test, the interpersonal performance test, and the role-played interaction. The behavioral approach test is most relevant to assessing simple phobia.

The behavioral approach test (BAT) dates to the early work of Lang and his colleagues (Lang & Lazovik, 1963) and has for nearly 20 years been a standard tool for evaluating phobia therapy outcome. There are various clinical reports of BATs in assessment of common phobias. Ritter (1969) developed a Height Avoidance Test to assess overt motor behavior among acrophobic patients. The test called for patients to climb an outdoor stairway with an assistant, pausing for at least 2 minutes at each of nine landings for situation-specific ratings of fear intensity to be made. Miller and Bernstein (1972) developed a behavioral test to assess overt motor behavior among claustrophobic patients. The test called for subjects to sit in a small, dark, closed chamber until they became sufficiently uncomfortable to terminate the test, or for 10 minutes, whichever came first. Subjects' heart rates and respiration while in the chamber and time to termination of the test were recorded. There also are clinical reports of behavioral approach tests in evaluating unique phobias. McGlynn and Linder (1971), for example, used a BAT to assess overt motor behavior in a woman who was intensely phobic vis-à-vis wooden kitchen matches. The test called for her to perform in the clinic a series of hierarchically ordered behaviors ranging from "observing a closed box of kitchen matches" to "barehanded, picking up a dirty, wet, and burned match."

There is certainly no guarantee that a patient's fear responses to a phobic stimulus during a contrived behavioral test will allow the therapist to predict directly the patient's responses to similar but inevitably different phobic stimuli encountered in the natural environment. However, when clinicians are aware of these limitations, contrived assessment of overt phobic behavior can be extremely valuable in understanding simple phobias. In general, performing a behavioral approach test involves providing the patient with a structured series of graduated overt performance tasks that culminates in contact with the phobic stimulus, then observing and recording details (e.g., time, self-reported fear, hesitations, terminations) of the patient's progress along the behavioral gradient. The accuracy of a contrived BAT in predicting naturalistic fear behaviors probably rests on how representative the contrivance is of the natural environment.

Naturalistic Assessment of Behavior

As noted, clinical assessment of phobic behaviors ideally will take place during adaptively significant interactions with problematic subsets of the patient's natural environment. More and more, therapists are going into problematic environments alongside their patients and recording behavioral observations. In other instances, graduate students, interns, or residents are used for such evaluations. Significant others (e.g., a spouse, parent, friend) are also being called upon more frequently. Naturalistic observation of conduct is not without validity problems (e.g., reactivity, content-sampling validity), but, if done carefully, it can serve as the bottom line in both treatment planning and outcome monitoring. Informants should not be used unless the patient agrees. The informant's attention should be focused on accurately described and specific situations. Probably, the informant should be provided with checklists of well-defined behaviors to observe.

Naturalistic contexts afford opportunities for evaluating physiological and private/cognitive fear behaviors as well as motoric ones. An example is seen in the

Patient's name: _____ Date: _____

Therapist's name: _____

Describe your location and task: _____

_____

_____

Exact starting time: _____

Heart rate before entry (2 x 30 sec. sample): _____

Respiration rate before entry (2 x 30 sec. sample): _____

SUDs rating before the trial: _____

Entry: YES/NO

Exposure duration: _____

Exact ending time: _____

Describe fear behaviors observed during the task: _____

_____

_____

Describe reasons for terminating the trial: _____

_____

_____

Figure 2. An example chart used in naturalistic assessment for stairway–elevator–calculus phobia.

treatment of a highly specific stairway–elevator–calculus phobia treated by McGlynn some years ago. Aside from a history of sleep disturbances and occasional somnambulism, the patient, who was a college freshman, had been symptom free until 6 weeks before the initial consultation. The phobia began with "feelings of relief" going down in the elevator after calculus class on Friday of the first full week in a fall semester. The following week feelings of relief seemed to continue and were accompanied by a "sense of tension and dislike" while ascending the elevator to class. During the fourth week of school the patient received an *F* on an unannounced quiz. Thereafter, the phobia quickly generalized to all means of getting to the calculus classroom. It had not yet generalized to elevators or stairways other than those governing access to the calculus class. Naturalistic assessment of behavioral, physiological, and private/subjective fear behaviors was assigned to a graduate student who was provided with checklists as in Figure 2 and was instructed to accompany the patient into his problematic environments and record his entry behaviors, his exposure durations, his SUDs ratings, his heart and respiration rates, and so forth.

Naturalistic Self-Monitoring

Reactivity and other problems are encountered when other persons observe a fearful patient's conduct in natural (as well as clinic and laboratory) settings. A general approach to minimizing the reactivity problem, and an approach that is economical, is seen in self-assessment of fear behavior. Self-monitoring of fear behaviors was used only infrequently until the advent of self-managed exposure (Marks, 1978, 1981) as an approach to treatment. In his popular self-help book for anxious persons, Marks (1978) provides standardized instructions and formats for self-assessment of anxiety. In general, they are structured to provide the same information that is sought when informants are used.

Assessment of Emotional Imagery

In the previous section, Self-Reports of Fear Intensity, we noted that therapists sometimes use imagery instructions to replace real-life objects in quantifying subjective fear intensity. This procedure can be broadened to become a clinical test of emotional/imaging behavior. First, the patient is given some instruction in muscular relaxation. Then instructions to continue relaxing are interspersed with instructions to imagine phobic and perhaps neutral situations or objects. During the imagery trials, the therapist assesses heart rate and respiration manually and watches for muscle tremors, grimaces, and so forth. At the end of imagery trials, patients rate their private/cognitive fear intensity during the various phobic imaging tasks.

Psychophysiological Assessment

For the not insignificant number of therapists who are suitably equipped, clinical assessment of simple phobia can be supplemented with psychophysiological measurement. This technology can be coupled to real or instructional regulation over the patients' phobic behaviors and might involve heart rate and skin conductance as well as various special purpose measures. (See Lader, 1975; Lang, 1971, 1977, for details on psychophysiological assessment of anxiety.) Clinicians are cautioned, however, that psychophysiological assessment of individual patients' fearful behavior is rendered complex by the profound idiosyncrasies of fearful behavior at the level of psychophysiology (cf. Lacey, 1967).

Choice of Treatment

The end result of early assessment is choice of the therapy modality. The choice is based on a characterization of the phobia in terms of its exact controlling stimuli; its specific physiological, motoric, and private/cognitive fear behaviors; and its instrumental consequences for the patients' behavior in the world. Accuracy in specifying clinically focal stimuli is required for differential diagnosis. For example, Dengrove (1972) reported an apparent agoraphobic who was really just afraid of dogs. Accuracy in characterizing fear behaviors points toward optimal treatments. For example, within an orthodox behavior therapy approach (used here), significant *autonomic* fear behaviors point toward relaxation/desensitization as a potentially valuable treatment mode, whereas significant *motoric* fear behaviors point more toward exposure-oriented methods. Assessment of the instrumental functions served by fearful behaviors points toward important adjunctive methods. For example, the calculus class–elevator–stairway phobic described previously was told during therapy not to go to the student union at all because the union was precisely where he went on 4 consecutive days of phobic avoidance.

Ordinarily, choice of nonoptimal treatment is not catastrophic. The empirical anchoring of orthodox behavior therapy practice will soon reveal ill-chosen methods. Ordinarily, too, therapy should proceed as soon as possible after the patient presents for treatment. For these reasons, therapists need not, and probably should not, do all of the assessments before beginning active intervention. Indeed, the first few sessions of behavior therapy for phobias will inevitably be a blend of assessment and treatment activities. For example, assessment of emotional imagery might be added to a session scheduled primarily for progressive relaxation training. For another example, homework assignments to monitor subjective fear intensity might be made early during self-managed exposure. In short, the assessment/therapy process ideally is continuous. At the same time, even a small amount of assessment information can point in particular directions for early treatment. Special case criteria for matching patients with treatments are summarized where appropriate later.

Treatment

Note on Muscular Relaxation Training

In the day-to-day practice of behavior therapy with anxious patients, therapists *often* need to know how to teach them the skill of voluntarily controlling or influencing levels of tension in the skeletal muscles. Space limitations precluded an overview here, but see the following sources for exact setting, preliminaries, and procedures (Bernstein & Borkovec, 1973; Goldfried & Davison, 1976; McGlynn, 1978; Rimm & Masters, 1979).

Systematic Desensitization

Uses

Systematic desensitization based on relaxation is the major orthodox behavior therapy approach to simple phobias. The list of fears to which desensitization has been applied is quite extensive (cf. Bandura, 1969). In brief, patients are taught to relax and, while maintaining relaxation, are instructed to calmly but clearly visualize a hierarchy of increasingly frightening scenarios based on their phobia(s).

In selecting patients for desensitization, seven questions are to be answered: (a) Can the phobic cues be described in concrete terms? (b) Does the anxiety persist even though there are no deficits in coping skills? (c) Does the patient suffer from four or fewer phobias? (d) Can the patient learn the skill of muscular relaxation? (e) Does the patient report clear imagery for phobic and related stimuli? (f) Does the patient report extreme subjective discomfort or show clear signs of autonomic responsivity while imaging aversive material? and (g) Is it impractical to arrange for regular *in vivo* encounters with therapeutically targeted phobic stimuli? In general, as positive answers are tallied, systematic desensitization is indicated as a suitable approach.

Procedure

The general format for conducting desensitization is very well known and is overviewed here. The first step entails four to six sessions of teaching voluntary muscular relaxation. The second and concurrent step is that of constructing one or more desensitization hierarchies, listings of increasingly frightening phobic scenarios. The third step is desensitization proper—the guided activities of relaxing and simultaneously imaging aversive scenarios from the hierarchy. The fourth and final step in systematic desensitization is structured self-exposure to phobic stimuli *in vivo*.

The most common types of desensitization hierarchies for simple phobias are spatiotemporal listings in which increasing aversiveness across items is produced by lowering progressively the time and/or distance to feared encounters or performances. However, seemingly different fears that have a common theme will sometimes form the bases of a hierarchy. For example, the separate fears of theaters, buses, and downtown city streets might be clustered as fears of crowds (simple phobia), as fears of being closed in (claustrophobia), as fears of scrutiny and ridicule (social phobia), or as settings for feared loss of control (agoraphobia). Hence the procedure of hierarchy construction for desensitization often guides differential diagnoses of phobia types and sometimes prompts shifts in the therapeutic approaches. Specific procedures for constructing hierarchies and a number of sample hierarchies are available in standard sources (e.g., Goldfried & Davison, 1976; Rimm & Masters, 1979; Wolpe, 1976, 1982).

There are two procedures for desensitization proper: the *orthodox* (Wolpe & Lazarus, 1966) and the *improved* (Wolpe, 1982) versions. They vary in detail but produce the common end result of prompting increasingly robust emotional imagery behaviors in the context of profound relaxing. In the orthodox procedure, the relaxed patient is first instructed to visualize the least aversive hierarchy scene and to signal by elevating an index finger if the imaging brings about discomfort. If the patient does not signal the presence of anxiety he or she is instructed to relax and, later, to imagine the scene once more. If there is likewise no signal of anxiety on the second imaging trial, a brief relaxing period ensues, and the next hierarchy item is presented. This process is repeated again and again until the most feared scenarios in the hierarchy are imaged without accompanying discomfort signals. In the improved procedure for systematic desensitization, the relaxed patient is instructed to visualize the appropriate hierarchy item and to elevate an index finger briefly during clear imaging. The therapist allows time after this signal for the patient to continue visualizing the scene, then instructs the patient to drop the image and report orally a SUDs rating of discomfort while imaging. This process is repeated until the patient visualizes the zenithal hierarchy item(s) and reports orally that no fear was experienced. Several important considerations involved in the use of both of these procedures are discussed elsewhere (McGlynn, 1978).

Graduated naturalistic exposure instructions are standard in clinical desensitization. Clinicians should, where possible, attempt to facilitate naturalistic exposure during desensitization therapy by *in vivo* tracking of imaginal progress.

Graduated Participant Modeling

Uses

Anytime it is possible and not inconvenient, patients with simple phobias should be considered seriously for treatment with graduated participant modeling procedures. Extremely fearful patients might require "pretreatment" with relaxation training or systematic desensitization. Moderately fearful patients can be treated successfully with partial versions of the package described here. The use of participant modeling in the natural environment parallels the use of therapist-assisted *in vivo* exposure. Hence, our narrative about modeling procedures is slanted toward the clinic setting.

Procedure

Graduated participant modeling (Bandura, 1971, 1976) is based on a hierarchy of increasingly aversive to-be-enacted behavioral performances involving lesser to greater contact with phobic stimuli. Once the behavioral gradient is set up, the fearless model (the therapist) performs each of the hierarchical activities while concurrently describing his or her various actions and pointing out the absence of adverse consequences for them. After these demonstrations, the therapist again performs the least aversive activity. Hopefully, the patient then does so as well. After the patient performs the least aversive step competently and calmly, the therapist again demonstrates the next step. The patient then imitates the therapist's second performance, and so on.

A number of supplementary tactics can be used to maximize clinical efficacy for graduated participant modeling. *Joint simultaneous performance* of the feared activity can be used initially in place of the successive modeling procedure just described. In this procedure, the patient and therapist simultaneously perform the aversive behavior after it has been demonstrated and before the patient attempts to perform the behavior alone. Joint performances might be undertaken at each step up the aversive behavioral gradient and can include continuous (comforting) body contact between the patient and therapist during the aversive performances (see Ritter, 1969). *Repeated modeling trials* can precede any attempt to get patients to imitate the modeled behavior. The use of "multiple models" is likely to be beneficial. This is true because varied and flexible coping behaviors will be acquired from observing several models do the aversive behaviors somewhat differently. *Graduated temporal intervals* can be used to enhance the likelihood of early imitative performances. Early on, requirements of very brief imitations might precede requirements of more protracted ones. *Arrangement of protective conditions* that minimize the likelihood of adverse consequences during demonstrative or imitative performances can prevent setbacks from accidents. For example, in the graduated participant modeling treatment of animal fears, the therapist should use target animals that are known to be docile and/or restrain the animals' movement.

Joint performances, repeated modeling trials, multiple models, graduated temporal intervals, and protective arrangements are referred to, collectively, as *response induction aides*. The purpose of these aides is that of prompting the patient to display approximations to the nonanxious performances that are sought. Two final adjunctive procedures round out the package. One of these is the *gradual withdrawal of performance aides*. The response-induction and protective aides used early on should be withdrawn gradually. There are no fixed rules governing withdrawal of these supports. Certainly, the aides should not be withdrawn so abruptly that the patient can no longer perform the targeted behaviors. Probably, the withdrawals should proceed up the hierarchy in sequence. The final adjunctive procedure is called *self-directed mastery* trials. In self-directed mastery, patients continue to practice mastered performances by themselves for relatively long periods of time. Self-directed mastery trials can take place within each step of the behavioral hierarchy or at the end of treatment. Self-directed mastery opportunities that are instituted after the withdrawal of supportive aides serve to provide for the autonomous and protracted patient performances that are sought.

Naturalistic Exposure Approaches

Naturalistic exposure methods were first used widely in the treatment of agoraphobic and obsessive-compulsive patients. Yet, they have also been applied with success to simple phobias. The methods of exposure therapy are difficult to pin down because the paradigm is not procedurally defined, aside from stipulating that exposure to be achieved. Practically anything that one might do to "persuade" (Marks, 1981) a phobic patient to confront his or her phobic situation is called *exposure therapy,* provided that it works.

Therapist-Assisted Exposure

Frequently, naturalistic exposure is undertaken with the assistance of a therapist. Marks (1978) reported a representative example of how assisted exposure might ordinarily proceed. The patient was a 20-year-old student who for several years had exhibited nightmare behaviors and checking rituals having to do with fear/avoidance of pigeons. At the time of treatment she avoided open windows, traversed circuitous paths around known pigeon hangouts, and so forth. In treatment, the patient was encouraged to "get used to pigeons by gradually coming closer to them, despite the terror that this inspired in her." Treatment began by instructing the patient to buy and hang pictures for her room and to buy and handle dummy birds. After this, the patient stroked and handled a pigeon that was being held by the therapist and spent some time alone in a room with a caged pigeon 3 feet away. In the next session the patient and therapist conjointly fed pigeons in the park and sat at a parkside table while pigeons flew about. On subsequent sessions the therapist-assisted naturalistic exposure was continued, and therapist assistance was gradually faded out.

Therapist-assisted naturalistic exposure can be similar to participant modeling, to flooding, or to several other paradigms depending on the details of how the patient is "persuaded" to confront feared cues. "Toleration" and "flooding" seem to be important and somewhat different themes within different assisted-exposure treatments. In a toleration approach, generically, an aversive stimulus is encountered in such small and finely graduated doses that significant emotionality never is produced (see Guthrie, 1935). Extrapolations can be made directly from the previous section on participant modeling in order to guide assisted-exposure treatments geared toward toleration. In a flooding approach, generically, an aversive stimulus is encountered in such large and continuous doses that significant emotionality is purposefully produced, then attenuated. Guidance of assisted-exposure treatments that are geared toward flooding comes from three specific goals: (a) to require full confrontation with phobic stimuli; (b) to ensure that the confrontation is not accompanied by painful or injurious consequences; and (c) to "prevent" psychological (e.g., dissociative) and motoric escape from the confrontation.

Self-Managed Exposure

Assisted naturalistic exposure often is accompanied by self-exposure homework assignments, wherein patients are instructed to tolerate or endure highly structured encounters with phobic stimuli. Forms such as that in Figure 2 are used to guide self-managed exposure activities (as well as self-assessment). As with the early history of exposure in general, most of the work reported on self-managed exposure relates to agoraphobic and, to a lesser degree, obsessive-compulsive individuals. However, it is appropriate to include it here if only to highlight the therapeutic implications of self-assessment procedures.

Marks (1978) provides an elaborate protocol for patients to use in assessing and managing their anxieties. Self-assessment entails answering 10 questions having to do with (a) depression; (b) alcohol/sedative use; (c) confirmed physical disease; (d) specific anxiety cues; (e) clarity of the problem; (f) specificity of self-management goals; (g) significance of overcoming the problem; (h) commitment to change; (i) need for co-therapists; and (j) availability of co-therapists. In general, different answers at each of the 10 test items guide the patient to different courses of action. For example, a patient who answers "yes" to Test 1 (about depression) is instructed to see a doctor, whereas a patient who answers "no" to Test 4 (about specific fear antecedents) is told that exposure treatment is not indicated.

Self-managed exposure therapy is presented by Marks (1978) as a five-step strategy. Step 1 is to work out exactly what one fears. The patient is assisted here with questionnaires vis-à-vis fears and the like. Step 2 is to write down specific problems/goals for immediate attention. Step 3 is to prepare a timetable for exposure to the things that trouble one and record what happened immediately after each session. The self-help narrative also encourages weekly replanning of exposures, long durations of exposure per trial, and 100-point self-ratings of anxiety after each exposure session. Step 4 is to learn to discriminate the onset of tension. This is done by working from a self-administered questionnaire about "what sensations do you have when you are frightened?" Step 5 is the choice and use of self-managed coping tactics. This is done by working from a list of 10 diverse "coping devices," for example, "I must breathe slowly and steadily . . . and gradually learn to deal with this situation"; "I have to stay here until I can tolerate this panic, even if it takes an hour. Meanwhile let me experience the fear as deliberately and fully as possible." Narratives concerning each of these steps are supplemented by rules and suggestions having to do with specific self-management areas, for example, rules for self-exposure sessions, special tactics for common special problems such as insomnia and anxiety about swallowing, and the like.

Comments on Cognitive Behavior Therapy

Simply put, the cognitive view of the phobia problem is that expectancies or other cognitions are responsible for binding together phobic stimuli and phobic responses. Accordingly, a major thrust of cognitive behavior therapy is modification of private/cognitive activities, and a major purpose of cognitive behavioral assessment is monitoring changes in those activities. A step-by-step review of cognitive behavioral methods is well beyond the scope of this chapter. Furthermore, in the treatment of simple phobias, cognitive behavioral methods are best used adjunctively along with orthodox behavior therapy. Hence, we will only overview cognitive behavioral methods here.

The special approaches to assessment that are required by adding cognitive behavior therapies depend largely on the specific cognitions thought to bind stimuli and responses (misconceptions, irrational beliefs, self-statements, performance-/nonperformance-outcome expectations, self-efficacy). By and large, these special techniques are based on standard assessment approaches (interviewing, contrived behavioral tests) that are slanted in new directions in the search for cognitive activities (for reviews see Hollon & Bemis, 1981; Kendall & Hollon, 1981). Specific approaches to cognitive behavior therapy likewise depend on differing interpretations of the nature of fearful cognitive behavior. The treatment packages offered by Beck and Emery (1979), Ellis and Grieger (1977), Mahoney (1974), and Meichenbaum (1977) are representative. The literatures generated by these packages and others have been reviewed (Barrios & Shigetomi, 1979; Mahoney & Arnkoff, 1978). Our narrative is about stress inoculation training (Meichenbaum, 1977; Meichenbaum & Cameron, 1974).

Stress Inoculation Training

Stress inoculation training has three phases. In an "education phase," the therapist begins by evaluating the things each patient says to himself or herself about phobic encounters and by articulating how these cognitive "self-statements" are related to other phobic behaviors. For example, a dog-phobic patient might be privately saying things like "If I go up that street the dog will surely bite me"; "If I go four blocks around, the dog won't see me"; or "If I start going up that street I will chicken out before I am all the way past the dog, and I will have to turn around and go the long way anyhow." During this "education phase," the therapist also articulates with the patient a plausible cognitive account of the phobia and how it can be overcome by altering self-statements. In a second or "rehearsal phase" of treatment, the patient is taught one or more activities that can be brought to bear in coping with anxiety, for example, muscular relaxation or private rehearsal of coping self-statements. During this phase the patient also is taught to discriminate the onset of tension/anxiety. In the final or "application phase" of treatment, the patient practices the newly acquired coping techniques while imaging and/or role playing and/or naturalistically experiencing a graded series of encounters with phobic stimuli.

Self-Managed Stress Inoculation

Usually, stress inoculation training is undertaken with the guidance of a therapist. Again, however, a self-management format is available and unfolds in an elaborate protocol with instructions for relaxing, for constructing graded hierarchies of stressful scenarios, and the like (see McKay, Davis, & Fanning, 1981). The program is broken down into four steps: (a) preparing for *in vivo* encounters with phobic stimulation; (b) confronting the situation(s); (c) coping with emotional arousal during *in vivo* encounters; and (d) self-reward for success *in vivo*. The McKay *et al.* manual provides "stress-coping thoughts" for use during each stage. For example, the preparation stage is facilitated by thinking "There's nothing to worry about," "I'm going to be alright," "I've succeeded with this before," whereas the confrontation stage is to be accompanied by thinking "Stay organized," "Take it step by step; don't rush," "I can get help if I need it," and so forth.

McKay *et al.* (1981) reported a representative example of how self-managed stress inoculation training might typically proceed. A ranger employed in a large regional park began treatment by constructing a hierarchy of SUDs ratings for situations involving various scenarios in his job and married life. Examples included "driving huge dump or water truck over narrow mountain roads" (25 SUDs); "fear that lightning will hit trees near house" (50 SUDs); "helping a snake-bite victim" (75 SUDs); "seeing a snake" (90 SUDs). Next, the ranger learned to relax and undertook imaginal desensitization of elaborately detailed scenes within the hierarchy. During imaginal desensitization, the ranger also learned to detect the onset of tension and to use tightness in particular muscles as a cue for practicing relaxation. Next, the ranger articulated his lists of "stress-coping thoughts." For example, "I'll take one thing at a time" and "I'll make a plan for coping" were to be used in the preparation phase, whereas "It will be over soon enough" and "I'll follow each step of my plan" were to be used during the confrontation phase. Finally, the ranger undertook hierarchical desensitization *in vivo* using both relaxation and stress-coping thoughts to cope with *in vivo* exposures.

Other Behavioral Techniques

An attempt has been made here to present procedural considerations fundamental to the task of treating simple-phobic individuals. Because the chapter length was limited, a number of approaches had to be omitted. In some instances, procedures were omitted because they are unnecessarily aversive. Foremost among procedures omitted for this reason are *in vivo* flooding, imaginal flooding, and implosive therapy (Marks, 1975; Stampfl & Levis, 1967). In other instances, procedures were omitted because their known ranges of application overlap entirely with the ranges of techniques that are herein described. Foremost among the techniques omitted for this reason are those in which fearful avoidance of phobic stimuli is overcome by positively reinforcing motoric approach behaviors (e.g., Leitenberg, 1972).

Some Problems and Limitations

Systematic Desensitization

The questions used in selecting patients for desensitization point to the major pitfalls in using desensitization. Phobias cannot be too many in number. The patient must be able to learn to relax. The patient should show signs of emotional arousal to instructional fear cues as well as to actual phobic stimuli. Conditions that point toward clinic or naturalistic modeling treatments should not hold. Problems might be encountered in the hierarchy-construction phase as hierarchies are based on homogeneous fear clusters, and fear clusters sometimes are hard to identify. Wolpe (1973), for example, described how 14 "different" psychoneurotic fears were grouped into the four categories of *acrophobia, agoraphobia, claustrophobia,* and *fears of illness and related occurrences.* Problems might be encountered also in the mechanics of desensitization, that is, what is to be done when the patient is "hung up" on a particular hierarchy item or when the patient reports anxiety out of proportion to the substance of the imaged scenario? Ways to deal with problems such as these have been summarized elsewhere (McGlynn, 1978).

Graduated Participant Modeling

Graduated participant modeling is basically an outpatient clinic treatment for phobias involving stimuli that are readily obtainable and portable to the clinic setting. The principal weakness in graduated participant modeling is its restricted range of convenient application. A second important weakness is that fear reduction wrought in the clinic might very well *not* transfer to adaptively significant naturalistic encounters with phobic stimuli unless structured *in vivo* practice is arranged. In such cases the clinic modeling procedures might be superfluous.

Naturalistic Exposure Approaches

As noted earlier, "exposure approaches" are not procedurally defined, and they sometimes seem similar to "flooding," but other times they seem similar to "toleration." Accordingly, their limitations and problems in specific instances are both vague and variable. All *in vivo* exposure formats are limited to phobic stimuli that can be confronted conveniently. We cannot produce thunderstorms to fit our schedules, and it might use up a half day or more to ride across town, park the car, walk to and ride in the adjustively significant bank of elevators with the patient for 40 to 60 minutes, debrief and reschedule the patient, and return to the office. All exposure formats likewise seem to possess at least some potential for exacerbating the patient's phobia—at least temporarily. Perhaps too much has been made of this historically, but it underscores the value of gradual, as opposed to, confrontive naturalistic exposure formats.

Some potential limitations in cost, convenience, and the like can be corrected by the self-managed exposure format, but other problems are therein introduced. First, there is added the general problem of assessing the patient in terms of suitability for a self-management effort. This is a complex evaluation involving skills assessments, evaluation of commitment, and so forth, and there is virtually no systematic empirical literature that can be brought directly to bear on the problem (Bellack & Schwartz, 1976). Second, there is the problem of insufficient data to justify regular use of a self-managed exposure approach to therapy for simple phobias.

Case Study

Background and Goals

The narrative that follows reports a case in which both systematic desensitization and assisted naturalistic exposure were used in the treatment of a 29-year-old, married, white female with an intense phobia for black males.

Behavioral interviewing (along the lines described previously) revealed a clear traumatic history for the phobia. In the patient's words:

> I worked in a convenience store. I was robbed and shot in the arm. I have bad dreams about this and have fears also. . . . I am scared of colored men now, where before I wasn't. I keep thinking that they'll try to hurt me again. . . . I need to be a better wife and mother because it has bothered my family.

In short, behavioral interviewing pointed toward motoric and private/cognitive fear behaviors that were under the control of black men, that had been traumatically acquired, and that were interfering with the smooth functioning of the patient's family.

Behavioral interviewing also pointed toward two goals for treatment. In the patient's words: (a) "I want to be able to testify in court with the three robbers looking at me"; (b) "I don't want to be scared to go to the store and some other places." Interviewing revealed no other problems and generated no other treatment goals, aside from some dissatisfaction in the area of conjugal sex. The patient did seem motivated to achieve her goals; she had no prior history of psychotherapy and readily understood several brief descriptions of possible behavior therapy scenarios.

Behavioral Assessment

During Sessions 2 to 4 behavioral assessment was undertaken along with other activities. In one assessment protocol, an intern accompanied the patient on two weekly tours around the health center complex in order to encounter black males in hallways, rooms, elevators, and enclosed stairways. The patient guided these tours herself. The intern recorded acts of escape/avoidance, monitored pulse rates manually during (or sometimes immediately after) the encounters, and recorded the patients SUDs ratings. In a second assessment protocol, the intern once accompanied the patient to/toward the superette where she had been shot and to other places that were problematic. Thematically, these were places where close proximity to black males was likely. Concretely, these were the grocery store, two public lakes in the area, several otherwise convenient gasoline stations, and the courthouse complex where the patient hoped to testify against her assailants.

During these assessments, the patient completely avoided (i.e., would not enter) one particular long hallway in the health center, even though she was accompanied by the intern. She also was clearly hesitant to enter and was quick to leave several other situations (e.g., the hospital cafeteria). Her heart rate was chronically elevated (90 to 95 BPM) from the beginning to the end of the three *in vivo* assessment sessions, and encounters with black males elevated her heart rate dramatically (e.g., 117 to 143 BPM). SUDs ratings that were recorded soon after various encounters and at other times during the assessments concurred in the picture of mild to moderate fearfulness throughout the trials, with intense fearfulness during encounters with black males.

As noted later, muscular relaxation training was undertaken routinely during the second session. This set the stage for emotional imagery assessment during the third. The patient was assisted in relaxation and was instructed to imagine various 30-second aversive and nonaversive scenarios interspersed with 30-second periods of relaxing and thinking of nothing at all. For example:

> Rest, relax, and think of nothing [*pause for 10 + 30 seconds*]; Imagine you are standing in the checkout line at the ———— supermarket. You are looking at the beauty magazines in the rack to your left. Two black males about 30 years of age wearing blue jeans and work shirts enter through the door in front of you. You feel your fear grow as your heart pounds heavily [*brief pause*]. They turn toward the grocery carts and move away toward the back of the store [*pause for 10 + 30 seconds*]. Rest, relax, and think of nothing [*pause for 10 + 30 seconds*]. Imagine you are standing in the backyard at your uncle's ———— farm. You are looking at the rustic smokehouse to your left. Your uncle is slowly leading a little pony that your sister's little girl is riding [*pause for 10 + 30 seconds*]. Rest, relax, and think of nothing [*pause for 10 + 30 seconds*]. Imagine you are walking up the steps of the courthouse on the day of the trial. You notice a group of black males standing at the top of the stairs off to the left. You try to ignore them, but you feel the fear rise up inside you [*pause for 10 + 30 seconds*]. Rest, relax, and think of nothing.

Heart beats were counted manually throughout the imagery assessment, excluding the 10-second periods right after instructions. Mean heart rates during the rest and relaxation periods (85 BPM) were about the same as during neutral imagery periods (82 BPM) and were markedly different from those during aversive imaging (109 BPM). Clear differences also were seen for retrospective SUDs ratings of aversive versus nonaversive imaging tasks.

Behavioral Treatments

In sum, the various assessments pointed to motoric, physiological, and private/cognitive fear behaviors that were responsive to both actual and instructional fear stimuli and that were imposing lost opportunities for reinforcement and other problems on the patient's life. There was some urgency in treating this patient as the traumatically acquired simple phobia seemed to be evolving into agoraphobia. Hence, therapist-assisted naturalistic exposure was chosen as the most efficient basic treatment mode for daily-living problems such as going to the grocery store, to the gas station, and so forth. However, the patient's robust heart rate responding during the test for emotional imagery, an adequate response to muscular relaxation training, and the impossibility of *in vivo* exposure to the assailants before the trial prompted the use of systematic desensitization for the goal of calmly testifying. The latter treatment is described first.

Muscular relaxation training is undertaken routinely during the second or third session in the senior author's practice of orthodox behavior therapy with anxious patients. In this case, muscular relaxation according to the 16 muscle group format was begun "live" during the second session. The relaxation training manual of Bernstein and Borkovec (1973) was used to guide these sessions. Relaxation was taught during Sessions 2 to 5, and the patient was also provided with a cassette player and tape with which to practice relaxation at home and with instructions to record and turn in a diary of the location, time, and success of each relaxation homework effort.

Hierarchy construction for desensitization was undertaken during Sessions 4 and 5 using SUDs ratings of items and would-be items that were imaged while the patient was unrelaxed. A 17-item spatiotemporal hierarchy was generated by successively reducing the times and/or distances involved in going to the courthouse and in testifying. The hierarchy was organized according to the following criteria: the initial item occasioned five SUDs; each successive item from 2 to 12 occasioned at least five additional SUDs; each successive item from 13 to 17 occasioned at most five additional SUDs; and the items sampled the situations and behaviors involved in the act of testifying. Each item within the hierarchy was also designed following explicit criteria. It was detailed with relatively fine-grain descriptions of things such as actual courthouse stimuli and actual behaviors the patient would likely have to exhibit. Each item was also designed to facilitate, then attenuate the emotionality of imaging. For example, Item 17 on the hierarchy said:

> You are sitting in the witness chair noticing its highly polished arm. You have been sworn in and the preliminaries are over. You are feeling pretty calm because the bailiff and the deputies are nearby protecting you. . . . The prosecutor turns toward you and smiles reassuringly. Now you know it is coming, and you tense up. For a brief instant you feel panicky, but the panic subsides. The prosecutor says to you that it is time to point your finger at the men who robbed and shot you. You point at them, and your panic subsides further. You have done it! You have pointed them out! You hear yourself saying they're the ones, they're the ones that shot me.

Desensitization proper was undertaken "live" during twice weekly Sessions 6 to 12 using the "orthodox" procedure with the restriction that no more than four items were to be rehearsed in any session. Four muscle group relaxation instructions (Bernstein & Borkovec, 1973) were used to lead into desensitization. The desensitization protocol allowed 20 seconds after instructions for scene visualization and 60 seconds after internuncial instructions to relax. The patient was encouraged to "track" the imaginal desensitization process with *in vivo* performances, to lag about 4 items behind imaginal desensitization, and to keep and turn in records of *in vivo* practice. This type of rehearsal was possible for the first 11 hierarchy items.

The stage for therapist-assisted naturalistic exposure therapy was set during the assisted naturalistic assessment. Because fear behaviors tend to be situation specific, the approach was to tackle *in vivo* each of the major problematic performances that impinged on the patient's day-to-day life: going to the superette, going to the grocery store, going to each of two gasoline stations and each of two recreational lakes, and going to her church (which was located in a racially mixed, mostly black neighborhood). These *in vivo* programs went on simultaneously. Going to the grocery store will be our example here. The intern was given the following instructions, among others.

(1) Each day ride with the patient from her home toward the grocery. Do this 4 days for each of the next 2 weeks as needed. Be supportive and praise all reports of calmness. (2) Each day, manually record the patient's pulse for 1 minute in her car before entering the store. (3) Each day, record the patient's SUDs as she contemplates entering the store. (4) Stay with the patient until the two of you have stayed in the store for 20 minutes on 2 consecutive days. (5) On the next trip, remain inside in the front of the store while the patient moves about for 20 minutes or longer. (6) As is feasible, fade yourself out of the picture while encouraging the patient to undertake self-exposure. Be sure to get the patient to monitor her pulse rates and SUDs before entering the store on her own.

Results

Methods of assessing the efficacy of treatment are spelled out in the next section. In general, the two therapy programs were successful. The patient did succeed in testifying against her assailants (and they, in turn, were convicted). The patient is able to go to the grocery store, and so forth. She sometimes catches herself trying to find excuses to not do things like going to the grocery, and she sometimes has rapid pulse while doing so. She knows from experience (and instruction), however, that the problem will get worse "if she gives an inch." Hence, she is gradually continuing a course of improvement brought on by a rough but completely autonomous course of self-managed naturalistic exposure.

Problems in the Case, Outcome Evaluation, Follow-Up

Problems

There were no problems with progressive relaxation training in the clinic. Instructions for tensing/relaxing the left forearm were omitted due to the still painful gunshot wound. Compliance with the relaxation homework was sporadic as was the reported quality of relaxation at home.

Desensitization unfolded routinely with significant problems involved only in the imaging of being sworn in while looking, for the first time, at the defendants (Item 16). Reality factors prevented *in vivo* tracking of hierarchy Items 12 to 17.

Therapist-assisted naturalistic exposure was punctuated by minor but possibly noteworthy problems. The patient tearfully refused to drive toward the superette where she had been shot and maintained her refusal until the other *in vivo* goals had been nearly accomplished. The initial plan of massed exposure daily for 2 weeks was extended for 1 full week just to meet the criterion of 20 minutes alone in the superette with the therapist outside. Even so, the criterion was first achieved only with much persuasive effort. The massed exposure protocol placed burdensome demands on the intern's time and necessitated that a second intern, an advanced practicum student, and the patient's husband be called upon to assist. All of these people had to be trained how to follow the instructions, provided with some *do's* and *don't's,* and so forth. During one exposure trial a fight ensued when the patient wanted to leave a favorite recreational lake and her husband who was assisting on that afternoon did not. In general, the course of assisted exposure was not smooth. Partially, at least, this mirrors the absence of consensually endorsed fine-grain procedures.

Outcome Evaluation

Desensitization effects were evaluated with a clinical test of emotional imagery that was done 2 days after the final desensitization session and that was very much like the test described previously except that Items 16 and 17 from the desensitization hierarchy were substituted as aversive scenarios. The patient's mean heart rates during phobic imaging (90 BPM) were higher than were her mean heart rates during neutral imaging (78 BPM), but they were substantially lower than were the aversive imaging heart-rate means during the initial test for emotional imaging (109 BPM). Retrospective SUDs ratings of the various imaging tasks concurred. The patient did calmly visualize all 17 items, and she reported tracking her imaginal progress *in vivo* insofar as possible. She did testify at the trial of her assailants.

Outcome evaluation is built into the protocol for exposure-oriented methods. Throughout the trials, the intern (or his replacement) used a chart similar to that in Figure 2 to record the patient's heart rate immediately before taking on the next unmastered task, to record her SUDs rating for that upcoming task, to record the duration of her stay in the setting, and to record where the therapist was stationed during the trial. With only occasional discrepancies, the heart rates, SUDs ratings, and durations of exposure all shifted dramatically as expected during the 2 weeks required to overcome most of her problems. During the additional week of exposure to the superette itself, heart rates were reduced and durations of exposure were increased, but SUDs ratings in the car outside the store remained at 80 to 90 SUDs.

Follow-Up

The patient was terminated with instructions to "not be surprised if the phobia tries to come back." She was told that it was not unusual for such things to happen and when it did she could either tackle the problem on her own by "gritting her teeth and going there" or return to the clinic for some "booster" help. She was telephoned 6 months after termination and reported no significant return of the problems—though she "allowed as how" she had "set her jaw" a few times. She was telephoned again after another 6 months. There was no phobic complaint remaining, but her marriage was falling apart and she did not know what to do. She was given the names of several colleagues who were experts in marital adjustment problems.

Summary

Simple phobias are specific anxiety disorders in which behavioral and/or physiological and/or private/cognitive fear behaviors are regulated by tangible states of affairs: commonly by high and closed-in places, by animals, by contemporary modes of travel, and by weather conditions. Behavioral models of the simple phobia problem have been proposed in both "conditioning" and "cognitive" terms. Herein a "multifaceted framework" is reiterated in which physiological, overt motor, and private/cognitive fear behaviors are seen as functional classes that have largely independent ontogenies and that might require separate interventions. Adequate assessment is fundamental to reliable therapeutic success. The goals of assessment are to pinpoint the controlling stimuli for phobic behaviors, to describe the fine grain of the phobic behaviors themselves and any instrumental functions they serve, and generally to formulate a realistic prognosis. The techniques to be used selectively are behaviorally oriented interviewing, fear questionnaires, self-reports of fear intensity, contrived behavioral tests, naturalistic assessment (including self-monitoring), assessment of emotional imagery, and psychophysiological assessment.

An orthodox behavior therapy approach to simple phobias rests on using one or more of these techniques: muscular relaxation training, systematic desensitization, graduated participant modeling, and assisted and/or self-managed naturalistic exposure. The cognitive therapy movement is providing supplementary approaches. A case was described in which a 29-year-old woman's traumatically acquired phobia concerning black males generated two sets of treatment targets and prompted two approaches to treatment.

References

American Psychiatric Association. (1980). *Diagnostic and statistical manual of mental disorders* (3rd ed.). Washington, DC: Author.

Bandura, A. (1969). *Principles of behavior modification.* New York: Holt, Rinehart & Winston.

Bandura, A. (1971). Psychotherapy based upon modeling principles. In A. E. Bergin & S. L. Garfield (Eds.), *Handbook of psychotherapy and behavior change: An empirical analysis* (pp. 653–708). New York: Wiley.

Bandura, A. (1976). Effecting change through participant modeling. In J. D. Krumboltz & C. E. Thoreson (Eds.), *Counseling methods* (pp. 248–265). New York: Holt, Rinehart & Winston.

Bandura, A. (1977). Self-efficacy: Toward a unifying theory of behavioral change. *Psychological Review, 84,* 191–215.

Barrios, B. A., & Shigetomi, C. C. (1979). Coping-skills training for the management of anxiety: A critical review. *Behavior Therapy, 10,* 491–522.

Beck, A. T., & Emery, G. (1979). *Cognitive therapy of anxiety.* Philadelphia: Center of Cognitive Therapy.

Bellack, A. S., & Schwartz, J. S. (1976). Assessment for self-control programs. In M. Hersen & A. S. Bellack (Eds.), *Behavioral assessment: A practical handbook* (pp. 111–142). New York: Pergamon Press.

Bernstein, D. A., & Borkovec, T. D. (1973). *Progressive relaxation training: A manual for the helping professions.* Champaign, IL: Research Press.

Bolles, R. C. (1970). Species-specific defense reactions and avoidance learning. *Psychological Review, 77,* 32–48.

Cameron, N. (1963). *Personality development and psychopathology: A dynamic approach.* Boston: Houghton Mifflin.

Carr, A. T. (1979). The psychopathology of fear. In W. Sluckin (Ed.), *Fear in animals and man* (pp. 199–235). New York: Van Nostrand Rheinhold.

Cronbach, L. J. (1970). *Essentials of psychological testing* (3rd ed.). New York: Harper & Row.

Delprato, D. J., & McGlynn, F. D. (1984). Behavioral theories of anxiety disorders. In S. M. Turner (Ed.), *Behavioral theories and treatment of anxiety disorders* (pp. 1–49). New York: Plenum Press.

Dengrove, E. (1972). Practical behavioral diagnosis. In A. A. Lazarus (Ed.), *Clinical behavior therapy* (pp. 73–86). New York: Brunner/Mazel.

Dollard, J., & Miller, N. E. (1950). *Personality and psychotherapy: An analysis in terms of learning, thinking, and culture.* New York: McGraw-Hill.

Ellis, A., & Grieger, R. (1977). *Handbook of rational-emotive therapy.* New York: Springer.

Eysenck, H. J. (1976). The learning theory model of neurosis: A new approach. *Behaviour Research and Therapy, 14,* 251–267.

Geer, J. H. (1965). The development of a scale to measure fear. *Behaviour Research and Therapy, 3,* 45–53.

Goldfried, M. R., & Davison, G. C. (1976). *Clinical behavior therapy.* New York: Holt, Rinehart & Winston.

Guthrie, E. R. (1935). *The psychology of learning.* New York: Harper & Row.

Herrnstein, R. J. (1969). Method and theory in the study of avoidance. *Psychological Review, 76,* 49–69.

Hollon, S. D., & Bemis, K. M. (1981). Self-report and the assessment of cognitive functions. In M. Hersen & A. S. Bellack (Eds.), *Behavioral assessment: A practical handbook* (2nd ed., pp. 125–174). New York: Pergamon Press.

Husek, T. R., & Alexander, S. (1963). The effectiveness of the anxiety differential in examination stress situations. *Educational and Psychological Measurement, 23,* 309–318.

Kendall, P. C., & Hollon, S. D. (1981). *Assessment strategies for cognitive-behavioral interventions.* New York: Academic Press.

Kleinknecht, R. A., Klepac, R. K., & Alexander, L. D. (1973). Origins and characteristics of fear of dentistry. *Journal of the American Dental Association, 86,* 842–848.

Kleinknecht, R. A., McGlynn, F. D., Thorndike, R. M., & Harkavy, J. (1984). Factor analysis of the dental fear survey with cross validation. *Journal of the American Dental Association, 108,* 59–61.

Lacey, J. I. (1967). Somatic response patterning and stress: Some revisions of activation theory. In M. H. Appley & R. Trumbull (Eds.), *Psychological stress: Issues in research* (pp. 14–42). New York: Appleton-Century-Crofts.

Lader, M. (1975). The psychophysiology of anxious and depressed patients. In D. C. Fowles (Ed.), *Clinical applications of psychophysiology* (pp. 12–41). New York: Columbia University Press.

Lang, P. J. (1971). The application of psychophysiological methods to the study of psychotherapy and behavior modification. In A. E. Bergin & S. L. Garfield (Eds.), *Handbook of psychotherapy and behavior change: An empirical analysis* (pp. 75–125). New York: Wiley.

Lang, P. J. (1977). Physiological assessment of anxiety and fear. In J. D. Cone & R. P. Hawkins (Eds.), *Behavioral assessment: New directions in clinical psychology* (pp. 178–195). New York: Brunner/Mazel.

Lang, P. J. (1978). Anxiety: Toward a psychophysiological definition. In H. S. Akiskal & W. L. Webb (Eds.), *Psychiatric diagnosis: Exploration of biological predictors* (pp. 365–389). New York: Spectrum.

Lang, P. J., & Lazovik, A. D. (1963). Experimental desensitization of a phobia. *Journal of Abnormal and Social Psychology, 66,* 519–525.

Lazarus, A. A. (1971). *Behavior therapy and beyond.* New York: McGraw-Hill.

Leitenberg, H. (1972). Positive reinforcement and extinction procedures. In W. S. Agras (Ed.), *Behavior modification: Principles and clinical applications* (pp. 27–57). Boston: Little, Brown.

Mahoney, M. J. (1974). *Cognition and behavior modification.* Cambridge, MA: Ballinger.

Mahoney, M. J., & Arnkoff, D. B. (1978). Cognitive and self-control therapies. In S. L. Garfield & A. E. Bergin (Eds.), *Handbook of psychotherapy and behavior change* (2nd ed., pp. 689–722). New York: Wiley.

Marks, I. M. (1975). Behavioral treatments of phobic and obsessive-compulsive disorders: A critical appraisal. In M. Hersen, R. M. Eisler, & P. M. Miller (Eds.), *Progress in behavior modification* (Vol. 1, pp. 65–158). New York: Academic Press.

Marks, I. M. (1978). *Living with fear.* New York: McGraw-Hill.

Marks, I. M. (1981). *Cure and care of neuroses.* New York: Wiley.

McGlynn, F. D. (1978). Adults with anxiety-based disorders. In M. Hersen & A. S. Bellack (Eds.), *Behavior therapy in the psychiatric setting* (pp. 259–285). Baltimore: Williams & Wilkins.

McGlynn, F. D., & Linder, L. H. (1971). The clinical application of analogue desensitization: A case study. *Behavior Therapy, 2,* 385–388.

McKay, M., Davis, M., & Fanning, P. (1981). *Thoughts & feelings: The art of cognitive stress intervention.* Richmond, CA: New Harbinger Publications.

Meichenbaum, D. (1977). *Cognitive-behavior modification: An integrative approach.* New York: Plenum Press.

Meichenbaum, D., & Cameron, R. (1974). The clinical potential of modifying what clients say to themselves. *Psychotherapy: Theory, Research, and Practice, 11,* 103–117.

Miller, B. V., & Bernstein, D. A. (1972). Instructional demand in a behavioral avoidance test for claustrophobic fears. *Journal of Abnormal Psychology, 80,* 206–210.

Mowrer, O. H. (1947). On the dual nature of learning: A re-interpretation of "conditioning" and "problem-solving." *Harvard Educational Review, 17,* 102–148.

Rachman, S. (1976). The passing of the two-stage theory of fear and avoidance: Fresh possibilities. *Behaviour Research and Therapy, 14,* 125–131.

Rachman, S. (1977). The conditioning theory of fear-acquisition: A critical examination. *Behaviour Research and Therapy, 15,* 375–387.

Rachman, S. (1978). *Fear and courage.* San Francisco: W. H. Freeman.

Reiss, S. (1980). Pavlovian conditioning and human fear: An expectancy model. *Behavior Therapy, 11,* 380–396.

Rimm, D. C., & Masters, J. C. (1979). *Behavior therapy* (2nd ed.). New York: Academic Press.

Ritter, B. (1969). The use of contact desensitization, demonstration-plus-participation, and demonstration alone in the treatment of acrophobia. *Behaviour Research and Therapy, 7,* 157–164.

Seligman, M. E. P., & Johnston, J. C. (1973). A cognitive theory of avoidance learning. In F. J. McGuigan & D. B. Lumsden (Eds.), *Contemporary approaches to conditioning and learning* (pp. 69–110). Washington, DC: V. H. Winston.

Spielberger, C. D., Gorsuch, R. L., & Lushene, R. E. (1970). *Manual for the State-Trait Anxiety Inventory.* Palo Alto, CA: Consulting Psychologist Press.

Stampfl, T. G., & Levis, D. J. (1967). Essentials of implosive therapy: A learning-theory-based psychodynamic behavioral therapy. *Journal of Abnormal Psychology, 72,* 496–503.

Walk, R. D. (1956). Self-ratings of fear in a fear-invoking situation. *Journal of Abnormal and Social Psychology, 52,* 171–178.

Wolpe, J. (1973). *The practice of behavior therapy (2nd ed.).* New York: Pergamon Press.

Wolpe, J. (1976). *Theme and variations: A behavior therapy casebook.* New York: Pergamon Press.

Wolpe, J. (1982). *The practice of behavior therapy* (3rd ed.). New York: Pergamon Press.

Wolpe, J., & Lazarus, A. A. (1966). *Behavior therapy techniques.* New York: Pergamon Press.

Agoraphobia

DIANNE L. CHAMBLESS

Introduction

The advances in the treatment of agoraphobia made since 1970 and the adoption of the new techniques by practitioners stand as a gratifying example of the potential benefits to be gained from persisting with clinical research, difficult though it be. By 1981 Barlow and Wolfe were able to report that across treatment centers 65 to 75% of agoraphobic clients were found to improve with fairly brief behavioral treatment. Prior to the advent of active therapies for this problem, agoraphobia tended to be a lifelong disabling disorder, from which Roberts (1964) found only 24% to recover with standard interventions. There is enough known about agoraphobia in 1984 to fill an entire volume; in fact, two have been written on the subject for professional audiences (Chambless & Goldstein, 1982; Mathews, Gelder, & Johnston, 1981). Because all of this material cannot be compacted into one chapter, the focus in this paper will be on those aspects of our knowledge most pertinent to service providers. The reader expecting to practice heavily in this area or to perform research on this topic would do well to consult these more extensive works.

Agoraphobia is most briefly described as a fear and avoidance of public places and of being away from home, based on the anticipation of experiencing noxious levels of anxiety or panic attacks. Within this general framework, people with this fear are found to avoid a wide variety of situations: public conveyances, shops, restaurants, theaters, journeys away from home, standing in lines, being in elevators, and even being home alone are common triggers for anxiety. There are two

DIANNE L. CHAMBLESS • Department of Psychology, The American University, Washington, District of Columbia 20016.

underlying, related themes. The agoraphobic fears any situation where one is confined with restricted freedom of movement or possibility for escape, whether by physical constraint or social convention. Consequently, she or he may avoid visits to the dentist, social engagements (the more formal, the more anxiety provoking), and elevators. Agoraphobia is not, therefore, the opposite of claustrophobia, as the dictionary would lead one to believe. In fact, on the average, these clients are more afraid of enclosed than of open spaces.

Agoraphobics fear that their anxiety levels will rise to panic in these situations and that they will be unable to escape. Their goal may be simply to escape the noxious situation or, commonly, to reach a situation where they feel safe. This introduces the second theme, which involves not so much the fear of being someplace in particular, but the fear of being away from people and places that give the agoraphobic person a relative sense of security. Thus, many agoraphobics are able to function much better if accompanied by a trusted companion, typically a spouse or other family member, but possibly any responsible figure, or if they remain in, or close to, their homes or other familiar places. There are variations on the safety theme. For example, intensely hypochondriacal agoraphobics may feel relatively safe anywhere near a hospital or doctor's office. Recalling these themes of being trapped and of being alone and cut off from support and security is most helpful in understanding an agoraphobic's idiosyncratic reactions. For example, some clients consistently feel trapped whenever presented with something that must be done. One woman became persistently panicky in her last trimester of an unwanted pregnancy because she then had no choice. She had to go through with the delivery. This sort of client may react adversely to being pushed strongly in treatment. A second client felt alone, "dead, cut off from the world," whenever she closed her eyes. Consequently, she had difficulty at the beauty parlor, not because she felt trapped, as many clients do, but because so many procedures required that she close her eyes to avoid damage from chemicals. Coping strategies for her symptoms had to be altered accordingly. Hence, although it is certainly crucial to obtain a list of the places clients avoid, it is also extremely important to remember that an agoraphobic's fears generalize not just along physical lines but also along cognitive ones.

Agoraphobic people vary widely in the size of their safety zones and in the degree to which a companion limits their anxiety. There is also considerable variability in the degree to which a particular agoraphobic is symptomatic on a given day or during a particular year. Some can vary from being almost asymptomatic to being housebound within a month (Buglass, Clarke, Henderson, Kreitman, & Presley, 1977), and some report having periods of remission over a number of years (Marks, 1970). This changeability bewilders and often frustrates not only the agoraphobic but also those in her or his life. These fluctuations in avoidance are generally based on the agoraphobic's perception of the likelihood of panic at a given time. Commonly, agoraphobics begin the day by monitoring their levels of anxiety and make or alter decisions about their activities accordingly. Panic attacks are quite variable in occurrence, and agoraphobic people may have periods of years without frequent panic and gradually begin to do more. However, when a series of panics is once again experienced, often associated with increased stress, a rapid acceleration in avoidance typically follows.

The problem of panic is, thus, central to the understanding of agoraphobia. Under conditions of extreme fear, most phobic clients report the symptoms of panic, which include rapid heart beat, chest pain, difficulty with breathing, dizziness, faintness, a sense of unreality, shaking, numbness or tingling in the extremities, and an urge to urinate or defecate. Particular symptoms are salient for different people. For the agoraphobic person the panic is accompanied by an intense urge to flee, a sense of doom, and thoughts of impending catastrophe. These attacks are all the more frightening in the case of agoraphobia, for, contrary to specific phobias, agoraphobic panic is rather unpredictable in nature, often striking without warning, seemingly without reason, and engendering a sense of helplessness. This erratic course of panic has led some to believe that these attacks reflect an endogenous disturbance, best treated with psychotropic medication (e.g., Sheehan, Ballenger, & Jacobsen, 1980). I find it more useful to conceive of panic as a reaction some people are prone to have when under stress, just as others might develop hypertension, ulcers, or migraines. There is increasingly good evidence that the panic reaction is familial in origin and more likely to develop in female family members (Crowe, Noyes, Pauls, & Slymen, 1983). Whatever its origin, the unpredictability of panic leads the agoraphobic to think of no place as being completely safe and to discount occasions when, on a sortie into the external world, the expected panic did not occur. The avoidance behavior thus is negatively reinforced on an intermittent basis and is, consequently, all the more resistant to alteration.

Panic attacks are highly noxious unconditioned stimuli. Places, thoughts, and feelings associated with panic quickly become anxiety provoking themselves. Consequently, although agoraphobia has been described as a fear of fear (Goldstein & Chambless, 1978), fear of many intense sensations that share component responses with panic may develop. Often, agoraphobics become fearful of anger, worrying that being upset will drive them to panic, and even of intense, presumably pleasant, sensations such as profound relaxation or orgasm because of the sense of loss of control accompanying these events. Almost all become hyperalert to the physiological sensations associated with their attacks and focus on these sensations, monitoring their bodies for any increase in these signs, and spiraling into panic or fleeing when the dreaded signals are detected. Finally, the agoraphobic's assessment of the possible consequences of panic is an important component of the phobic response. Almost all believe that some catastrophe will result. There are two general categories of these catastrophes: physiological events such as having a heart attack, fainting, and vomiting; and social/behavioral events such as losing control, screaming, babbling, and becoming insane. During the panic state, most strongly believe these events are imminent. When calm, fewer hold these beliefs fixedly despite all medical and psychological reassurance, but the majority continue to have some concerns that spring back to full force when anxiety next increases. These doubts about mental and physical integrity are pervasively demoralizing and serve to drive the agoraphobic's anxiety quickly higher when the thoughts occur.

In summary, we can see that although panic attacks may initially strike "out of the blue" as a nonspecific response to stress, the agoraphobic's response to the panic serves to perpetuate the stress and to make the likelihood of continued attacks all the higher.

Whether community samples or clinical populations are studied, agoraphobia is found to be about four times more prevalent in women than men (reviewed by Chambless, 1982; Weissman, 1983). In recent community studies reviewed by Weissman, generally 2–4/100 women were diagnosed as agoraphobic. The problem is most likely to begin in late adolescence and young adulthood (Marks, 1970), although many clients report having had similar feelings for circumscribed periods during childhood, often taking the form of school phobia or panic attacks without subsequent phobic complications.

Any number of stressors have been listed as the final precipitants of panic attacks. These stressors do not necessarily have any particular attributes, but most often they relate to the themes of being trapped and/or alone. Late adolescent onset generally is related to separation issues such as leaving home, going to college, taking a job, and leaving behind childhood. Onset in the 20s may pertain to moving away from parental attachments into adult relationships. For example, one client, raised in a conservative Catholic home, had decided that as she approached 30 she would like to move out of her parents' home and share an apartment with her boyfriend. In the months of frantic quarrels that followed, her mother threatened that the client would cause her to have a nervous breakdown by such wicked behavior. The client remained in the parental home but became agoraphobic, feeling trapped but unable to break the bond with her mother. A final example of this issue is the young married woman with children who is unhappy with her relationship but feels trapped in her marriage. She feels unable to leave due to her own fears of being alone and most often also due to the very real difficulties a female, single parent faces: inadequate child support, economic discrimination, poor vocational training, and isolation with the burdens of raising children alone. Women may be particularly prone to agoraphobia because they are shaped to be more emotionally dependent on relationships than are men and because of their economic dependence on men. (For a more complete discussion of these issues see Chambless, 1982.) Other common precipitants include bereavement and moving (both again involving separation), physical illness or surgery, and the assumption of new responsibilities such as those brought on by a promotion. Similar events may exacerbate the symptoms of one who is already agoraphobic.

Even once we have added in the ingredient of a familial predisposition to have panic attacks when under stress, we have not solved the problem of the onset of agoraphobia because not everyone who develops panic attacks becomes phobic. In part, this may reflect modeling because families of agoraphobics are more likely to have all sorts of phobias than are families of probands with panic disorder (Harris, Noyes, Crowe, & Chaudhry, 1983). Elsewhere (Chambless & Goldstein, 1981; Goldstein & Chambless, 1978), we have argued that other important contributing factors are (a) a tendency to misattribute the source of panic, looking to physical situations or some disease process as the cause of distress rather than the pertinent stressors; (b) a vulnerability to separation whether through overprotection, neglect, or childhood separation trauma, which is related to (c) a sense of being inadequate to care for oneself and function as an autonomous adult. All of these characteristics point to important therapeutic issues to be resolved in the treatment of an agoraphobic client.

Associated Problems

Part of the complexity of treating agoraphobics should be apparent from the list of problem areas requiring attention that has been presented so far. There are, however, additional complicating factors that need to be addressed. Only the most common will be touched on here (see Chambless, 1982, for a more complete treatment). Depression is so often associated with agoraphobia that there have been attempts, now largely abandoned, to categorize this disorder as *atypical depression*. The great majority of these clients are mildly to moderately severely depressed. Depression is frequently part of the initial sense of being abandoned, helpless, and overwhelmed that the person is already undergoing when the panic attacks begin or recur. Once panic attacks have begun and avoidance behavior is established, even if the external crisis is resolved, depression is still likely, now a result of the agoraphobic symptoms. Not only is the distress associated with panic related to increased depression, avoidance is strongly related to higher levels of depression. Being dysfunctional when faced with the most mundane task, like grocery shopping, is destructive to self-esteem. Moreover, the restrictions of being agoraphobic cut one off from many of the most powerful reinforcers in our society: social contact, avocational interests, and career advancement.

Agoraphobics are characterized by very high levels of chronic anxiety. Many report having always been "high strung," which fits with a prevalent familial pattern of anxiety problems as well as phobias (Harris *et al.*, 1983). Their tension no doubt increases their tendency to develop panic attacks. This propensity to be a "worrier" may be associated with their tendency toward hypochondriasis, which is particularly pronounced in the men. Their anxiety and avoidance is typically increased by even mild illnesses, and they often "catastrophize" that any physical symptom is a sign of impending major, perhaps fatal, illness. Although they may, if able to reach and wait in a physician's office or emergency room, seek repeated assurance about their health, they are generally loathe to accept medical treatment, being terrified that the prescribed medication will drive them out of control or cause life-threatening side effects.

Finally, a significant problem for the great majority of agoraphobics is social anxiety, which is generally related to a strong fear of others' negative evaluations. It has been previously noted that interpersonal relationships are extremely important to these clients. They are easily distressed by loss of approval or even temporary withdrawal of affection and are greatly disturbed at being the target of another's anger. As a result, they are often unassertive, particularly in intimate relationships, and allow themselves to be manipulated or bullied. These tendencies are worsened by the development of agoraphobia, in that the increased dependency associated with the disorder causes them to fear offending significant others even more. In addition, the associated loss of self-esteem increases their sense of inadequacy in interpersonal situations, and their fears that their anxiety will be noticed by others (it generally is not) may cause them to avoid formerly satisfying social contacts.

Assessment

In the last decade there has been an increasing amount of publicity about agoraphobia, resulting in a large number of such clients who seek treatment from therapists known to use specific techniques for treating this fear. These clients, and indeed many who refer them, have a rather imprecise notion of what agoraphobia is, often using the term to refer to severe nonphobic anxiety states, other phobias, or any problem that leads one to avoid leaving the house. Typically, they have fixed their attention on one aspect of an article or television report that matched their own symptoms and have ignored the discrepancies. Consequently, the first task of assessment will be the determination of whether a client is agoraphobic. Apart from this decision, an important function of assessment is treatment planning.

To quantify relevant information and to gather material in an efficient, economical fashion I send clients a packet of questionnaires to fill out before they come in for their intake interview. The questionnaires I currently use are the Beck Depression Inventory (Beck, Ward, Mendelson, Mock, & Erbaugh, 1961), the Trait Anxiety form of the State-Trait Anxiety Inventory (Spielberger, Gorsuch, & Lushene, 1970), the Michigan Alcoholism Screening Test (Selzer, 1971), the Fear Questionnaire (Marks & Mathews, 1979), the Mobility Inventory for Agoraphobia (Chambless, Caputo, Jasin, Gracely, & Williams, 1983), the Agoraphobic Cognitions Questionnaire and Body Sensations Questionnaire (Chambless, Caputo, Bright, & Gallagher, 1983), and a semantic differential measure of marital dissatisfaction (Bland & Hallam, 1981). The Fear Questionnaire is a fairly brief questionnaire useful for general phobia screening. It has three factors of five items each representing the phobias for which clients most frequently seek treatment: agoraphobia ($M = 21.31$, $SD = 10.06$), social phobia (M for agoraphobics $= 15.94$, $SD = 9.99$), and blood and injury phobia. Additional write-in items allow clients to list particular fears of concern or specific phobias. The need to assess social phobia, depression, and chronic anxiety should be apparent from the section on associated problems.

The Mobility Inventory is comprised of 26 situations commonly feared by agoraphobics that are rated on 1–5 scales for avoidance alone ($M = 3.37$, $SD = 1.05$) and accompanied ($M = 2.64$, $SD = 0.89$), with higher ratings indicating greater severity. The total scores are averages of individual item ratings. Discomfort ratings are generally so highly correlated with avoidance ratings as to be unnecessary to take separately. However, if a client reports being fearful but not avoidant, the scales can be administered with instructions to rate for the amount of fear in these situations instead. This inventory is used in addition to the Fear Questionnaire because it taps a much broader range of functioning and is more useful for treatment planning. A final item on the Mobility Inventory asks for the frequency of panic attacks in the previous week (median = 2.00).

The Agoraphobic Cognitions Questionnaire (M = 2.32, SD = 0.07) and the Body Sensations Questionnaire (M = 3.05, SD = 0.86) are used to measure important aspects of fear of fear: the particular catastrophes a given client thinks will result from anxiety and the physiological signs of anxiety that the client finds most disturbing. These measures, also on 1–5 scales, are helpful in assessing the severity of fear of fear and in cuing the therapist to the particular thoughts and sensations a client must learn to cope with in treatment.

The Michigan Alcoholism Screening Test is a brief questionnaire that is highly functional as an initial assessment of problematical drinking. False positives are fairly common, but false negatives are rare. I have had several clients deny drinking problems after receiving positive scores on the MAST, only to reveal serious alcohol abuse later in treatment. I began to use the scale in the last year and follow up suspicious cases and find that 10% of agoraphobic clients applying for treatment are actively abusing alcohol or are recovered alcoholics, whose recovery, of course, is not always stable. Because these clients are apt to use alcohol in part to cope with anxiety, it is an important factor to be aware of.

Finally, the Spouse–Partner Description Questionnaire is a semantic differential rating form using five adjectives that Bland and Hallam (1981) found to be sensitive indicators of marital dissatisfaction. Marital dissatisfaction has frequently been found to predict poorer response to treatment for agoraphobia and is consequently important to assess. No real norms exist on this form, but I prefer it to marital dissatisfaction inventories because of its greater subtlety. The average score for an agoraphobic population is 5.42 (SD = 4.20). As marital problems are such a common feature of agoraphobia, any score at or above the mean should probably be viewed as clinically significant.

In my view, psychophysiological assessment and formalized pretreatment behavioral avoidance measures are not useful or economically viable procedures in ordinary clinical treatment. However, they might be appropriate for particular research designs or for the therapist preparing court testimony for insurance cases and such. Informally, the therapist will certainly want to observe the client's behavior and ask for reports of thoughts, images, and feelings, particularly during initial exposure sessions, to gain a further understanding of that client's phobic response. It is helpful to train the client to report anxiety levels using a 0–100 scale. This allows therapist and client finer levels of discrimination in the anxiety response than clients are wont to make spontaneously. It requires a bit of practice with the scale, assisted by feedback from the therapist (e.g., "You look considerably more tense than a 30 would indicate right now. Do you mean to say you're only mildly uncomfortable?") to obtain consistent data. As will be illustrated, these *in vivo* observations may lead to a change in diagnosis or in the treatment plan.

In the case of physiological monitoring, most therapists will not have the necessary equipment available to them, and it is extremely difficult, even with excellent equipment, to get reliable and valid psychophysiological measures for agoraphobic clients. Nevertheless, it is inexpensive and relatively easy to occasionally measure heart rate, should that seem advisable, by taking the client's pulse. Although not everyone responds to anxiety with increased heart rate, it is the index most consistently linked with self-reported fear. Also, a great many reactions are readily observable to the perceptive observer: blanching, flushing, sweating, trembling, postural rigidity, and the like. There are two common reasons to monitor pulse rate. First would be the case of a client who appears to do everything easily but reports a high anxiety level. Finding a rapid heart beat helps to confirm the client's perception. The absence of a rapid pulse proves little because not only is the measure unreliable, but also the client may not be a person who responds to anxiety with increased heart rate. The absence may, nevertheless, encourage the therapist to probe the client's anxiety report more carefully, checking for possible operants maintaining the behavior or for unrealistic expectations, for example, that one should be completely calm on an expressway at rush hour. If all fails, however, we are ultimately dependent on clients' reports about their experience of fear.

Diagnosis

Several other conditions may lead to avoidance of leaving the home or of being in public places alone. These are most easily discerned through an interview wherein the patterns of the client's avoidance behavior are explored, as are the reasons for staying home. Some clients with thought disorders fear persecution of some sort if they go out to public places or loss of control over unacceptable sexual or aggressive impulses. In the great majority of cases, these clients may be quickly picked out during the course of an interview by their affect and thought progression. If not, the nature of the material they provide when asked what they anticipate happening in the phobic situation and a history of what has happened to them in these situations in the past generally resolve the question. When there is any doubt, a thorough psychiatric history is advisable, as are records of prior treatments. In a few cases, I have known of such clients slipping through a screening, particularly when initial interviews were conducted by relatively inexperienced people, and decompensating during treatment. If the therapist has a sense that the client is withholding information when asked about fears and behavior in the phobic situation, further assessment *in vivo* should be planned using mildly to moderately stressful situations and probing the client's reactions while he or she is frightened and less defensive. This step is crucial if the client is to be turned over to a trainee or paraprofessional for subsequent *in vivo* exposure work.

Severe depression may lead to apathy and withdrawal or extreme agitation with a sense of inability to cope with any demands. In these cases, one may see clients who do not, for the duration of the depression, leave their homes much, but who, once the depression lifts, again become completely mobile. Scores above 40 on the Beck Depression Inventory are one clue to this type of case. However, agoraphobic clients may become very depressed and often become more phobic when they do, making the decision more difficult. A detailed history of prior episodes of depression and the relationship of avoidance behavior to these episodes is clarifying. Also a careful discussion with the client about how it is that she or he comes to stay at home so much is important. For example, one woman with a Beck score of 45 reported having several periods of major depression with clear vegetative signs that lasted for several months during which she rarely left the house. Her behavior was normal between these episodes. When asked what happened to prevent or discourage her from leaving home during the episodes of depression such as the current one, she reported having no energy, finding that it took her until late afternoon to get out of bed, get dressed, and have breakfast. By this time she would often have missed the planned appointment or would decide it was really too late to go out anyway. She described no fear of panic attacks or concerns that anything negative would happen to her once she did get out of the house. In fact, she often felt better once having done so. Clearly, treatment for depression, not agoraphobia, was in order.

Clients with severe hypochondriasis may appear very similar to agoraphobic clients in behavior. Some avoid going out, quit work, and may even confine themselves to bed because they cannot tolerate one or more physical symptoms that they fear indicate serious illness. They differ from agoraphobic clients in having no concern about place (except perhaps distance from medical care), being trapped, or being alone. Their focus is solely on minimizing the feared symptom. On the Mobility Inventory, these clients may give extreme ratings on all items—an unusual repsonse. Their scores may approach 5 on the Body Sensations Inventory as well. A common case is that of the "cardiac neurotic" client. One client, a healthy athlete, quit his team and all other effortful work, convinced he was close to a heart attack. He monitored his pulse constantly and avoided walking on the street, standing in lines, and such because the exertion increased his heart beat. I could bring on his full anxiety response by having him run in place in my office. Going anyplace in particular was irrelevant. These clients can be successfully integrated into treatment groups with agoraphobic clients, but it is essential that the therapist recognize their difference and alter the treatment accordingly. For example, when asking agoraphobic clients to walk several blocks, I make a point of saying they are to do it slowly, rather than rushing through to end the anxiety as quickly as possible. With the cardiac neurotic case, however, I asked him to walk briskly, increasing his speed over the sessions to expose him to the feared response of accelerated heart beat.

Obsessive-compulsive clients may become housebound by lengthy rituals or by their attempts to avoid contamination if the contaminants are widespread. This is generally readily apparent on interview by asking the client about her or his concerns about leaving home and by the ritualistic behavior. In one case where the client explicitly denied rituals, the pattern was discerned on an exploratory *in vivo* session carried out because she seemed to be withholding something and did not describe the same concerns as agoraphobic or socially phobic clients. Her rituals were triggered by activities like shopping, and she feared others would notice them. She eventually explained that she had read so much about agoraphobia, she thought it was acceptable, but she feared the rituals were a sign of insanity that would lead to her rejection from treatment. For those occasional clients who seem both obsessive-compulsive and agoraphobic, it is wise to treat the ritualistic behavior first.

The *Diagnostic and Statistical Manual of Mental Disorders* (DSM-III) (American Psychiatric Association, 1980) description of *social phobia* is that of a fear of one type of situation or interaction. This does not fit with the clinical presentation of these people, and there are plans afoot to revise the DSM accordingly. In many cases, social anxiety is generalized; in fact, after agoraphobia this is the most common kind of generalized fear for which people seek treatment. This common characteristic can result in confusion of these problems, particularly because most agoraphobic clients are also socially phobic. Most often, the cases can be fairly easily distinguished with a bit of care. The Social Phobia Factor on the Fear Questionnaire will be high and the Agoraphobia factor fairly low. On the Mobility Inventory a pattern emerges of high ratings on situations involving social exchange, for example, parties and restaurants, and lower ratings on other items such as tunnels and driving. These clients report avoiding situations where they fear they will be perceived as socially inadequate and/or where others will see their anxiety: awkward speech, trembling hands, blushing, sweating, and the like. In very severe cases some socially phobic clients may avoid going out to some degree to avoid public scrutiny.

Here is an example of the sort of confusing picture a therapist may be confronted with. Ms. L. was a 27-year-old law student with a Social Phobia factor score of 34 and an Agoraphobia factor score of 17. One might initially hypothesize moderate agoraphobia and severe social phobia. Here the broader range of items on the Mobility Inventory was useful. Her overall scores were 1.88 Alone and 1.84 Accompanied, which are rather low. Her individual item scores were almost all 1s (never avoid) except for theaters, department stores, buses, subways, standing in line, parties, and other social gatherings. She added on "talking to people" and "sitting in front of the classroom." On the Agoraphobic Cognitions Questionnaire her concerns were social in nature: acting foolish, losing control, and babbling—overall score 2.21. Items given high ratings on the Body Sensations were sweating, having a knot in her stomach, and feeling confused—overall score a rather low 2.0. The items most salient for agoraphobics (e.g., heart palpitations, dizziness) were low. Her scores on depression (35) and chronic anxiety (69) were both quite high. The picture was one of severe social phobia, but the items concerning public transportation were confusing. Excerpts of the intake interview follow.

T: Tell me what happens to you when you get an anxiety attack. What's that experience like?

C: Well, I get very, very nervous and I feel like I have to escape, and you can see I start sweating.

T: As I can see? What am I supposed to see?

C: Well, I feel like I'm sweating now.

T: Okay, I really don't see, but that's what it feels like, huh?

C: Right. It's not just new situations; it can be old ones.

T: What is it about this situation right now that you think you are responding to?

C: I just feel very warm. Very hot. Maybe it's because you're new to me.

T: Sitting and talking to a new person is hard for you?

C: That's part of it. Uh, also with old people. I really don't know that triggers it.

T: OK.

C: [*Describing onset*] Well, I'm in law school and I really feel like I don't belong there. I felt that everybody was superior as far as intelligence, and they were brighter and it [*the anxiety*] happened so much in school. It was a very tense time for me [*beginning school*].

T: Yes, it was a lot of stress. Is this your first year in law school?

C: Yes. And after the first semester I didn't want to go back. Academically, I did very poorly. I got two D's and a C. But half the time I wasn't there; I mean I would be there in body but not in mind. I was just waiting for a panic attack to come, and so it was very difficult for me to concentrate on what was actually going on in the classroom.

T: Uh huh. So the whole time you were in school you were constantly around people that you're putting yourself down in reference to.

C: Yes, that's true. [*Goes on to describe her refusal to do oral presentations in class because she fears she won't be able to express herself well, even if she knows the material.*]

C: [*Asked about other phobic situations*] Well, uh, I haven't been on a bus in the summer in 2, if not more, years. Once I get on the bus, if I feel like I can ride to the end of the line, I could stay there. But if I have to get off, say, midway, I can't do it because my clothes will be soaking wet. All the clothes, skirt, blouse, everything, my face. I'll be so nervous I'll feel like I want to escape, but I'm afraid to actually get off the bus.

T: Because . . .

C: Because I don't want people to see me with wet clothes.

T: People would notice . . .

C: Yeah, that something is wrong. In the wintertime I can ride the bus. I have my coat on or a jacket and it doesn't bother me; I can get off at midway. I can get off anywhere, at the beginning of the line, or at the end. But, I guess I'm very conscious of the fact of sweating.

T: So, in the summertime you are more likely to sweat, and then you are going to worry about sweating.

C: Well, I sweat in the winter, but it's not so obvious in the winter. You wear darker clothes.

T: Is that always what you get concerned about, that people would notice how anxious you are?

C: Yes.

T: Any other concerns that you have at that time?

C: In what respect?

T: About when you get anxious.

C: Just other people's feelings about me, how they will react, and what they will think about me in the future.

T: Uh huh, uh huh.

C: And, and, uh, if it happens more than once when I'm talking to the same person, that's really more of a concern because I'm afraid that "well, it happened yesterday, and now it's happening again, and, I'm wondering what this person's doing here in law school, or at work."

Subsequently, I learned that the client had begun having some difficulty in junior high school, but it stayed at a mild level, although she never dated much. Several years after receiving her bachelor's degree, watching her friends become professionals, Ms. L. decided she should overcome her general insecurity, quit working in clerical positions, and apply to law school. She secretly hoped she would not be admitted but entered a predominantly white law school when accepted. (The client is black and from a background of poverty, and social phobia is often associated with upward mobility [Amies, Gelder, & Shaw, 1983].) The soft-spoken, quiet Ms. L. quickly felt overwhelmed by aggressive, competitive fellow students and the demands for verbal debate. She became increasingly anxious in class, and the heightened anxiety then spread to all encounters with people except family members and a few close friends. Unlike agoraphobic people, she did not fear riding the bus because she could not quickly get out and get home. Rather, she feared enforced contact with people who would see her typical sign of anxiety—sweating. If, in fact, it was so hot that everyone was sweating, the client was no longer very uncomfortable. *In vivo* exposure would not be the treatment of choice for this client. Instead, a program of anxiety management training and assertiveness training would probably be in order as first steps in her treatment.

Finally, rape victims and other victims of violence may become reluctant to go out because of fear of being assaulted again (see Chambless & Goldstein, 1980, for an example of an interview with such a client). The history of onset of the fears and the clients' reports of what they fear on the street is diagnostic here. Also, the pattern of fears will be different, with fewer concerns about enclosed spaces, social settings, actually being on public transportation (as opposed to waiting for it), and stores. Because so many rape victims do not volunteer information about sexual assault, anytime the pattern does not fit an agoraphobic one, the therapist should inquire. It is also important to recognize that assault can be a final stressor that leads to the development of true agoraphobia as well.

Other Anxiety Disorders

Because most people with generalized phobias are agoraphobic, clients with multiple phobias are often misdiagnosed as agoraphobic, particularly because these people are often generally anxious individuals who consequently acquire fears easily. The agoraphobic cluster of fears will be missing, however. For example, such clients may be afraid of driving because someone might collide with them, of fires in upper stories of hotels, of accidents on planes, and of dogs, which might bite. These clients are pervasively fearful of harm, but from an external source, not from their own panic as would be the case of agoraphobic clients. The consistent nature of their phobic avoidant responses serves to distinguish them from the pervasively anxious individual who diffusely sees danger and misfortune lurking everywhere. The latter are currently labeled as having *generalized anxiety disorder.* When the element of panic attacks is added to chronic anxiety, thus earning the diagnosis of *panic disorder,* we have a case commonly confused with agoraphobia because of the salience of panic attacks in the latter syndrome. There is, in fact, considerable overlap between these disorders and their treatments. The clearest case of panic disorder is someone who reports panic attacks on the Mobility Inventory, high Trait Anxiety, often moderately high depression on the Beck, but who is not found to be avoidant on the Mobility Inventory.

There is an increasing number of clients applying for treatment who are mildly avoidant in a typical agoraphobic pattern or who are fearful according to the agoraphobic pattern but do not permit themselves to avoid. They often describe having read about agoraphobia fairly extensively and, having realized that there was no real danger to them in facing their fears, they simply continued to go out. Moreover, they describe being comforted by learning their panic attacks were a sign of anxiety and finding that they were less likely to continue having attacks once having acquired this knowledge. In some treatment centers, these clients are labeled *agoraphobic* and in others as having *panic disorder*. For treatment and conceptual purposes, I find it most useful to consider them to be mildly agoraphobic.

Types of Agoraphobia

In a 1978 paper, Goldstein and Chambless proposed that for treatment planning and research it was useful to conceptualize agoraphobics as falling into two, albeit imperfect, categories: *simple* and *complex* agoraphobia. The simple cases are delightful to treat and account for most reports of miracle cures of agoraphobia. These people are free of most of the associated problems of agoraphobia and typically develop panic attacks due to some sort of physical illness or bad experiences with prescribed or street drugs. Once this event has passed, there are few panic attacks that occur outside of the phobic situation. Although distressed by any restrictions, they are generally not chronically anxious, depressed, or socially phobic. One has the sense of a basically healthy person who, but for some chance event, would not have become agoraphobic. Perhaps 5% of cases in my experience fit this description.

In the case of complex agoraphobia, the phobic symptoms seem only part of a wide range of problems the person faces. The phobia is intertwined with personal, interpersonal, and situational difficulties in a way that makes treatment much more difficult and ultimately less successful for most. Except for therapists who do time-limited, didactic style groups limited to discussions of fear, most clinicians confronted with a case of complex agoraphobia will find themselves addressing many different issues requiring a variety of treatment techniques. Two case examples will help to illustrate these differences.

Ms. N. is a 37-year-old married woman with no children. She has a graduate degree in her field and holds a high-level job. She sought treatment for agoraphobia of 15 years duration when new job responsibilities made her restrictions more awkward. She had previously seen various intrapsychically oriented therapists with whom she became impatient and terminated after several sessions and one behavior therapist who treated her with systematic desensitization, which was somewhat helpful.

Ms. N. had a Mobility Inventory Alone score of 3.08, indicating considerable avoidance, but could go most places if accompanied by her husband, the only person who knew of her fears. Her Accompanied score was 1.84. She reported no panic attacks in recent years, was a calm person (Trait Anxiety = 24), and showed no evidence of depression (Beck = 1) or alcoholism (MAST = 0). She had some anxiety in formal social functions where she could not escape being the focus of attention but was otherwise socially comfortable (Social Phobia factor = 8). She had low scores overall on the Agoraphobic Cognitions Questionnaire (1.36) and the Body Sensations Questionnaire (1.88) but had high scores on individual items concerning passing out, dizziness, blurred vision, wobbly legs, and feeling disoriented and confused. She reported that she feared going out alone because of these symptoms. As is common for many agoraphobic women sensitive to dizziness, the client avoided wearing high heels that gave her a feeling that she was dizzy and might fall. She also carried an umbrella at all times to use like a cane should her legs become wobbly.

Ms. N. stated her attacks began when she was under a considerable amount of stress. She was being sexually harassed at her job, and her parents were in opposition to her plans for marriage. It is noteworthy that the client has two siblings with anxiety problems, one of whom is mildly agoraphobic. Otherwise, her family history was unremarkable, without the usual family history of depression and alcoholism.

The client had persisted in marrying the man she had chosen, was quite happy in her marriage (Spouse Dissatisfaction = 3) and her friendships, and excited about her new duties at work. Her phobias had gradually improved over the last 10 years but still formed a major source of dissatisfaction in her life. Her husband was quite supportive, had moved with her wherever necessary for her career advancement, and uncomplainingly assisted her in getting about the city. Although Ms. N. does not have the most typical onset picture for simple agoraphobia, she nonetheless fits this category well in the pattern of her symptoms.

Ms. H. is a 50-year-old married woman with three children who range in age from 16 to 21. She is middle class, college educated, and holds a job requiring presentations to groups. Ordinarily, during the 10 years she has been agoraphobic, work has been a safe place for her. In the past 2 months before intake, she has been distressed to see her panic attacks (three in the last 7 days on the Mobility Inventory) spread to her job. Her Avoidance Alone and Accompanied scores were both high, 3.85 and 3.21, respectively, indicating widespread avoidance. A safety zone of 10 to 15 minutes' drive from her home was indicated. On the Agoraphobic Cognitions Questionnaire, her overall score was 2.36, with 5s (the highest score) on passing out, acting foolish, and losing control. Extreme scores on the Body Sensations Inventory were on items concerning dizziness, wobbly legs, sweating, and heart palpitations, with a total score of 2.71. She scored as being moderately socially phobic (17), extremely anxious (69), and moderately depressed (19). Significant marital distress was indicated by a Spouse Dissatisfaction score of 9. Excerpts from her intake interview follow:

> [*The client has begun talking before the tape recorder is turned on and has begun to describe how her problem began when her husband was diagnosed as having cancer.*]
>
> C: . . . which was very, I mean, everything was fine, and he's been well since then . . . but about 3 months after that, it started.
> T: You still seem pretty shaky from driving here and talking about this.
> C: Yeah, and talking about this whole thing.
> T: Uh huh, it's upsetting talking about this whole thing.
> C: I'm highly motivated, very ambitious, and this is screwing up. . . [*waves hands*].
> T: Uh huh, just interfering with your life.
> C: Yes! And I've seen shrinks [*blowing nose*], I mean, up to here [*holds hand at level of nose*]. It's all very nice. I know the *how*'s and the *why*'s, but I don't know how to stop doing what I'm doing.

T: Yeah, So you have come to sort of an understanding you think of how it got going and what's happening to you.

C: I'm a classic. I think maybe you talked about it in the article about you in the paper, about people who have had problems with parents and the childhood, leaving them you know.

T: Uh huh.

C: My mother was exactly like me, she . . . well, rather I'm exactly like her. She had a heart problem all the time and, myself and my siblings always used to go at night to check if she's still breathing.

T: Uh huh. So she was real scared that she was going to die.

C: I don't know how scared she was; she sure as hell made us scared.

T: Made you scared. Uh huh.

C: So, I was always, you know, living under the shadow. She's going to leave me. She's going to die.

T: Uh huh. Was she actually physically ill or had anxiety attacks?

C: No. She had a bad heart.

T: Uh huh. She actually had a bad heart.

C: Yeah. And, uh . . . I, uh, I'm not American born. I was born and grew up in a country where there was warfare. My father would be called out on patrol.

T: Yes.

C: And I would lie down as a child, we lived opposite the emergency room of the hospital at the time, and I remember lying as a child looking to see if the men then were being brought wounded, if they were my father.

T: Yeah.

C: So, I mean. It's a classic.

T: So you didn't have a whole lot of security, huh?

C: No, and then when my husband, getting cancer, when he was going to leave me [*i.e., die*]. Again, you know. . . .

T: Uh huh, just set all that stuff off again. . . . OK.

C: And then he had another episode with heart trouble. And it turned out to be a false alarm and, and, so, you know . . . they're leaving me. And recently my children left home for college, so, everybody is leaving me again, you know, so I understand, and the shrink explained to me that I wanted to have power and hold them, so I'm going to have this, this tyranny [*referring to her phobia*] and, and . . . I understand that whole shit, I just don't know how to stop it!

C: Well, I read Dr. Weeks and what she said made a lot of sense.

T: Uh huh.

C: [*At this point client is pacing around the room.*] I'm getting up because it's easier.

T: Yes, that's fine. Tell me what you're experiencing right now. What it feels like to you to be really anxious right now?

C: Oh, I'm afraid of passing out all the time.

T: OK.

C: And I've never passed out in my life.

T: Uh huh. But you fear it now.

C: That's the biggest fear.

Ms. H., as she indicates, is indeed a classic example of agoraphobia preceded by childhood insecurity and activated by separation threats in adult life. Her agoraphobia has worsened with each successive threat to her emotional attachments. This history and the associated problems also make her a classic example of the category of complex agoraphobia. This will become even clearer as we use additional excerpts from her tape in our discussion of treatment planning.

Medical Issues

Finally, the client's physical condition needs to be discussed. Of importance here are debilitating conditions such as chronic heart disease or severe asthma that may require alterations in the treatment approach. Furthermore, conditions that can mimic or exacerbate anxiety symptoms should be discussed. Problems such as hypoglycemia, diabetes, and paroxysmal tachycardia need to be under control. Caffeinism should also be ruled out.

Much has been made recently of the connection between a diagnosis of agoraphobia or panic disorder and the usually benign congenital heart defect of mitral valve prolapse (MVP). About 25% or more of clients with these particular anxiety disorders are found to have MVP. The prolapse seems to account for the reduced exercise tolerance noted in anxious clients. It is easy to get the impression that a substantial proportion of clients with panic attacks suffer instead from MVP and require some different form of treatment. The best evidence to date, however, indicates that panic attacks and MVP happen to run in the same families (Crowe, Pauls, Slymen, & Noyes, 1980), probably due to their association with some as yet unknown third factor, and that the link is not a causal one. Indeed, most people with MVP are never aware of any symptoms from it. In research on treatment response, agoraphobics with MVP have improved on panic attacks despite unchanged cardiac functioning (Mavissakalian, Salerni, Thompson, & Michelson, 1983). Thus, a diagnosis of MVP does not seem to change the course of treatment (unless vigorous exercise is anticipated) but may require special reassurance for confused clients. The one complicating factor is iatrogenic. Clients with MVP may be prescribed beta-adrenergic-blocking drugs if they complain of heart palpitations. The effect of such drugs will be considered in the treatment section.

Treatment Planning

It is difficult to discuss treatment planning without alluding to treatment approaches. Consequently, some techniques will be briefly mentioned in this section; more detailed explanations will follow in the treatment section. There are several central decisions to be made at this juncture: what kind of treatment is needed for the phobias; how urgent the need for intervention is; what other issues, if any, must be addressed for the resolution of the phobias; and whether any physical or emotional factors contraindicate treatment.

By this time we have diagnosed the client as agoraphobic, but this includes a range of clients from those who do not avoid but are fearful to those who are totally housebound. Not surprisingly, different treatment approaches are advisable according to the severity of the case. Clients who are not avoidant and those who are mildly avoidant (1s–3s on Mobility Inventory individual items) may not require treatment with therapist-assisted *in vivo* exposure. In these cases, training in anxiety and panic management techniques coupled with clear instructions for self-directed exposure may be adequate. When clients are more severely avoidant, individual or group *in vivo* exposure is advisable. Those who avoid many situations can be placed in a group and treated more economically in that fashion. If a client is very avoidant of only a few situations, it is important to determine whether he or she will be able to get adequate practice on those items in a group situation. Otherwise, individual treatment is more efficient. A common example of this is the client who has most difficulty with driving, where individualized attention is often necessary.

In the cases of both Ms. N. and Ms. H. the clients' Mobility Inventory scores indicated generalized, strong avoidance. Ms. H. was socially anxious but certainly not to the degree that group treatment was ill advised; consequently, both clients could be assigned to either group or individual exposure. At the time of intake these two clients were concerned about the effect of the phobias on their job performance. However, neither was in a crisis. Several weeks passed between intake and the beginning of treatment for Ms. H. During this time she continued to deteriorate. Her panic attacks became much more frequent; she dropped all voluntary activities and began running out of meetings at work to take a tranquilizer. The thought of her work being disrupted was extremely distressing for her, and she demanded something be done immediately to stop her panics. She refused to begin exposure treatment until we got rid of her anxiety and rejected introductory explanations of coping strategies as not working quickly enough. In light of the changed situation, Ms. H. was sent for psychiatric consultation to switch her from minor tranquilizers to a more effective antipanic drug. She was very eager to try a pharmacotherapeutic approach and accepted this suggestion readily.

In the case of Ms. N. and other cases of simple agoraphobia, intervention for the phobias is all that is required. For Ms. H. and other clients with complex agoraphobia, the situation is much more complicated. Therapy for additional issues is usually required. In some cases the issues are fairly clear at intake. In others, clients insist that their lives would be rapturous if not for the phobias, and the assoicated difficulties only emerge during the course of treatment. Excerpts from Ms. H.'s intake session will be used to illustrate some of the other issues that frequently require attention. The childhood separation threats were clear in the excerpt already presented. There are, however, additional issues that come to light.

C: All the time, I'm so extremely embarrassed about it [*her symptoms*]. [*Client describes how competitive her workplace is, how she fears discovery and dismissal because of her problem.*]
T: What a terrible pressure to be under, to feel like you have to hide all the time.
C: Right, right, right. I'm in a panic all the time that they will find out. I don't know if the "they" is really my colleagues, or if the "they" is the world. Or if the "they" is the people who told me when I was young that I must always be wonderful.
T: Yeah.
C: Any my house is always spotless, and every assignment I get, God knows how long I work. So . . . there is your perfection [*referring again to the article she read*].
T: Uh huh. So as hard as you work you're not perfect enough 'cause you have this problem. [*Client tells how her employers questioned whether she should get a long-term contract for her job because she lacked the appropriate degree. She has gotten much worse since then, even though ultimately the decision was made to retain her.*]

T: Just having it questioned was very traumatic for you.

C: Just finding me less than perfect, that was a very bad situation.

T: So, what you're afraid of is passing out and embarrassing yourself in front of these people whose criticism you fear?

C: I'm afraid . . . I'm afraid to walk on the street, too.

T: Uh huh, even people you don't know, you'd be embarrassed.

C: I . . . I don't even know what it is I'm afraid of all the time. I couldn't go anywhere this summer because I was . . . just like . . . a rag [*after her job was questioned*]. The night [*after the issue of possibly terminating client was raised*] I was driving home from a ballet class, it was about 9:30–10 o'clock at night, and I was on the road and all of a sudden I couldn't drive. I just couldn't drive.

T: You were really frozen, huh.

C: I was . . . like that [*demonstrates*].

T: Uh huh.

C: And I drove in pieces. Finally I made it to a shopping center near home, and this psychologist who was seeing me said, "What a treat!"; my husband jogged to the shopping center to rescue me. I mean, I want Dave to show me. . . . There is my, I forget what they call it, the uh, the . . .

T: Secondary gain?

C: Secondary gain, yeah. He drives me. Wonderful.

T: Uh huh. So that's a way that he can show he cares for you. And he has trouble doing that in other ways?

C: Yeah, he, uh, he's . . . I mean . . . he's an extremely loyal man. He just doesn't know how to give love. [*Client rapidly begins talking about symptoms again, and client and therapist explore the extent of them. She forces herself to go a number of places alone in her safety zone but otherwise must be accompanied. Also explored are issues that have increased her anxiety such as a child who has a birth defect and feeling alone in America as a foreigner.*]

C: But, also there are a lot of times when I feel like saying just the hell with it. I'm staying home.

T: Yeah.

C: I just went out [*to come to the appointment*] in the midst of a real bad attack. What happened was Sunday we decided to come here on a dry run to see where it was. And it was just incredible. I got such a terrible attack. And I don't know if it was coming here, I guess . . . because this morning I was also shaking coming in [*client drove with husband following behind and leaving her at my office*] 'cause there were a lot of painful things that we mentioned.

T: Yeah. How is it for you also to meet a new person and to be talking with a new person about your life? Is that difficult for you?

C: Yeah. You are also very young.

T: How old are you now?

C: 50, 51 next December.

T: And you have a sense of really becoming older now that you haven't had before? What's changed, do you think?

C: Uh, I think the children leaving home.

T: It feels like a real marker for you?

C: Yeah.

T: Uh huh. What's it like for you with them gone?

C: It's more lonely. It's a hell of a lot easier, physically, to take care of the house.

T: Yeah.

C: There's almost a Dr. Jekyll, Mr. Hyde kind of situation, because when I am feeling "normal" I do reach out for people a lot. And, uh, basically, I . . . I . . . I . . . I want people all the time. My husband is an extreme loner.

T: Yeah.

C: And I think he's the stronger of the two of us, and I think that's why I had to invent my tyranny. And, uh, after living years with someone who, I'll say, "Let's have a dinner party," and he'll say, "What for?" And then I'd have to sit down and show him that we owe many invitations, and then he'd be willing to consider it. In other words, uh . . .

T: It's not enough that you want people around.

C: Yes, it's hard for me to now know what I am like anymore because I have adjusted so much. Where I come from, it's always outgoing. My parents used to go out at least three, four times a week. And you come to the suburbs, and if you're lucky, you go out once a week, so I . . . I, there's so many adjustments that I have made that sometimes I don't know the real me, and what I really wanted, or what I want now.

T: That's true; in long-term relationships you do change.

C: Right.

T: Um, you adjust to the other person, you develop different patterns. How long have you been married now?

C: 26 years.

T: How did you happen to marry someone so different from you in so many ways?

C: [Laughing] I don't know, I was 27, and at that time the pressure on me, on a woman, to marry was much stronger.

T: You were well overdue by that point.

C: Oh, boy, I mean, I was just a total failure. And I met him, and he wanted to marry me. That was it. I think I really fell in love later. I was rather hoping to take him back home, but he wouldn't, I guess he couldn't, take off, also. And that was that.

T: How are things between you now?

C: Good. He went recently. . . . See, that may well be the fruit of my tyranny, or my sickness. Went twice to the opera with me. Normally he wouldn't.

T: You mean he went because you couldn't go alone?

C: He went because he realizes that we are doing an awful lot of things his way. He's uh, extremely tight with money, and uh, I'm more inclined to go out and spend money, and he, uh . . .

T: So there are a number of conflicts around affection and spending time with people and spending money and just kind of going out. What are the parts that sustain you and keep you together all these years?

C: [Laughing] I'm not sure. I love him. And he loves me very much. Uh, there's a certain dependence. Uh.

Although Ms. H. describes her marriage as good, her Spouse Dissatisfaction Questionnarie and her own report during the interview indicate there are significant problem areas. From prior therapists, Ms. H. has learned to see her phobia as an attempt to manipulate her husband for more attention. There may be some truth to this, but such an explanation is only partially correct and has served to further diminish Ms. H.'s self-esteem. This analysis overlooks the loneliness the client feels within this marriage and the positive relationship of marital dissatisfaction to the incidence of panic attacks. Fear of the attacks is the more proximal factor related to her avoidance behavior. The loneliness theme is continued with her feelings about living in the United States and about her children's leaving home. Clearly, couples therapy is of top prioroity in this case. It is quite likely that if Mr. H. were asked by the therapist to come in for sessions to help his wife rather than because he needed therapy himself, he would be willing to come.

As is common for agoraphobic clients, when Ms. H. touched on sensitive issues during intake she dropped them quickly and began describing or experiencing her anxiety symptoms, illustrating the cognitive set where symptom focus rather than problem solving predominates. This is also well depicted in the scene she describes where, riding in the car with her husband, she suddenly has a severe panic attack under circumstances where she is ordinarily comfortable. She first attaches her panic to riding in the car and, with continued discussion, begins to see the relationship between her anxiety and her own feelings. Continued work on her attentional set and attribution needs to be part of her therapy as well.

Finally, the excerpt demonstrates a theme that pervaded the session with this client: her perfectionism and extreme sensitivity to criticism. On the one hand, she was very proud of her accomplishments, whereas on the other she was terrified of someone's finding fault with her work. Although she was ultimately granted a long-term contract, the idea that anyone questioned renewing her contract had so unsettled her that she had begun a severe downward spiral and could hardly face her colleagues. Losing some of her physical attractiveness in aging made her very jealous and uneasy around younger women and having a brain-damaged child who could never be an academic star was excruciating. These concerns also served to keep Ms. H. highly chronically anxious and thus more likely to panic and be avoidant.

Comprehensive treatment of such cases will require concurrent focus on these problems as well as the agoraphobic symptoms. This is not to suggest that one cannot treat agoraphobia without addressing every problem such clients face. Rather, it is important to look at the web of relationships among problems and to treat those that feed into anxiety and other phobic symptoms.

Finally, factors that contraindicate the proposed treatment program need to be considered. If group treatment is planned, the usual considerations apply as to whether a client can function appropriately in a group. Clients with severe social phobia may be unable to make use of a group, or worse, they may be further sensitized in such a setting. Clients who became housebound at an early age may be so unsocialized as to need extensive individual work before they are ready for group. Chronic physical illness may require alterations in the treatment plan; the energy required for an ordinary *in vivo* exposure program may be lacking, and a gentler, shaping approach is called for. Consultation with the client's physician is highly advisable in these cases. Most often, the physician will encourage pushing the client much harder than the latter thinks is physically healthy, but there are exceptions.

Finally the therapist needs to assess whether additional problems faced by the client are so severe as to preclude a therapeutic response to an exposure-based treatment. Severe depression is one such case. In this situation, the client may fail to habituate to phobic situations and also may be so distraught as to have difficulty cooperating with a demanding treatment program. Because most agoraphobics are depressed and their depression usually lifts with treatment, it is a judgment call as to when the depression must be addressed first. Beck scores over 40 indicate this should be considered along with the clinical assessment that the client is too dysfunctional to cooperate with treatment. Similarly, crises that prevent the client's devoting time and attention to the treatment program may well require postponement of treatment.

A last problem is substance abuse. About 1 of 20 agoraphobics applying for treatment has a serious, current alcohol-abuse problem. A smaller number may be addicted to other substances, such as high doses of minor tranquilizers. Exposure treatment has not been effective, in my experience, as long as the substance abuse continues. It does present a tricky problem in that most agoraphobics are afraid of being away from home and trapped in an inpatient facility for detoxification and treatment and swear that, if only their anxiety could be reduced, they would stop drinking or taking drugs. For similar reasons, Alcoholics Anonymous meetings are likely to be anathema to these clients. Central nervous system depressants make change so difficult, however, that I find reducing their anxiety first to be impossible and require these clients to get treatment initially for the substance abuse.

Treatment Techniques

In Vivo *Exposure*

The keystone to treatment of agoraphobia is *in vivo* exposure: the deliberate practice in reality of those things a client has been avoiding. In extensive empirical validation, this treatment has been found to lead to at least 50% improvement on avoidance behavior in 60 to 70% of the agoraphobic clients treated (Jannson & Öst, 1982). Exposure works not only to increase approach behavior but also to decrease subjective anxiety, panic attacks, and the depression associated with agoraphobic restrictions. This approach is coupled with an explanation of how anxiety works in the phobic situation: that anxiety will rise to some maximum point and then decrease. If one stays in the phobic situation until a decrease occurs, on subsequent occasions the anxiety response will be weaker and shorter lived, until the fear is largely overcome. Clients are reassured that none of their feared catastrophes will occur if they remain until habituation, rather than fleeing as is their wont. *In vivo* exposure has come to replace systematic desensitization with agoraphobic clients, as the latter has not proved to be a powerful intervention with this population (reviewed by Goldstein & Chambless, 1978).

Exposure has been carried out in a number of different ways: a flooding approach where the client is pushed into highly anxiety-provoking situations from the start, a shaping approach where the client retreats every time anxiety begins to rise and then enters the situation again, and a graduated approach where a rough heirarchy is used, but the client is encouraged to enter and remain in situations that are anxiety provoking and to increase task difficulty as soon as possible. All three approaches have been effective in research trials (reviewed by Emmelkamp, 1982). However, in practice it is very difficult to persuade clients to adopt the flooding approach, as well as it is unnecessarily painful for them, and the shaping approach is slow and unwieldy to apply in situations where free access to come and go many times is not feasible (e.g., a concert or restaurant). Consequently, when the term in vivo *exposure* is used, it typically refers to graduated exposure, with individual therapists varying in how quickly they urge clients to challenge difficult situations.

In over a decade of research on *in vivo* exposure with agoraphobia, a number of important parameters have been discerned (see Emmelkamp, 1982). First, exposure needs to be long and continuous. Many clients attempt to enter their phobic situation, at least on occasion, and question why they have not improved if this technique is effective. The answer is that they usually leave the situation as quickly as possible and before habituation has occurred and that they avoid returning to the situation for as long as they possibly can. Not only are prolonged sessions required, but repeated sessions are also necessary because of spontaneous recovery of anxiety. An exposure session typically lasts from 1 1/2 to 2 hours. If a shorter time must be used, then the hierarchy should be approached in finer gradations so that high levels of anxiety are not generated. As massed practice (every day) is more effective than spaced practice (every week), sessions should be scheduled as frequently as possible. It is very difficult to make progress if sessions are less frequent than once weekly, unless the client is assiduous about homework practice sessions.

Feedback about performance over a number of efforts in a similar situation is important. As clients can do more with successive trials, this information serves to reinforce progress and to let the client see concretely the beneficial effects of exposure. The therapist's assistance in making tasks more manageable and promoting mastery is also of significant benefit and undercuts much of what is often seen as client resistance but is in fact a reflection of high anxiety. These therapist behaviors include breaking particularly difficult tasks into small steps, breaking up defensive postures such as freezing, and accompanying the client on early trials (Williams, Dooseman, & Kleifield, 1984). Clients' sense that they have mastered the situation (not merely that they have done it) is strongly related to their predilection to try that task again.

There are a number of ways that exposure treatments can be delivered. Overall, clients seem to do as well in group as in individual treatment provided the staff/client ratio is not too low. Exposure can be carried out by the therapist, or the client may be given careful homework instructions instead. Good studies comparing the effectiveness of these approaches are lacking; however, it is clear that progress can be made with treatment manuals and explicit weekly contracts for self-directed exposure. Therapist-assisted exposure is more rapid, but some workers in the field (e.g., Hafner, 1982) think this rapidity may be detrimental in the stress it may place on a family system that has adjusted to the agoraphobia. Nevertheless, highly avoidant clients may be unwilling to change their behavior without the reassurance of the therapist's presence, and the rapidity of change with therapist-assisted treatment is reinforcing and builds confidence in one's ability to overcome the phobia. Ultimately, however, clients must begin to practice alone. The cost of therapist-assisted exposure treatment may be reduced through the use of paraprofessional workers. Relatively inexperienced people can provide beneficial treatment as long as they are closely supervised.

Treatment may be home based or clinic based. Mathews *et al.* (1981) have devised a program to deliver treatment economically in the home through the use of treatment manuals for the clients and a few visits by the therapist to make sure the treatment plan is being appropriately followed. This is particularly advantageous for this population whose ability to reach treatment facilities is limited. Mathews *et al.* have also constructed a manual for spouses of agoraphobic clients who may be enlisted to assist in the exposure process. In two studies, treatment has been found to be equally effective whether or not the spouse was included (Boisvert, Marchand, & Gaudette, 1983; Cobb, Mathews, Childs-Clarke, & Blowers, 1983). Barlow, O'Brien, and Last (1984), however, found a small positive effect of including the spouse in exposure homework for couples who were maritally distressed. The benefit seemed to be in helping the spouse become more understanding of the agoraphobic symptoms and more supportive. Nevertheless, the use of the spouse as an exposure cotherapist should be carefully considered lest the therapist inadvertently reinforce the client's dependence on significant others. Perhaps because ongoing support is beneficial, clients who are treated in groups according to the neighborhood they live in seem to do somewhat better in treatment (Sinnott, Jones, Scott-Fordham, & Woodward, 1981). If all else fails, treatment can be provided with manuals through the mail with phone or letter contacts to monitor homework assignments. This sort of treatment may be all that is possible for clients living in remote areas. It is, unfortunately, of limited effectiveness and may have no impact on the severely housebound.

In some situations, it may be difficult to carry out an *in vivo* exposure program because it is not feasible to practice the target behavior frequently (e.g., long trips away from home), too expensive to do (e.g., traveling in airplanes), or the precise conditions are hard to arrange at will (e.g., driving in a snowstorm at rush hour). At these times, imaginal exposure may be employed, following the same parameters as for *in vivo* exposure, if the client can imagine clearly and experiences the anxiety response with imagery. There is some disagreement in the literature as to how effective imaginal exposure is when compared to *in vivo* exposure (see Emmelkamp, 1982). The effects of *in vivo* seem to be more consistent; indeed, imaginal exposure may work in an indirect fashion by potentiating self-directed *in vivo* exposure. As a result, it seems wise to use the *in vivo* approach when possible. There are additional advantages. *In vivo* work obviates the need for training clients in imagery, with which some clients have great difficulty. Moreover, it can be quite difficult to monitor avoidance in imagery (e.g., the client loses the image and cannot retrieve it), making it harder to ensure prolonged, continuous exposure.

Panic Management Strategies

The central importance of panic attacks and the fear of fear to the development and maintenance of agoraphobia has already been emphasized. Exposure serves to mobilize clients, but if they continue to experience panic attacks, treatment gains will often be reversed. Thus, it should come as no surprise that clients with higher frequencies of panic pretreatment tend to fare worse. Two approaches to this problem have developed: psychotherapeutic interventions and psychopharmacological ones.

Psychotherapeutic Strategies

Coping with Panic. A number of interventions have been devised for handling panic when it begins to occur. Among them are cognitive restructuring, paradoxical intention, and attention manipulation. In cognitive restructuring, the clients' maladaptive thoughts about anxiety are systematically challenged. This includes educating the clients about the nature of anxiety (this is basic to all exposure approaches) and training clients to provide reassurance to themselves, when anxious, that anxiety is not in fact life threatening, that they will not lose control, faint, become insane, and so forth.

Agoraphobics are usually convinced that their anxiety is apparent to all and that they are not only feeling strange but acting strangely. Thus, in the cases of Ms. H. and Ms. N., the clients were convinced they wobbled terribly when walking in the open, and Ms. H. was very concerned that others would notice. In reality, neither had a noticeable change in gait. Unless clients are so convinced of the danger of falling that they hug the walls when walking, actual changes in appearance are confined to clients who hyperventilate so much as to blur vision and cause dizziness. Repeated feedback to the client while the client is anxious and thinks the symptoms are apparent helps to correct these misperceptions.

Another important cognition to challenge is the impression that anxiety is all pervasive and forever. Agoraphobics tend to remember the worst part of an excursion as how it was the entire time and to fear if they do not leave a situation where they are anxious the anxiety will go on and on. For this reason as well as for the therapist's information in assessing progress, it is very useful to teach them to rate their anxiety on a 0–100 scale ranging from calm to panic. There is often some resistance to doing this, as clients fear they will become more anxious if they think about how they are feeling. Once they learn to do it, however, they are generally surprised to see how brief a period of time they were actually very uncomfortable, how often the anticipation was actually worse than the doing, and how their anxiety levels typically declined after some time, even though they did not flee.

Agoraphobics tend to believe that anxiety or tension is an abnormal state, that they should be perfectly calm at all times, in all situations. It is certainly true that they experience an abnormal amount of anxiety compared to most people in, for example, stores. However, their expectation that everyone else is completely calm and their assessment that something is terribly wrong if they feel low levels of tension in such places is erroneous and maladaptive. These beliefs increase fear of fear and avoidance. An important task for the therapist is to consistently communicate that some anxiety is a normal part of life, that anxiety may be unpleasant but not terrible, and that anxiety is to be confronted and mastered, not avoided. For example, an upcoming event such as a trip the client is dreading should be reframed as an opportunity for practicing new skills. Anxiety experienced during exposure sessions, similarly, is not failure but is a chance to learn that dreaded consequences will not befall one and is an occasion to see oneself mastering the unpleasant feelings.

A somewhat different approach that may be used in combination with cognitive restructuring is attention manipulation. Agoraphobics, as has been noted, heighten their anxiety response by focusing on it and "catastrophizing" about it. Their attention is concentrated on the threatening aspects of a situation or of their feelings, and their thoughts are preoccupied with how they will behave, will feel, or will be harmed. Consequently, they are out of touch with the complete present reality and are fantasizing about a future, much more unpleasant time. Needless to say, this is not a reassuring approach to one's anxiety. Zane (1978) has emphasized the importance of keeping the client in the present as a way of cutting into this anxiety spiral and has suggested a number of useful techniques. One is having clients broaden their present awareness by focusing on concrete nonthreatening aspects of the situation that they have been excluding from awareness: the sound of the therapist's voice, the colors and textures of objects around them, and the sense of their feet touching the floor. This is not to be confused with distraction, which is countertherapeutic. With distraction, clients attempt to avoid realizing where they are and how they feel by fantasizing being elsewhere, engaging in endless conversation, or always carrying a book or magazine to read. The idea is not to deny one's anxiety but to also be aware of the total context, which is much more than anxiety and which is not filled with danger. Because the present situation is never dangerous in the way the client fears, only the fantasized future situation, the continued practice of having clients cut off future-oriented thoughts (e.g., "I better get out of here, or I'll faint") and concentrate on present ones (e.g., "I'm tense, but I'm conscious. I can tell because I see this, and I feel that") reduces the anxiety response considerably. This takes much practice and vigilance on the client's part. When approaching a threatening task or when discussing doing one, the therapist can anticipate the client is imagining future catastrophe, ask "where the client is," and call the client back to the present. After many repetitions, the process is internalized. Some clients find it useful to aid the thought stopping by wearing a rubber band on the wrist, snapping it to help break up a concentration on the negative, and then concentrating on the present.

A rather different approach but one that is well in keeping with the overall message that anxiety is not threatening is *paradoxical intention* (see Chambless & Goldstein, 1980). Clients are asked to exaggerate or to deliberately try to bring on their feared anxiety symptom or consequence. The woman afraid of wobbling is asked to wobble; the person embarrased by sweating to sweat buckets; and the man with shaking hands to shake them like leaves. The client fearful of rapid heart beat is asked to concentrate on his or her heart and to speed it up even faster, and the woman afraid of fainting is asked to faint while the therapist is there to catch her. The client fearful of insanity is urged to take the opportunity to go insane with a therapist who will handle the situation. In the case of symptoms under voluntary control (for example, trembling hands) the therapist may model the exaggerated behavior.

Paradoxical intention serves several purposes. First, it communicates that the therapist is not worried about the client's symptoms and does not believe that something awful will happen. Second, it helps the client break into the cycle of fighting anxiety and becoming even more tense from the effort. The client learns that nothing terrible happens even when one does not struggle to dampen the anxiety. In this way, paradoxical intention is a more active variation on Weekes's (1976) suggestion that one "float with anxiety" rather than fight it. The active aspect of paradoxical intention is easier for many clients than the passive approach of floating. Third, it injects a note of humor into the therapy that in itself counteracts anxiety. This can be used particularly effectively in a group where clients can play with their symptoms and gain distance from them by labeling various group members according to their predominant symptom (e.g., *The Choker*).

It is of the utmost importance that this approach only be used with compassion, lest the client think the therapist does not understand how painful and frightening the symptoms are. It is not necessary to use paradoxical intention in a manipulative fashion, that is, without explaining the purposes of the techniques to the client as well as the reasons it seems to work. This is an extremely effective technique with most symptoms but is commonly frightening for clients to attempt, as they fear that the dreaded catastrophe just might befall them. Consequently, it is easiest to use attention manipulation first, then resorting to paradoxical intention if the former fails. Symptoms that do not respond well to being focused on directly are dizziness, nausea, and feelings of unreality. Such sensations may be increased by focusing on them. If the client cannot in fact vomit on command (I have never had a client be frightened of nausea who could in fact vomit at will), the appropriate paradoxical instruction is "go ahead and vomit." The dizzy client may be encouraged to faint if this is a feared catastrophe. Focusing on present stimuli is usually more productive for feelings of unreality than is paradoxical intention, but if necessary the client can be instructed to float as far away from the situation as possible, see how that feels, and then when that is comfortable, to return. Dizziness, numbness in the extremities, problems with breathing, and feelings of unreality primarily result from hyperventilation. Thus, it is only necessary to use other coping techniques if proper breathing has been established but the symptoms continue.

A final coping technique is *proper breathing*. Agoraphobics generate or exacerbate a number of their symptoms through hyperventilation. Others may stop breathing for short periods at times of great anxiety. Under less anxiety-provoking situations, most still breathe in a shallow, rapid fashion rather than from the diaphragm. A calming breathing pattern is to take slow, even breaths from the diaphragm. In learning this technique, it helps to place one hand on the diaphragm and another on the chest, seeking to keep the latter stationary while the former rises with inhalation and falls with exhalation. Some clients may have to practice this technique initially in a supine position before they can accomplish it sitting and standing. Clients are requested to practice several times daily for about 5 to 10 minutes and to monitor their breathing when entering an anxiety-provoking situation. The therapist also should watch for maladaptive breathing during exposure sessions and prompt the client to use the new method. Should the client become very frightened and begin to hyperventilate, she or he should be instructed to close the mouth and breathe only through the nose, as it is very difficult to hyperventilate without gasping for air. Clients who return from a task reporting they are unable to get their breath have often been hyperventilating. The instruction to blow out all air in the lungs before attempting to breathe again not only has a paradoxical effect but also helps correct overoxygenation.

Empirical research on cognitive restructuring and paradoxical intention indicates that, combined with homework instructions, these techniques are effective in the treatment of mildly to moderately avoidant agoraphobic clients (Mavissakalian, Michelson, Greenwald, Kornblith, & Greenwald, 1983). The former works more slowly but eventually is as effective as the latter. In the treatment of more severely avoidant clients, Emmelkamp and his colleagues failed to find any positive effects of adding cognitive restructuring to therapist-directed *in vivo* exposure (see Emmelkamp, 1982). Research using paradoxical intention plus exposure versus the exposure alone is still in progress. Based on my experience in using *in vivo* exposure without cognitive restructuring or other coping techniques, I would interpret Emmelkamp's findings in the following way: once clients manage to enter and stay in their phobic situations for an adequate length of time, they do just as well on the whole, regardless of the addition of cognitive restructuring. Getting them to enter and remain in the phobic situations without some promise of relief through coping strategies (even if this ultimately turns out to be superstitious belief) is very difficult. Thus, training in panic management cuts down on avoidance during treatment and on dropouts. I also think it is difficult to test these coping mechanisms in group designs because different strategies work for different clients, making it nonproductive to use a prepackaged intervention.

Reducing the Propensity to Panic. It has been noted that agoraphobics are highly chronically anxious people. This high daily tension level keeps the agoraphobic in a state of excitation from which the anxiety may easily escalate into panic. A sudden loud noise may be a sufficient trigger. Once clients become more mobile and less anxious in anticipation of encountering a phobic situation, they are ready to turn their attention to treatment directed at lowering this chronic tension. Anxiety management training has proved effective with these clients in reducing the frequency of panic attacks as well as the severity of anxious mood (Jannoun, Oppenheimer, & Gelder, 1982) Clients are first trained in progressive relaxation and cognitive restructuring, if this has not been previously taught during exposure. Because becoming profoundly relaxed may be frightening to some clients (see Heide & Borkovec, 1984), the therapist may have to proceed slowly with relaxation training. Once they have acquired these skills, the next step is practicing the application of these technqiues as they imagine situations of all sorts that make them feel tense. In the third step, clients apply their skills throughout the day in situations where they feel uncomfortable as a coping skill. Anxiety management training differs from systematic desensitization in that it is not a technique to use in a therapist's office with a particular hierarchy but is a skill for use in the daily environment, whatever the distressing stimuli, to cope with (not eliminate) anxiety. Some clients also seem to benefit from exercise programs and training in problem-solving strategies as other ways to reduce tension.

A final strategy involves training clients to identify accurately the type of emotion they are experiencing and the source of their distress. As has been earlier explained, many types of intense affect may come to be interpreted by agoraphobics as anxiety. Moreover, when anxious about other events in their lives, the agoraphobic may label the source of his or her anxiety to be the shopping mall or expressway, rather than attending to the actual distressing event. Probing for the antecedents of panic can be done retrospectively in the therapist's office or during *in vivo* exposure sessions. In the case of Ms. H., we saw that when she discussed her unhappiness with her spouse she consistently switched to a focus on her anxiety symptoms. With the therapist's persistently bringing her back to the topic of what was happening when she panicked under unusual circumstances (riding in the city with her husband was usually a "safe" activity), she was able to identify part of her distress as being attributable to her loneliness in the marriage.

Clients can be trained to keep records of panic attacks that seem to occur out of the blue and to identify sources of discomfort that are most often interpersonal. Often they will draw a blank and have much more difficulty than Ms. H. It may be necessary to ask for a brief review of the day's events and especially contacts with people the therapist knows to be troublesome to the client before the pertinent events come to light. One client, for example, came to a session having panicked severely during the week, losing all the progress she had made during several previous weeks on her driving. She denied any problems during the week. When pressed to recall how long she felt strong and positive about her changes (the state in which she left the prior session), she eventually pinpointed a conversation with her husband, with whom she had a difficult relationship. He was quite controlling and rigid in his expectations for her in general. Observing her progress, her spouse announced that because she was getting better, they could now start on the family that he wanted but that the client definitely did not want. The client reported feeling trapped, condemned by him as a failure if she remained agoraphobic but subject to relentless pressure to meet his expectations if she improved. Subsequent to this conversation, she became panicky again driving short distances and lost motivation to continue practicing. It was important that she see that her anxiety was an understandable response to what seemed to be irresolvable conflict rather than a property of driving and that she needed to find ways of dealing with her anger and resentment in her relationship.

It is easier to intervene if this attribution training can be done in the *in vivo* session itself. The therapist can then more readily identify feelings being mislabeled as *anxiety*. A client was working on riding subways without the therapist, who waited at the end of the line. She returned to meet the therapist, eyes brimming with tears and face full of sorrow. Left without the opportunity of escape when she had parted from the therapist at the other end of the line, she found that beyond the panic was a feeling she found even more difficult and fought to reject: a sense of overwhelming isolation and sorrow. Although this was hard for her to experience, she ceased to fear panic and began to confront her terrible loneliness and her history of abandonments in her therapy. Staying in touch with core feelings and aware of causes of distress seems to be highly effective in reducing so-called *spontaneous panic attacks*. Anxiety management training is still advisable, however, for reducing the chronic generalized anxiety levels.

Psychopharmacological Intervention

A very different approach to the control of panic is the use of psychotropic medication. A considerable amount of research has been conducted on the effects of various medications on clients who have panic attacks, including those with agoraphobia (see review by Liebowitz & Klein, 1982). Major tranquilizers, such as the phenothiazines, seem to exacerbate the symptoms, whereas minor tranquilizers help control the chronic anxiety for a time but seldom adequately control panic. Nevertheless, most clients with agoraphobia have a long history of minor tranquilizer use. Typically, they avoid large amounts of these drugs but take them when panicky or when forced to confront a difficult situation. A few, however, become addicted.

As the role of the tricyclic antidepressants in controlling panic has received considerable publicity in recent, years, more and more agoraphobic clients have had experience with these drugs. Monoamine oxidase (MAO) inhibitors (e.g., Nardil) have similar effects but are not widely used in the United States because of potentially serious side effects. These drugs have a therapeutic effect in the treatment of agoraphobia. The results of various treatment centers vary as to whether they add to the effects of *in vivo* exposure. Data from the most carefully conducted research indicate the answer is "no" but that these drugs combined with education and systematically followed homework instructions do constitute an effective treatment in the absence of therapist-assisted exposure (Mavissakalian & Michelson, 1983). Agoraphobic clients have often had bad experiences with a tricyclic because the drug was prescribed by a physician unfamiliar with their use in anxiety disorders rather than depression. Agoraphobic people are extremely sensitive to and frightened by the drug's side effects (e.g., heart palpitations, hand tremors) and many become very agitated and discontinue the medication unless they are built up slowly on the drug in 10- or 25-mg increments. Paradoxical effects of the drug are common, making it rather difficult to know if the client is agitated because the dosage is too high or too low. The most common therapeutic dose of imipramine (Tofranil) is 150 mg daily. However, about one-fourth of agoraphobic people have been found to be so sensitive to the drug that they reach a therapeutic level on as little as 75 mg. Clients are continued on the medication for about a year once good results are reached before withdrawal is attempted. If panic attacks begin again, the drug is reintroduced.

Propranolol (Inderal), a beta-adrenergic blocker often used to control high blood pressure, has been tested on agoraphobic clients with mixed results. It seems to effectively control some of the physical sensations of anxiety (e.g., rapid heart beat, trembling hands) but to be ineffective for the psychological aspects. For clients whose main concern is rapid heart beat, however, the drug may be quite beneficial. It is sometimes combined with imipramine to reduce the noxious heart palpitations some clients have with that drug, is often used with paroxysmal tachycardia, and is increasingly prescribed to clients with mitral valve prolapse. Consequently, it is beneficial to be aware of the drug and its effects.

Finally, a highly touted new drug has appeared on the scene that is said to have antipanic properties—alprazolam (Xanax). As its name would suggest, it is closely akin to diazepam (Valium). From its chemical properties, it is difficult to discern why this drug should be more effective than Valium with panic. Moreover, the same potential for abuse and for decreasing effectiveness of the drug over the space of a few months would seem to apply to this new compound. Nevertheless, it is being eagerly received, for it is much more difficult to get clients adjusted on the tricyclics and to get them to stay on them than it is to take a drug that has an immediate sedating effect and fewer unpleasant side effects. The drug may have potential as a short-term treatment for panic attacks during a limited period of stress (although its effectiveness needs to be demonstrated in controlled trials, which are currently being conducted), but it does not seem appropriate for long-term use with a chronic disorder such as agoraphobia.

There are drawbacks as well as benefits to the use of these drugs. The long-term disadvantage to tricyclics, MAO inhibitors, and propranolol is the tendency for relapse once the drug is withdrawn. Anecdotally, this is the case for alprazolam as well. This is understandable in that the clients have learned no other ways of controlling their panic and attribute their improvements to the drug. Furthermore, there is about a 20% initial refusal rate by clients who are afraid of ill effects from the drug or loss of control associated with a foreign substance in the body (see Telch, Tearnan, & Taylor, 1983). In addition, with the tricyclics, the drug class of the most documented effectiveness, there is an average of a 40% dropout rate due to side effects. Last, agoraphobia most often begins in women of childbearing years, and none of these drugs is considered safe to take during pregnancy. Moreover, the long-term risk of damaging side effects remains unknown.

For all of these reasons, I do not see pharmacotherapy as the first-line treatment of choice, unless there is urgent need for rapid control of frequent panic. Nevertheless, it may be the only effective treatment for agoraphobic people isolated in areas where behavioral treatment is not available or for those who cannot obtain treatment at a fee they can afford. I do describe pharmacotherapy as an alternative to clients applying for treatment, but it is unusual that they opt for trying this approach first. If a client has not made substantial progress in 3 to 6 months of behavior therapy despite genuine efforts on her or his part, we discuss the use of medication again at that time. At times, the medication makes a dramatic difference. Unfortunately, the same factors that predict poor response to exposure (high depression and high frequency of panic) also predict poor results with imipramine (Zitrin, Klein, & Woerner, 1980).

The Process of Treatment

Throughout this chapter, I have emphasized the multiple problems clients with complex agoraphobia bring into treatment. Because many therapeutic strategies and techniques not specific to the treatment of agoraphobia are required for comprehensive treatment, I will most often, in this section, have space only to point out the problems that need to be addressed and how they are likely to occur.

The client's depression interacts with his or her response to treatment, requiring the therapist to intervene when maladaptive behavior common to depressed clients surfaces. For example, it is common for a client to downplay or ignore gains made during a session unless the therapist encourages the client to recognize and acknowledge such efforts by verbalizing them to the group or to the therapist. Similarly, clients lose track of the progress they have made and persist in thinking they have not changed over the weeks of treatment. Having them keep records of progress is helpful, particularly in the face of the setbacks that are bound to occur. Because losing ground after a particularly bad panic attack is such a common event, we encourage clients to make sure to have a setback while they are still in treatment. This does not prevent clients from feeling helpless when the relapse occurs, but, when reminded of what we told them, they do bounce back more quickly. Clients often are distressed because their expectations of therapy were unrealistic; they hoped the anxiety would be "cured." We stress the importance of viewing therapy not as a cure but as a way to learn to cope. It is an unusual client who never has a panic attack again after termination.

As clients change in treatment and as they learn to identify sources of tension and unhappiness in their lives, they need therapy focused on the other identified problem areas as well. Because these problems often interfere with exposure treatment if ignored, it is preferable to conduct this treatment concurrently with the exposure work (see Chambless & Goldstein, 1981, for an extensive description of this format). Many therapists have been caught in the trap of trying to resolve the other issues first and then turn to the exposure. This is a road to nowhere in that the client is generally unwilling, and indeed unable, to focus on other problem areas while so distressed by phobias and panic. Moreover, until awareness is developed through treatment, the client may be unaware that there is a connection between other life events and agoraphobia. Certainly, multiple sessions weekly are costly; however, if desirable, costs may be held down through using trained paraprofessionals for the exposure work (see Zane & Seif, 1982).

The most common problem that emerges is the agoraphobic person's difficulty in recognizing and expressing feelings and needs in significant personal relationships. Communications training is important, but the larger proportion of the work lies in helping the person to sort out what she or he wants or feels and to believe that she or he is entitled to these feelings and their expression. Gestalt therapy techniques are often extremely useful in this way. Because of the agoraphobic's extreme sensitivity to others' reactions, desensitization to anger and withdrawal may be required.

Couples or family sessions are almost always desirable in the treatment of agoraphobia, if only to provide the significant others with information about how to support the agoraphobic person through the change process. Commonly, however, the work needs to go beyond simple information. After prolonged agoraphobia, couples and families may interact extensively around the symptoms and need help finding healthier ways to relate as the client improves. Most importantly, the agoraphobic person's sense of being trapped and/or alone is generally, at least in part, a reflection of how she or he feels in these intimate relationships. Assisting the couple or family in developing mutually supportive relationships that also allow individuation is a central therapeutic task.

Rehabilitation counseling may be required for clients who have been out of the work force for a prolonged period due to their phobias. Vocational counseling is also important for the female client who is considering entering the work force after caring for young children. Some sort of meaningful involvement outside the home is particularly important for these clients, not only to help them stay mobile but also to give them a sense of connection with the external world. It is particularly beneficial for them to know they could be financially self-sustaining, as this fosters their feeling more powerful in their marital relationship.

I have emphasized the importance of separation and threats of separation in the history of agoraphobic clients. Many times, these clients have unresolved grief reactions that surface when they are alone and that spur their avoidance of this situation. Others may have images of especially painful memories, such as those reported by Ms. H., who stayed awake as a child at night monitoring her mother's breathing and watching the hospital door to see if her father was among the wounded. Psychological resolution of these issues is vitally important if the fears of being alone are to be overcome. Imaginal flooding may be used to expose the client to these images and memories within the safe context of the therapist's office. Repeated exposure sessions are necessary in this case, just as they are for the phobic stimuli. Examples of this sort of treatment have been provided by Chambless and Goldstein (1980, 1981) and Ramsey (1977). A study by Mawson, Marks, Ramm, and Stern (1981) has demonstrated the empirical effectiveness of this approach, sometimes called *guided mourning* when bereavement is concerned.

This multifaceted approach to treatment, combining work on associated problems with exposure, results in improvement in a broader group of clients. With this approach, clients who fare poorly with exposure alone (those starting treatment with higher depression and marital dissatisfaction and a greater frequency of panic attacks) have an equally good chance of responding well to treatment (Chambless, Goldstein, Gallagher, & Bright, in press). Furthermore, a higher rate of overall improvement is noted. On broad ranges of agoraphobic avoidance, only a 39% overall improvement rate has been reported (Agoraphobia factor on the Fear Survey Schedule, Hafner & Ross, 1983) with exposure alone, whereas this multitherapeutic approach results in a 55.5% improvement rate on the even broader Mobility Inventory.

Treatment Limitations

Although great strides have been made in the behavioral treatment of agoraphobia, there remains a notable proportion of clients who do not improve with treatment. Using an intensive approach to treatment, combining exposure with attention to the other problems that have been described, we (Chambless *et al.*, in press) still find 14% of clients to be treatment failures (i.e., they improve less than 25% on measures of phobic avoidance and panic attacks). With less than optimal treatment, the failure rate is even higher. As has been noted, at a group level the addition of pharmacotherapy seems to add little to the effectiveness of behavior therapy, although it might make some difference for individual clients. The broader approach to treatment advocated here does negate the effects of statistically documented predictors of failure with treatment by exposure and pharmacotherapy. Nonetheless, there are several common problems that crop up and remain unresolved.

The first is the client who is enmeshed in personally destructive relationships and who refuses to acknowledge and work on these problems in therapy or who is unwilling to consider leaving a relationship in which the other will not bend. A second example is the client who refuses to take any responsibility for his or her improvement. This client, despite every direct or indirect effort on the therapist's part, does not do homework assignments and is generally unwilling to tolerate even moderate levels of discomfort during treatment, expecting the therapist to magically remove all obstacles. Usually these clients have been very spoiled and babied in their families of origin and are often wealthy, so that they can lead comfortable lives within their restrictions. Yet a third type of case is exemplified by those clients who fixedly believe that some catastrophe will befall them from a panic attack and who are therefore unwilling to take risks during treatment. Although some of these clients have seemed to be of low intelligence, this is not the case for all. The most puzzling case of all is the occasional client who works hard in treatment but, despite repeated exposure sessions, does not show the predictable pattern of within- and across-session habituation (see Foa & Chambless, 1978). Fortunately, these are clients who seem to respond well to medication.

In working with clients in less fortunate circumstances, the problems are multiplied. Not only must the frequency and comprehensiveness of treatment be reduced in most facilities, but also the client's life circumstances serve to keep her or his anxiety level extremely high, fostering panic attacks and inhibiting inhibition. Thus, social problems such as poverty, unemployment, inadequate housing, poor medical care, drug abuse by one's children, and so forth all have a profound impact on the client's emotional status but can hardly be resolved by the behavior therapist. Time and time again, these clients struggle to improve in therapy, only to be knocked flat by the next crisis in their lives. Moreover, poverty-level clients often attend treatment irregularly and follow through poorly on homework instructions. Data reviewed by Weissman (1983) indicate that agoraphobic people are disproportionately likely to be poorly educated and minority group members. These clients are not represented in most research trials. Consequently, the improvement rates for exposure are undoubtedly an overestimate for this group. Cognitive coping strategies that were devised in interaction with educated, verbal clients may also be less useful for lower-class clients.

Complex Agoraphobia

Treatment of a case of complex agoraphobia is considerably more demanding and multifaceted than is the case with simple agoraphobia, as will be illustrated by the case of Ms. J. This client first sought treatment for agoraphobia of 4 years' duration at age 22. Ms. J. was a secretary with a high-school education. She came from a blue-collar family, was single, and lived with her parents and two brothers. An older brother was married and out of the household. Ms. J. described her mother as a very nervous person and her father as a weekend alcoholic who physically abused his wife but not his children. One of the client's brothers had severe learning disabilities; another had psychotic episodes, occasionally attempted suicide, and had been arrested for criminal acts. Ms. J. was the good child who was protective of her parents, caused no trouble, and was, she thought, consequently ignored.

Ms. J. was very close to her mother as a young child but lost her when the latter began evening shift work, thus leaving the house when the client was just returning from school. Ms. J. reported feeling extremely isolated and abandoned, particularly because she feared her father—his angry outbursts and his overly affectionate behavior when intoxicated. The family's attention seemed primarily focused on the troublesome brothers. When Ms. J. was about 13 years old, her mother became a member of a fundamentalist religious group and involved the client in this religion as well. Feeling this to be her only connection with her mother, Ms. J. became very involved in this church, which taught that members were not to associate with people outside the faith and that all nonmembers were eternally damned. Controls over sexual behavior were particularly rigid. As Ms. J. approached adulthood, it became time for her to be confirmed as a full member of the church. She had considerable qualms about this, as she secretly disagreed with many of the teachings. Nevertheless, the church was her sole social system and her bridge to her mother. Also, she truly feared that leaving the church, whose members would no longer be allowed to speak to her, would result in her damnation. It was in this climate that the client began having panic attacks while traveling to her job in downtown Philadelphia from the semirural area where she lived. Unable to overcome the attacks, she relinquished her job and also began avoiding trapped situations in general: public transportation, elevators, restaurants, and beauty parlors. In addition, she became afraid of being more than 30 minutes from her home. She was confirmed in the church and found a position close to home.

Before being referred to me, Ms. J. had been in individual psychotherapy for about 9 months and had irregularly attended an *in vivo* exposure group for about 6 months. During that time, she had begun to examine herself and her needs and to separate from the church temporarily despite condemnation by her mother. She was involved in a fairly positive relationship with a man who was not a church member. Sexual contact with her boyfriend was greatly limited by sexual phobias as well as continued confusion about the morality of extramarital sexual relationships. The client's avoidance behavior was relatively unimproved (Alone score = 2.42; Accompanied = 2.21). It appeared that her exposure group was composed of clients who were much more limited; consequently, most group time was devoted to situations like shopping malls with which the client had little difficulty. Being extremely unassertive, she had never complained to the exposure group therapist. Moreover, during the exposure group treatment the client actually became even more socially phobic than before treatment. Group exercises used by the therapist to foster support and intimacy were instead sensitizing to this very shy client who was phobic of physical contact. She had improved somewhat on her catastrophic thinking (score of 2.00) but little on her fear of body sensations (score of 3.00). She was moderately severely depressed (Beck = 22), chronically anxious (score of 54), and extremely unassertive on an assertiveness inventory.

Ms. J. began treatment with me when the former therapist moved away. She was somewhat agitated, feeling angry and abandoned, but quickly formed a relationship with me. Her financial situation and the long distance from her home (her boyfriend had to bring her) to the clinic precluded more than one session weekly. Because the exposure group had not been helpful, we agreed she would drop group and have weekly individual sessions. Identified treatment targets were increasing her mobility, reducing her social anxiety, clarifying her feelings about church and family, and resolving her conflicts about her relationship with her boyfriend. Sexuality and intimacy in general were difficult issues for her.

Initially, homework assignments were used for *in vivo* exposure, with the client being accompanied by her boyfriend, who was very willing to be helpful. The pair worked on beauty parlors and riding trains, although their attempts were more sporadic than desirable. This approach was taken because the client strongly needed treatment for the other target areas and because her work schedule and distant location made arranging therapist-assisted exposure sessions quite difficult. As Ms. J. conquered a situation in her boyfriend's company, she next attempted to do it on her own. This step required forceful persuasion not only because of her fearfulness but also because of this couple's pattern of spending every available moment together. When the client seemed stuck on a plateau, occasional therapist-assisted *in vivo* sessions (a total of six over 9 months) were interspersed with homework assignments. These were particularly needed for train trips to unfamiliar suburbs or cities. Although more such sessions would have been desirable and would have led to quicker and more extensive change, substantial changes were apparent. The posttreatment Avoidance Alone score was 1.89, and Avoidance Accompanied was 1.80. Some residual avoidance of public transportation remained, and Ms. J. gave high ratings to forms of transport that she had not had occasion to attempt—boats and airplanes. She became completely mobile when traveling by automobile and was able to regularly make the 90-minute drive to the clinic alone and to take trips with friends. Her Body Sensations Questionnaire score was down to 1.53 (the normal sample mean), with some remaining concern about heart palpitations and being short of breath. Further improvement was also apparent on the Agoraphobic Cognitions Questionnaire, where her score was 1.57 (close to the normal sample mean of 1.38). Some fear of acting foolish and loss of control remained.

In work on the other related issues, one focus was on exploring the client's values and helping her to clarify her own beliefs versus the teachings of the church. Readings about ethics and values were also suggested. Ms. J. found these both frightening and important to her, as she struggled between her desire to follow her own conscience and her fear of being damned and cut off from the fellowship of the church. Although unable to make a permanent break from the church, she decided she could not follow its teachings and became more assertive when members questioned or criticized her behavior. In particular, she decided she wanted to have a sexual relationship with her boyfriend. Discussion, readings, homework assignments, and films for desensitization were used to help reduce her anxiety about sexual activity and her intense discomfort with her body.

A central issue for Ms. J., as for almost all agoraphobics, was being alone. Although she never complained of this problem, it became clear to her as treatment progressed that she could not tolerate being alone even to the extent of being in her room with the door closed while other family members were downstairs. Thus, although she felt increasingly stifled by her relationship with her boyfriend, she spent all her evenings with him and developed no other internal or external resources. Through homework assignments, halting and difficult progress was made on spending time in her room alone reading and seeking friends to socialize with. During evenings alone in her room, she became fully aware of her sense of isolation in her family and in the world in general without the church and had a number of episodes of severe panic. Anger at her parents became an important issue at this time. The client resolved to obtain her own apartment but, frightened of doing so, she precipitously moved in with her boyfriend instead. Once she had done so, she felt even more suffocated by the relationship and angry at her boyfriend for his clinging behavior. With great difficulty, she became more assertive about spending time apart from him, but this was a continual struggle.

Assertiveness training was also important in working on Ms. J.'s relationships with other people whom she cut out of her life if ever they hurt her feelings. Through homework assignments, she began to speak more to her co-workers rather than isolating herself, to take evening classes to broaden her contacts, and to develop her interests by becoming a volunteer at a social service agency. She also began to explore career options other than her secretarial position, which she found boring and poorly paid.

After 8 months of working with Ms. J., I accepted a position in another city and let her know I would be leaving in 3 months' time. Our therapeutic relationship had been a particularly close one, and Ms. J. became extremely panicky, agitated and severely depressed in response to this impending change. Over a number of sessions she was gradually able to express some anger at my abandoning her but continued to deteriorate, developing problems with eating, sleeping, and had suicidal impulses. Eventually, she barely spoke during her sessions; rather she sobbed for most of the hour. After a month with no movement toward resolution, we decided it might help if Ms. J. began to form a connection at that time with the therapist who would see her on my departure. She approached her new therapist, a particularly warm and supportive woman, with considerable hostility but eventually decided to trust her and to meet with her regularly. Daily telephone contact was maintained with the new therapist until her suicidal impulses subsided. Ms. J. and I also continued to meet during this period to deal with her anger and grief.

The crisis continued for several months after I moved. Ms. J. and I exchanged letters and had occasional telephone contact as well. With her new therapist, she was gradually able to explore how this situation opened up her feelings about her mother's earlier abandonment of her and her decision at that time never to care for anyone again. She struggled extremely hard not to end our relationship by cutting me off as she had all others. Through this process, the client began to open up once again to her family and to reestablish an affectionate relationship with her mother. Her letters to me became less frequent and contact with me less painful.

In her continued therapy, Ms. J. has had no further *in vivo* exposure but at 18-month follow-up had maintained her gains on mobility, cognitions, and fear of body sensations. During this treatment, she has continued to work on autonomy, intimacy, and sexuality. She moved to her own apartment, established closer relationships with her parents, and continued to build social contacts and friendships. Testing on social anxiety inventories indicated her social phobia was improved by 50% and her fears of criticism were reduced to the normal range. Her chronic anxiety score was much lower, although still elevated compared to population norms (Trait Anxiety = 44), and her depression score was low in the mildly depressed range (Beck = 11). At this time, she reports that her life seems enough in order that she can devote some of her treatment time to making further gains on mobility.

Summary

In reading the behavioral research literature on the treatment of agoraphobia, one has the impression that all these clients need is a few sessions of exposure to resolve their problems. This is sometimes the case, as was illustrated by the report on Ms. N. More often, however, agoraphobics have a host of problems that the practitioner will need to address for comprehensive treatment of the whole person. Ms. J. represents a case at the other end of the continuum in complexity and length of treatment. In practice, most clients require 6 to 18 months of treatment, more than the brief intervention used with Ms. N., although the exposure part of treatment is generally over in the first 3 to 6 months. Thus, unless the therapist strictly delimits the treatment program to covering only phobic avoidance behavior, a broad range of skills is required for treating these clients. This makes treatment challenging and seldom boring for the therapist.

Because agoraphobics react so strongly to the tenor of interpersonal relationships, it is particularly important that therapists be warm, accepting figures who are also able to be firm and insistent in a treatment that is often frightening. Additionally, the therapist needs to have a high frustration tolerance for missed appointments and noncompliance. Too many are ready to write these clients off as not being motivated or ready for treatment, when they are, in fact, most often simply being what they are, that is, phobic. The therapist, consequently, has to take an active and directive role, especially in the early part of treatment. Although this role is a familiar, comfortable role to behavior therapists, it may be initially awkward to those approaching this work from different theoretical perspectives.

Working with agoraphobic clients can be the most rewarding task I know of in that one has the opportunity to help someone make dramatic changes in her or his life. The clarity of change or failure with agoraphobic clients provides concrete feedback of efficacy that is often lacking in our profession. The failures are still too many, but the successes are truly gratifying.

ACKNOWLEDGMENTS

The author wishes to thank Alan Goldstein and the clients and staff of the Agoraphobia and Anxiety Program of Temple University Medical School for their contributions to the ideas and information presented in this chapter.

American Psychiatric Association. (1980). *Diagnostic and statistical manual of mental disorders* (3rd ed.). Washington, DC: Author.

Amies, P. L., Gelder, M. G., & Shaw, P. M. (1983). Social phobia: A comparative clinical study. *British Journal of Psychiatry, 142,* 174–179.

Barlow, D. H., O'Brien, G. T., & Last, C. G. (1984). Couples treatment of agoraphobia. *Behavior Therapy, 15,* 41–58.

Barlow, D. H., & Wolfe, B. E. (1981). Behavioral approaches to anxiety disorders: A report on the NIMH-SUNY, Albany Research Conference. *Journal of Consulting and Clinical Psychology, 49,* 448–454.

Beck, A. T., Ward, C. H., Mendelson, M., Mock, J., & Erbaugh, J. (1961). An inventory for measuring depression. *Archives of General Psychiatry, 4,* 561–571.

Bland, K., & Hallam, R. S. (1981). Relationship between response to graded exposure and marital satisfaction in agoraphobics. *Behaviour Research and Therapy, 19,* 335–338.

Boisvert, J. M., Marchand, A., & Gaudette, G. (1983, December). *Group treatment of agoraphobia with or without partners.* Paper presented at the meeting of the Association for the Advancement of Behavior Therapy, Washington, DC.

Buglass, D., Clarke, J., Henderson, A. S., Kreitman, N., & Presley, A. S. (1977). A study of agoraphobic housewives. *Psychological Medicine, 7,* 73–86.

Chambless, D. L. (1982). Characteristics of agoraphobics. In D. L. Chambless & A. J. Goldstein (Eds.), *Agoraphobia: Multiple perspectives on theory and treatment* (pp. 1–18). New York: Wiley.

Chambless, D. L., & Goldstein, A. J. (1980). Agoraphobia. In A. J. Goldstein & E. B. Foa (Eds.), *Handbook of behavioral interventions* (pp. 322–415). New York: Wiley.

Chambless, D. L., & Goldstein, A. J. (1981). Clinical treatment of agoraphobia. In M. Mavissakalian & D. Barlow (Eds.), *Phobia: Psychological and pharmacological treatment* (pp. 103–144). New York: Guilford Press.

Chambless, D. L., & Goldstein, A. J. (Eds.) (1982). *Agoraphobia: Multiple perspectives on theory and treatment.* New York: Wiley.

Chambless, D L., Caputo, G. C., Bright, P., & Gallagher, R. (1983). *Assessment of fear of fear in agoraphobics: The Agoraphobic Cognitions Questionnaire and the Body Sensations Questionnaire.* Manuscript submitted for publication.

Chambless, D. L., Caputo, G. C., Jasin, S. E., Gracely, E., & Williams, C. (1983). *The Mobility Inventory for Agoraphobia.* Manuscript submitted for publication.

Chambless, D. L., Goldstein, A. J., Gallagher, R., & Bright, P. (in press). A multitherapeutic approach to the treatment of agoraphobia. *Psychotherapy.*

Cobb, J. P., Mathews, A. M., Childs-Clarke, A., & Blowers, C. M. (1983). *The spouse as co-therapist in the treatment of agoraphobia.* Manuscript submitted for publication.

Crowe, R. R., Noyes, R., Pauls, D. L., & Slymen, D. (1983). A family study of panic disorder. *Archives of General Psychiatry, 40,* 1065–1069.

Crowe, R. R., Pauls, D. L., Slymen, D. J., & Noyes, R. (1980). A family study of anxiety neurosis. *Archives of General Psychiatry, 37,* 77–79.

Emmelkamp, P. M. G. (1982). *In vivo* exposure treatment of agoraphobia. In D. L. Chambless & A. J. Goldstein (Eds.), *Agoraphobia: Multiple perspectives on theory and treatment* (pp. 43–75). New York: Wiley.

Foa, E. B., & Chambless, D. L. (1978). Habituation of subjective anxiety during flooding in imagery. *Behaviour Research and Therapy, 16,* 391–399.

Goldstein, A. J., & Chambless, D. L. (1978). A reanalysis of agoraphobia. *Behavior Therapy, 9,* 47–59.

Hafner, R. J. (1982). The marital context of agoraphobia. In D. L. Chambless & A. J. Goldstein (Eds.), *Agoraphobia: Multiple perspectives on theory and treatment* (pp. 77–117). New York: Wiley.

Hafner, R. J., & Ross, M. W. (1983). Predicting the outcome of behaviour therapy for agoraphobia. *Behaviour Research and Therapy, 21,* 375–382.

Harris, E. L., Noyes, R., Jr., Crowe, R. R., & Chaudhry, D. R. (1983). Family study of agoraphobia. *Archives of General Psychiatry, 40,* 1061–1064.

Heide, F. J., & Borkovec, T. D. (1984). Relaxation-induced anxiety: Mechanisms and theoretical implications. *Behaviour Research and Therapy, 22,* 1–12.

Jannoun, L., Oppenheimer, C., & Gelder, M. (1982). A self-help treatment program for anxiety state patients. *Behavior Therapy, 13,* 103–111.

Jansson, L., & Öst, L. G. (1982). Behavioral treatments for agoraphobia: An evaluative review. *Clinical Psychology Review, 2,* 311–336.

Liebowitz, M. R., & Klein, D. F. (1982). Agoraphobia: Clinical features, pathophysiology, and treatment. In D. L. Chambless & A. J. Goldstein (Eds.), *Agoraphobia: Multiple perspectives on theory and treatment* (pp. 153–181). New York: Wiley.

Marks, I. M. (1970). Agoraphobic syndrome (phobic anxiety state). *Archives of General Psychiatry, 23,* 538–553.

Marks, I. M., & Mathews, A. M. (1979). Brief standard self-rating scale for phobic patients. *Behaviour Research and Therapy, 17,* 263–267.

Mathews, A. M., Gelder, M. G., & Johnston, D. W. (1981). *Agoraphobia: Nature and treatment.* New York: Guilford Press.

Mavissakalian, M., & Michelson, L. (1983). Agoraphobia: Behavioral and pharmacological treatment. *Psychopharmacology Bulletin, 19,* 116–118.

Mavissakalian, M., Michelson, L., Greenwald, D., Kornblith, S., & Greenwald, M. (1983). Cognitive-behavioral treatment of agoraphobia: Paradoxical intention vs. Self-statement training. *Behaviour Research and Therapy, 21,* 75–86.

Mavissakalian, M., Salerni, R., Thompson, M. E., & Michelson, L. (1983). Mitral valve prolapse and agoraphobia. *American Journal of Psychiatry, 140,* 1612–1614.

Mawson, D., Marks, I. M., Ramm, L., & Stern. R. S. (1981). Guided mourning for morbid grief: A controlled study. *British Journal of Psychiatry, 138,* 185–193.

Ramsay, R. W. (1977). Behavioural approaches to bereavement. *Behaviour Research and Therapy, 15,* 131–135.

Roberts, A. H. (1964). Housebound housewives: A follow-up study of phobic anxiety states. *British Journal of Psychiatry, 110,* 191–197.

Selzer, M. L. (1971). Michigan Alcoholism Screening Test. *American Journal of Psychiatry, 127,* 89–64.

Sheehan, D. V., Ballenger, J., & Jacobsen, G. (1980). Treatment of endogenous anxiety with phobic, hysterical and hypochondriacal symptoms. *Archives of General Psychiatry, 37,* 51–59.

Sinnott, A., Jones, R. B., Scott-Fordham, A., & Woodward, R. (1981). Augmentation of *in vivo* exposure treatment for agoraphobia by the formation of neighborhood self-help groups. *Behaviour Research and Therapy, 19,* 339–347.

Spielberger, C., Gorsuch, A., & Lushene, R. (1970). *The State-Trait Anxiety Inventory.* Palo Alto, CA: Consulting Psychologists Press.

Telch, M. J., Tearnan, B. H., & Taylor, C. B. (1983). Antidepressant medication in the treatment of agoraphobia: A critical review. *Behaviour Research and Therapy, 21,* 505–517.

Weekes, C. (1976). *Simple effective treatment for agoraphobia.* New York: Hawthorn.

Weissman, M. M. (1983, September). *The epidemiology of anxiety disorders: Rates, risks, and familial patterns.* Paper presented at the National Institute of Mental Health Conference on Anxiety and Anxiety Disorders, Tuxedo, NY.

Williams, S. L., Dooseman, G., & Kleifield, E. (1984). Comparative effectiveness of mastery and exposure treatments for intractable phobias. *Journal of Consulting & Clinical Psychology, 52,* 505–518.

Zane, M. D. (1978). Contextual analysis and treatment of phobic behavior as it changes. *American Journal of Psychotherapy, 32,* 338–356.

Zane, M. D., & Seif, M. N. (1983). Agoraphobia: Contextual analysis and treatment. In D. L. Chambless & A. J. Goldstein (Eds.), *Agoraphobia: Multiple perspectives on theory and treatment* (pp. 119–152). New York: Wiley.

Zitrin, C. M., Klein, D. F., & Woerner, M. G. (1980). Treatment of agoraphobia with group exposure in vivo and imipramine. *Archives of General Psychiatry, 37,* 63–72.

Stress and Generalized Anxiety

ROBERT L. WOOLFOLK AND PAUL M. LEHRER

Introduction

For the behavior therapist, the treatment of stress and generalized anxiety offers both comforts and frustrations. On the one hand, behavioral methods would seem ideally adapted to dysfunctions in which anxiety and physiological arousal are central. Early clinical behavior therapy was fashioned as a treatment for anxiety-related disorders. The most compelling and best documented successes of outpatient behavior therapy have come in the area of fear reduction. Yet, on the other hand, stress and generalized anxiety are not in all respects analogous to those phobic and obsessional syndromes with which behavior therapy has been so effective.

Anxiety has been central to conceptions of psychopathology since classical times. Theorists as diverse as Freud, Sullivan, Binswanger, and Wolpe have made anxiety the cornerstone of their theories of emotional dysfunction. Population surveys suggest that clinically significant anxiety symptoms are ubiquituous phenomena, being observed in approximately one-third of all individuals (Salkind, 1973; Taylor & Chave, 1964). One survey indicated that anxiety ranked behind only preventative examination, hypertension, lacerations and trauma, and pharyngitis and tonsilitis as reasons for appointments with primary care physicians. Anxiety-related symptoms probably account for between 10 and 30% of visits to primary care physicians (Pitts, 1971; Shepherd, Cooper, Brown, & Kalton, 1966). Anxiety also may be associated with another disorder that is the primary reason for an initial consultation. For example, Mullaney and Trippett (1979) found that more than a third

ROBERT L. WOOLFOLK • Department of Psychology, Busch Campus, Rutgers University, New Brunswick, New Jersey 08903. PAUL M. LEHRER • Department of Psychology, Rutgers Medical School, University of Medicine and Dentistry of New Jersey, Piscataway, New Jersey 08854.

of the patients coming to a clinic for problem drinking were also self-medicating for anxiety.

The prevalence of anxiety is further attested to by the frequency with which antianxiety drugs are prescribed. General practitioners in the United Kingdom give these drugs to 15.8% of all female patients and to 7.4% of all male patients (Skegg, Doll, & Perry, 1977). By 1972, diazepam (Valium) was prescribed more often than any other drug in the United States, with its close relative chlordiazepoxide (Librium) being the third most frequently prescribed (Blackwell, 1973). These two anxiolytics accounted for more than half of all psychotropic drugs prescribed. In just one 12-month period in the United States retail pharmacies filled 77 million prescriptions for these drugs and other benzodiazepines (Greenblatt & Shader, 1974).

Assessment

The medical literature distinguishes between pure "anxiety states" and other emotional disorders. Phobias are almost universally differentiated from pure "anxiety states": those in which symptoms do not appear related to specific stimuli. Lader and Marx (1971) have argued that, in fact, on a psychophysiological level, anxiety states and agoraphobia are rather similar and that both show more autonomic reactivity than do the simple phobias. Sheehan (1983) has argued that all problems involving seemingly spontaneous panic attacks result from a single psychobiological disorder and should carry the same diagnosis—*endogenous anxiety*. Other emotional problems that often are associated with anxiety but that usually receive separate diagnoses are obsessive-compulsive problems, depression, and manic-depressive disorder. Anxiety, however, is present to some degree in almost all classifications of psychiatric disorder, as, indeed it is a part of "normal" existence.

Lang (1968) has provided a useful conceptualization of fear and anxiety as composed of events in three response systems: *phenomenological, behavioral, and physiological*. These response systems correspond to the categories employed in the operational definition of anxiety. Phenomenological dimensions of anxiety are mapped by self-report questionnaires or clinical interviews that explore the subjective, experiential domain. Lehrer and Woolfolk (1982) devised a paper-and-pencil test that differentiates among these three dimensions. Measuring the behavioral aspects of fear usually involves some objective assessment of avoidance. Physiological assessment typically involves obtaining psychophysiological measures (e.g., surface EMG, skin conductance, heart rate). Behavioral, subjective, and physiological measures of stress tend to be imperfectly correlated, and no one system can be regarded as adequately mapping the domain of stress and anxiety. The three response systems are functionally interrelated in highly complex ways that still are poorly understood.

The standard *Diagnostic and Statistical Manual of Mental Disorders* (DSM-III) (American Psychiatric Association, 1980) distinguishes between the *phobic disorders* and the *anxiety reactions*. The former include agoraphobia (with and without panic attacks), social phobia, and simple phobia. The latter, which are the addressed in this chapter, include panic disorders, generalized anxiety disorders, posttraumatic stress disorders, and, oddly, obsessive-compulsive disorder (in which anxiety symptoms often are minimal). The criteria for panic disorder include panic attacks with a frequency of at least three in a 3-week period, with multiple somatic symptoms (including dyspnea, palpitations, chest pain, choking, dizziness, feelings of unreality, paresthesias, hot and cold flashes, sweating, faintness, and trembling). Generalized anxiety disorders manifest similar symptoms but without acute and sudden panic disorders. Historically, this set of symptoms has been recognized and given various labels: *irritable heart of the soldier* (Da Costa, 1871), *effort syndrome* (Lewis, 1919), *cardiac neurosis* (Schnur, 1939), *neurocirculatory asthenia* (Oppenheimer, Levine, Morison, Rothchild, St. Lawrence, & Wilson, 1918), *neurasthenia* (Savill, 1907), *hyperventilation syndrome* (Lowry, 1967), and *autonomic imbalance* (Kessel & Hyman, 1923).

Proper assessment is an important precursor to successful clinical treatment of stress and anxiety. It is also a safeguard against inappropriate and potentially harmful errors in matching clinical strategems and presenting disorders. A number of questions should be answered rather early in the diagnostic activities of the therapist. The most important of these are given next.

1. *Does the emotional arousal have a direct organic cause requiring medical treatment?* There are realistic concerns that some patients suffering symptoms of anxiety actually have a definable physical problem that is best treated medically. Lader and Marx (1971) include alcoholism, epilepsy, paroxysmal tachycardia, pheochromocytoma, and thyrotoxicosis as disorders that often produce anxious symptomatology. To these we may add epilepsy, caffeine intoxication (Greden, 1974), hypoglycemia, the well-known effects of taking or withdrawing from various drugs, mitro valve prolapse (Szmuilowicz & Flannery, 1980; Wooley, 1976), and various disorders of the inner ear (Jacob, 1983).

A client complaining of stress and tension was being interviewed during a first session. The client described his symptoms, which consisted primarily of cognitive arousal, distractability, and a feeling of agitation.

T: When did you first begin experiencing these feelings?
C: About 3 weeks ago.
T: Have your life circumstances changed in any way recently, say within the last few months?
C: I can't really think of anything?

The client was asked to keep a diary in which he recorded both symptoms and daily activities (at least one entry every half hour) during the week before the second session. An inspection of this record revealed no mention of any midday meal.

T: Do you eat lunch?
C: I haven't recently.
T: Any particular reason?
C: Well, I've been trying to lose some weight.

It turned out that the patient had been on an extremely low-calorie (400 per day) diet for a period of time that roughly corresponded with the duration of the anxiety. After returning to a more reasonable pattern of food consumption, the client reported feeling more like his "old self." Two sessions later he terminated and 1 year later reported no return of his difficulties.

2. *Should drugs be utilized as an adjunct to treatment?* Pharmacological intervention by far is the most prevalent clinical treatment modality for anxiety. This is understood even more clearly if, to the multitude of individuals holding prescriptions from their physicians for anxiolytic agents, we add the millions who self-medicate with either alcohol or illegal substances. Of course, the use of drugs to control anxiety has many drawbacks, including the possibility of psychological or physical dependency, negative side effects, the direct and indirect hazards of excessive use, and often questionable efficacy. Drugs do, however, have an important role in the behavioral treatment of anxiety.

Clients may enter therapy with anxiety severe enough to preclude the learning of behavioral methods of relaxation or any other meaningful participation in therapy. Thus, when emotional arousal is so intense and pervasive as to prevent the normal clinical activities, psychotropic medication has been used in order to reduce anxiety to levels that will allow therapy to proceed productively. High levels of chronic anxiety are most often treated by anxiolytics with a relatively long half-life, such as diazepam (Lader, 1984). Panic episodes are more effectively controlled by a fast-acting agent with a rapid absorption rate, such as lorazepam (Ativan), even after their onset. The mere ready availability of a rapid and reliable means of controlling panic attacks can dispel some of the secondary "fear of fear" that often is found in panic disorders.

Some recent studies, however, raise cautions about the common use of some of the minor tranquilizers, particularly the benzodiazepines, the most common of which are best known by their trade names: Librium, Valium, Ativan, and so forth. Although the short-term effects of these medications appear to be positive, there is some indication that chronic anxiety conditions may be worsened by courses of benzodiazepine treatment (cf. Lavallee, Lamontagne, Pinard, Annable, & Tetreault, 1977). These potent drugs appear to create a psychological dependence on taking at least some sort of medication to relieve problems. People who are prescribed them at some point in treatment tend to be less cooperative in following behavioral regimens, preferring to seek relief through medication. Over time, the benzodiazepines can even lead to actual physiological dependency. Tolerance to them is developed, and larger doses are required to produce therapeutic effects. Thus, use of the benzodiazepines as a long-term treatment for chronic states is a questionable practice.

Antidepressants, such as the tricyclics and MAO inhibitors, have shown some promise in controlling panic episodes and have enhanced the effect of behavioral interventions in some instances. Therefore, it is particularly important to determine whether panic attacks actually do occur—for these medications usually have less impact on other anxiety symptoms. Even more promising in this regard has been the recent use of the drug alprazolam (Xanax), which has both antianxiety and antidepressant effects. Although initial experience suggests that alprazolam has stronger effects on controlling panic attacks than do the antidepressants (without the negative effects of the benzodiazepines), there as yet has been insufficient research on it to be certain of all its short- and long-term effects.

Patients with symptoms entirely mediated by the beta division of the sympathetic nervous system (e.g., palpitations, trembling, and gastrointestinal upset) may be helped by administration of propranolol (Inderal) or another of the beta-adrenoceptor antagonists. These medications have almost exclusively peripheral physiological effects and should not be expected to help individuals who may have components of worry or behavioral avoidance in their conditions. Anxiety attacks in the absence of cognitive or behavioral components have sometimes been labeled *hyper beta adrenergic states* (Lader & Marx, 1971, p. 27) because of their dissimilarity to most generalized anxiety reactions. Beta blockers recently have been used in the treatment of musicians suffering from stage fright, who feel in good cognitive and behavioral control, but whose sympathetic autonomic arousal interferes with their ability to play their instruments on stage (Brantigan, Brantigan, & Neil, 1979).

In most cases the adjunctive use of drugs will be temporary, with the pharmacological agent being faded as behavioral methods become effective in ameliorating the presenting problems.

3. *Are there additional psychological or social factors that will complicate treatment?* Woolfolk and Lazarus (1979) have discussed a number of the factors that may impede treatment of clinical fears by straightforward behavioral intervention. Among these are reinforcement from the environment for anxious behavior ("secondary gain"), family systems factors, client resistance, interaction of clinical fears with complex skill deficits, and presence of severe psychopathology. The "whole person" must be taken into account in behavioral treatment. An analysis of the client's overall life situation, goals, values, and attitudes is therefore an essential part of any broadly applicable and viable form of behavioral treatment.

Anxiety is often associated with feelings of guilt, frustration, and/or conflict (Meyer & Crisp, 1970). These observed associations led Freud and his psychoanalytic followers to incorrectly posit that such factors were almost always the cause of neurotic anxiety (Freud, 1936). Eysenck and Rachman (1965) concluded that "approach/avoidance" conflicts are generally productive of anxiety. Stimuli and thoughts that may even vaguely remind us of our faults, our conflicts, or our true feelings may, at times, evoke anxiety. Inability to understand or to cope with the demands of the environment also can produce anxiety. Thus, anxiety is often at its height during periods of transition in one's life (e.g., adolescence, leaving home for the first time, marriage, a new job, etc.). At these times necessary understanding and coping skills have not yet been developed. When the individual is under performance pressure and when the probability of failure or rejection in a significant area of life is elevated, anxiety is often increased. Frequently the individual is unaware that such factors are the source of the emotional discomfort. Thus, an important preliminary step in therapy is to identify life stresses and to assist the client to understand their significance in his or her life and how to cope more effectively with them.

An executive described severe tension accompanied by stomach pains that began each morning during his commute by train to Manhattan. He experienced minimal discomfort on weekends and vacations.

T: Are you having some difficulties at work?
C: No more than anyone else.
T: What do you mean?
C: I get paid a lot of money for what I do. I'm expected to produce.

As it developed, the client's conception of a normal amount of job stress was somewhat distorted. He expected that he should never make a mistake, always succeed in everything he did, have subordinates who were as competent as he, and work for a just and rational boss. His morning bouts of tension eventually began to improve when cognitive therapy resulted in his altering his expectations of himself and his work environment.

Another client, a married woman in her mid-40s, reported sleep onset insomnia, restlessness, inability to concentrate, and feelings of dread.

T: Otherwise, how are things going in your life?
C: That's what is really perplexing. I have absolutely nothing to complain about.

Further investigation revealed that the woman's youngest child would be going away to college in 5 months and that she and her husband were having sex less frequently than in past years. I met with the husband and wife together and with the husband alone. During my individual session with the husband, he revealed to me that he was planning to leave his wife to live with a woman with whom he had been having an affair. The husband eventually separated from his wife and her amorphous fears were diminished and became focused upon her uncertain future as a single woman. Therapy was directed toward aiding her in coping with her changed situation.

Mark, a 21-year-old first-year graduate student, came to the student health service complaining of acute chest pains, dizziness, difficulty in breathing, and anxiety. He was given a physical examination, which revealed no abnormalities. He was referred to the mental health service. Upon the therapist's inquiry about his general adjustment, Mark reported that he had never before experienced these feelings. The therapist attempted to fashion a picture of the client's current life situation by asking open-ended questions and for elaboration of the answers to those questions. It emerged that Mark recently had been given a warning by his department that his grades were not quite up to par. He felt overwhelmed by the demands of graduate study and did not know what directions his studies should take. Also, for the first time in his life, he was living thousands of miles from friends and family. He had always been relatively introverted. Although he had always maintained a few close friendships, he did not make new friends easily. He was lonely and felt unsure of himself socially. He had not dated since coming to graduate school. During the first session, the therapist listened quietly and sympathetically to Mark's problems, gently probing about various aspects of his daily functioning. At the end of the session, Mike said: "Gee, I didn't realize that I had so much to be anxious about." By the next session, he already seemed visibly less nervous. Three sessions of counseling involved some assertion training, cognitive therapy, and nondirective reflection of feelings. A minor tranquilizer (Librium) was also prescribed by a consulting physician. Although he continued to experience some anxiety during the rest of the year, it gradually diminished as he started work on his master's thesis, made new friends, and began to date.

Where life circumstances, skill deficits, or interpersonal relationships prove to be central factors, they must be addressed in therapy. Just as organic factors must be ruled out before embarking upon behavioral treatment, so must the presence of more severe forms of psychopathology. Occasionally, psychotic or borderline patients will present with anxiety ostensibly as their primary symptom. For such individuals, direct behavioral treatment targeting the anxiety is not indicated as an initial intervention. Although some relaxation techniques (most particularly meditation) have been employed with such patients (Glueck & Stroebel, 1975), this is a questionable approach outside of a closely supervised hospital environment.

4. *Is anxiety tied to specific enough stimuli to permit exposure based methods?* The complexity and lack of specificity manifested by many anxiety states is a potential source of frustration for the behavior therapist who has available a number of demonstrably effective techniques for ameliorating fears tied to specific stimuli. Many patients manifesting generalized stress and anxiety, however, will report either subsidiary phobic or obsessive-compulsive patterns. Responses to particular stimulus configurations can and should be treated with exposure methods. In these instances either direct exposure methods (flooding or graduated exposure *in vivo*) or indirect exposure (systematic desensitization or imaginal flooding) should target the specific fear involved.

Techniques

Various forms of relaxation training, including progressive relaxation, biofeedback, and meditation have been found to ameliorate stress and anxiety states, although a number of factors seem to mediate the therapeutic effect. Relaxation strategies have been rather extensively researched and have proven to be effective treatments for such stress-related problems as anxiety, phobias, and psychosomatic disorders. Particularly convincing evidence has been amassed for the effectiveness of these techniques in treating hypertension, insomnia, and headaches (see review by Lehrer & Woolfolk, 1984).

The relaxation procedure most frequently employed by behavior therapists is progressive muscle relaxation. Progressive relaxation is not, as is commonly thought, a unitary technique. There are two major varieties that, although similar, have important differences. Jacobson's (1938) original procedure is designed to instruct clients in the complete reduction of tonic muscle tension. The trainee is taught to identify extremely low levels of muscle tonus by tensing each muscle only to the extent required to produce proprioceptive "control" sensations. Successively, diminishing levels of client-produced tension are utilized until extreme sensitivity to muscle tension is developed. Training in the classical Jacobsonian method is usually rather lengthy, often requiring more than 20 sessions in which over 40 muscle groups are individually addressed. Jacobson's original method contrasts with the modified procedures that have wide currency in behavior therapy (Bernstein & Borkovec, 1973; Paul, 1966; Wolpe & Lazarus, 1966). These methods are highly abbreviated and attempt to produce an overall feeling of deep relaxation very early in training. Rather liberal use is made of suggestion, with patients typically being told what sensations they will experience after each muscle contraction and release of tension. In contrast, the Jacobsonian procedure emphasizes the gradual production of profound somatic effects rather than an immediate psychological sense of calm and assiduously avoids the use of suggestion. Only two studies have examined the relative efficacy of the two forms of training. Turner (1978) found the Jacobsonian procedure to be marginally superior, whereas another study (Snow, 1978) found no differences between techniques.

Two reviews (Borkovec & Sides, 1979; Lehrer, 1982) have identified procedural elements that may be critical in the production of clinical effects. Of especial importance seems to be therapist administration of training. Tape-recorded training appears to produce weaker physiological effects that do not generalize beyond the treatment session. Although Borkovec and Sides (1979) found that studies using five or more sessions of training produced better results than studies using fewer sessions, Lehrer's (1982) review did not confirm this. It is probable that the intensity and care involved in training is more important than the actual number of training sessions. Lehrer's review also found that EMG biofeedback appears to have no beneficial effects when combined with live progressive relaxation training. Also, it is generally less effective than the latter when used separately. EMG biofeedback, however, appears to be more effective than relaxation training administered by tape, and, when combined with taped relaxation, renders the latter a more effective technique. Other forms of biofeedback have had less satisfactory results. Although there are a few studies showing positive effects for finger temperature warming, there is no firm evidence that biofeedback for heart rate or EEG alpha produces any beneficial effect on anxiety. Combinations of cognitive therapy and relaxation therapy tend to have better results than either technique alone in reducing anxiety. Although the various relaxation methods reduce many of the manifestations of anxiety, they do not appear to represent a sufficient treatment for panic disorders (Raskin, Johnson, & Rondestvedt, 1973). In such cases they may reduce the levels of many ancillary anxiety symptoms, such as headaches, insomnia, situational anxiety, and the like, but they do not totally eliminate panic attacks. Thus, although we personally have had some success with these and other behavioral techniques in treating panic disorders, we recommend that adjunctive use of medication be seriously considered for such conditions.

With the advent of transcendental meditation (TM), meditation became somewhat Westernized though not totally stripped of its esoteric trappings. The complete secularization of meditation was realized in Benson's (1975) method, Woolfolk's clinical meditation technique (Woolfolk, Carr-Kaffashan, McNulty, & Lehrer, 1976; Woolfolk & Richardson, 1978), and Carrington's "clinically standardized meditation" (1977). Although these methods of meditation vary, they have a number of features in common. Among these are avoidance of discursive, ruminative thought and the attempt to deploy attention in a nonanalytical way. Similarly, each method requires the meditator to concentrate on a repetitive or recurring stimulus, usually a verbal mantra and/or a bodily process, while reclining or sitting in a comfortable position.

Meditation has shown considerable promise as a treatment for stress and anxiety (Lehrer, Woolfolk, Rooney, McCann, & Carrington, 1983; Woolfolk, Lehrer, McCann, & Rooney, 1982). A 1984 review by Holmes suggests that brief training in meditation may be less efficacious that earlier research indicated in reducing physiological arousal relative to simple rest or unsystematic self-initiated attempts to relax. Thus far, an inadequate number of studies have assessed meditation as a treatment for chronic anxiety of clinical proportions. Research by Heide and Borkovec (1983) indicates that meditation may be more likely than progressive relaxation to produce negative side effects: "relaxation-induced anxiety," or paradoxical anxiety experienced by the client while employing a relaxation strategy. This finding is consistent with other reports indicating occasional adverse reactions to meditation (Carrington, 1977).

The viability of cognitive interventions for stress and anxiety is suggested by cognitive theories of emotion that emphasize the role of cognitive appraisal in the generation of dysfunctional affective states (e.g., Lazarus, 1982). Also supportive is the work of Beck, Laude, and Bohnert (1974), who employed a structured interview in ascertaining that the images and patterns of thought of anxious patients revolved around the twin themes of physical danger and psychosocial threat.

All forms of cognitive therapy have in common the attempt to alter or restructure the client's thoughts, imagery, or beliefs in such a fashion as will alleviate emotional distress. Although there is much overlap among the following forms of cognitive therapy, each has its distinctive emphasis. Meichenbaum's (1977) approach emphasizes the systematic modification of self-verbalization and the substitution of salutary self-talk for the anxiety-generating mentation and worry characteristic of many anxiety states.

Beck's (1976, 1984) approach tends to focus on identifying and changing the forms of faulty thinking and the styles of cognition that lead to anxiety and stress through a Socratic dialectical exchange between patient and therapist. Among the targets of Beck's (Beck & Emery, 1979; Bedrosian & Beck, 1980) therapy are:

1. Polarized thinking (dichotomous, black/white reasoning)
2. Personification (false self-referent ideation)
3. Magnification and exaggeration (catastrophizing and emphasizing the most negative possibilities)
4. Overgeneralization (faulty induction)
5. Selective abstraction (missing the significance of the total situation because of focusing on a single element)
6. Incorrect appraisals of danger and safety
7. Arbitrary inference (various forms of unsound reasoning)

Ellis's (1962) approach is a persuasive, didactic effort oriented toward modifying the content of cognitions that seeks to identify and eradicate "irrational" beliefs and attitudes (especially those having to do with moralism and perfectionism) and substitute for them a certain outlook on life characterized by the following (Ellis, 1973):

1. Self-direction (assuming responsibility for one's own life)
2. Self-interest (long-range hedonism and rational egoism)
3. Acceptance of uncertainty (accepting the contingent nature of the human situation)
4. Tolerance (accepting one's own and other's fallibility and the suspension of blame)
5. Scientific thinking (rational, objective thinking)
6. Flexibility (openness to change and novelty)
7. Risk taking (to risk failure in attempting change)
8. Self-acceptance
9. Commitment (involvement in someone or something outside oneself)

Very little controlled research has studied the effects of cognitive therapy on generalized anxiety, although these approaches have been relatively effective in the treatment of social anxiety, performance anxiety, and depression (Kendall & Hollon, 1979). Woodward and Jones (1980) treated generally anxious clients with cognitive therapy, systematic desensitization, or their combination and found the combined treatment to be the most effective. Novaco (1975) found that cognitive therapy was an effective treatment for chronic anger. Cognitive strategies have been successful in ameliorating adverse effects of a variety of stressors (Meichenbaum & Jaremko, 1983).

Compliance, Resistance, Generalization

Of all the difficulties that confront behavior therapists involved in treating stress and anxiety disorders, perhaps none is more bothersome than that of patient noncompliance. Behavioral self-regulation techniques are effective when employed but only if employed. Unfortunately, a rather large percentage of clients troubled by stress and anxiety either: (a) are reluctant or unwilling to attempt a program of stress management, and (b) begin such a program but fail to persist in their efforts over time.

Behavioral treatment typically requires the active participation of the client outside of the consulting room both in practice and in the direct application of the methods of self-regulation in the stressful environment of daily life. Deep relaxation and peace of mind are often readily obtained in the somewhat tranquil and protected confines of the consulting room. In order for these states to generalize to the outside, much work must be done by the client outside in his or her normal living environment.

Having effective techniques avails us little if our clients do not invest the homework time and effort required to learn how to effectively apply the methods to the stresses that confront them. The following recommendations are based on our own clinical experience and that of numerous colleagues.

1. *Client Responsibility.* The essence of behavioral methods that require homework between therapeutic sessions is the proposition that the client is the one responsible for taking the skills and knowledge learned in therapy and applying these in everyday life. The client must understand that managing stress and anxiety must be learned as is any other skill, and that it must be practiced religiously during the early stages to be acquired with any level of proficiency. In this regard, there is an analogy with various athletic or artistic pursuits. The patient should be cognizant that the gains to be derived from stress management techniques are proportional to the amount of practice one engages in. "It doesn't work if you don't do it" is a message that must be communicated unambiguously to clients prior to undertaking to train them in relaxation and stress reduction techniques.

2. *A Knowledgeable Client.* Although it is neither feasible nor desirable for the client to become an expert in the physiological, biochemical, and psychological dimensions of stress, a small amount of education can facilitate instilling in the client a sense of informed participation in the project therapy. A basic model of stress and anxiety and a rationale for why the particular treatment employed is valuable in combating stress can both create faith in the method and lend some increased sense of purpose to the participation required of the client. The therapist should answer all questions related to the nature of the dysfunction, provided the questions are not being asked by the occasional obsessional client who seems to prefer a seminar on stress to therapy for it. An open therapist, manifesting minimal defensiveness, is likely to be one with whom problems related to homework can be discussed fruitfully.

3. *Compatibility of Technique.* In order to facilitate the patient's active participation, the therapist should strive to match the client with a clinical strategy that holds some appeal for him or her. In cases where the client comes into treatment with some clear attraction or dislike preference for one or more methods, the task of the therapist is made easier. The client can be exposed initially to several procedures by means of brief handouts, videotaped depictions of the method, or by a short *in vivo* demonstration. The initial client preference for a particular method, however, may decrease following actual experience with it. A client should never continue to practice any technique of stress control that is experienced as aversive.

4. *Individualized Techniques.* Adjustments aimed at individualization in frequency of meetings with the therapist, in practice schedules, and in the techniques themselves are often beneficial. Individual tailoring of this kind is, in fact, essential to therapeutic efficacy. In meditation, for example, some people find the normal 20-minute, twice-a-day routine unfeasible. We have found that variations in this pattern do not destroy the benefits of meditative practice. Carrington, Collings, Benson, Robinson, Wood, Lehrer, Woolfolk, and Cole (1980) observed the same self-reported benefits from meditation and progressive relaxation among those subjects whose practice schedules deviated from the customary routine as were found for those who practiced as prescribed. Similarly, although meditation pro-

cedures derived from yoga are practiced with the eyes closed, some individuals find it difficult to keep their eyes shut. Meditating with the eyes open or half open is an effective alternative that has the ancient Zen tradition to recommend it as a legitimate alternative. Although some rather high degree of therapist experience and expertise with a technique may be necessary to make effective modifications, this is the essence of therapeutic artistry. Adjustments in the standardized approaches, however, do require that extraordinarily careful attention be paid to the ongoing evaluation of therapeutic progress.

5. *Planning and Rehearsal.* One of the frequent errors made by beginning therapists is to allow clients to leave an initial relaxation training session without having discussed the particulars of how they will integrate the routines of practice into their daily lives. The investment of a few minutes to anticipate possible pitfalls and to schedule the practice times can result in more regular practice. It is a good idea to have the patient commit to a specific place and time for each practice session and to schedule the time and place on his or her weekly calendar. Practice must be accorded such a high priority by the client that it is assumed that it always will be carried out, unless an emergency occurs. Getting the client to imagine relaxing in the environment he or she has selected can point out potential problems with that environment as a place to relax. The client should be questioned about features of the chosen time and place that might be problematic.

A common therapeutic mistake is to train a client with a self-regulation method, such as progressive relaxation, and then merely tell him or her to employ the procedure whenever under stress. This approach will invariably produce less satisfactory results (Lehrer & Woolfolk, 1984). When clients develop proficiency with a stress reduction technique, therapists and clients, working together, must anticipate recurrent episodes of anxiety in their lives and begin to practice the technique. Using either role playing or imagery to generate some approximation of the life situation, the client can practice coping efforts in the consulting room. Follow-up *in vivo* practice should be planned systematically and its effects evaluated. Predictable environmental stressors or internal sensations thus can become cues to initiate self-regulatory procedures.

In applying the technique of progressive relaxation, even instructing the client to use the relaxation skills in his or her daily life often is not sufficient to insure generalization. The method of "differential relaxation" is often employed (Jacobson, 1970). In the office, the client is specifically trained to discuss emotionally charged topics: for example, to role-play an argument with a spouse, or the like. This is done while keeping all skeletal muscles relaxed that are not needed to perform the task at hand, such as talking or sitting erect.

C: Everything is piling up on me. I have work deadlines I can't meet. I'm not with my kids or my wife enough, and I'm being a lousy father and husband. I'm at loose ends, and I can't think straight about what I should do to make things better. My head hurts . . .

T: I understand your feelings of frustration and your anger at yourself for not being able to do well all the things you feel you should be able to. But notice that while you talk about these things, your forearm muscles are tensing up, you are grasping the arms of the chair, your fingers are turning white, your shoulders and forehead are tight, and, I'll bet, lots of other muscles in your body are also tense. You have already been trained in progressive relaxation. Use it now. If you deliberately relax your muscles while you think and talk about these problems, maybe some solutions will come to you. You will feel less anxious, more clearheaded, and will get rid of your headache. Would you attempt this as an exercise, here and now?

6. *Involvement of Significant Others.* Sabotage by significant others can render ineffective the most artfully engineered program of behavioral treatment. Conversely, the supportive involvement of family members in a program of behavior change can have a beneficial effect. A cooperative spouse can enhance the client's therapeutic progress in a number of ways. He or she can provide support and encouragement, function as a buffer between the patient and family demands during practice times, and can give the therapist an extra source of information about the client's progress. Embarking on a comprehensive program of behavioral treatment occasionally can prove disruptive to stable patterns of family dynamics and thus may result in a high emotional price for the client. Coordination with the client's spouse can be of help in preventing such negative side effects of treatment.

7. *Evaluation of Progress.* The therapist must make a systematic attempt to evaluate the client's progress. This includes some evaluation of how well the client has carried out assignments and how proficient in relaxation or cognitive self-management strategies he or she has become. Also, improvement or deterioration in the client's target symptoms should be monitored. Client self-monitoring can be helpful in evaluation, although the therapist must understand that self-monitoring is subject to noncompliance just as are all other assignments.

A therapist should never give therapeutic homework without later determining whether it has been done. Failure to check up on the client after an intervention may suggest to the client that the assignment was not important and that no consequences are contingent on its completion or lack of completion. An active, involved therapist who keeps abreast of the client's efforts between treatment sessions is better able to direct the course of therapy. Also, such a therapist displays a high level of commitment to the client and reinforces in him or her a sense of accountability to the therapeutic endeavor.

In this same vein, the scheduling of "booster sessions," at intervals of 3 and 6 months following termination has some useful effects. Such sessions can serve as incentives to continue utilization of the strategies learned in therapy. Such sessions are also useful in "trouble shooting" and "fine tuning" the client's coping skills.

8. *Realistic Expectations.* Clients with stress and problems often enter therapy with unrealistically high expectations. They seek quick total "cures" for the debilitating problems that have brought them into therapy. Inordinately high hopes of this sort are usually met with disappointment. Generalized stress and anxiety disorders are not analogous to diseases for which a complete cure is attainable. Clients should be taught by their therapists to eventually expect to manage stress rather than to eliminate it entirely. Acquisition of self-regulation skills is rarely rapid and almost never free of setbacks. Clients should be prepared to expect these setbacks and understand that progress toward effective coping will not be uninterrupted. Some discomfort, uncertainty, and tragedy are inevitable aspects of human exis-.

tence. Indeed, if it were possible to eradicate stress and anxiety from life, it would mean that most passion, loyalty, freedom, ambition, caring, and commitment to higher ideals also would disappear from the human experience. The instilling of some philosophical acceptance of the inevitable stress of life is an important accompaniment to behavioral treatment.

Case Study (Treated by R. W.)

The client, Mrs. J., was a 27-year-old woman referred by her family physician for behavioral treatment of anxiety. The referring physician described Mrs. J. as "generally anxious" and suggested that her anxiety could be "desensitized." He had prescribed Valium at a dosage of 20 mg/day for temporary relief of symptoms.

My first session with Mrs. J. reveal her principal area of concern to be the relatively frequent episodes of "weakness" and "light headedness" that seemed to her unpredictable and tied to no identifiable circumstances or antecedents. I attempted to determine the exact nature of these anxiety episodes.

T: Let's try to get as specific as possible about these anxiety episodes. I'd like to know everything that happens to you at these times: what you feel and think, how you behave, and what your bodily reaction is. Let's start with what your body does at those times.

C: I feel really shaky. I guess the best way to describe the feeling would be that I get shaky and panicy.

T: Does your body actually shake or tremble?

C: I'm not sure.

T: What about your heart? Do you notice any changes in the way it beats?

C: Yes. My heart definitely beats faster and stronger.

The client went on to report a pattern of physical symptoms that included dizziness, light headedness, and tingling extremities.

T: What sorts of thoughts do you have at these times?

C: I start to panic.

T: What sorts of "panicky" ideas run through your head?

C: At the beginning it's something like, "Oh, no! Not again." But then it always starts to intensify. Then I start getting very worried.

T: And what do you think then?

C: I think that I can't control what's happening to me. I sometimes think I may pass out. Sometimes I think I'm going to die. You know. Have a heart attack.

T: Do you just imagine this verbally or are there mental pictures that go along with the words?

C: Sometimes I see myself passing out, falling down in front of other people. Everybody rushes to help me.

T: Did anything like that ever really happen to you?

C: Only once. It was a few years ago.

The client went on to relate how she had once, at a social gathering, consumed an alcoholic punch that had caused her, a very infrequent drinker, to become somewhat disoriented. She had begun to panic, was unable to catch her breath, and had briefly lost consciousness. She described the incident as "embarrasing in the extreme" and "humiliating." The image of herself as a helpless object of public sympathy was both powerful and almost unbearably aversive for the client.

Further discussion revealed Mrs. J. to be less than forthcoming about areas of her life not obviously related to her presenting problem. She described herself as happily married with no children and her husband as "very supportive." She told me that she had left high-school teaching 2 years previously because of the emotional strain inherent in the practice of her profession. My overall impression of Mrs. J. was that of a superficially cooperative but rather intensely formal, private, and highly controlled individual.

At the close of the session, I told her that during the next session (scheduled for 5 days later) we would begin to instruct her in techniques aimed at alleviating her anxiety. I also gave her a copy of the Lehrer-Woolfolk Anxiety Inventory to complete at home and asked to monitor both her heart rate and respiration during any future episodes of intense anxiety.

At the beginning of the second session, Mrs. J. described three anxiety episodes that had occurred since the first session. One of the incidents she described as "as bad as they come." On all three occasions her pulse rate had been elevated to above 110 beats per minute for at least 1 hour.

During the second session, I began relaxation training with Mrs. J. She was unfamiliar with any systematic method of relaxation instruction but did understand and accept the rationale presented. She indicated a willingness to practice for an hour a day between sessions. Because I had a hunch that Mrs. J. would grow impatient with a relaxation procedure that did not produce an immediate and powerful effect, I used a method that typically generates an intense initial effect. Employing the modified progressive relaxation procedure (Bernstein & Borkovec, 1973), I utilized two tension-release cycles with each of the following muscle groups: lower arms, upper arms, shoulders, chest, abdomen, thighs, and calves. Afterward, I gave Mrs. J. some quasi-hypnotic (Barber, 1984) suggestions of relaxation that she followed by 10 minutes of abdominal breathing (Patel, 1984). She then was given some calming scenes to imagine. Toward the end of the procedure the client was virtually motionless. Her breathing became slow and rhythmical and deepened substantially. She later reported a profound experience of tranquility and well-being. Her initial reaction to relaxation portended well for its utility in treating her anxiety.

Given an array of reactions that suggested a hyperventilation syndrome, I asked the client to practice very slow, consciously regulated abdominal breathing whenever she experienced signs of anxiety. Immediately after the session, I consulted with Mrs. J.'s physician and informed him of the symptomatology and my plan to use relaxation training as the initial therapeutic intervention.

Sessions 3 and 4 were devoted almost exclusively to training in the abbreviated version of progressive muscle relaxation. Over the course of training, it became clear that the client, although a conscientious student, reported that the procedure of going through each muscle group gave her too much time to think and was the occasion for much worry. She volunteered that the method I had employed during our second session had been much more effective and enjoyable. Given her preference and her favorable response to the relaxation strategy employed initially, I immediately consolidated the individual muscle groups to four and returned to a more hypnotic approach. Because the client found abdominal breathing to be "soothing" and of some help during panic episodes, I again had her breathe abdominally after relaxing her muscles. After experimenting with several calm scenes, none of which seemed to produce the intended effect, the client was given a mantra to couple with her breathing.

T: I'd like you to try linking your breathing with a mantra. It will give you something to focus your thoughts upon while your are relaxing and some people find that it deepens their sense of quietude.

C: Is this like TM?

T: Sort of. We like to draw from the best of various methods of producing relaxation. Let's start with the English words *in* and *out*. As you inhale silently, say the word *in,* and when you exhale, say the word *out.* Draw out or extend the enunciation of each word so that the whole time you are inhaling you are saying *in* and the entire time you are breathing out you are saying the word *out.* We'll start by doing this together. I'll say the mantra aloud slowly. You repeat along with me. Gradually my voice will fade out, but you just keep right on silently with the mantra as you breathe in and out.

Over the next two sessions, the client and I worked on enhancing her ability to relax, teaching her to let go of muscle tension without producing muscle contractions, and generalizing the effects of training. The generalization training involved having the client self-monitor and release tension throughout the day and utilize an abbreviated version of the technique we had created for her when anxiety levels became more severe. Although the client reported fewer panic episodes, less fear of fear, greater general comfort and well-being, and enhanced ability to cope with panic episodes, she continued to have frequent protracted periods of elevated heart rate. After consulting with her physician, it was decided that he would prescribe propranolol. Her response to the drug was immediate with the cardiac symptoms essentially disappearing after beginning drug treatment.

After eight sessions, Mrs. J.'s panic episodes were under control and she felt more comfortable throughout the day. We then began four sessions of desensitization to the image of her collapsing in a public place after an anxiety attack. The client's catastrophic cognitions in this area also were discussed and, after some initial resistance, became more rational. She began to say reasonable and calming things to herself rather than the alarmist self-verbalizations previously employed.

As is often the case with clients who obtain relief in one acute area of discomfort, Mrs. J.'s other difficulties began to emerge as her immediate distress subsided. I also felt that she had decided she could trust me. She began to "open up" somewhat, revealing that she suffered from severe social anxiety and was rather frustrated with many aspects of her marital relationship. Further therapy focused on communication skills training. After six sessions devoted to assertion training with homework assignments interspersed, seven conjoint sessions with her husband addressed topics of sex and intimacy. I referred this client to group therapy at this point while continuing to see her individually every 3 weeks. The client was withdrawn from maintenance on propranolol 6 months after beginning medication. Two episodes of tachycardia ensued over the next 2 months, but these were not deemed serious enough by either the client or her physician to require a return to the previous pharmacological regimen. The client terminated after 13 months of therapy. She left the group a short time later. At 1-year follow-up she reported no recurrence of the cardiac symptoms, a circumstance she attributed to beginning aerobic dancing. She had returned to teaching and was finding the work very stressful, although she found the students much easier to cope with as a result of her newfound ability to assert herself.

C: I'm not sure what I expected at first. I guess I thought I would be completely cured, but I still get worried, and there are times when I feel just like I used too. Not the panic attacks but really uptight.

T: When does this happen?

C: Mainly at school. Do you think I need more therapy?

T: What do you think?

C: Some part of me thinks it would be a good idea to come back, but I'd really like to beat this on my own. I wonder if anybody ever gets to the point when they are never anxious?

T: I sincerely doubt it.

Summary

Stress and anxiety are significant factors in a large proportion of individuals treated by psychotherapists. Proper assessment of stress and generalized anxiety is a necessary precursor to effective behavioral treatment and requires investigation of organic factors, the advisability of adjunctive pharmacological intervention, an examination of the client's broader life situation, and identification of targets for exposure-based methods. The two groups of behavioral methods most widely employed in the treatment of generalized anxiety are arousal reduction methods (e.g., progressive relaxation) and various cognitive interventions. Critical to effective behavioral treatment is the artful use of behavioral techniques and an effective cooperative liaison between therapist and client.

References

American Psychiatric Association. (1980). *Diagnostic and statistical manual of mental disorders* (3rd ed.). Washington, DC: Author.

Barber, T. X. (1984). Hypnosis, deep relaxation, and active relaxation: Data, theory, and clinical applications. In R. L. Woolfolk & P. M. Lehrer (Eds.), *Principles and practice of stress management* (pp. 142–187). New York: Guilford Press.

Beck, A. T. (1976). *Cognitive therapy and the emotional disorders*. New York: International Universities Press.

Beck, A. T. (1984). Cognitive approaches to stress. In R. L. Woolfolk & P. M. Lehrer (Eds.), *Principles and practice of stress management* (pp. 255–305). New York: Guilford Press.

Beck, A. T., & Emery, G. (1979). *Cognitive therapy of anxiety and phobic disorders*. Philadelphia: Center for Cognitive Therapy.

Beck, A. T., Laude, R., & Bohnert, M. (1974). Ideational components of anxiety neurosis. *Archives of General Psychiatry, 31,* 319–325.

Bedrosian, R. C., & Beck, A. T. (1980). Principles of cognitive therapy. In M. J. Mahoney (Ed.), *Psychotherapy process* (pp. 127–152). New York: Plenum Press.

Benson, H. (1975). *The relaxation response.* New York: Morrow.

Bernstein, D. A., & Borkovec, T. D. (1973). *Progressive relaxation training.* Champaign, IL: Research Press.

Blackwell, B. (1973). The role of diazepam in medical practice. *Journal of the American Medical Association, 225,* 1637–1641.

Borkovec, T. D., & Sides, K. (1979). Critical procedural variables related to the physiological effects of progressive relaxation: A review. *Behaviour Research and Therapy, 17,* 119–126.

Brantigan, C., Brantigan, T. A., & Neil, J. (1979). The effect of beta blockade on stage fright. *Rocky Mountain Medical Journal, 7,* 227–232.

Carrington, P. (1977). *Freedom in meditation.* Anchor Press/Doubleday.

Carrington, P., Collings, G. H., Benson, H., Robinson, H., Wood, L. W., Lehrer, P. M., Woolfolk, R. L., & Cole, J. W. (1980). The use of meditation-relaxation techniques for the management of stress in a working population. *Journal of Occupational Medicine, 22,* 221–231.

Da Costa, J. M. (1871). On irritable heart: A clinical study of a functional cardiac disorder and its consequences. *American Journal of Medical Science, 61,* 17–52.

Ellis, A. (1962). *Reason and emotion in psychotherapy.* New York: Lyle Stuart.

Ellis, A. (1973). *Humanistic psychotherapy: The rational-emotive approach.* New York: McGraw-Hill.

Eysenck, H. J., & Rachman, S. (1965). *The causes and cures of neurosis.* San Diego: Robert R. Knapp.

Glueck, B. C., & Stroebel, C. F. (1975). Biofeedback and meditation in the treatment of psychiatric illness. *Comprehensive Psychiatry, 16,* 303–321.

Freud, S. (1936). *The problem of anxiety.* New York: Norton.

Greden, J. F. (1974). Anxiety or caffeinism: A diagnostic dilemma. *American Journal of Psychiatry, 131,* 1089–1092.

Greenblatt, D. J., & Shader, R. I. (1974). Drug therapy: Benzodiazapines. *New England Journal of Medicine, 291,* 1011–1015.

Heide, F. J., & Borkovec, T. D. (1983). Relaxation-induced anxiety: Paradoxical anxiety enhancement due to relaxation training. *Journal of Consulting and Clinical Psychology, 51,* 171–182.

Holmes, D. S. (1984). Meditation and somatic arousal reduction. *American Psychologist, 39,* 1–10.

Jacob, R. G. (1983, December). *Oto-vestibular dysfunction in panic disorder or agoraphobia with panic attack.* Paper presented at the annual meeting of the Association for the Advancement of Behavior Therapy, Washington, DC.

Jacobson, E. (1938). *Progressive relaxation.* Chicago: University of Chicago Press.

Jacobson, E. (1970). *Modern treatment of tense patients.* Springfield, IL: Charles C Thomas.

Kendall, P. C., & Hollon, S. D. (Eds.). (1979). *Cognitive-behavioral interventions: Theory, research, and procedures.* New York: Academic Press.

Kessel, L., & Hyman, H. T. (1923). Studies of Grave's syndrome and the involuntary nervous system. II: The clinical manifestations of disturbances of the involuntary nervous system (autonomic imbalance). *American Journal of Medical Sciences, 165,* 513–530.

Lader, M. (1984). Pharmacological methods. In R. L. Woolfolk & P. M. Lehrer (Eds.), *Principles and practice of stress management* (pp. 306–333). New York: Guilford Press.

Lader, M., & Marx, I. (1971). *Clinical anxiety.* London: Heinemann.

Lang, P. J. (1968). Fear reduction and fear behavior: Problems in treating a construct. In J. M. Schlien (Ed.), *Research in psychotherapy* (Vol 3). Washington, DC: American Psychological Association.

Lavallee, Y. J., Lamontangne, G., Pinard, G., Annable, L., & Tetreault, L. (1977). Effects of EMG biofeedback, diazepam and their combination on chronic anxiety. *Journal of Psychosomatic Research, 21,* 65–71.

Lazarus, R. S. (1982), Thoughts on the relations between emotion and cognition. *American Psychologist, 37,* 1019–1024.

Lehrer, P. M. (1982). How to relax and how not to relax: A re-evaluation of the work of Edmund Jacobson. *Behaviour Research and Therapy, 20,* 417–428.

Lehrer, P. M., & Woolfolk, R. L. (1982). Cognitive, behavioral, and physiological dimensions of anxiety. *Behavioral Assessment, 4,* 167–177.

Lehrer, P. M., & Woolfolk, R. L. (1984). Are stress reduction techniques interchangeable or do they have specific effects?: A review of the comparative empirical literature. In R. L. Woolfolk & P. M. Lehrer (Eds.), *Principles and practice of stress management.* New York: Guilford Press.

Lehrer, P. M., Woolfolk, R. L., Rooney, A. J., McCann, B. S., & Carrington, P. (1983). Progressive relaxation and meditation: A study of psychophysiological and therapeutic differences between the two techniques. *Behaviour Research and Therapy, 21,* 651–662.

Lewis, T. (1919). *The soldier's heart and the effort syndrome.* London: Shaw.

Lowry, T. P. (1967). *Hyperventilation and hysteria.* Springfield, IL: Charles C Thomas.

Meichenbaum, D. (1977). *Cognitive-behavior modification: An integrative approach.* New York: Plenum Press.

Meichenbaum, D., & Jaremko, M. E. (Eds.). (1983). *Stress reduction and prevention.* New York: Plenum Press.

Meyer, V., & Crisp, A. H. (1970). Phobias. In C. G. Costello (Ed.), *Symptoms of psychopathology: A handbook* (pp. 263–301). New York: Wiley.

Mullaney, J. A., & Trippett, C. J. (1979). Alcohol dependency and phobias: Clinical description and relevance. *British Journal of Psychiatry, 135,* 565–573.

Novaco, R. W. (1975). *Anger control: The development and evaluation of an experimental treatment.* Lexington, MA: D. C. Heath.

Oppenheimer, B. S., Levine, S. A., Morison, R. A., Rothchild, M. A., St. Lawrence, W., & Wilson, F. N. (1918). Report on neurocirculatory asthenia and its management. *Military Surgeon, 42,* 409–426.

Patel, C. (1984). Yogic therapy. In R. L. Woolfolk & P. M. Lehrer (Eds.), *Principles and practice of stress management.* New York: Guilford Press.

Paul, G. L. (1966). *Insight vs. desensitization in psychotherapy.* Stanford, CA: Stanford University Press.

Pitts, F. N. (1971). Biochemical factors in anxiety neurosis. *Behavior Science, 16,* 82–91.

Raskin, M., Johnson, G., & Rondestvedt, J. W. (1973). Chronic anxiety treated by feedback-induced muscle relaxation. *Archives of General Psychiatry, 28,* 263–267.

Salkind, M. R. (1973). *The construction and validation of a self-rating anxiety inventory.* Unpublished doctoral dissertation, University of London.

Savill, T. (1907). *Clinical lectures on neurasthenia.* New York: William Wood.

Schnur, S. (1939). Cardiac neurosis associated with organic heart disease. *American Heart Journal, 18,* 153–165.

Sheehan, D. V. (1983). *The anxiety disease.* New York: Charles Scribner's.

Shepherd, M., Cooper, B., Brown, A. C., & Kalton, G. W. (1966). *Psychiatric illness in general practice.* London: Oxford University Press.

Skegg, D. C. G., Doll, R., & Perry, J. (1979). Use of medicine in general practice. *British Medical Journal, 607b,* 1561–1563.

Snow, W. G. (1978). The physiological and subjective effects of several brief relaxation training procedures (Doctoral dissertation, York University, Canada, 1978). *Dissertation Abstracts International, 40,* 3458B.

Szmuilowicz, J., & Flannery, J. G. (1980). Mitral valve prolapse syndrome and psychological disturbance. *Psychosomatics, 21,* 419–421.

Taylor, L., & Chave, S. (1964). *Mental health and the environment.* London: Longman.

Turner, P. E. (1978). A psychophysiological assessment of selected relaxation strategies (Doctoral dissertation, University of Mississippi, 1978). *Dissertation Abstracts International, 39,* 3010B.

Wolpe, J., & Lazarus, A. A. (1966). *Behavior therapy techniques.* New York: Pergamon.

Wood, P. (1941). Da Costa's syndrome (or effort syndrome). *British Medical Journal, 1,* 767–772.

Woodward, R., & Jones, R. B. (1980). Cognitive restructuring treatment: A controlled trial with anxious patients. *Behaviour Research and Therapy, 18,* 401–407.

Wooley, C. F. (1976). Where are the diseases of yesteryear? Da Costa's syndrome, soldier's heart, the effort syndrome, neurocirculatory asthenia, and the mitral valve prolapse syndrome. *Circulation, 53,* 749–751.

Woolfolk, R. L., & Lazarus, A. A. (1979). Between laboratory and clinic: Paving the two-way street. *Cognitive Therapy and Research, 3,* 239–244.

Woolfolk, R. L., & Richardson, F. C. (1978). *Stress, sanity and survival.* New York: Simon & Schuster.

Woolfolk, R. L., Carr-Kaffashan, L., McNulty, T., & Lehrer, P. M. (1976). Meditation training as a treatment for insomnia. *Behavior Therapy, 7,* 359–365.

Woolfolk, R. L., Lehrer, P. M., McCann, B. S., & Rooney, A. J. (1982). Effects of progressive relaxation and meditation on cognitive and somatic manifestations of daily stress. *Behaviour Research and Therapy, 20,* 461–468.

Social Anxiety

Susan R. Walen

Social anxiety has as its common theme a discomfort, often acute and quite immobilizing, in interpersonal relationships and other social situations. Although the idiosyncratic statement of the fear can vary quite widely from patient to patient, the central core of social anxiety is that one will be judged poorly by others and eventually—in some form—be rejected. In addition, most patients who suffer from social anxiety add another layer to their troubles and become embarrassed (that is, socially anxious) about their anxiety. In fact, this second layer of anxiety may be worse than or even outlive the original focus of the initial anxiety. In what one might think of as extremely creative patients, a third layer may emerge: patients may examine their social track records and conclude that they are hopeless social failures doomed to a life of loneliness and social isolation, thereby creating the additional stress of depression. I have referred to these subsequent emotional problems elsewhere as *symptom stress* (Walen, DiGiuseppe, & Wessler, 1980) and often find them responsible for greater personal pain than the original issues.

Incidence of Social Anxiety

Social anxiety has been studied by Zimbardo and his associates under the label of *shyness* (e.g., Zimbardo, 1977). Based on large-scale studies of over 7,000 people, Zimbardo reports that 80% of responders say that they were shy at some time in their lives, and over 40% consider themselves currently shy. Projecting to the general population, Zimbardo estimates that 87 million Americans would describe themselves as shy (Zimbardo & Radl, 1979).

SUSAN R. WALEN • Baltimore Center for Cognitive Therapy, 6303 Greenspring Avenue, Baltimore, Maryland 21209.

Social anxiety can occur at all ages, across all socioeconomic groups, and in men as well as women, although dating anxiety in particular seems to occur somewhat more often in men, a finding that may well relate to sex-role expectations (Arkowitz, Hinton, Perl, & Himadi, 1978). For example, even with the increased liberation of women from rigid sexual scripts, there is some evidence that in the overwhelming majority of cases, it is still the man who makes the first major sexual advance, whereas the woman remains passive (Lipton & Nelson, 1980). Although ethological data collected in singles' bars suggests that women initiate heterosocial encounters by subtle, typically nonverbal signals (Morris, 1977), it is usually the man who asks for a date. In one large dating study conducted on two different college campuses, male–female pairs of students were given each others' names and phone numbers and individually told to arrange to contact the other to set up a practice date; in over 90% of the cases it was the male who made the telephone call (Arkowitz *et al.*, 1978).

As McEwan (1983) points out in discussing dating behaviors, there is a "naturally occurring shyness or mild anxiety associated with opposite sex interactions," (p. 100). For example, large-scale studies of college students at various campuses have indicated that about one-third of those sampled reported themselves to be "somewhat" or "very" anxious about dating, and about half of those surveyed expressed interest in participating in a program to increase dating comfort (Arkowitz *et al.*, 1978; Zimbardo, Pilkonis, & Norwood, 1975). At issue, then, is not *whether* one experiences social anxiety, but more relevantly, how much anxiety is experienced, how long the anxiety episode lasts, how frequently the anxiety recurs, how much dysfunctional avoidance behavior is precipitated by the anxiety, and perhaps most importantly, how the anxiety is evaluated by the individual experiencing it.

Assessment of Social Anxiety

Anxiety can be a somewhat tricky state to measure, in part because it can refer to events in any one or more of three domains: *somatic, behavioral,* and *cognitive.* Somatic symptoms of anxiety refer primarily to physiologic events of the autonomic nervous system and may be indexed as changes in galvanic skin response, blood pressure, heart rate, muscle tension, breathing, peripheral skin temperature, and so forth. Monitoring a patient's anxiety in this dimension can be problematic for a number of reasons, most obviously because many (if not most) practitioners do not have access to the apparatus required, nor do they have the technological sophistication to deal with complex electrophysiologic assessments. In addition, typically more than one arousal index is required because measures of different physiologic channels often correlate very poorly with each other. For readers wishing a more detailed overview of psychophysiologic measures of anxiety, I would recommend the writing of Nietzel and Bernstein (1981).

Behavioral measures of anxiety typically involve recording either motoric behaviors assumed to result from anxiety (e.g., trembling, speech dysfluencies, eye contact, etc.) or avoidance behaviors. Among the problems encountered in coding anxiety this way are the demand characteristics of the measurement procedures, the generalizability from the clinically sampled behavior to "real life" situations, and the core problem of "reactivity"—the changes that can be induced by the knowledge that one is being observed. A somewhat more subtle problem occurs when the anxiety is actually being controlled by the patient via successful avoidance behaviors. For example, the highly accomplished businessman who devotes his time to work or work-related social contacts may not acknowledge that he is anxious in heterosocial situations, in part, because he has avoided placing himself in such situations.

Similar problems arise in considering behavioral measures of social skills and skill deficits; measurement,, in itself, is an invasive procedure. Too, there is no current agreement on a definition of social skills (Bellack, 1983). Not only do we have little in the way of "normative" data, but social skills are known to be highly situation specific. Consider, for example, the issue of eye contact, or more accurately, direction of gaze. In a typical social conversation, gaze direction shifts on a moment-to-moment basis; the speaker most frequently looks away when speaking or gathering thoughts, whereas the listener watches the speaker. An individual may be judged as less skilled either because she or he avoids gaze when speaking or stares unblinkingly when speaking. A similar bidirectionality of dysfunction would be so for other behavioral indexes (e.g., voice volume, speech latency, etc.). The important point about the rating of social skills is that because norms are minimal, deviations may be subtle, and the ultimate arbiter of social acceptibility may be the personal distress of a specific *rater*.

The cognitive or self-report measure of anxiety is the third major assessment strategy, accomplished by formal psychological testing or less formal interventions. (This chapter will emphasize the latter; the reader interested in a more detailed review of formal self-report instruments may find the chapter by Arkowitz, 1981, quite helpful.) Self-report measures are certainly vulnerable to criticisms of bias due to social desirability and other demand characteristics, yet they provide us with perhaps the most direct and potentially relevant measures of the cognitive as well as the emotive aspects of anxiety.

The most obvious assessment strategy for obtaining self-report data is the clinical interview. Quite typically, the individual with social anxiety will be anxious about the first meeting with the therapist, thus providing an *in vivo* opportunity to sample the affect and cognitions of the distress while they are "fresh." For example, an early question I ask new patients is how they felt about coming in to see me. Were they aware of any particular feelings as they drove to the session or sat in the waiting room? Can they identify any particular thoughts they were having or any expectations they may have held? I might follow up by inquiring if the anxiety they felt is typical of them in new situations and if the cognitions they report are good examples of how they usually think in such instances. If social anxiety is identified as a problematic theme, the interviewer at some point in the session will do well to stop discussing it as a general issue and focus the interchange by asking for one or two recent examples when the client can recall feeling socially anxious. A detailed content analysis of the most recent illustrations, even if these examples are not the most traumatic episodes, may be preferable because the client can usually recall the thoughts and feelings with less difficulty and distortion than older episodes.

In eliciting the client's affective experiences, the therapist may question whether the affect is correctly labeled. Often clients will use loosely defined words (e.g., "I was so upset") to label their emotions, so that aversive affective states may be intertwined or indistinguishable. Is the problem one of anxiety, or would it more properly be labeled one of *depression* or *anger* or *guilt*—or some admixture of these? In helping clients discriminate affective states, I find that I often use their cognitions as roadmaps. I listen for self-downing (depression), self-damning (guilt), other-damning (anger), or danger-signaling (fear) themes in the client's report. I then use one of a number of reflection strategies to validate my hypothesis: for example, "It sounds like you were really experiencing both guilt and anxiety, Mary" or "The way you describe it, Tom, I think I'd be feeling very anxious! Were you?"

The discrimination between depression and anxiety may be particularly difficult; for example, the patient may complain that he just cannot bring himself or herself to get out of bed in the morning and go to work. Is this patient suffering the energy and fatigue of a moderately severe depression or is he or she, perhaps without awareness, avoiding some anticipated unpleasantness at the job site? Among the clues one can use in making this discrimination are (a) consistency of affect; (b) self-concept of the patient; and (c) response to therapeutic prodding. Anxiety is usually associated with a specific concern, and if that concern passes, the patient will experience a mood shift; depression, on the other hand, tends to be more pansituational and involves a general sense of hopelessness and diminution in performance (Young & Epstein, 1982). Similarly, in anxiety the patient's negative self-concept tends to be limited to the problem area, whereas it tends to be more globally negative in depression. With therapeutic prodding to push oneself to do what one is not doing, the affect may become clearer to the patient; by agreeing to go to work as "an experiment," the avoidant client may discover it was not as difficult as she or he predicted and thus feel relieved, or he or she may be flooded by fearsome images and thus experience an exacerbation of the anxiety. Frequently, behavioral challenges tend to alleviate the distress in depression, whereas behavioral challenges may temporarily increase the distress in anxiety.

Another strategy to help clients more accurately assess the nature of their emotional reactions is to change the task from an essay inquiry into a multiple-choice inquiry. For the client who is not socialized to the world of his or her feelings, a question such as "What were you feeling?" or "What was your emotional reaction?" may fail to elicit meaningful material. With a client who is not very "psychologically minded" and who needs an "affective education," I will ask the question in a more concrete way. For example:

> You know, Joel, people come into my office and tell me about the various problems that they might be having with their work, or their marriage, or their school, and so forth. And when I listen to them, I'm sifting through those external problems to see what their *emotional* reactions are. Generally, I find that

people react to life stresses with one of four troublesome emotions: anger, depression, guilt, or anxiety. Of these four, which one (or ones) do you think *you* were experiencing during this incident you were just telling me about?

When I write this list of four affects on my chalkboard, I find that such patients frequently glance at the list as prompts in our discussion, thus aiding their learning and our communication.

In addition to identifying the affect, the client can also provide self-report data on its itensity. A general strategy for measuring the intensity of fear is to use pencil-and-paper devices such as the Social Avoidance and Distress Scale (Watson & Friend, 1969). Arkowitz (1981) reviews a number of such instruments. Clinically, however, I rely on the frequent use of a SUDs scale (Wolpe & Lazarus, 1966), an acronym for Subjective Units of Disturbance Scale. The client is instructed to imagine an emotional thermometer with a scale that runs from 0 (no anxiety at all) to 100, which represents a time in their lives when they were at their most anxious, perhaps near panic. After a moment or two, while the client is allowed to ponder this subjective range, she or he is asked for a number between 0 and 100 that describes how much anxiety was being experienced during the moment under discussion. Clients seem to readily adapt to this scaling procedure and quickly socialize to this communication strategy, so that later, when I ask "How anxious were you?" they respond with numbers. The SUDs scale is also particularly useful for ongoing *in vivo* assessment of the anxiety level. I might ask a client for such an instant "readout" a number of times during the course of a clinical encounter; any major shifts upward or downward can help to focus the discussion on a proximal cause for the shift, such as the introduction of a particular topic, a rush of imagery, or an awareness of a troubling thought.

In addition to assessing affect, the therapist may need to help the client learn to collect cognitions. Many clients, particularly those new to cognitive-behavioral therapies, seem nonplussed when asked to record what they were thinking at the time of anxiety. In part, their confusion may come from simply not understanding what a cognition is. A simple strategy that I use to get such a client started is to engage them in a dialogue in which they describe a recent example and, as the story unfolds, I take notes that primarily consist of a listing of their cognitions (as opposed to descriptions of the realities of the external situation or their affective reactions). Then I simply hand the notes to the client and point out that "these are some of the thoughts that seemed to be running through your head at the time." Such modeling may be sufficient, but often I will have clients practice collecting their cognitions in session by asking *them* to take the notes and cuing them when, in the course of a dialogue, they are verbalizing cognitions. It might sound something like this:

T: OK, Lillian, now before we really get into a discussion of that office party last night, let me give *you* the note pad so you can get some practice collecting the thoughts, ok?
C: OK.
T: Now . . . tell me about the party. How was it for you when you walked in?
C: It was really bad. I just knew I wasn't going to be able to think of anything to say to anyone.

T: All right! Now there's a heavy-duty thought. Let's catch that one on paper.

C: [*Writes, and then looks up*] It's true. I can talk about profit-and-loss statements and things in the business that I know about, but that's not what people talk about at parties.

T: Good [*Points to the paper*]. Sounds like you're aware of two more thoughts you held: that you can only talk about business matters that you know about and that others do not discuss business at parties. Can you tell me what else you were thinking as you walked into the party?

In addition to the automatic thoughts that a client may have in approaching a social situation, the therapist will want to tap into broader, more philosophical assumptions of the client. To illustrate, the client may believe that without love, life is not meaningful. If the therapist and client collude in a scramble to get the client out into dating and love relationships as a route to happiness—without examining the philosophy embedded in that very move—the core problems may be exacerbated. Potentially troublesome cognitive philosophies are embedded in our culture's songs, stories, and films: for example,

1. People who need people are the luckiest....
2. Love is a many splendored thing.
3. Love means never having to say you're sorry.
4. Love makes the world go 'round.
5. You know when it's the real thing.
6. What the world needs now is love....

In fact, because many of these unexamined assumptions are pervasive in our society, the therapist may want to consider his or her own value system as well.

During the interview assessment, the client can also be asked to report on specific external cues that precede the anxiety as well as on specific external consequences that follow the experience of anxiety. Obtaining a historical perspective on the problem will also be important; when was the client first aware of feeling such anxiety, and was its appearance related to any developmental landmarks in the client's life? Are there any conditions under which the anxiety seems to worsen? Are there any strategies that the client has observed previously that seem to temporarily alleviate the anxiety?

A very important assessment strategy, which can also have therapeutic ramifications, is to ask the client to generate and then bring in new examples of the clinical problem that she or he will self-monitor between therapy visits. Instructions to the client might be:

> All right, John, during this week let's hope that you can have at least one good anxiety attack in a social situation so that you can use it to collect information for us about your SUDs level and what you hear going on in your head at the time. In fact, if you could have at least *two* anxiety episodes, that would be even better!

The paradoxical nature of such an assessment request serves a number of functions, the most helpful of which may be to take the "sting" out of the anxiety or to reduce the symptom stress.

Finally, an assessment would do well to include a clear statement of the goals of treatment. Is a successful outcome a marriage, a Saturday night date, or the ability not to worry about either? One could measure many aspects of the client's functioning, and any number of outcomes could be satisfactory, so that the decision of the criteria for "success" will need to be clarified and negotiated with the individual client. Just as the ability to be assertive does not mandate that one must always or even often be so, the ability to be socially comfortable need not presume that one must frequently socialize. The "bottom line" may be attaining a level of social ease that allows one the choice.

Theoretical Models of Social Anxiety

Four major models of social anxiety have been described in the literature. These models, however, should not be assumed to be orthogonal or unrelated to each other. The four etiologic models are outlined in Table 1.

In the SOCIAL SKILLS DEFICIT MODEL, the assumption is made that the anxiety is a natural outgrowth of deficits/excesses in the individual's behavioral repertoire. These skill problems are assumed to result in negative outcomes both in terms of self-evaluations and evaluations by others, with consequent rejections and failures leading to further avoidance patterns. A number of studies have empirically tested the assumption that dating skills are more poorly developed in dating-anxious than in nonanxious individuals. However, no clear pattern of social skill deficits has been found (Arkowitz, Lichtenstein, McGovern, & Hines, 1975; Borkovec, Stone, O'Brien, & Kaloupek, 1974; Glaskow & Arkowitz, 1975).

In the CONDITIONED ANXIETY MODEL, the internal stress is assumed to be acquired in the manner of a classically conditioned phobia. Presumably, either direct or vicarious classical conditioning experiences have paired social situation cues with the experience of anxiety.

Whether the anxiety is established via classical conditioning or not, there is clear evidence that dating-competent versus dating-avoidant individuals are discriminable on the amount of anxiety they report (Arkowitz *et al.*, 1978).

In COGNITIVE MODELS the anxiety is assumed to arise from dysfunctional cognitions. Included in such cognitive styles would be (a) excessively high performance

Table 1. Models of Social Anxiety

Designation	Etiology	Anxiety appropriate	Treatment
Skill deficit model	Problems in social skills	Yes	Social skills training
Conditioned anxiety model	Classically conditioned anxiety	No	Anxiety reduction techniques
Cognitive model	Dysfunctional thinking	No	Cognitive restructuring
Physical attractiveness model	Physical unattractiveness	Yes	Training to improve appearance and attractiveness

standards; (b) negative self-statements; and (c) selective attention to and memory for negative input about one's performance. For example, Clark and Arkowitz (1975) demonstrated that low-frequency daters are characterized by overly negative self-evaluations. Thus, the individual may erroneously perceive a social situation as a potential failure experience and may exaggerate the importance of the anticipated failure, thereby approaching it with undue trepidation. Together, distortions of perception and exaggerated evaluations lead to anxiety that, in turn, may lead to avoidance behaviors that effectively prevent the individual from correcting the distortions.

Finally, a PHYSICAL ATTRACTIVENESS MODEL suggests that there is a strong relationship between one's physical attractiveness and (a) how others see us; and (b) how they react to us. More positive characteristics are attributed to more attractive people, and others are more likely to behave positively toward them as well (Berscheid & Walster, 1973). Glaskow and Arkowitz (1975) found that dating-anxious subjects were rated as significantly less physically attractive than nonanxious subjects, thus lending support to the reality issues in this model and suggesting the possibility of relevant therapeutic interventions to increase attractiveness.

Each of the theoretical models may have something to suggest to the clinician who is designing an antianxiety program for a specific client. In collaboration with the patient, the therapist may want to include treatment strategies that will focus on (a) coping with the anxiety itself; (b) challenging dysfunctional cognitions; (c) polishing certain social skills; and (d) improving one's attractiveness. However, my clinical experience suggests that before one begins working on a social program, certain preliminary steps may need to be taken. Typically, the patient has a fairly long history of social isolation and carries a view of himself or herself as a wallflower, and this poor self-image leads to an often chronic overlay of dysphoria. Intuitive logic would suggest that these individuals would be in a better position to present themselves socially and to offer their hands in friendship when they have achieved more *self-acceptance* and have learned to create some happiness for themselves while engaged in solitary pursuits. If the individual's dysphoria is too quickly lifted by the sudden appearance of a new friend or lover—often one just as desperately hungry for social nurturance as the patient—the "cure" may be a fragile one, hinging dangerously on the availability and desire of the other. The patient may thereby not only lose the control but also the opportunity to learn some valuable lessons in the fine art of self-acceptance.

Learning to Like Yourself

A core premise in this stage of therapy is that once the individuals have overcome their superordinate mood problems and have, in essence, learned to find happiness within themselves, they will be in better shape to go off and find others with whom to share it. They will look for a relationship not because they *have* to but because they *want* to.

Much of the client's dysphoric mood may result from the belief that most activities are not really enjoyable unless they are done with someone else, and because the someone else is not present, there is little point in planning enjoyable activities. This kind of self-fulfilling prophecy may have resulted in such a restricted set of recreational activities that it may be difficult for the individual to discriminate between dysphoria and simple boredom. It is not hard to find examples of people who make elaborate and frequent plans to do enjoyable activities as long as they have a lover or mate with whom to do them; they plan outings, have dinner parties, buy tickets to shows, and so forth. When alone, however, those same individuals stop planning and eke out a meager recreational existence.

A strategy to help such an individual challenge the dysfunctional belief and counteract the resulting inertia could be framed as a set of experiments to be done. For example, the patient and therapist in discussion could construct a list of activities that the patient has found to be even somewhat enjoyable/relaxing in the present or past. Commonplace activities should not be overlooked. A sample Pleasant/ Relaxing Activities list might look like this one: (a) reading Sunday comics; (b) weeding garden; (c) playing squash; (d) taking bubble bath; (e) having glass of wine; (f) watching football game; (g) reading in the library; and (h) fishing.

Each activity can then be coded as to whether it can be enjoyed alone (A), whether it requires money ($), and whether it takes much time (T). The frequency with which the client has engaged in that activity within the past week (or month) can also be noted. Frequently, clients are surprised at how many of the activities that they had found to be reinforcing do not involve the presence of others, nor do they require significant outlays of time or money. They may also increase their awareness of the "starvation diet" they have put themselves on and may be more willing to program these activities back into their lives.

Similarly, the pleasure-predicting method (Burns, 1980) may be a useful experiment. Table 2, adapted from Burns's book *Feeling Good,* illustrates how the technique could be used by a client. Before engaging in a particular activity at work or play, the client logs it in using the first columns, noting whether it involves themselves or others and then making a prediction (between 0 and 100%) about the amount of satisfaction they anticipate the activity will bring. At the conclusion of the activity, the actual amount of satisfaction is recorded. Each entry is thus an experiment, and the client is encouraged to do perhaps 40 to 50 such experiments over a 2- to 3-week period. Again, the data from such charts typically come as a surprise to many patients and often serve not only to correct the belief that pleasure is only possible with others but may also help the client develop a schedule of activities that can provide an optimal amount of pleasure.

Table 2. Pleasure Predicting Sheet

Activity	Companion	Satisfaction	
Schedule Activities with Potential for Pleasure or Personal Growth	(If Alone, Specify Self)	Predicted (0–100) (Record This *Before* Each Activity)	Actual (0–100 (Record This *After* Each Activity)
Making dinner	Self	20%	60%
Going to movie	Jim	80%	75%

Note. From *Intimate Connections* (p. 284) By D. Burns, 1984, New York: Morrow. Copyright 1984 by David D. Burns. Reprinted by permission.

Some clients, on the other hand, engage in a seemingly frenzied amount of activity, either social or work related, often without much enjoyment; when questioned, they may not be aware of their fear of quiet times at home alone. The fear of loneliness, in fact, also keeps many such people in quite dysfunctional relationships. A useful strategy, therefore, may be to review (cognitively and behaviorally) with the client the important difference between "alone" and "lonely." Upon reflection, most people can quickly identify important times of aloneness that may have been qualitatively very positive and restorative. Similarly, loneliness can be experienced even when one is in a crowd of people. Loneliness seems to be a phenomenological experience composed of a perception of one's isolation coupled with a deep conviction of one's unworthiness, which arises from an intense focus on the discrepancy between evaluations of the social relationships one has and those that one believes she or he "should" have (Perlman & Peplau, 1981). Among the cognitive distortions that follow from such thinking are (a) negative distortions of the relationships one does have; (b) negative views of past and future relationships; (c) negative views of oneself; and (d) negative beliefs in one's ability to tolerate discomfort.

Strategically, it may be therapeutic to have the client plan to remain alone for specific (and perhaps gradually increasing) intervals of time, which may provide some desensitization experiences. During these practice "alone" times, the client can be on the watch for the dysfunctional cognitions mentioned previously and work to combat them. For example, the client might draw up a list of the advantages of being alone. Or, the client might challenge the notion that she or he is, in some absolutistic sense, truly alone. Milgram (1967) reported that the average American has anywhere from 500 to 2500 acquaintances and associations; clients have probably discounted their relatives, acquaintances, colleagues, neighbors, and others who know them. Keeping a running tally of the different people with whom one comes in contact during a 30-day period and reviewing that list at times of loneliness may help challenge the perception of isolation.

A program of learning to like oneself may be conducted as a group enrichment experience such as that described by Primakoff (1983). She describes a 10-session model that includes meetings devoted to love/sex/approval "needs," daily domestic living, being at home with oneself, going out with oneself, developing a physical and sensual relationship with oneself, and discussions of the unique advantages and opportunities of the single life-style. To motivate themselves, clients are asked to consider the following questions: "If I'm bored and unhappy with myself, what do I have to offer to anyone else? How can I make a genuine commitment to someone else if I have not made one to myself?"

Dealing with the Anxiety

For many clients, the experience of anxiety is particularly distressing because of their sense of helplessness in dealing with it. Providing the client with some coping strategies that can be immediately rehearsed and practiced as skills may counteract this source of distress.

Dietary strategies may be an important first step in helping to curtail the sensations of anxiety, particularly because some patients may be misconstruing physiological arousal as anxiety and thereby setting up a vicious cycle of worry. Clients can be cautioned to limit the amount of caffeine they ingest daily in coffee, tea, and cola drinks; to limit their intake of alcohol, particularly in stressful situations; and to monitor their eating patterns so that they avoid the anxietylike symptoms of hypoglycemia. One client, a slender young woman who was very concerned about maintaining her weight, would fast at least all day before going out on a dinner date; the tremulous sensations she experienced, which faded after the first round of cocktails, convinced her that not only was she socially incompetent but that she was in danger of becoming an alcoholic. She experimented with less drastic eating patterns and also discovered that a glass of warm milk before a date increased her comfort level.

Distraction strategies may provide a temporary source of relief. For example, the client may be encouraged to focus attention on very specific details of the physical environment (e.g., by pretending that she or he is a reporter from a home fashion magazine doing an article on the room) or to attend to a distracting cognitive task (e.g., doing mental arithmetic or subvocal poetry recitation). One young man developed music as a distractor; whenever feasible, he would very quietly hum or sing a song he was trying to learn. He felt that this strategy not only diverted his attention from ruminative self-doubts but projected an image of confidence to others.

Relaxation strategies may also be useful as a distractor as well as a physiological tension-reduction strategy. Techniques such as use of Benson's Relaxation Response (Benson, 1975), Jacobson's Relaxation Procedures (Jacobson, 1938), or Sensory Awareness Training (Goldfried & Davison, 1976) may be introduced to the patient as skills that if well practiced, may provide a portable relief mechanism when in an anxiety-arousing situation. More elaborately, the relaxation component may be combined with presentation of a graduated series of stressful images in a program of *systematic desensitization* (Wolpe, 1969). Patient and therapist work together to develop a series of images of social-evaluative situations graded in a hierarchy from least to most stressful and, while the patient tries to practice maintaining a relaxed sense of calm, the therapist presents the lowest item repeatedly until the client reports little anxiety as it is imaged. Successive rungs of the hierarchy are similarly rehearsed. Such a sequence may serve many purposes: rehearsal of nonexaggerated social scenarios, repetition of imagery, reduction of psychophysiologic hyperarousal, practice in distraction, and acquisition of a sense of coping skills.

Acceptance of the anxiety—even actively courting it—may produce the most profound changes. As a first step in acceptance, the patient may need to understand more about anxiety: where it comes from, how it is expressed, its course, and its immediate prognosis. Among the "myths" of anxiety that the therapist may need to correct are the following:

1. Anxiety is dangerous: I could have a heart attack.
2. I could lose control or blow up in some way.

3. I must be going crazy.
4. The attack will never pass.
5. Other people do not experience it like I do.
6. It is a sign of weakness.

A number of educative sources may be called upon to dispute these erroneous notions, including the therapist's experience, the experience of others, the client's own experience, and information available in books (e.g., Weeks, 1978). A gathering of such information will reveal that anxiety is not dangerous but in fact is a natural biological reaction to prepare the body for action and to maximize oxygen intake and delivery. The anxiety has a "life cycle," and after reaching its peak, it will begin to subside; it has a cyclical nature and may facilitate certain performances. It is experienced in varying degrees by virtually everyone and does not reflect "characteriological flaws" nor lead to mental illness (Walen, 1984). Corrective information may be pooled into a self-instruction script that the client may want to consult and rehearse before confronting stressors. Here, for example, is one client's script:

> OK. Here comes my old friend, anxiety. It's now a ———— [numerical rating], and I know it will drop soon. It won't hurt me. It will pass. It's normal. I can still function despite it.

Be on the lookout for *emotional reasoning* in the client (Burns, 1980, p. 40); this cognitive distortion is common in anxiety and consists of using the affect to validate a "danger" cognition. In essence, the client is saying: "I'm feeling so anxious, therefore something terrible will happen." Illogically, the client has put the cart before the horse and more correctly is feeling anxious *because* she or he has defined the situation as dangerous. Clients can learn to recognize and challenge this belief as well as its corollary: "I've got to get out of here!"

Ultimately, the client will need to stop running from the anxiety and learn to run toward it. *In vivo desensitization,* in which the client repeatedly confronts the stressor, experiences the anxiety, and practices living through it has proven to be an effective technique. Clients readily see the logic in this step, by analogy, as in the following dialogue:

T: John, if your little brother were afraid to ride his bike, and you wanted to help him get over his fear, you know that reassurances probably aren't going to do the trick, right?
C: Right.
T: Eventually, what does he *have* to do . . . in order to stop being afraid of riding the bike?
C: Well, he has to get on it and ride it.
T: Right. And doesn't the same thing apply if you want to get a small child over their fear of the water? When you take them to the beach. What's the procedure?
C: I guess they have to get their feet wet. Just talking about it on the sand won't do the trick. You take them in little by little.
T: Right. So, to get over a fear, you just have to do it. If we want to get you over your fear of meeting new women and asking for a date . . .?
C: [*Smiling*] Guess I'd better take the plunge too, huh?

Thus, rather than taking the pulse of the anxiety as a signal to run, clients may cognitively restructure the experience of it and view it as a signal that they are *successfully* confronting the stressor and thereby working at the problem. In addition, the stress reaction may be looked at as a valuable learning experience for it provides an opportunity for retrieval of the anxiety-arousing, dysfunctional cognitions at a time when they are most accessible.

Dealing with Dysfunctional Cognitions

The socially anxious individual typically terrorizes himself or herself with a number of kinds of dysfunctional cognitions; among the most paralyzing are those that are *critical of the self*. The patient may be scanning himself or herself, making derogatory comments on any personal aspect, ranging from physical appearance to personality or intellectual functioning. Sometimes these thoughts emerge as projections; the patient believes that others see him or her in these negative ways. For example, a 35-year-old woman who was separated from her husband had begun a program of taking new social risks, one of which was to go out to eat by herself. At the entrance to the restaurant she had chosen, she asked to see the menu, and, while peeking over the edge of it to scan the crowd of diners, she became aware of a flood of thoughts:

> I couldn't possibly sit down and eat by myself! They'll all be wondering what's the matter with me. How come she has to eat alone? She probably doesn't have any friends. No wonder she doesn't have a date; she's so chubby. The poor thing!

Occasionally, the anxious individual will take this negative focus and turn it outward, reporting bitterly *critical views of others*. Often, the patients who are the most lonely and isolated, who express the hungriest need for others, are also the most embittered. They speak with great disdain and disparagement of others as individuals and collectively as groups. Although such negative attitudes may serve a defensive purpose, they are obviously incompatible with the client's stated goals of affiliation. Nonetheless, such clients may "prophylactically" reject others by setting unreasonably high expectations of them, by devaluing them, and by making snap negative judgments of them. For example, in a recent singles' discussion group, three young men, each of whom spent much of his recreational time in bars, discovered that they operated under similar principles. They would enter the bar feeling very anxious, would order a drink, typically would not engage in conversation with anyone, and would negatively judge their surroundings. One spent his time mentally criticizing the looks of the women; one eavesdropped and concluded that people in bars were capable of only the most superficial of conversations; and all believed that they could never establish a relationship with a woman that they picked up in a bar!

A third class of dysfunctional cognitions that appear prominently are *negative predictions*, which unfortunately may become self-fulfilling prophecies. When clients learn to monitor their thoughts, they become aware that they usually enter a social situation after giving themselves the equivalent of a "locker room pep talk" in reverse. One client recorded the following train of thinking as he prepared to go to his first formal cocktail party:

> I should probably stay home. I won't be able to think of anything to say to anybody. I won't even know anybody to say hello to. I can just see me now, walking around with a drink in my hand, trying to find someplace to stand. Everybody will be in little groups. I just have this feeling that if I go up to a group, they'll close their ranks or turn and look at me like I'm some sorta nut. God, I'll probably have to spend the whole evening alone in that crowd.

Another way clients can defeat themselves socially is by holding *unrealistic expectations*. For example, they may expect that others do not feel any anxiety and that they should be placid themselves. They may expect that others easily and often have social successes and that if they themselves take a social risk it should rapidly, effectively and painlessly "pay off." They may, in other words, display very low tolerances for frustration (Ellis & Becker, 1982, p. 109).

Among the general strategies useful for challenging these dysfunctional cognitive sets is the skill of *shifting focus*. Rather than continuing to ruminate about themselves, clients can be encouraged to experiment with attending to others in the situation. One client used this strategy to advantage in a feared task—that of interviewing people on the street about her company's product. She reported that it was helpful in her task if she vigorously and frequently reminded herself to keep her focus off herself and onto the interviewees; her "watchword" was *focus out!* In addition, clients can use the opportunity to carefully attend to the behavior, speech patterns, clothing, and conduct of the others for purposes of modeling or countermodeling.

A second general strategy might be called *reality checks*. For example, rather than trying to read minds, the client can be actively encouraged to gather data. Are the others anxious also? Does the client appear to be anxious to others? What do the others think about people whose anxiety shows? Often the answers to these questions are surprising to the socially anxious individual who truly may not have realized that others are empathic, caring, kindly, or merely indifferent.

Finally, clients can be encouraged to *evaluate their evaluations*. The socially anxious individual not only assumes the worst about his or her behavior, display of affect, and impact on others but evaluates these negative impressions as highly significant and quite horrific. Instead, the client can be helped to develop an antiembarrassment attitude about expressing anxiety. Were there behaviors about which the client used to feel embarrassed but that have now been put into perspective? How was this perspective achieved? Could those same reevaluative strategies be applied to the current problem? With rethinking, each subsequent anxiety episode can be viewed as a chance to be open about it, to discuss it with others, and to thereby confront the embarrassment. More generally, the client can work on shame-attacking assignments (Ellis & Becker, 1982, p. 50).

It is useful to review the reasons why it is dysfunctional to place too much emphasis on how others evaluate us; for example, a list of advantages and disadvantages of living a life mainly to please others may be drawn up. Behaviorally, the client can practice doing specific things that she or he fears will not earn approval simply in order to practice managing without it.

Dealing with Social Skills

The determination of social skills problems is difficult, and often the patient may be inaccurately assessing himself or herself as deficient when an external observer might not agree. This point was vigorously brought home to me a number of years ago. I had been working with a young woman who repeatedly assured me that she was a social dud whose ineptitude would be patently obvious to anyone. Not long after, she and I met at a large fund-raising party, during which I had the opportunity to observe her social interactions from varying distances. She was consistently interacting with others, in large and small groups, smiling, chatting, and appearing more at ease than most. Thus, a useful strategy for validating whether a skills deficit is present is to devise methods of observation, the most economical of which may be to have the patient poll others in the environment for their honest and very specific feedback. The patient may ask, for example, "Did I look anxious? In what way? What specific things did I do [or not do] that gave you that impression? Prompts may help: "Was there anything awkward about my posture/voice/facial expression/conversation skills?"

When a social behavior problem is pinpointed, a next question may be to evaluate whether the problem really lies in the behavior *per se* or in the match between the behavior and the current environment. Consider the issue of self-disclosure and intimate verbal sharing, for which one former client had been repeatedly reprimanded or rebuffed in his social group. In our discussions, we placed conversations along a dimension running from "things" to "stuff." At the *thing* end of the spectrum are topics that one could discuss with any stranger—things such as the weather, cars, politics, soap powders, and so forth. At the other end of the continuum is the *stuff* of intimacy, topics that some people find very difficult to share—"stuff" like our aspirations, our fears, our sex lives, our self-doubts, and so forth. After much discussion, my client decided that he was just one of those people who prefers to talk about stuff and that his current friends simply did not match him on this dimension. Three subsequent decisions emerged from this conceptualization: (a) that there was nothing wrong with him for being a "stuff man"; (b) that he could be more tolerant of his friends' rejecting behavior by understanding it as their discomfort; and (c) that he wanted to search out new friends who also appreciated stuff talk.

If the patient and therapist agree that there are specific behaviors that could use some polishing, an important first step may be to ensure that the patient can separate the behavior from his or her sense of self. Awareness of how one is behaving and adjusting one's behavior is an important element in social skills and need have no relationship to (unnecessary and typically negative) global evaluations of oneself.

Much of the research literature on social anxiety has focused on social skills training, which is often conducted in small groups and involves using role playing, modeling, coaching, feedback, and homework assignments. Although such formal social skills training packages have been demonstrated to be effective (for example, see review by Curran, 1977), it is not clear whether changes are due more to the anxiety reduction that occurred because of the behavioral rehearsal or to the removal of presumed deficits in behavioral repertoires (Arkowitz *et al.*, 1978). In addition, the problems of expense of treatment and ensuring generalization from the office setting to the natural environment have been noted. For perhaps most outpatient work, a somewhat less elaborate yet programmatic approach to specific behavior change may be sufficient. Consider smiling behavior, for example; many socially anxious individuals do not frequently smile at others. One such patient that I saw would sit glumly in the waiting room, avoiding eye contact with anyone, and when I came to greet her, despite weeks of good rapport building, she would look up at me without any sign of recognition or change in affect. Together we discussed this style of hers and its probable impact on others around her, and she agreed to begin to work on a program of "smile practice" as an experiment in social relations. Because she stated that smiling at strangers would be very difficult for her, we followed a suggestion of Dave Burns (personal communication, 1983) and developed a plan in which she would first practice smiling at inanimate objects, next at animals and small children, later at older people, and finally at women and men in her age bracket. In addition, she deliberately practiced smiling into her mirror and noticing the pattern of muscle tension in her face when she found the most pleasant expressions. Similarly, a client who had been given feedback about his tendency to be "verbally negative" decided to work on this as a bad habit—one that he did almost unconsciously. Accordingly, we agreed that I and others in his social world were to become helpers in his change plan by signaling him when we became aware of negatives; the signal was *G & D*, shorthand for "gloom and doom!" Simply by focusing on specific behavior(s) a straightforward self-monitoring plan was found to be helpful in such cases.

Dealing with Physical Appearance

Not long ago in my city, there was a bar that had a "selectrocution" device; each person who entered the bar received pin-on initials coated in florescent paint. Throughout the evening, others in the bar would mark these initials down in a rank order on a computer card, and at the end of the evening the cards would be fed to the computers that printed out each patron's mean ranking for the night. The lowest ranked person was declared to be "selectrocuted!" Although these numerical ratings were quite uncomfortable for many, they did provide a dependent variable for an experiment by an undergraduate student of mine. On successive weeks this coed and her roommate went to the selectrocution dressed either in a somewhat slinky, low-cut dress or in a plain, high-necked wool dress; the dresses were switched in counterbalanced order, and the data were clear: no matter which coed wore the slinky dress, her rankings for the evening were always significantly higher. Clothes, in other words, do indeed make the (wo)man.

Another case in which appearance was a key factor was one that involved a young woman's trying to decide whether or not to stay in a relationship that she found unsatisfying but comfortable. One of her dilemmas was that other men, although they seemed to enjoy her company, were not rushing to fill her social calendar. After a number of sessions in which we dealt with various facets of her presenting issue, I finally found an opportunity to discuss grooming with her. She was a lovely and healthy-looking young woman, slim and extremely athletic, always clean and impeccably dressed—yet her appearance sent out confusing sexual signals at best. For instance, she wore "sensible" shoes, man-tailored suits complete with string ties, no makeup, and very short hair. Again, as an experiment, she decided to vary her wardrobe and grooming routines and see if others noticed, commented, or changed their behavior toward her. They did.

Many times clients are aware that they have avoided taking steps to improve their appearance; helping the client to uncover and examine the cognitions that have blocked them from doing so will be important. The following are some thoughts collected by one woman who had decided to make an appointment with a cosmetologist and then had backed out of the commitment:

> People will just think "there goes that ugly person *with* makeup." They'll laugh at me: "Why are you wearing makeup. . . . It's not going to help." If I don't try and don't succeed, it's not so much a *personal* blow. But if I really try— lose weight, wear makeup, buy new clothes—and then I don't succeed, then I have to conclude that it's some terrible fatal flaw that makes me undesirable. If I don't play the game, I'm safe. I could always convince myself that if I *did* play the game I'd win. If I play and then don't win, I am defenseless. I'd conclude that I *am* a flop.

A stream of negative assumptions and self-defeating illogic such as the preceding clearly would need attention before a self-improvement suggestion could be taken. It may take a bit of extra courage on the part of the counselor to bring up such items as cleanliness, personal hygiene, dress, skin and teeth care, and so forth. Failure to do so, however, may leave the client's repertoire of social skills untended and may reflect more about the therapist's level of social comfort than a wise therapeutic choice. Strategies to improve physical attractiveness have been increasingly acknowledged in the literature on social anxiety as valid and important elements of treatment (cf. Arkowitz, 1977).

The Importance of Practice

Research (e.g., Arkowitz *et al.*, 1978) and clinical experience suggest that typically the most important ingredient in producing change in social anxiety is real-life practice, provided, of course, that the patient views these social risks as just that—practice. For example, the goal of asking someone out for a date is to acquire experience in initiations, accepting refusals, and practice in dating; the goal had better not be to find one's ideal mate nor to impress the dating partner.

In socializing, as in fishing, the process is really more significant than the product, and each of these activities can easily be ruined by taking it too seriously. To continue the analogy: it is often necessary to cast a line many, many times before a fish is caught, and although one might catch a fish in any body of water, the chances are increased if the fisherman goes where the fish are known to be schooling. Analogies such as the preceding are an example of a strategy to help clients identify and challenge inflated ideas they may hold of the success rates they should be achieving in a social anxiety program. Clients frequently block or devalue their practice efforts by holding perfectionistic standards, so that the therapist will need to alternate frequently between the use of behavioral strategies and cognitive strategies to maximize psychotherapeutic benefits.

Julia's Case

Julia was an attractive 25-year-old medical secretary who entered therapy with Barbara Mandell, a supervisee of mine. Julia was experiencing a mild clinical depression and described problems in her current romantic relationship as well as relationships with family members and difficulties pursuing her career goals; she accurately labeled herself as having *little self-confidence*. Julia and her younger siblings had been raised by her mother after her parents' divorce. While she was still quite young, her mother remarried a man who was both verbally and physically abusive. Eventually that marriage ended, and by her late teens, Julia had been placed in charge of her younger sibs while her mother searched for another mate. The third partner that the mother married was from Europe, to which the couple returned, leaving Julia to finish the job of raising the remaining children. At the point that she entered therapy, she was living alone for the first time and was contemplating whether or not to move in with her boyfriend, Tony, with whom she had a conflicted yet very dependent relationship. Aside from Tony, her social contacts were very limited, primarily because her self-doubts and fear of rejection prevented her from reaching out to others.

A number of areas of her life were examined in the course of several months of therapy. As is often true of adults who survived years of life as an abused child, certain cognitive assumptions about oneself and about relationships to others needed to be reexamined. Both cognitively and behaviorally, Julia challenged the notion that she was totally responsible for others' bad moods and bad treatment of her and that if she were just more perfect in her behavior, everything would be fine. She examined the lessons she had learned from her mother as a model of a woman who did not feel capable of running her life successfully without a man; she learned to profit from her mother's mistakes without hating her mother for making them. She learned to recognize and to express her thoughts and feelings, first just to her therapist, and later to others that she decided to trust. She examined the notion that she needed the approval of others in order to feel good about herself. As she began to accept herself with her imperfections, she began to take more social risks. The following dialogue segment was transcribed from a session in which Julia was telling her therapist about a party she had attempted to attend the previous week and how she had finally wrestled successfully with her anxiety.

C: I was just thinking of last weekend. I went to a party, and it was a small party, with people I didn't really know, and the host was someone I wasn't particularly crazy about. But I wasn't feeling up to par, just like what we had talked about. About going to a party where you don't really look as good as you'd like to and still see how it would work out.

T: Um hum.

C: I didn't keep those thoughts in my head. I was there maybe 10 or 15 minutes and I just felt terrible. There were people there that I didn't know so I didn't try to talk to anyone. And I just left. I just couldn't handle it.

T: What couldn't you handle?

C: Uh, well, I couldn't handle the fact that I thought . . . well, like there were three girls there that are airline stewardesses, and I just looked . . . well, I didn't look as good as I could've. And I just felt about this tall [gestures].

T: Because you didn't look good?

C: Yeah, I felt like I didn't. And I just went on with all those negative thoughts. Ugly. Unattractive. And I didn't feel like I had anything to say.

T: Why was that?

C: Because I was feeling very uncomfortable. I didn't feel good about myself. You know . . . I wouldn't have been able to carry on a conversation.

T: Because you were too busy thinking about what you looked like?

C: Yeah.

T: Did you get any feedback from people around you?

C: Well, a couple of the girls kinda looked me up and down and I took it to heart. I didn't stay there long enough to get too much feedback. I left and just went walking around and went to a telephone booth and called up a girlfriend. I just wanted her to come and get me. And when I talked it out with her—got my feelings out—I decided I was being kind of foolish, and I started thinking about some of our therapy sessions. So I did the hardest thing. I knew it wouldn't be easy, but I went back.

T: Good for you!

C: [Chuckles] Well, see, my whole attitude changed after I talked to her and talked it out.

T: That's great, and you know, it shows that you took your therapy skills . . . took them outside of therapy and used them outside. And you used somebody else as a sounding board.

C: Yeah.

T: And if you were really desperate and you didn't have a sounding board, what could you do?

C: I could just . . . well, I could talk it out to myself . . .

T: Or you could . . . ?

C: Write it out . . .

T: That's right.

C: Um hum.

T: That's great! What did you tell yourself to change things?

C: Well, I thought about Tony; they were Tony's friends and I'd kind of ruin things for him if I left the party for good and didn't go back. Well, I told myself: I don't even know these people. I'm not going to go there and get all of them to *love* me. It doesn't matter.

T: It doesn't matter if they don't love you?

C: Yeah. I'm who I am . . . and that's OK.

T: OK!

C: That I'm doing well . . . you know . . . I'm getting back on the right track in steps that I've made.

T: You feel good about many of the things you've been doing?

C: Yeah. And I wasn't going to let anything that I thought they would think bother me.

T: If they don't like the way you look, or think you're an unattractive person, it's not going to bother you.

C: Right.

T: And you were able to convince yourself of that?

C: [*Nods*]

T: And what happened when you went back?

C: It was fine. And I felt good that I didn't have to try to get these people to like me. It was *my* choice. I mean, if I wanted to, fine, and if I didn't . . . so what? And I was more at ease too when I went back. I did talk to them.

T: Cause the pressure was off, right?

C: Right.

T: That's great.

C: Yeah. I've been thinking about it; it felt good.

Cautions and Problems

In the multifaceted assessment and treatment program outlined in this chapter, there are a number of potential trouble spots that should be avoided. Among these pitfalls are misdiagnoses, missed diagnoses, and misattributions on the part of the therapist.

Misdiagnoses

In making an assessment of social anxiety, the therapist will be examining three major elements: (a) the situation; (b) the client's perceptions and cognitions about the situation; and (c) the client's affective and behavioral reactions to the situation. Misdiagnoses could occur in any of these channels. For example, problems in social interaction could be assumed to lie within the client, whereas in fact, they may lie in the social environment or the mismatch between the client's behavior and the environment. Similarly, it may be assumed that the client has a deficit in social skills when, in fact, this assumption is merely a product of the client's unremittingly negative self-perceptions rather than an objective assessment. Finally, inaccurate or incomplete assessment of the affective problem may lead to derailed treatment. Strategies useful in combating anxiety may be only tangentially relevant to alleviation of depression, or guilt, or hostility.

Missed Diagnoses

At the risk of belaboring the obvious, I would remind the reader that assessment of any presenting problem entails a differential diagnosis. At the most basic level we try to assess whether the problem is one of "I can't" versus "I won't." Included in the former category, of course, would be biologic and/or psychopathologic conditions that would interfere with competent social conduct, such as psychotic processes, character disorders, substance abuse, and so forth. A complete clinical evaluation, including a formal mental status examination if it seems warranted, will help to prevent treatment failures due to missed evidence.

The second category ("I won't") would include a variety of cognitive, affective, or behavioral blocks to change. For example, the client may indeed have the social skills necessary for adequate functioning but may be stopped by incompatible values or belief systems, such as "It's not ladylike to do that" or "All good things come to those who stand and wait." A detailed cognitive assessment will help in uncovering such attitudes.

Similarly, the problem may be an imagery one. After extensively working up and rehearsing a more assertive communication with one female client, I then happened to ask if she could see herself actually saying those words to her spouse. "No," she replied, and she meant it literally. Subsequent experiences have convinced me that just as it seems to be important in athletic competition for the athlete to be able to visualize the completed performance, visual rehearsal seems to be important in verbal/interpersonal skills. Recognizing such a deficit and using imagery tactics of rehearsal may help this problem.

Misattributions

In this category, I place the therapist error of letting personal values, moralities, and *shoulds* interfere with assessment and treatment. A basic example would be in the area of aesthetic preference: the therapist's notions of what are attractive clothing styles or attractive interpersonal styles may reflect a narrow personal bias. More appropriately, the therapist's voice could be one of many that the client might poll for advice. It is as important as it is obvious to remember that the world has lots of room in it for all styles of people. Each of us can find a socioecological niche.

Sometimes therapists expose and impose their values before they have sufficient information. For example, one young man in my practice had a very serious kidney disease resulting from a complicated and exhausting fight with diabetes; 3 days a week he was on kidney dialysis. On those days and often on the surrounding days he experienced overwhelming fatigue. During a brief hospitalization, the psychiatric resident who was called in for a consultation did a detailed social history on my patient. He was asked not only did he have a girlfriend and a sex life, but also, accusitorily, why not? My client now had a new problem with which to cope: the flashes of guilt and self-doubt elicited by the doctor's probing questions. Unfortunately, the doctor had not bothered to find out the medical details; had he done so, he would quickly have seen that his expectations were unrealistic.

Perhaps the most difficult *should* to recognize is the one that prevents the therapist from "giving up"—or, more accurately—from changing the treatment goals. Let me give a concrete example. Years ago I treated a gentleman who had multiple problems, all quite serious. He was a medicated schizophrenic whose life consisted of days spent at the V.A. poolroom and day hospital and whose nights consisted of looking for a woman friend. He had very limited spending money. He suffered angina on exertion. His conversation was stilted, his clothing and home furnishings were meager at best, and he was not an attractive man. To make matters worse, he had a sexual problem; the presenting complaint, in fact, was inability to ejaculate, a problem that was compounded by the angina and was anathema to the prostitutes to whom he turned for sexual service and companionship. His other socializing attempts had netted poor results. He regularly attended singles' events and just as regularly received multiple rejections in the course of an evening. Previous therapists had worked with his social skills, his assertiveness skills, his social anxiety, and had encouraged him to continue to play the dating game. The issue that this case raised for me was a values clarification one: Was it really an act of kindness to continue to encourage the client to go out into the social fray? Considering the range of his social and sexual handicaps, was it wise for him to continue a painful and potentially fruitless pursuit? We debated these issues at some length and agreed that for the time being he could take a respite from the battle. The ending of the story is a strange but happy one. My client returned some months later and scolded me for not having thought of it myself. He now had a sex partner, one who was always accepting and comforting, and who was patient with him when he took a long time to reach a climax. He had purchased an expensive, life-sized, inflatable doll; he was content.

Bibliotherapy

Quite a number of excellent self-help books are available for the socially anxious individual; many of these books offer valuable suggestions for coping with and enjoying living alone, caring for oneself, learning to conquer emotional distress, and reaching out to others. The following list contains items that some of my clients have found useful, and new materials can be found frequently in popular periodicals, local newspapers, and more updated self-help literature.

1. *Single Blessedness,* by M. Adams (Basic Books, 1976)
2. *Single,* by P. J. Stein (Prentice-Hall, 1976)
3. *First Person Singular,* by S. M. Johnson (Signet Books, 1977)
4. *Love and Addiction,* by S. Peele (Signet Books, 1976)
5. *Sex and the Liberated Man,* by A. Ellis (Lyle Stuart, 1976)
6. *The Intelligent Woman's Guide to Dating and Mating,* by A. Ellis (Lyle Stuart, 1979)
7. *The Challenge of Being Single,* by M. Edwards and E. Hoover (New American Library, 1974)
8. *Cooking for One is Fun,* by H. L. Creel (Quadrangle, 1976)
9. *Living in One Room,* by J. Naar and M. Siple (Vintage, 1976)
10. *Liberating Masturbation: A Meditation of Self-Love,* by B. Dodson (Bodysex Designs, 1974)
11. *A New Guide to Rational Living,* by A. Ellis and R. Harper (Wilshire, 1975)
12. *Feeling Good,* by D. Burns (Morrow, 1980)

Summary

Social anxiety is seen as having cognitive, emotive, and behavioral components, each of which the therapist would do well to assess and address prescriptively. As preliminary measures, however, the presence of "symptom stress" and lack of self-acceptance may need attention. The social-evaluative aspect of the anxiety problem can then be challenged at the level of coping with the anxiety, the philosophical level of reevaluating the need for the approval of others, and the behavioral level of enjoying being alone, reaching out to others, and deepening existing relationships.

References

Arkowitz, H. (1977). Measurement and modification of minimal dating behavior. In M. Hersen, R. Eisler, & P. Miller (Eds.), *Progress in behavior modification* (Vol. 5, pp. 1–61). New York: Academic Press.

Arkowitz, H. (1981). Assessment of social skills. In M. Hersen & A. S. Bellack (Eds.), *Behavioral assessment.* New York: Pergamon Press.

Arkowitz, H., Lichtenstein, E., McGovern, K., & Hines, P. (1975). The behavioral assessment of social competence in males. *Behavior Therapy, 6,* 3–13.

Arkowitz, H., Hinton, R., Perl, J., & Himadi, W. (1978). Treatment strategies for dating anxiety in college men based on real-life practice. *The Counseling Psychologist, 7,* 41–46.

Bellack, A. S. (1983). Recurrent problems in the behavioral assessment of social skill. *Behaviour Research and Therapy, 21,* 29–41.

Benson, H. (1975). *The relaxation response.* New York: Avon Books.

Berscheid, E., & Walster, E. (1973). Physical attractiveness. In L. Berkowitz (Ed.), *Advances in experimental and social psychology* (Vol. 7). New York: Academic Press.

Borkovec, T. D., Stone, N. M., O'Brien, G. T., & Kaloupek, D. G. (1974). Evaluation of a clinically relevant target behavior for analogue outcome research. *Behavior Therapy, 5,* 503–511.

Burns, D. (1980). *Feeling good.* New York: Morrow.

Burns, D. *Intimate connections.* (1984). New York: Morrow.

Clark, J., & Arkowitz, H. (1975). Social anxiety and self-evaluation of interpersonal performance. *Psychological Reports, 36,* 211–221.

Curran, J. P. (1977). Social skill training as an approach to the treatment of heterosexual social anxiety. *Psychological Bulletin, 84,* 140–157.

Ellis, A., & Becker, I. (1982). *A guide to personal happiness.* North Hollywood, CA: Wilshire.

Glasgow, R., & Arkowitz, H. (1975). The behavioral assessment of male and female social competence in dyadic heterosexual interactions. *Behavior Therapy, 6,* 488–498.

Goldfried, M. R., & Davison, G. C. (1976). *Clinical behavior therapy,* New York: Holt, Rinehart & Winston.

Jacobson, E. (1938). *Progressive relaxation.* Chicago: University of Chicago Press.

Lipton, D. N., & Nelson, R. O. (1980). The contribution of initiation behaviors to dating frequency. *Behavior Therapy, 11,* 59–67.

McEwan, K. L. (1983). Perhaps it's time to leave minimal daters alone. *The Behavior Therapist, 6,* 100–101.

Milgram, S. (1967, May). The small world problem. *Psychology Today,* pp. 61–67.

Morris, D. (1977). *Manwatching: A field guide to human behavior.* New York: Harry N. Abrams.

Nietzel, M. T., & Bernstein, D. A. (1981). Assessment of anxiety and fear. In M. Hersen & A. S. Bellack (Eds.), *Behavioral assessment: A practical handbook.* New York: Pergamon Press.

Perlman, D., & Peplau, L. A. (1981). Toward a social psychology of loneliness. In R. Gilmour & S. Duck (Eds.), *Personal relationships in disorder.* London: Academic Press.

Primakoff, L. (1983). One's company; two's a crowd: Skills in living alone groups. In A. Freeman (Ed.), *Cognitive therapy with couples and groups.* New York: Plenum Press.

Walen, S. R. (1983). Phrenophobia. *Cognitive Therapy and Research, 6,* 399–407.

Walen, S. R., DiGiuseppe, R., & Wessler, R. (1980). *A practitioner's guide to rational-emotive therapy.* New York: Oxford University Press.

Watson, D., & Friend, R. (1969). Measurement of social-evaluative anxiety. *Journal of Consulting and Clinical Psychology, 33,* 448–457.

Weeks, C. (1978). *Hope and help for your nerves.* New York: Bantam.

Wolpe, J. (1969). *The practice of behavior therapy.* New York: Pergamon Press.

Wolpe, J., & Lazarus, A. A. (1966). *Behavior therapy techniques.* New York: Pergamon Press.

Young, J. (1981). Cognitive therapy and loneliness. In G. Emery, S. D. Hollon, & R. C. Bedrosian (Eds.), *New directions in cognitive therapy.* New York: Guilford Press.

Young, J., & Epstein, N. (1982). Assessment and treatment of avoidance in anxiety disorders. *Cognitive Behavior Therapy Newsletter, 4,* 4–6.

Zimbardo, P. G. (1977). *Shyness: What it is, what to do about it.* Reading, MA: Addison-Wesley.

Zimbardo, P. G., & Radl, S. L. (1979). *The shyness workbook.* New York: A & W Publishers.

Zimbardo, P., Pilkonis, P., & Norwood, R. (1975). The silent prison of shyness. *Psychology Today, 8,* 69–72.

Obsessive-Compulsive Disorder

Jonathan B. Grayson, Edna B. Foa, and Gail Steketee

Introduction

Definition and Description

Obsessive-compulsive symptoms have been described and discussed for over 100 years but the clinical picture has changed little over time. Indeed, the *Diagnostic and Statistical Manual of Mental Disorders* (DSM-III) (1980) definition includes the classical criteria of persistent, intrusive, recurrent thoughts or images that are unacceptable and cannot be dismissed voluntarily, and repetitive ritualistic actions that the individual feels compelled to carry out.

It is customary to refer to thoughts, images, and impulses as *obsessions,* whereas repetitious behaviors are labeled *compulsions.* This modality-based classification poses conceptual as well as practical problems, which have been discussed at length by Foa and Tillmans (1980). These authors proposed a definition of obsession and compulsions based on the functional relationship between the symptoms and anxiety. According to this model, "obsessions" or "ruminations" are thoughts, images, or actions that *generate* anxiety/discomfort; by contrast, "compulsions" are attempts to *ameliorate* that anxiety through overt actions or thoughts (i.e., "neutralizing" cognitions, Rachman, 1976).

Obsessive-compulsive disorders have usually been classified according to the nature of the ritualistic behavior (i.e., washing and cleaning, checking, ordering, etc.); the most common of these are washing compulsions, with checking rituals

JONATHAN B. GRAYSON and EDNA B. FOA • Department of Psychiatry, Behavior Therapy Section, Eastern EPPI, 3300 Henry Avenue, Philadelphia, Pennsylvania 19129. GAIL STEKETEE • Department of Psychiatry, Temple University, Philadelphia, Pennsylvania 19122. Preparation of this chapter was supported by grant MH 31634 awarded to Edna B. Foa by the National Institute of Mental Health.

comprising most of the remainder. Washers are patients who feel contaminated by contact with certain objects or thoughts. Their ritualistic behavior consists mainly of washing themselves and/or cleaning the environment around them. Checkers tend to fear some future disaster, and their compulsive activities (checking, counting, praying) represent attempts to ward off feared consequences. Although the relationship of the ritual to the fear is usually quite direct, such as washing to remove dirt or checking the stove to make sure it is off, in other cases the relationship between obsessions and compulsions is obscure. Four cases (two washers and two checkers) are described next to demonstrate the complexity of this disorder.

Case 1

Alice is a 42-year-old married housewife with three children. For the last 10 years she suffered from feelings of contamination (a nonspecific feeling of being dirty accompanied by extreme anxiety and discomfort) when in contact with lice, feces, and public bathrooms, objects and places that she took pains to avoid. She also avoided touching things or places that may have had direct or indirect contact with her feared objects, including hair, combs, pillows, backs of chairs, bathing caps, towels, toilets, genitals, and people. When walking outside, Alice constantly watched her steps to avoid any discoloration on the pavement for fear it might be dog feces. Food shopping also posed difficulty because she thought the products might have been handled by a person who had neglected to wash his or her hands after using the toilet. Whenever possible, Alice washed her hands and arms up to the elbows immediately after contact with contaminants. In addition, she carried disposable hand-cleaning towelettes, which she would use if running water was unavailable. Finally, she engaged in subtle hand washing, such as wetting her hands with water from a fountain or a glass. Alice carried out these compulsive actions to protect herself from lice or a fatal disease and from spreading contamination to others, who, in turn, might further contaminate her.

Case 2

Jane is a 36-year-old married housewife who was afraid of flammable substances, such as gasoline, grease, cooking oil, or butter. She avoided contact with these substances as well as with the stove, which might contain their residue. Worrying about the safety of her children, Jane did not permit them to play near cars or around spots that looked like oil or gas. Although she knew that her concerns were greatly exaggerated, she banned cooking in her house in order to prevent fire. Like Alice, Jane washed her hands repeatedly; she scrubbed so vigorously that her skin became raw, shiny, and extremely sensitive to touch.

Case 3

Tom was a 38-year-old married man with a 6-year duration of excessive checking rituals, which he performed in order to achieve perfection in every activity. He felt that once something was finished, it became irreversible; if he failed to do it correctly the first time, he would have to live with the error forever. He also reported a compulsion to remember all steps of each activity in order to ensure that he would be able to repeat it successfully in the future (e.g., fixing a faucet, adjusting the heat registers for winter). In an effort to reach perfection, Tom repeated each action over and over again. The definition of perfection changed for each task. Screws were not to be too tight; pictures had to be leveled perfectly; letters had to be perfectly written. In order to "minimize" repetitions, Tom did not permit noisy activities around him to interfere with his concentration while he was working. Prior to treatment, even a simple activity such as changing a light bulb required 2 to 3 hours. After completing a task (e.g., food shopping, changing a light bulb), Tom would sit at the kitchen table for hours, trying to recall the exact details of what he had done to verify that he had performed the action perfectly. At the time of treatment, Tom could barely function; he was unable to complete more than two or three simple tasks per day because of his extensive repeating rituals and because he avoided many activities for fear that he would start to ritualize.

Case 4

Sara was a 32-year-old clerk who had a fear that she might hit somebody accidentally while driving. She constantly looked in the rear view mirror to verify that there were no injured persons lying behind on the street. Often, Sara would drive back to a place where she feared she might have hit a person, and while retracing her route, would imagine that she hit other people. Upon arrival at home she would spend between 1 and 2 hours examining the car for any evidence that somebody might have been hit by it. She also read the newspaper and watched the news on television in order to make sure that no hit-and-run accidents had occurred where she had been driving that day.

Classification

A shortcoming inherent in traditional classifications of obsessive-compulsives is their failure to bear on treatment. To overcome this flaw, Foa, Steketee, and Ozarow (in press) proposed a classification system based on the types of cues that evoke anxiety and the type of activity (cognitive or overt) that reduces it. This classification will be briefly discussed here, and its implications for treatment will be considered later in the chapter.

All obsessive-compulsives manifest *internal fear cues:* that is, intrusive thoughts, images, or impulses. These may be triggered by contact with *external cues,* such as a contaminated object or driving a car, or they may also arise without apparent external events. A further distinction can be made with respect to the presence or absence of fears of *disastrous consequences.* For example, the thought "Did I tighten the screw too much?" may be related to a concern that serious damage may ensue; the urge to stab one's child may elicit a fear of actually killing him or her. On the other hand, the intrusive thought "Is my hand contaminated?" often elicits discomfort in absence of any concern with possible aversive consequences.

Thus, obsessions can be divided into several kinds: (a) presence of intrusive cognitive material, external fear cues, and fears of disasters; (b) presence of intrusive material and external cues (in the absence of disasters); and (c) presence of intrusive material and fear of disasters (in the absence of external cues). A fourth type, intrusive cognitive material with neither external cues nor fear of disasters, is theoretically possible, but we have not observed patients with such obsessions, nor have we come across such reports in the literature.

How can compulsions be classified? If all compulsive actions are anxiety reducing, the type of ritual (e.g., washing, checking) becomes unimportant. A more useful approach is to categorize compulsions on the basis of their mode, cognitive or behavioral, because they carry different treatment implications. For an extensive discussion, see Foa, Steketee, and Ozarow (in press).

The feared cues give rise to much anxiety, which can be reduced in two ways. The first is simply to avoid the fear cues. For example, if the thought "I will kill my wife" is elicited by certain situations such as the news or violent movies, these will be avoided. For obsessive-compulsives, when such *passive* avoidance fails, active avoidance patterns (i.e., cognitive or overt compulsions) are then activated. Examples of active avoidance for the cases described earlier include the self-statement "God forgive me," which counteracts the thought "I will kill my wife," washing one's hands repeatedly to "erase" previous contact with feces, and repeatedly turning the stove on and off to make sure it is off. In general, the rituals of washers tend to be restorative; after being confronted with a contaminant, the function of washing is to bring back the former state of noncontamination. The rituals of checkers, on the other hand, tend to be preventative (e.g., one checks the stove to make sure that the house will not burn down in the future). Whether the avoidance is active or passive, patients typically report an immediate reduction of anxiety/ discomfort. In the rare cases where amelioration of fear does not follow the emission of a compulsion, such patients report a belief that nonperformance of the ritual will lead to worsening of anxiety. This belief may serve to reinforce ritualistic behavior. Indeed, Herrnstein (1969) found that with animals, behaviors were reinforced by an aversive event that was less aversive than its alternative. Marlatt and Donovan (1982) have found that at the onset of a drinking binge, alcoholics believe that drinking will make them feel better, although they often feel miserable once they are drunk. Similarly, many obsessive-compulsives believe that the repetition of a compulsive act will result in relief from discomfort.

Theoretical Models

Behavioral theories of fear and avoidance behavior have been commonly adopted to explain phobic and obsessive-compulsive disorders. Elaborating on Mowrer's (1939) two-stage theory, Dollard and Miller (1950) proposed that obsessive-compulsive symptoms are acquired via a process of classical conditioning. That is, through an associative process, concrete objects as well as thoughts and images acquire the capacity to produce discomfort. In the second stage of symptom development, escape or avoidance responses are developed to reduce the anxiety or discomfort evoked by the various conditioned stimuli and are maintained by their success in doing so. Because of extensive generalization, passive avoidance behaviors, such as those utilized by phobics, are rendered ineffective in controlling anxiety. Active avoidance patterns in the form of ritualistic behaviors are then developed.

The inadequacy of this model in accounting for the acquisition of fear has been discussed by several authors (e.g., Rachman & Wilson, 1980). Although the majority of patients cannot recall conditioning events associated with symptom onset, they often report preceding stressful life events. This led Watts (1971) to suggest that these events may serve to sensitize the individual to cues that have an innate tendency to elicit fear. Teasdale (1974) proposed that anxiety responses learned during early experiences may be enhanced by stress. Similarly, Rachman (1971) posited that for obsessive-compulsives, a state of heightened arousal could lead to sensitization of thoughts that have special significance for the individual. It follows that individuals who are highly arousable physiologically may be more prone to developing anxiety disorders. There is evidence to suggest that obsessive-compulsives are, indeed, more physiologically reactive to threat anticipation than normals (Boulougouris, 1977). However, these data were obtained after symptom onset, and arousability may have been the consequence rather than the cause of the obsessive-compulsive disorder. It is conceivable, then, that heightened physiological arousal when combined with a general stressor and with specific fear cues may produce such symptoms.

Whereas factors related to the acquisition of an obsessive-compulsive disorder are still largely unclear, there is experimental evidence to support the clinical observations that obsessions give rise to anxiety/discomfort and that compulsions reduce it. Ruminative thoughts were found to increase heart rate and deflection of skin conductance more than neutral thoughts (Boulougouris, Rabavillas, & Stefanis, 1977; Rabavilas & Boulougouris, 1974). Likewise, contact with contaminated objects resulted in increased heart rate and subjective anxiety (Hodgson & Rachman, 1972) as well as skin conductance level (Hornsveld, Kraaimaat, & van Dam Baggen, 1979). A series of experiments with washers and checkers indicated that, with few exceptions, anxiety decreased following the performance of a ritual after confrontation with cues that provoked an urge to ritualize (Hodgson, Rachman, & Marks, 1972; Hornsveld *et al.*, 1979; Roper, Rachman, & Hodgson, 1973; Roper & Rachman, 1976).

Cognitive Theories

A cognitive explanation of obsessive-compulsive symptoms has been advanced by Carr (1974), who proposed that obsessionals have abnormally high expectations of unpleasant outcome (i.e., they overestimate the risk of negative consequences for a variety of actions). Carr noted that obsessional content often included exaggerations of the normal concerns about health, death, others' welfare, sex, religious matters, performance at work, and the like. The erroneous beliefs of obsessive-compulsives were also stressed by McFall and Wollersheim (1979). These included the idea that one must be perfectly competent in all endeavors to be worthwhile, the belief that failure to live up to perfectionistic ideals should be punished, and that certain magical rituals can prevent catastrophes. These mistaken beliefs, according to the authors, lead to erroneous perceptions of threat, which in turn provoke anxiety. The obsessive-compulsives' lack of belief in their ability to cope effectively with such threats compounds the dysfunctional process. The resulting feelings of uncertainty, discomfort, and helplessness are ameliorated through the emission of rituals, which in the patients' view constitute the sole method available to them to reduce the perceived threat.

The preceding assertions have received support from several investigations. Obsessive-compulsives were found to be deficient in their ability to link concepts integratively. They catalogued events discretely, thus creating "islands of certainty" amidst confusion in an attempt to control and predict events (Makhlouf-Norris & Norris, 1972; Makhlouf-Norris, Jones, & Norris, 1970). Observing the performance of obsessive-compulsives on a series of cognitive tasks, Reed (1969) concluded that their thinking was characterized by underinclusion or overspecification of concepts. He attributed their doubt and indecision to a distrust of their own perceptions (Reed, 1968). Consistent with these findings, Persons and Foa (1984) observed that ritualizers utilized overly specific concepts in their thought patterns with respect to both obsessional and neutral cues. An analog study of college students who scored high on the MOC checking subscale indicated that such individuals had poorer recall for prior actions and greater difficulty distinguishing real from imagined events than did subjects who had low scores (Sher, Frost, & Otto, 1983). These findings suggest that memory deficits in checkers may motivate repetitious checking behavior. Congruent with this study is the observation that obsessive-compulsives have a greater tendency than other psychiatric patients to request a repetition of information before rendering a decision (Milner, Beech, & Walker, 1971).

The preceding finding suggests that obsessive-compulsives are more rigid, perfectionistic, and doubting, requiring excessive amounts of information to make a decision, only to distrust their choice. These observations must be interpreted with some caution, however, because several of the studies included individuals with compulsive personality style rather than an obsessive-compulsive disorder.

Foa and Kozak (1984) conceptualized *anxiety disorders* as specific impairments in affective memory networks. They viewed *fear* according to a bioinformational theory of emotions advanced by Lang (1979), in which affective memory was hypothesized to include information about feared *stimuli,* fear *responses,* and their *meanings.* Foa and Kozak proposed that neurotic fears differ structurally from normal fears, with the former characterized by the presence of erroneous estimates of threat, an unusually high negative valence for the threatening event, and excessive response elements (e.g., physiological, avoidance, etc.). In addition, neurotic fear structures are distinguished by their resistance to modification. This persistence may reflect failure to access the fear network, either because of active avoidance or because the content of the fear network precludes spontaneous encounters with situations that evoke anxiety in everyday life. Anxiety may also persist because of some impairment in the mechanism of change. Cognitive defenses, excessive arousal with failure to habituate, faulty premises, and erroneous rules of inference are all impairments that would hinder the processing of information necessary for changing the fear structure of the obsessive-compulsive.

Ideally, assessment of obsessive-compulsive symptomatology should involve separate evaluations of obsessions and compulsions. Assessment of obsessions should include information about external fear cues, internal fear cues (thoughts, images, or impulses), and thoughts of disastrous consequences. The degree of discomfort/anxiety associated with obsessional content should also be measured on physiological and cognitive indexes. The amount of passive avoidance behavior associated with obsessional thoughts must also be appraised. Additionally, both overt and cognitive compulsions should be separately assessed.

Although global measures of obsessive-compulsive symptoms have proven useful in assessing treatment effects (e.g., Foa, Steketee, Grayson, & Doppelt, 1983; Marks, Stern, Mawson, Cobb, & McDonald, 1980), measures of specific manifestations are essential to better understand the mechanisms underlying various treatment procedures. Several instruments to assess obsessions, anxiety, avoidance, and compulsions have been developed, largely for research purposes (for a review, see Steketee & Foa, 1984). However, they are of limited value for the clinician whose assessment is geared toward designing treatment programs. For example, in examining the Minnesota Multiphasic Personality Inventory (MMPI), a cluster analysis was used to divide patients into three groups (Doppelt, 1981). Examination of the clusters suggested that the groups differed in their level of general pathology, but group membership did not predict outcome.

The major vehicle for assessing the obsessive-compulsive symptoms is the clinical interview. An outline of the topics to be covered during the assessment interview are presented in Appendix A and is illustrated later.

We have suggested that obsessions are defined by specific anxiety-evoking cues that are classified as external cues (e.g., tangible objects), internal cues (e.g., images and impulses), and worries about future consequences. In addition, obsessive-compulsive patients show both passive and active (ritualistic) patterns of avoidance. Compulsion can be subdivided into *overt* and *covert* (cognitive) forms. As will be discussed later, information pertaining to each of these dimensions will determine the treatment procedure to be used.

External Fear Cues

For the vast majority of obsessive-compulsives, certain external cues generate anxiety. The interviewer should solicit highly specific information about such cues in an attempt to identify the basic sources of concern. Contamination "travels," and objects become contaminants through contact (which may be quite remote) with the source of contamination. It is impossible to understand the patient who fears walking in the woods, sitting near people who have just returned from a visit to the zoo, and sitting near their fireplace (where a bat was found 2 years ago) without knowing that they all represented potential contact with rabies.

Identification of the source of fear is important not only in comprehending the patient's conceptual structure but also in determining treatment. To achieve a successful outcome, confrontation with the source of fear is important. Often, when treatment does not include confrontation with this source, a relapse will occur. For example, a patient who feared contact with her mother was treated with systematic exposure to items that had been contaminated by "indirect" contact with her mother such as the mail. But because she lived so far from her mother, direct exposure was not implemented. Within a year, new items associated with her mother started to disturb her again, until a complete relapse was evident. It was not until she was repeatedly exposed (for prolonged periods) to her mother that she experienced lasting improvement.

Internal Fear Cues

Anxiety/discomfort may be generated by internal cues, that is, thoughts, images, or impulses that are shameful, disgusting, or fearful. Such cues may include number sequences, impulses to stab one's child (which may be triggered, in turn, by external cues such as knives or scissors), thoughts that one's spouse may have an auto accident on the way home, images of having sex with Christ, or impulses to expose one's genitals. Some obsessive-compulsives may respond with anxiety to bodily sensations such as minor pains or swallowing if these are interpreted as signals for physical disease (e.g., choking, cancer). When the latter concerns are accompanied by elaborate checking rituals, they are classified as obsessive-compulsive; when patients who are concerned with physical illness confine their efforts to reduce anxiety to frequent contact with physicians, they are diagnosed as hypochondriacal.

Patients who are reluctant to disclose their "shameful" obsessions can be encouraged with direct questions, a matter-of-fact attitude, and reassurance that many normal individuals also have unwanted ideas.

Fears of Harm

Often the external and internal cues for discomfort are associated with anticipated harm, which for some may be the primary source of discomfort. Many washers fear disease, physical debilitation, or death to themselves or others. Most checkers seek to avoid being responsible for an error that will lead to either physical harm (e.g., leaving the car in neutral and finding that it has rolled over a child) or psychological harm (e.g., making a mistake and eliciting criticism from others; writing "My husband is a homosexual" in letters to friends and thereby losing others' respect). Those with repeating rituals are often concerned that their upsetting thoughts will come to pass (e.g, an accident's happening, losing control and stabbing someone, punishment from God).

Many neurotic patients have not considered what harm they seek to avoid; such information may require careful questioning by the therapist. Others do not fear disastrous consequences. Tom (Case 3) ritualized merely to avoid being highly anxious. Others fear that they will "go crazy" as a result of continuous anxiety. However, for most obsessive-compulsives the feared consequences of exposure are connected to external sources (e.g., fear of disease from contamination).

As the dialogue demonstrates, the relationship between external cues and the associated feared consequences should be carefully explored. The patient was a young married male who spent hours checking his mouth for lumps that might be cancerous.

T: So what would happen if you found a lump?
C: I would go to the doctor to find out if it was cancer.
T: Then what would happen?
C: I don't know.
T: Well, suppose you had cancer, would that be the worst that could happen?
C: That would be horrible, but I wouldn't be afraid the same way.
T: What do you mean?
C: That would be a real fear; I don't think I'd have the same intense anxiety I have when I go to find out whether or not I have cancer. I rehearse my description of the lump for hours, so that the doctor will take my concern seriously.
T: Do you feel relieved when the doctor tells you that you don't have cancer?
C: No, because he may have missed something, or because I drew his attention to a particular area of my mouth, he may have ignored other areas where a real problem exists.
T: If I understand you correctly, it makes you more anxious to not be sure whether or not you have cancer than actually having cancer?
C: Yes, I think you are right.

As is apparent from the dialogue, the patient was also concerned that the failure to diagnose his cancer would somehow be his fault, either because he failed to identify the lump or because his presentation somehow affected the doctor's examination. His failure to communicate signs of his illness and being uncertain about a diagnosis of cancer turned out to be the focus of his fear rather than actually having cancer.

Strength of the Belief in Harm

Foa (1979) has observed that the assignment of high probabilities to feared consequences (i.e., having "overvalued ideas") was associated with failure. Therefore, information about the strength of the belief becomes important when one considers treatment. Although most obsessive-compulsives are aware that their fears are senseless, few will assert that the disastrous consequences they anticipate (e.g., dying from contact with a leukemic patient's garment) will, in fact, occur. Overvalued ideators may require cognitive manipulations to correct their misconceptions and to convince them of the need to accept the seemingly high risk in exchange for a normal life-style.

Avoidance and Compulsions

Having identified fear cues, the therapist should inquire about behavior symptoms. Whenever possible, obsessive-compulsives, like phobics, may engage in passive avoidance in an attempt to avoid situations that lead to discomfort. Such avoidance can be quite obvious, such as refraining from using public restrooms or refusing to drive to avoid injuring people. Avoidance may take more bizarre forms and become extremely debilitating. In order to avoid contamination of her house, one patient required all family members to remove their clothes upon entering the house, go straight to the bathroom to take a shower, after which they put on decontaminated clothing. In addition, the family lived in their finished basement and were not allowed upstairs in order to "simplify" the patient's effort to keep the home decontaminated. Another patient who had obsessive thoughts that he might attack his wife refrained from watching TV or reading the newspaper for fear he would encounter references to violence that would trigger his obsessions. He also avoided the kitchen where the sight of knives or forks could trigger impulses to stab his wife.

Active avoidance patterns take the form of ritualistic behaviors, which, as discussed earlier, are attempts to cope with anxiety or discomfort. It is important that the therapist collect detailed information about the ritual in order to plan response prevention as well as to instill confidence in the patient that the therapist understands his or her problem. The therapist will inquire into the length of each washing and the manner and method by which the hands are washed (i.e., washing to the elbows, using Lysol, soap, hot water, etc.). Obsessive-compulsives often have difficulty deciding when to stop ritualizing. The therapist should identify the circumstances that lead to repetitions of compulsive actions. At times, this may be due to a feeling that the ritual has not yet accomplished its purpose (e.g., a checker may not feel certain that the stove is really off or that there are not dents on the car that could have resulted from a hit-and-run). At other times, repetitions may result from a sense that the ritual was not carried out properly.

For most patients, ritualistic behavior consists of washing, cleaning (including wiping with alcohol or spraying with Lysol), checking, repeating actions, placing objects in a precise order, and repeatedly requesting reassurance. For some, anxiety is also reduced by cognitive rituals, such as praying, thinking "good" thoughts, and mentally listing events. The functional relationship of each ritual to the fear cues and to passive avoidance behaviors should be ascertained. If a relationship cannot be identified, then the diagnosis of obsessive-compulsive disorder should be questioned, and the possibility of psychotic thinking processes should be considered. Stereotyped ritualistic behavior is sometimes observed in schizophrenics.

Mood State

Both depression and high background anxiety have been identified as prognostic factors in the outcome of behavioral treatment with obsessive-compulsives (Foa, 1979; Foa *et al.*, 1983). Patients with severe depression were less likely to benefit from treatment and evidenced more relapse than mildly depressed patients. With regard to general anxiety, those who showed low anxiety benefited from treatment; patients with severe anxiety were equally likely to succeed or fail (Foa *et al.*, 1983). Because of their relationship to treatment outcome, mood states (especially depression) should be carefully assessed. Reduction of depression before treatment (either by drugs or psychological means) may enhance the efficacy of the treatment program. Depression can be assessed by administering the Beck Depression Inventory (Beck & Beamsderfer, 1974) or The Hamilton Depression Scale (Hamilton, 1960). A variety of inventories are available to measure anxious mood state, including the Spielberger State-Trait Inventory (Spielberger, Gorsuch, & Lushene, 1970) and the Taylor Manifest Anxiety Scale (Taylor, 1953).

Family Relationships

Often the family has been heavily incorporated into the patient's symptomatology. Family involvement may range from compliance to every demand made by the patient (as in the case of the family who stripped off their clothing as soon as they entered the house and went to the shower) to constant battling over compliance with the patient's unreasonable requests. The therapist should arrange a family session if possible to assess their willingness and/or ability to assist with treatment. Significant family difficulties may hinder success and may lead to a decision to remove the patient from his or her familial environment.

The preceding strategy of assessment not only provides the therapist with information necessary for designing a treatment program, but it also helps to educate patients and family members about their symptoms. The assessment process teaches them to break the obsessive-compulsive symptomatology into segments that can be more readily understood. This assists in building trust in the therapist's understanding of their problems and improves expectations of overcoming them.

Treatment: Review of Procedures

Obsessive-compulsive disorders have long been considered among the most intractable of the neurotic disorders. "Most of us are agreed that the treatment of obsessional states is one of the most difficult tasks confronting the psychiatrist and many of us consider it hopeless," Breitner stated (1960, p. 32). Indeed, the results of traditional psychotherapy have been quite disappointing. In a sample of 90 inpatients, Kringlen (1965) found that only 20% had improved at a 13- to 20-year follow-up. Somewhat more favorable results were reported by Grimshaw (1965): Forty percent of an outpatient sample were improved at a 1- to 14-year follow-up.

Early Forms of Behavioral Treatment

Some improvement in the prognostic picture emerged with the application of treatments derived from learning theories. These treatments can be categorized into two classes: (a) exposure procedures aimed at reducing the anxiety/discomfort associated with obsessions; and (b) blocking or suppression techniques directed at reducing the frequency of either obsessions or compulsions.

Procedures aiming at both have been developed. Anxiety-reducing techniques have included systematic desensitization (a series of brief presentations of fear-evoking material) as well as variants of prolonged exposure to feared situations (e.g., paradoxical intention, imaginal flooding, satiation, aversion relief). Limited success has been achieved with either desensitization or flooding, 30 to 40% with the former (e.g., Beech & Vaughn, 1978) and 40 to 60% with the latter (e.g., Emmelkamp & Kwee, 1977; Steketee, Foa, & Grayson, 1982).

If obsessive-compulsive symptomology is composed of obsessions that evoke anxiety and compulsions that reduce it, then treatment should consist of techniques that are directed at decreasing the former and blocking the latter. Interventions directed at both symptoms simultaneously would be expected to yield a more successful outcome. A treatment program that addresses both obsessions and compulsions—exposure and response prevention—has proven highly successful and has become the treatment of choice for this disorder. We shall now summarize the findings on this program.

Exposure and Response Prevention

Employing prolonged exposure to obsessional cues with strict prevention of ritualistic behavior, Meyer (1966) reported a successful outcome with two obsessive-compulsive washers. Later reports indicated that this treatment regimen was highly successful in 10 of 15 cases and moderately so in the remaining 5; only two relapses occurred after a 5- to 6-year period (Meyer & Levy, 1973; Meyer, Levy, & Schnurer, 1974). These reports investigated a series of controlled and uncontrolled studies using variants of this program. Findings have been remarkably consistent. Approximately 65 to 75% of more than 200 patients who were studied were improved and stayed so at follow-up (see Foa, Steketee, & Ozarow, in press; Rachman & Hodgson, 1980, for detailed reviews of these studies).

Briefly, the treatment consists of repeatedly exposing the patient for prolonged periods (45 minutes to 2 hours) to circumstances that provoke discomfort. Typically, exposure is graded so that moderately disturbing situations precede more anxiety-provoking ones. Ten to 20 daily sessions are held. Patients with washing rituals are required to touch their particular "contaminated" objects; those with checking compulsions are presented with situations in which they have an urge to check (e.g., driving a car, using the stove). They are instructed to refrain from ritualizing regardless of the strength of their urges to do so. The combination of exposure and response prevention has been demonstrated to yield results superior to either procedure alone (Foa, Steketee, & Milby, 1980; Foa, Steketee, Grayson, Turner, & Latimer, Steketee *et al.* 1982).

The advantage of exposing patients to feared circumstances in actual practice (i.e., *in vivo*) rather than in imagination has been demonstrated for simple phobics. For obsessive-compulsives, the picture is less clear; if *in vivo* exposure is superior, it is only marginally so. Foa, Steketee, Turner, and Fisher (1980) tested the effects of combined *in vivo* and imaginal exposure versus *in vivo* exposure only with checkers. Although at the end of treatment no differences between groups were observed, the combined treatment was superior in maintaining gains. It seems, then, that for checkers who have thoughts of future harm as an important feature of their obsessive ideation, the addition of imaginal exposure that readily permits exposure to such fears is indicated.

It is commonly noted that obsessive-compulsive symptoms produce a decline in the patient's general functioning. They interfere with work, home management, social, and leisure activities, and often produce conflict in marital relationships. Studying effects of marital therapy and exposure/response prevention treatment in obsessive-compulsives with disturbed marriages, Cobb, McDonald, Marks, and Stern (1980) found that marital treatment improved only the marital relationship, whereas exposure treatment improved both the obsessive-compulsive symptoms and the marriage.

Assertiveness training has also been employed with six patients who reported obsessions about harming others that were hypothesized to reflect social anxiety (Emmelkamp & Van de Heyden, 1980). It was found to be as effective as thought stopping. However, given the generally poor results with the latter procedure and the specificity of the obsessions selected for this study, the general utility of assertiveness training as a treatment for obsessive-compulsive symptoms is questionable.

Cognitive Psychotherapy

Cognitive therapy is founded on the assumption that thoughts and beliefs play a causal role in emotion and behavior. Accordingly, cognitive interventions aim at changing thoughts, belief systems, and irrational ideas and are for the most part delivered in conversationlike form. Only one study investigated the effects of cognitive therapy with obsessive-compulsives. Studying 15 patients, Emmelkamp, van der Helm, van Zanten, and Plochy (1980) compared graded exposure *in vivo* with exposure preceded by self-instructional training. Treatment produced significant improvement in both groups; no differences between conditions were found at posttreatment or at follow-up. The authors concluded that the cognitive technique did not enhance the efficacy of exposure. The failure of the procedure employed in the aforementioned study should not discourage attempts to implement cognitive treatment methods with obsessive-compulsives. If Foa and Kozak (1984) are correct in proposing that these patients have impairments in the rules by which they process information, then one might expect cognitive techniques to be beneficial. Such techniques, however, should be tailored to the specific cognitive deficits of this disorder.

In summary, the literature on exposure and response prevention with obsessive-compulsives clearly indicates that its efficacy exceeds that of any other psychotherapeutic procedure. At present, then, it constitutes the preferred treatment for this disorder.

Treatment: Implementation of Exposure and Response Prevention

In the following section we will discuss how to conduct exposure and response prevention, which has become the treatment of choice for obsessive-compulsive ritualizers.

Overview

The treatment program consists of three stages: an information gathering period, an intensive exposure/response prevention phase, and a follow-up maintenance period.

Assessment Period

For most patients, 3 to 6 hours are sufficient for collecting information about their obsessions and compulsions and for planning the treatment program. The treatment program should be discussed in sufficient detail with the patient so that he or she is not surprised during the active treatment phase by implementation of exposure and response prevention.

During these preliminary sessions, the therapist delineates the content of imaginal flooding scenes, the objects or situations to be confronted *in vivo,* and the rituals to be prevented. The setting (home or hospital) is determined, and individuals are designated to assist the patients in their assignments and to support them when difficulties arise between sessions. It is important that those who are assigned as helpers demonstrate a supportive attitude toward the treatment undertaking. Similarly, in the hospital only those nurses, aides, or other medical personnel with whom the patient feels most comfortable should be selected as assistants. It is important that the therapist instruct the aides in the patients' presence in order to avoid misunderstandings.

Treatment Period

When patients manifest several rituals and several sources of anxiety, treatment should aim at one or two major rituals and associated obsessions for maximal gain; remaining symptoms can be treated later. In our program, patients are usually seen for 15 treatment sessions scheduled every weekday. Because clinical observations indicate that massed sessions produce better results than spaced sessions, we suggest a minimum of three sessions per week. Treatment may be extended if significant progress is evident and the remaining discomfort is expected to decrease with 1 or 2 weeks of further therapy. There is a point, however, where the therapeutic efforts have diminishing returns. Rachman, Cobb, Grey, McDonald, Mawson, Sartory, and Stern (1979) observed that 30 sessions were only slightly better than 15 sessions of exposure. If 20 treatment sessions produce minimal results, it is doubtful that additional sessions will be of benefit.

A typical therapy session proceeds as follows: the first few minutes are spent in discussion of the patient's current mood, urges to ritualize, and prior homework assignment. Unexpected upsetting events are also attended to at the beginning of the session. In the remaining time, procedures directed at anxiety reduction are implemented. First, the patient is exposed in fantasy to descriptions of the situations, objects, or thoughts (including thoughts of future harm) that provoke fear and discomfort. In successive sessions, more disturbing items are added to previous ones; the most anxiety-provoking situations are typically presented by the sixth session.

For washers, all nonessential washing and cleaning is eliminated except for one 10-minute shower every fifth day. Dishwashing and other activities that necessitate contact with water should be conducted with gloves or assigned to someone else during the intensive phase of treatment. Checkers are permitted one check only of items that are normally checked after use, such as stoves and door locks. Other objects judged not to require routine checking (e.g., unused electrical appliances, discarded envelopes) may not be checked. Infractions of these rules are to be recorded on the daily self-monitoring form and are discussed in the beginning of the next session.

In the last few sessions of treatment, the patient should be introduced to rules of "normal" washing, cleaning, or checking. Response prevention requirements are relaxed to enable the patient to return to what we consider to be a normal routine. For washers, this would include one 10-minute shower daily and hand-washing before meals, after bathroom use, and after handling grimy, greasy, or sticky objects. Initially, any washing should be followed immediately by reexposure to contaminants. Also, the therapist may wish to continue some restriction, particularly when strong urges to wash are still present. For example, patients whose obsessions were focused on bathroom germs may be allowed to wash normally except after bathroom use for several weeks after completion of intensive treatment.

Maintenance Period

Following the intensive treatment phase, the therapist may prescribe a self-exposure maintenance regimen to ensure periodic contact with previously avoided situations and to prevent a return to former avoidance patterns. For many patients, normal work and/or leisure activities have been severely impaired by the obsessive avoidance patterns. These must be reestablished and new ones developed to fill the time that becomes available when hours of ritualizing are decreased to only a few minutes per day. This may entail interpersonal skills training for those who are deficient in this area. Marital or family therapy may be required by some patients to improve communication patterns. Partners who have participated in the ritualistic behavior of the patients need to rehearse refusal of such requests while, at the same time, encouraging and supporting the patient. Such maintenance treatment typically requires weekly sessions for periods varying from a few weeks to more than a year, depending on the level of pretreatment functioning.

Let us now describe in detail the three components of treatment: *in vivo* exposure, imaginal exposure, and response prevention.

Exposure In Vivo

The exposure *in vivo* program usually begins confronting the patient to items or situations that evoke 40 to 50 SUDs (Subjective Units of Discomfort on a 0–100 scale). By the sixth day, the most fearful item is approached. The remaining treatment sessions are devoted to repetitions of all items as well as to situations and objects that were not identified during the assessment period.

Exposure hierarchies for washers tend to be more straightforward than those for checkers. A typical hierarchy for a washer whose contaminants are urine and feces will be as follows: general floors, bathroom doorknobs and light switches, bathroom faucets, objects that have been in contact with the bathroom floor, the bathroom floor itself, toilets, urine, and feces. The hierarchies are more varied for checkers. If the individual is concerned with the dangers embedded in unsuccessfully turning things off, the hierarchy will focus on those objects that the patient finds most important to be off (e.g., faucets, lights, stove). If the individual is afraid of hitting a pedestrian, then the hierarchy will be driving on a deserted country road, driving in the suburbs, driving in the city, driving by a school at dismissal time, and so forth.

Obviously, the extent of contact and its manner will depend upon the patient's problem. As a rule, washers should handle the contaminant continuously during therapy, touching themselves with it all over. Although modeling has not been shown to enhance outcome in controlled studies, our clinical impressions as well as those of Rachman and Hodgson (1980) suggest that for some patients this procedure clearly helps. Through modeling, the therapist demonstrates the desirable manner of exposure. For example, in modeling exposure to a toilet rim the therapist will touch the rim with *both* hands and *rub them* on the rim. He or she then will rub his or her hands over his or her clothes, face, lips, hair, and so forth. The patient is then asked to follow the therapist's actions. It should be noted that patients should not be physically forced into contact they fear. Verbal persuasion and coaching will overcome resistance in most cases. However, in the face of persistent refusal to comply with exposure instructions, treatment should be discontinued. Out of more than 125 patients treated in our center, only a handful have dropped out during treatment. More often, patients refuse to enter treatment; once committed, however, they rarely refuse to follow exposure instructions.

Patients are requested to expose themselves to their main contaminants or feared situations. For example, patients who are afraid of feces will be asked to touch a piece of toilet paper with a small residue of his or her own feces on it. Clinical observation suggests that failure to directly contact the most feared situation is likely to result in relapse.

Exposure with checkers requires somewhat greater ingenuity. If the individual is afraid that switches and stoves are not actually turned off or that doors are not locked, we do *not* have them repeatedly turn switches on and off or lock and unlock doors because this is what they usually do. Instead, we may have them do each activity once, but "incorrectly," and then move immediately to another activity. For example, a patient will be asked to turn the stove on and off without inspecting the stove and then leave. It is important that the therapist also refrain from inspecting the stove because a checker may then assign responsibility to the therapist for checking the stove properly. If the patient is an orderer, then exposure involves changing the order of things in the home, placing objects in disturbing positions.

Although obsessive-compulsives tend to be honest in their reports, they often engage in minor avoidances. The therapist should be alert to the manner in which exposure is carried out. Does the patient touch the contaminant with *both hands*?

Does he or she wipe his or her hands *on the same part* of his or her body before continuing to contaminate the rest of himself or herself?

After each session, the patient is assigned 4 hours of homework that consists of repeating what had been accomplished during the session. If the patient cannot devote a single block of 4 hours, he or she may engage in exposure exercises for 2 hours at a time because long exposures have been found more effective than short ones. For a washer, homework assignments consist of holding contaminated objects and touching other household items with them (e.g., clothing, dishes, doors, family members, etc.) as well as carrying a contaminated object in his or her pocket. For a checker, homework might entail improperly checking the house and then leaving or driving without looking in the rearview mirror.

How difficult a patient will find exposure *in vivo* is somewhat hard to predict. Some patients with a 50-year history of severe checking or washing rituals have reported little discomfort during treatment. Others become highly anxious. When patients complain about their suffering, the therapist can acknowledge the difficulty of the treatment and reinforce their continued efforts at confrontation. A reminder that anxiety eventually decreases is helpful in maintaining motivation. It is important that the patient sense that the therapist is aware of and sympathetic to the degree of pain he or she is experiencing. Many patients will note that the exposure requirements do not correspond to "normal" behavior. The therapist should agree with the patient's observations and reexplain the treatment rationale (see later example).

Patients may request reassurance that their disastrous consequences will not occur. If such questions take a form of ritualist requests for reassurance, they should not be reinforced. Instead, the therapist should inform the patient that his feared disastrous consequence could, in fact, occur but emphasize that the likelihood of such an occurrence is low. Repeated questioning following such a discussion should be ignored in order to extinguish this ritual.

Exposure in Imagination

Many patients expend great effort to avoid fearful thoughts and images. Some who are capable of describing in considerable detail their daily rituals and avoidances are loath to describe their feared disasters. If a patient is afraid of harming her family, she might have the thought "I might stab my children," yet spend no time in elaborating on this thought. Similarly, if a patient is afraid of his house burning down with his family in it, he may never have imagined such a scenerio in detail. The main purpose of imaginal exposure is to expose the patient to the imagined feared consequences of exposure.

As with *in vivo* exposure, imaginal scenes are presented in a hierarchical order. The scenes should include as much detail as possible to make them realistic and vivid. The therapist may want to use the patient's *in vivo* homework as a starting point. The scene usually includes a description of the physical setting and circumstances and all of the patient's real and imagined disasters, his or her physiological anxiety reactions, and the kinds of thoughts he or she might have during the situation. A single scene is repeated for at least 40 minutes during a treatment session. It is described by the therapist and is taped so the patient can listen to it between sessions. At 10-minute intervals the therapist interrupts the scene to ask for an anxiety rating (0 to 100) and to have the patient describe the scene. This procedure encourages the patient to pay closer attention to the scene and provides the therapist with the opportunity to learn whether the presented image matches his or her internal fear concepts. The therapist can then use this information to enhance the vividness and validity of the scene for the patient.

Some patients report little anxiety during imaginal exposure, whereas others will report considerable discomfort, showing signs of distress such as shaking or crying. For most patients, anxiety elicited by the scenes decreases within and across sessions, and this decrement is related to outcome. But a number of patients who have benefited from imaginal exposure have responded atypically. A few patients treated with imaginal exposure alone did not habituate within or between sessions, yet they reported lasting reductions in ritualistic behavior and in the anxiety elicited by real-life situations. One patient reported using imaginal exposure as a coping response. That is, whenever confronted by the urge to ritualize, he would engage in imaginal exposure until the urge left him. Over time, he reported that he was no longer anxious when confronted with feared situations. Another client found that the imaginal exposure helped her to realize the absurdity of her rituals, and this realization removed both her anxiety and her urge to ritualize. High levels of anxiety typically indicate good attention and reduction of discomfort within a session and usually indicate processing of the scenes, whereas boredom experienced in later scenes is indicative of habituation across sessions.

What follow are segments of scenes from two patients. The first scene was constructed for the patient described earlier who frequently checked his mouth for cancerous lumps and who feared uncertainty regarding having cancer.

> You are sitting at the breakfast table. While you are eating you accidentally feel a lump on your cheek. You want to check it again, but remember that you have agreed not to do so. As you are sitting at the table you can feel your heart begin to speed up and your hands begin to sweat. You think to yourself, "What if I really have cancer. If I don't check this lump now, I might have cancer. And later the doctor will tell me how stupid I was for not coming sooner. But no, I can't allow myself to check again, even if it means I do have cancer. I wish I knew whether or not this is cancer. If I have cancer on my cheek, they may have to cut away part of my face."
>
> Two weeks have passed, and you still have not checked the lump on your cheek. You are in a state of constant panic, always thinking, "I really should check it. If I do maybe the fear will go away. No, I can't do that, because I remember how much worse I was before treatment. I just have to take the risk. Even though today is my scheduled yearly dental appointment I won't mention the lump I felt 2 weeks ago. I've been so conscious of it; it even feels like it hurts."
>
> In the scene the patient eventually sits in the dentist's chair where the dentist says, "My God! Why didn't you come in sooner? You have a lump on your cheek. Does it hurt at all?" You reply, "Yes." "Well, I think we should order a biopsy, because this lump looks suspicious. You should have come sooner. I don't understand how you could be so irresponsible. If it is cancer, I hope it

isn't too late. You should have called sooner." You feel your heart pounding in your chest. So many thoughts are going through your mind that you are having difficulty thinking. "Do I have cancer? What if they have to operate. Will the surgery be major or minor." You ask the dentist, "Do you think it is cancer and if so how serious?" "All I can say," he replies, "Is that it might be. As to how serious, well, if it is, you'll have to consult with a specialist."

The following scene was presented to a washer who was afraid of contracting and spreading disease after contact with feces.

You are walking down the street in front of your house. You are looking at the big weeping willow tree on your lawn when all of a sudden you feel your foot step on something soft; it's dog feces. You look down and see your dirty shoe and think to yourself, "Why didn't I look where I was walking. If I had been more careful this would never have happened." Your first impulse is to throw the shoes away and go home and shower. You can feel your anxiety rising. It is hard to remember the things that you learned in treatment. You start to think, "If I don't clean this off properly, my children will get sick, and it will be my fault. If only I had been looking where I was going! But no, I've got to take the risk. I'm only allowed to wipe my shoes on the grass like everyone else." You wipe your shoe on the grass and can't see any feces on your shoe. Rather than being relieved, this makes you more upset since you now have no good reason to wash the shoes. You go home and walk into your house. Just as you enter, your son, Stevie, comes running to greet you and trips over your contaminated shoe and lands on the floor where you just walked. You can feel your heart beginning to speed up and your palms are sweating. Your anxiety level continues to rise. You want to clean your son's hands but know you can't. Before you have the chance to say anything, he gets up and hugs you with his now contaminated hands. You think to yourself, "What if he gets sick, it will be my fault. Should I watch him to see what he touches?" But it is already too late. He has run off to another room. You suddenly realize that you were so distracted and worried that you took off the coat he contaminated and hung it in the closet. You desperately try to remember if you touched the spots he contaminated. "What if he gets sick because of my stepping in the dog feces? Did I touch that spot on my coat?" You remember that during treatment you would have actually had to touch your shoe. You feel so anxious and don't want to do this, but you realize that for the way you're thinking you need to do this. You take the shoe off and hold it with both hands and then proceed to go and make dinner. Throughout dinner you feel sick. With every bite all you can think about is the dog feces. You watch your family eat, but you stop because you feel nauseous. That night, time passes so slowly because you are so anxious you can't fall asleep. About two o'clock in the morning you hear your son begin to moan. You go into his room and feel his head. It is hot and sweaty. You begin to panic. The anxiety is so painful that you are having difficulty thinking straight. You don't know what to do. You run to your bedroom to get your husband. You go to wake him up and find that he also is hot and sweaty. Even worse, he doesn't respond to your shaking him. You think that you should have thrown those shoes away because look what is happening now. You feel very upset. You wonder whether it will help washing your hands now. You start to try to think of everything you've touched since you came in the house. You remember hanging your coat in the closet. Suddenly, you realize that your family is sick and you, instead of helping them, have been obsessing. Should you check their condition or should you call an ambulance? You can't think straight. Should you wash your hands before you touch the phone?

Response prevention is employed to block overt rituals. For covert rituals, patients are encouraged to turn their thoughts to the internal fear cues and engage in imaginal exposure. Response prevention is a procedure that requires that the patient stop engaging in any ritualistic activity. Because obsessive-compulsives can often delay their rituals for some time, it is important that response prevention be very strict and prolonged. A typical protocol for a washer is as follows:

1. The patient should take one 10-minute shower every 5 days. Immediately following the shower, the patient is to recontaminate himself or herself.
2. Clothing must be worn for at least 2 consecutive days; underwear may be changed daily.
3. The patient is not to engage in any handwashing; this means no washing of hands after contact wtih contaminants as well as after using the bathroom or before meals.
4. Illegal handwashes are to be followed by exposure to the contaminant that elicited it.
5. No cleaning of anything to prevent contamination is permitted.
6. The family is no longer permitted to engage in avoidance behavior or ritualistic activities formerly carried out at the patient's request.

Other types of grooming activities will be restricted only if they are of a ritualistic nature. For example, use of deodorant is permitted unless body odor is an obsession. Likewise, if washing the laundry is not a compulsion, the patient may engage in it. However, the patient will not be allowed to directly touch wet clothing because this might provide some relief from contamination.

The application of response prevention to checkers is less standardized and requires more ingenuity. The patient who checks continually in the rearview mirror should drive without using it; the patient who is afraid he will accidentally write "I am a homosexual" on his checks and therefore opens and closes the envelopes repeatedly before mailing them is required to write many checks, enclose them in their envelopes, and send them without reopening them.

Many patients comply readily with response prevention instructions. However, because of the stress it creates, it is desirable to designate a supervisor who will provide support when the patient experiences strong urges to ritualize. The role of the supervisor, then, is *not* to physically stop the patient from ritualizing but to encourage him or her to follow the treatment procedures. Most patients do not cheat. When patients do fail to comply with response prevention restrictions, they typically admit it to the therapist. Both the therapist and home supervisors should assume a supporting role rather than policing the patient's conduct.

Treatment of Washing Rituals: The Case of Susan

Susan was a 27-year-old white married woman, mother to a 2-year-old daughter. At the time that she sought treatment in our center, she had not been working in her profession as a registered nurse for 18 months due to obsessive-compulsive systems. She also reported marital difficulties that she attributed in part to her symptoms and in part to her husband's failure to establish himself in a career; he was employed as a janitor.

Assessment

The first session focused primarily on delineating the nature of the main complaint. Questions are thus directed at the presenting problem, that is, the fear cues, the avoidance patterns, and the relationship between them. An example of such an inquiry is given next.

T: Why don't we start with what brings you here.
C: I wash my hands all of the time—I don't know why I do it. It doesn't make any sense at all, but I just can't stop myself.
T: What kinds of things make you wash?
C: Too many things. It's all crazy. I'm embarrassed to talk about it—it's so stupid.
T: Do you wash because certain things make you feel uneasy, dirty?
C: Yes.
T: What kinds of things?
C: Anything that can have a disease called *pseudomonis*.
T: What is pseudomonis?
C: It's a very contagious disease. I learned about it as a nurse. You have to take all kinds of sanitary precautions if you work around it. But I never used to be worried about it. I don't know what has happened to me. I do all these strange things, and I can't stop myself. Do you know why I do these things?
T: If you mean do I know how it all started, the answer is no. If you are asking why do you keep doing these things, I think I can explain it. I assume that whenever you come into contact with something that you think is contaminated with pseudomonis, you become very anxious.
C: [*Nods*] Yes.
T: We all have learned that when we come in contact with a contagious disease we need to wash ourselves. When you think you have been infected with pseudomonis, and you get extremely anxious, you wash and then you feel safer and less fearful. In this way you have learned that washing reduces your anxiety. You wash even when you know it is senseless in order to feel better.
C: But isn't it crazy for me to become so anxious?
T: Do you mean crazy like you are going to lose complete control of yourself and lose touch with reality?
C: Yes, I'm so afraid that I won't be able to handle the anxiety. I feel like I'm going to explode.
T: I can answer you that you are not crazy. In fact, your washing makes perfect sense in view of your belief that you'll go crazy if you will be very anxious. Also, if you believe that pseudomonis can be contracted by indirect contact no matter how remote the contact is, it is no surprise that you feel threatened and therefore wash so much.

The rest of the session was spent exploring Susan's rituals and some of the stimuli that elicited them. Briefly, whenever she felt contaminated, Susan would wash her hands up to her elbows. Before washing she would first clean the faucets and the sink that she had contaminated with her "dirty" hands. She would then scrub her hands, one finger at a time, slowly working her way up to the elbows. When the ritual was uninterrupted, the entire procedure would be completed in 20 minutes. On "bad days" or when her concentration during the ritual was interrupted, Susan would have to start over and over again, finding herself washing as much as 3 hours continuously. This excessive washing caused extensive damage to her hands and forearms.

At the end of the first session, Susan was given a number of questionnaires, including the Beck Depression Inventory, to be completed at home. She was also asked to compile a list of situations and objects that elicited an urge to wash.

During Sessions 2 and 3, a brief psychiatric history was obtained as well as information about the onset of symptoms. Part of these sessions as well as Session 4 were devoted to planning the treatment. This included establishing a hierarchy of situations for exposure and identifying the avoidance responses to be blocked. A partial list of these situations and the corresponding anxiety discomfort (SUDs) ratings are given next.

Anything belonging to a pseudomonis patient	100
Hospital staff working with pseudomonis patients	95
Being in a hospital or touching objects from a hospital	90
Public restrooms	80
Restaurants	75
Food stores	70
Fresh produce	60
Canned foods	50
Nonfood items from a supermarket	40
The park two blocks from her house	30

The treatment program was discussed with Susan.

T: Well, let's talk about what we need to do during treatment.

C: Do you think I'm hopeless?

T: No, but treatment will be quite difficult. As I describe the treatment you may feel that you could not possibly go through it. I think you will find that you are much stronger than you believe. Let me first describe how treatment works, okay? Let me start with an example of a problem different from yours. Suppose you were afraid of cats and . . .

C: I wish I was, that seems so much easier.

T: Cat phobics may feel just as bad. Other people's problems always seem better. Anyway, every time you saw a cat you would become frightened. Now, a "natural" way to handle this fear is to run every time you find yourself near a cat. The only problem with this solution is that you keep on running away. With time the problem might get worse. You may grow to fear not only cats 2 feet away from you but also ones that are two blocks away. Eventually, you find yourself devoting much of your energy to searching for cats to run away from. Now suppose I take a cat and put it in your lap. What would happen?

C: I'd hit the ceiling.

T: Right, because you haven't been within two blocks of a cat for quite some time, and now you are sitting here with a cat in your lap. You are going to be pretty anxious. You have two choices: you can throw the cat off your lap and run away. Or, you could decide to sit there with the cat in your lap. Sooner or later, the anxiety will drop. The problem is that anxiety usually gets worse before it gets better. Basically, you will suffer a lot in the short run, but in the long run you won't have to have your life so restricted.

C: You really think I can do this?

T: Yes.

C: What happens if I refuse to touch something?

T: You will continue to have your problem. I know the treatment is very difficult. Therefore, I will give you my home and my office number and you can call anytime, day or night, whenever you need my help to overcome difficult moments.

C: I appreciate that. [*Smiles*] I hope you don't mind calls at three o'clock in the morning.

The three components of treatment were then described. Susan was given the rules for response prevention as described earlier, and the planned schedule of exposures was discussed. The imaginal scenes were hierarchically arranged. In the early scenes, she imagined that she and her daughter *might* have pseudomonis. In the most anxiety-provoking fantasy, Susan was asked to imagine that she and her daughter had actually contracted the disease due to her negligence. In this last image her daughter dies, and she is close to death.

After describing the treatment, the therapist discussed the expected results after 3 weeks of intensive treatment.

T: After the 3 weeks you will get used to not washing. However, you may still have some obsessive thoughts that make you feel somewhat anxious. These will become less frequent over time. For some people this process takes 2 months; others report that it takes a year. It will be very important for you to continue to use the techniques you learned in treatment. Whenever you need it, I can see you periodically to help you make further progress.

C: Will I ever be completely free of my symptoms?

T: It is possible, but for some the symptoms periodically reappear. You can, however, prevent it from controlling your life. Patients seem to slip in ways similar to alcoholics. One day they are hit by terrible anxiety and find themselves ritualizing. Rather than applying what they learned in treatment they say to themselves: "I'm back where I started, so I may as well give up." This, of course, doesn't make sense. Of course you can overcome the problem again, but the longer you wait the harder you will have to work to regain control.

C: So I will always be a sickie.

T: That's not what I said. You will have periods of being symptom free, but there may be times when the symptoms return to some degree.

Treatment

In the first session, Susan's anxiety during imaginal exposure went as high as 70 and dropped to 40 by the end of the exposure. The interchange at the beginning of the first *in vivo* session went as follows:

C: I'm really anxious. My SUDs is about 80 even before we start.

T: Starting is really difficult because you don't know what to expect and how you'll feel during or after the exposure. Are you ready? Let's start with the nonfood products from the store. I have a package of paper plates and a can opener. Ready?

C: Okay?

The therapist handled the unwashed package of plates and the can opener. He touched the items to his hair, face, and clothing and then gave them to Susan.

T: Now you do exactly what I did. [*She does so*] What's your level of anxiety?

C: About 35.

T: What happened to the 80?

C: It wasn't as bad as I thought it would be.

T: That's good. Many people find that to be the case. Anticipating exposure is usually worse than the actual event. I will keep pointing this out to you, since it is anticipatory fear that leads to extreme avoidance behavior.

By the end of the session, Susan had exposed herself to canned foods and boxed foods. That is, the containers were opened, and she touched the contents. Food was more frightening because she felt it would provide a medium for the germs to grow in. She considered boxed foods to be worse because boxes are more permeable than cans. For homework she was asked to listen to the taped imaginal exposure from that day's session and to expose everything in her house, including her daugher, to the contaminated food for another 3 hours.

Sessions 2 through 4 were uneventful. Susan's responses to imaginal exposure typically rose to a level of 80 to 90 and then dropped to a level of 20 to 35. The content of the scenes moved from suspicions that she and her daughter had pseudomonis to having very mild cases to having severe cases. She reported one "illegal" handwash that lasted for 5 minutes. This occurred after going to the bathroom to urinate. After some coaxing by her husband, she agreed to recontaminate herself by touching her genitals with both hands. Exposure *in vivo* progressed from food items to eating a meal in a restaurant, to touching the water inside public restrooms in gas stations. Homework involved taking the most contaminated object she could find in each situation and bringing it home to contaminate everything.

The plan for Session 5 had been to omit the imaginal exposure in order to allow more time for exposure to the hospital parking lot to which the therapist drove with the patient.

C: I can't do this. I'm too anxious.

T: How anxious are you?

C: One hundred.

T: You couldn't be more anxious than you are now?

C: No, I couldn't.

T: How about the days you used to spend sitting in bed naked, paralyzed with fear? Are you that anxious?

C: No.

T: Then you can't be 100.

C: Then I'm 95. What's the difference? I'm never going to get over this. This is a hospital. You can't guarantee that I won't get pseudomonis.

T: That's right, I can't. On the other hand, I don't know how much your precautions protect you. What I do know is that you can get over this problem.

C: I don't want to have anything to do with hospitals. Why don't we just work on other things. I can live a normal life that way.

T: No you can't. If you don't try to conquer this, sooner or later the fear of contamination will spread, and you will lose all that you have gained. Or perhaps your daughter will have to go the hospital for a broken leg or a tonsillectomy, and you won't be able to be there to support her. We are a block away, would you be able to get out of my car and just stand here?

C: Yes.
T: Well, then let's do it [*Susan and the therapist got out of the car*]. Can you take one step closer to the parking lot?

After 20 minutes of progressing in this manner Susan was able to walk on the parking lot.

Because of Susan's high level of anxiety, exposing her to a pseudomonis patient was delayed to Session 8 as opposed to our usual procedure of reaching the highest item by Session 5 or 6. For each session, there was a repeat of the dialogue presented before in Session 5, but coaxing required less and less time. Convincing her to touch a pseudomonis patient took only 15 minutes. Because she had become quite competent at making her own flooding tapes, we decided that she could spend 1 hour of her homework time either making or listening to her own flooding tapes.

During the remaining sessions, Susan and her therapist went to different hospitals looking for pseudomonis patients, touching hospital toilets, eating in hospital cafeterias, and so on. By the end of treatment, these situations elicited an anxiety level of only 20. She had experienced very little difficulty with the implementation of response prevention procedures throughout treatment.

At the end of the third week of treatment, the therapist visited Susan's home twice, contaminating the entire house with items from hospitals. A daily posttreatment routine was programmed. Susan was allowed to take a daily 10-minute shower and was to contaminate herself as soon as she was done. She was also permitted five handwashes per day lasting for no more than 30 seconds. These, too, were to be followed by some kind of contamination. She was not allowed to wash any food with the exception of fresh produce.

Follow-Up

Susan decided to be seen weekly to help maintain her treatment gains. After the intensive part of treatment, she found that her behavior was under control, but she still obsessed about pseudomonis and had mild urges to ritualize. The intensity of these symptoms was further reduced over time. During this follow-up period she also worked on assertiveness. Four months after the intensive part of treatment, Susan decided to divorce her husband. During the first 2 weeks of separation she reported a flare up of obsessive-compulsive symptoms; for 2 days she engaged in very severe washing after which response prevention and exposure were instituted.

Complications during Treatment

Potential problems and difficulties in the implementation of treatment by exposure and response prevention are discussed in this section.

Noncompliance

Despite patients' initial concerns about their ability to tolerate confrontation with contaminants and at the same time comply with the demands of response prevention, they must follow the treatment regimen. Although only a few patients fail to abide by the agreed-upon rules, a larger number try to bend them. Failure to resist rituals and persistence in avoidance patterns lead, of course, to poor outcome.

It is quite rare for a patient to actively conceal ritualistic activity from the therapist. If ritualizing continues, the patient should be confronted with the implications of this conduct for treatment outcome. If noncompliance persists, treatment should be discontinued with the understanding that the patient may return when he or she is prepared to follow the treatment regimen. It is preferable to stop treatment than to continue under unfavorable conditions where failure is likely to occur, leaving the patient hopeless about future prospects for improvement.

Although direct violation of response prevention instructions is relatively rare, the replacement of prohibited rituals with less obvious avoidance patterns is quite common. For example, one man found that use of deodorant served to "decontaminate" him almost as successfully as actual washing. Inadvertently, he disclosed the anxiety-reducing properties of the deodorant to the therapist who, of course, banned its use. Other examples of replacement rituals include brushing off hands and "blowing off" germs. These can be discovered by direct questioning. Although they may be only minimally intrusive, these rituals must be prevented in order for the patient to learn that anxiety decreases in the *total absence* of rituals.

Another problem is posed by individuals who carry out the required exposure without ritualizing but continue to engage in unreported and sometimes unnoticed passive avoidance behaviors. Examples include placing "contaminated" clothing back in the closet for a second wearing but making certain it does not touch the clean garments and delaying entry or departure from a public bathroom until another person heads for the door, thereby eliminating the need to touch the doorknob. Such behaviors reflect an ambivalent attitude toward treatment, and in this respect they are predictors for failure. Their persistence hinders habituation of anxiety to feared situations and may leave the patient with the erroneous belief that such avoidance protects him or her from harm. Failure to give up avoidance patterns also calls for a reevaluation of continuation in treatment.

Familial Patterns

Family members have typically experienced years of frustration with the patient's symptomatology. It is not surprising that some are impatient, expecting treatment to result in total symptom remission; when this does not happen, they are disappointed and angry. Conversely, some family members continue to protect the patient from formerly upsetting situations. Years of accommodation to the patient's peculiar requests have established habits that are hard to break. Maintaining such familial patterns may offset progress in treatment or interfere with maintenance of gains and may require the application of family therapy.

Many obsessive-compulsives have become nonfunctional as their symptomatology occupies an increasing proportion of their time. Successful treatment leaves them with a considerable void in their daily routine. Assistance in the development of new skills and the planning of both social and occupational activities should be the focus of follow-up therapy in these cases.

A complicating factor is the patient's concern that the new ventures may fail, which often prevents him or her from acquiring necessary skills or making needed overtures. Failure to resume a functional life-style would most likely have resulted in relapse.

Depression

Marked depression is likely to interfere with the ability of some to habituate to feared situations, perhaps by heightening their anxiety during exposure (Foa *et al.*, 1983). It may be that when patients are exceedingly fearful, they are incapable of processing the information that is inherent in the exposure situation, and thus discomfort persists unabated (Foa & Kozak, 1984). High general anxiety was also found to hinder treatment efficacy for some individuals, although not for others. Given the present state of knowledge, we suggest that if patients are highly depressed and do not evidence anxiety reduction during the first two or three sessions of exposure treatment, antidepressant medications should be tried.

Overvalued Ideation

The patient's belief system regarding the likelihood that the feared consequences will in fact materialize may also interfere with improvement during treatment. Those who firmly believe that their worst fears will come to pass if they fail to protect themselves by ritualizing have been observed not to habituate to feared contaminants across exposure treatment sessions (Foa, 1979). Unfortunately, adequate measures of the degree of conviction have not yet been developed, and little is known about effective treatment manipulations for this difficulty. Perhaps the most difficult task is to have patients accept the fact that they may have some residual symptoms.

Lack of Maintenance Program

Most patients improved markedly immediately after treatment. A sizable portion evidenced some degree of relapse and some (about 20%) lost their gains entirely. In searching for predictors of relapse, we have found that those who improved only partially are more likely to relapse than the very successful patients. Also, patients from out of town did not maintain their gains as well as those living locally. Perhaps the latter had more access to booster treatments and therefore evidenced less relapse.

Many patients report slips (i.e., instances of avoidance or ritualizing). It appears that slips are a necessary but not sufficient condition for relapse. Patients who initiate exposure and response prevention to counteract the slip, either on their own or with the help of others, do not relapse. Therefore, patients should be prepared for such brief return of symptoms.

Summary

The treatment program described here effects marked improvement in most obsessive-compulsive ritualizers. The example provided in this chapter was that of a washer, largely because the description of that treatment program is more straightforward. The results with checkers are not less favorable, although planning a therapy program for them requires some ingenuity. A problem specific to checkers arises when their rituals are performed only in an environment for which they feel responsible and other places do not trigger urges to ritualize. Therefore, treatment with them should often be conducted in their natural settings.

In evaluating the state of the art in the treatment of obsessive-compulsives, we should remember that patients rarely find themselves entirely symptom free at the completion of this regimen. Maintenance of gains is problematic for about 20% of patients (Foa *et al.*, 1983). Relapse is most common among patients who have only improved partially at the end of treatment. Implementation of drugs, specifically antidepressants, in combination with behavioral treatment may improve the prognosis of patients who manifested severe depression at the beginning of treatment. Most importantly, we need to develop maintenance programs that will focus on the patients' interpersonal and occupational adjustment and provide support in their efforts to change from a nonfunctional life-style to a healthy exsistence.

References

American Psychiatric Association. (1980). *Diagnostic and statistical manual of mental disorders* (3rd ed.). Washington, DC: Author.

Beck, A. T., & Beamesderfer, A. (1974). Assessment of depression: The depression inventory. In P. Pichot (Ed.), *Psychological measures in psychopharmacology.* (Reprinted from *Modern Problems in Pharmacopsychiatry,* 1974, *7,* 151–169.

Beech, H., & Vaughan, M. (1978). *Behavioral treatment of obsessional states.* New York: Wiley.

Boulougouris, J. C. (1977). Variables affecting the behavior modifications of obsessive-compulsive patients treated by flooding. In J. C. Boulougouris & A. D. Rabavilas (Eds.), *The treatment of phobic and obsessive-compulsive disorders* (pp. 73–84). Oxford: Pergamon Press.

Boulougouris, J., Rabavilas, A., & Stefanis, C. (1977). Psychophysiological responses in obsessive-compulsive neurosis. *Behaviour Research and Therapy, 15,* 221–230.

Breitner, C. (1960). Drug therapy in obsessional states and other psychiatric problems. *Diseases of the Nervous System,* 31–35.

Carr, A. T. (1974). Compulsive neurosis: A review of the literature. *Psychological Bulletin, 81,* 311–318.

Cobb, J. P., McDonald, R., Marks, I. M., & Stern, R. S. (1980). Marital versus exposure treatment for marital plus phobic-obsessive problems. *European Journal of Behavioral Analysis and Modification, 4,* 3–17.

Dollard, J., & Miller, N. E. (1950). *Personality and psychotherapy: An analysis in terms of learning, thinking and culture.* New York: McGraw-Hill.

Doppelt, H. G. (1981). *Personality variables as predictors of treatment outcome of obsessive-compulsives.* Unpublished manuscript.

Emmelkamp, P. M. G., & Kwee, K. G. (1977). Obsessional ruminations: A comparison between thought-stopping and prolonged exposure in imagination. *Behaviour Research and Therapy, 15,* 441–444.

Emmelkamp, P. M. G., & van der Heyden, H. (1980). The treatment of harming obsessions. *Behavioural Analysis and Modification, 4,* 28–35.

Emmelkamp, P. M. G., van der Helm, van Zanten, B. L., & Plochy, I. (1980). Contributions of self-instructional training to the effectiveness of exposure *in vivo:* A comparison with obsessive-compulsive patients. *Behaviour Research and Therapy, 18,* 61–66.

Foa, E. B. (1979). Treatment of obsessive-compulsives with prolonged exposure and strict response prevention. *Archives of Greek Association for Behavioral Modification and Research, 1,* 5–17.

Foa, E. B., & Kozak, M. J. (1984). *Emotional processing of fear: Exposure to corrective information.* Unpublished manuscript.

Foa, E. B., Steketee, G., & Milby, J. B. (1980). Differential effect of exposure and response prevention in obsessive-compulsive washers. *Journal of Consulting and Clinical Psychology, 48,* 71–79.

Foa, E. B., Steketee, G., Turner, R. M., & Fischer, S. C. (1980). Effects of imaginal exposure to feared disasters in obsessive-compulsive checkers. *Behaviour Research and Therapy, 18,* 449–455.

Foa, E. B., Steketee, G., Grayson, J. B., & Doppelt, H. G. (1983). Treatment of obsessive-compulsives: When do we fail? In E. B. Foa & P. M. G. Emmelkamp (Eds.), *Failures in behavior therapy* (pp. 10–34). New York: Wiley.

Foa, E. B., Steketee, G., Grayson, J. B., Turner, R. M., & Latimer, P. (1984). Deliberate exposure and blocking of obsessive-compulsive rituals: Immediate and long term effects. *Behavior Therapy, 15,* 450–472.

Foa, E. B., Steketee, G., & Ozarow, B. J. (in press). Behavior therapy with obsessive-compulsives: From theory to treatment. In M. Mavissakalian (Ed.), *Obsessive-compulsive disorders: Psychological and pharmacological treatment* (pp. 49–129). New York: Plenum Press.

Grimshaw, L. (1965). The outcome of obsessional disorder, a follow-up study of 100 cases. *British Journal of Psychiatry, 111,* 1051–1056.

Hamilton, M. (1960). A rating scale for depression. *Journal of Neurological and Neurosurgical Psychiatry, 23,* 56–62.

Herrnstein, R. J. (1969). Method and theory in the study of avoidance. *Psychological Review, 76,* 49–69.

Hodgson, R., & Rachman, S. (1972). The effects of contamination and washing in obsessional patients. *Behaviour Research and Therapy, 10,* 111–117.

Hodgson, R., Rachman, S., & Marks, I. M. (1972). The treatment of chronic obsessive-compulsive neurosis: Follow-up and further findings. *Behaviour Research and Therapy, 10,* 181–189.

Hornsveld, R. H. J., Kraaimaat, F. W., & van Dam Baggen, R. M. J. (1979). Anxiety/discomfort and handwashing in obsessive-compulsive and psychiatric control patients. *Behaviour Research and Therapy, 17,* 223–228.

Kringlen, E. (1965). Obsessional neurotics, a long term follow-up. *British Journal of Psychiatry, 111,* 709–722.

Lang, P. J. (1979). A bio-informational theory of emotional imagery. *Psychophysiology, 6,* 495–511.

Makhlouf-Norris, F., & Norris, H. (1972). The obsessive-compulsive syndrome as a neurotic device for the reduction of self-uncertainty. *British Journal of Psychiatry, 121,* 277–288.

Makhlouf-Norris, F., Jones, H. G., & Norris, H. (1970). Articulation of the conceptual structure in obsessional neurosis. *British Journal of Social and Clinical Psychology, 9,* 264–274.

Marks, I. M., Stern, R. S., Mawson, D., Cobb, J., & McDonald, R. (1980). Clomipramine and exposure for obsessive-compulsive rituals. *British Journal of Psychiatry, 136,* 1–25.

Marlatt, G. A., & Donovan, D. M. (1982). Behavioral psychology approaches to alcoholism. In E. M. Pattison & E. Kaufman (Eds.), *Encyclopedic handbook of alcoholism* (pp. 560–580). New York: Gardner Press.

McFall, M. E., & Wollersheim, J. P. (1979). Obsessive-compulsive neurosis: A cognitive behavioral formulation and approach to treatment. *Cognitive Therapy and Research, 3,* 333–348.

Meyer, V. (1966). Modification of expectancies in cases with obsessional rituals. *Behaviour Research and Therapy, 4,* 273–280.

Meyer, V., & Levy, R. (1973). Modification of behavior in obsessive-compulsive disorders. In H. E. Adams & P. Unikel (Eds.), *Issues and trends in behavior therapy* (pp. 77–137). Springfield, IL: Charles C Thomas.

Meyer, V., Levy, R., & Schnurer, A. (1974). The behavioral treatment of obsessive-compulsive disorders. In H. R. Beech (Ed.), *Obsessional states* (pp. 233–259). London: Methuen.

Milner, A. D., Beech, H. R., & Walker, V. J. (1971). Decision processes and obsessional behaviour. *British Journal of Social and Clinical Psychology, 10,* 88–89.

Mowrer, O. (1939). A stimulus-response analysis of anxiety and its role as a reinforcing agent. *Psychological Review, 46,* 553–565.

Persons, J. B., & Foa, E. B. (1984). Thinking processes in obsessive compulsives. *Behaviour Research and Therapy, 22,* 259–265.

Rabavilas, A. D., & Boulougouris, J. C. (1974). Physiological accompaniments of ruminations, flooding and thought-stopping in obsessive patients. *Behaviour Research and Therapy, 12,* 239–243.

Rachman, S. (1971). Obsessional ruminations. *Behaviour Research and Therapy, 9,* 229–235.

Rachman, S. (1976). Obsessional-compulsive checking. *Behaviour Research and Therapy, 14,* 269–277.

Rachman, S., & Hodgson, R. (1980). *Obsessions and compulsions.* Englewood Cliffs, NJ: Prentice-Hall.

Rachman, S. J., & Wilson, G. T. (1980). *The effects of psychological therapy.* Oxford: Pergamon Press.

Rachman, S. J., Cobb, J., Grey, S., McDonald, B., Mawson, D., Sartory, G., & Stern, R. (1979). The behavioral treatment of obsessional-compulsive disorders with and without clomipramine. *Behaviour Research and Therapy, 17,* 467–478.

Reed, G. F. (1968). Some formal qualities of obsessional thinking. *Psychiatria Clinica, 1,* 382–392.

Reed, G. F. (1969). "Underinclusion"—A characteristic of obsessional personality disorder, II. *British Journal of Psychiatry, 115,* 787–790.

Roper, G., & Rachman, S. (1976). Obsessional-compulsive checking: Experimental replication and development. *Behaviour Research and Therapy, 14,* 25–32.

Roper, G., Rachman, S., & Hodgson, R. (1973). An experiment on obsessional checking. *Behaviour Research and Therapy, 11,* 271–277.

Sher, K. K., Frost, R. O., & Otto, R. (1983). Cognitive deficits in compulsive checkers: An exploratory study. *Behaviour Research and Therapy, 21,* 357–364.

Spielberger, C. D., Gorsuch, R. L., & Lushene, R. G. (1970). *The State-Trait Anxiety Inventory.* Palo Alto, CA: Consulting Psychologists Press.

Steketee, G., & Foa, E. B. (1984). Behavioral treatment of obsessive-compulsive disorders. In D. Barlow (Ed.), *Behavioral treatment of adult disorders* (pp. 69–144). New York: Guilford Press.

Steketee, G., Foa, E. B., & Grayson, J. B. (1982). Recent advances in the behavioral treatment of obsessive compulsives. *Archives of General Psychiatry, 39,* 1365–1371.

Taylor, J. A. (1953). A personality scale of manifest anxiety. *The Journal of Abnormal and Social Psychology, 48,* 285–290.

Teasdale, Y. D. (1974). Learning models of obsessional-compulsive disorder. In H. R. Beech (Ed.), *Obsessional states* (pp. 197–232). London: Methuen.

Watts, F. (1971). *An investigation of imaginal desensitization as an habituation process.* Unpublished doctoral dissertation, University of London.

Guidelines for Planning a Treatment Program

I. *Information Gathering*
  1. *Obsessions*
     a. *External Cues*
        Specifically elicit information about objects or situations which provoke high anxiety or discomfort—e.g., urine, pesticides, locking a door.
     b. *Internal Cues*
        1) Inquire about *thoughts, images, or impulses* that provoke anxiety, shame, or disgust—e.g., images of Christ's penis, numbers, impulses to stab one's child.
        2) Inquire about *bodily sensations* that disturb the patient—e.g., tachycardia, pains, swallowing.
     c. *Consequences of External and Internal Cues*
        1) Elicit information about possible harm that can be caused by the *external object or situation*—e.g., disease from touching a contaminated object, burglary if a door is not properly locked.
        2) Elicit fears about harm caused by *internal cues*—from:
           a) Thoughts, images, or impulses, e.g., "God will punish me. I may actually stab my child."
           b) Bodily sensations, e.g., "I'll lose control."
           c) From the long-term experience of high anxiety, e.g., "This anxiety will never go away and I'll always be highly upset."
           d) *Strength of Belief System*—Assess the degree to which the patient believes that the feared consequences may actually occur. What is the objective probability that confrontation with feared cues will actually result in psychological or physical harm?
  2. *Avoidance Patterns*
     a. *Passive Avoidance*
        Gather a list of all situations or objects that are avoided—e.g., using public bathrooms, stepping on brown spots on the sidewalk, carrying one's child on a concrete floor, driving. Attend to subtle avoidance practices, e.g., touching doorknobs on the least used surface, driving at times of least traffic.
     b. *Rituals*
        List all ritualistic behaviors including washing, cleaning, checking, repeating an action, ordering objects, requesting reassurance, and cognitive ritual (such as

praying, neutralizing thoughts, "good" numbers). Many patients exhibit more than one type of compulsion.

Pay attention to subtle rituals such as the use of "handiwipes" or lotion to decontaminate hands. Wiping as a short version of a washing ritual.

   c. *Relationship between Avoidance Behaviors and Fear Cues*

   Ascertain the functional relationship between the fear cues and the avoidance associated with it.

  3. *History of the Main Complaint*

    a. Events associated with onset.

    b. Fluctuations in the course of symptoms and events associated with remission and recurrence of symptoms.

    c. Prior coping with symptoms, prior treatment efforts, and resultant effects.

  4. *Mood State*

    a. *Depression*

    Assess the level of depression by clinical interviews and inventory (e.g., Beck Depression Inventory or Hamilton Depression Rating).

    Consider antidepressant medication or cognitive therapy for depressed ratings prior to behavioral treatment.

    b. *Anxiety*

    Consider ameliorating procedures such as anxiolytic drugs. If used, fade their use near the end of treatment.

  5. *General History*

   Include information about relationship with parents, siblings and peers, educational achievements, employment history, dating history, sexual experiences, marital relationship, and medical history.

II. *Treatment Program*

  1. *Decision to Hospitalize*

   During intensive treatment the patient is likely to be temporarily under high stress. Hospitalization should be considered for those who live alone or are in a stressful familial relationship.

  2. *The Use of Prolonged Exposure*

    a. In vivo *exposure for external objects or situations that evoke high levels of anxiety.*

    b. *Imaginal Exposure*

     1) When *in vivo* exposure is practically impossible.

     2) When the feared catastrophes constitute a major component of the patient's fear model. In these cases imaginal exposure is used in combination with *in vivo* exposure.

    c) *Suggestions for Exposure Treatment*

     1) All designated exposure items are arranged hierarchically according to the SUDs (Subjective Units of Discomfort) levels they evoke and are presented in ascending order beginning midway. That is, if the top item evokes 100 SUDs, exposure commences with items at a 50-SUD level; if the top item evokes 80 SUDs, a 40-SUD item is presented first.

     2) A given item should be presented until the anxiety level provoked is reduced by half.

     3) An exposure item should be repeated until it evokes no more than minimal anxiety.

     4) Frequent sessions should be implemented preferably three or more times per week.

     5) Ideally, the intensive treatment program should be terminated when the most feared item has been confronted and provokes only mild anxiety. If substantial gains are not evident after 15 sessions, continuation of intensive treatment should be questioned.

6) Regularly scheduled follow-up sessions are recommended to consolidate treatment gains.

7) For motivated patients, detailed instructions for self-exposure may be sufficient. If the relationship between spouses or family members is good, they can be actively involved in the treatment program.

III. *Homework*

A total of 4 hours of exposure homework are assigned. For patients whose treatment includes imaginal exposure, a tape of that day's fantasy exposure is made for later replay at home; an additional 3 hours of *in vivo* exposure is also assigned.

IV. *Response Prevention*

a. Washers are usually permitted one 10-minute shower every fifth day and no handwashing except under unusual circumstances during the first 2 weeks of treatment. Thereafter, to facilitate learning of normal washing, the therapist may permit one 10-minute shower per day and 30-second handwashings after bathroom use, before meals, and when hands are visibly dirty or greasy.

b. Checkers are allowed one brief check of items that are normally checked after use (e.g., stove, door locks) and no checking of items that are not typically checked by most people.

c. Supervisors at home or in the hospital should not use force to prevent ritualizing but report infractions to the therapist.

III

Depression

Cognitive Approaches

STEVEN D. HOLLON AND VIRGINIA JACOBSON

Introduction

In this chapter, we will outline a cognitive approach to the treatment of clinical depression. In particular, we will focus on cognitive therapy (Beck, 1970; Beck, Rush, Shaw, & Emery, 1979), a time-limited, focused intervention targeted at changing the maladaptive beliefs and dysfunctional attitudes posited by cognitive theorists to be causal and/or maintaining factors in depression.

Cognitive therapy is, despite its name, an integration of behavioral and cognitive change strategies (Hollon & Beck, 1979). As described in the comprehensive treatment manual provided by Beck and colleagues (Beck *et al.,* 1979), the basic thrust of the approach is that the client is encouraged to treat his or her beliefs as hypotheses to be tested, typically utilizing his or her own behaviors to test the validity of those beliefs. In essence, the therapist attempts to engage the client in a process of *collaborative empiricism,* in which the client's own experiences with a series of behavioral "experiments" are utilized to evaluate the accuracy of those beliefs. Conceptually, the approach overlaps to some extent with the more exclusively cognitive *Rational Emotive Therapy* (RET) (Ellis, 1962), although this latter approach appears to rely more heavily on verbal persuasion. The approach also overlaps with the more exclusively behavioral operant, social skills training, and self-control approaches (e.g., Hersen, Eisler, Alford, & Agras, 1973; Lewinsohn,

STEVEN D. HOLLON • Department of Psychology, University of Minnesota and St. Paul-Ramsey Medical Center, Minneapolis, Minnesota 55455. VIRGINIA JACOBSON • Ramsey County Adult Mental Health Center, St. Paul, Minnesota 55101. Presentation of this chapter was supported, in part, by a grant from the National Institute of Mental Health (RO1-MH33209) to the Department of Psychology, University of Minnesota, and to the St. Paul-Ramsey Hospital Medical Education and Research Foundation, Grant No. 6287.

1974; Lewinsohn, Biglan, & Zeiss, 1976; Lewinsohn, Munoz, Youngren, & Zeiss, 1978; Rehm, 1977), particularly in its use of explicit behavioral engineering strategies, but is more likely to tie behavioral change strategies to the hypothesis testing of presumed underlying cognitive mediators. The approach is, in short, an integrated hybrid of behavioral and cognitive change techniques, unified by an underlying cognitive theory of change.

Despite being only recently developed, cognitive therapy has fared well in several carefully controlled clinical trials. Beginning with early trials with depressed student populations (Shaw, 1977; Taylor & Marshall, 1977) and continuing through trials with clinically depressed outpatients (Blackburn, Bishop, Glen, Whalley, & Christie, 1981; Murphy, Simons, Wetzel, & Lustman, 1984; Rush, Beck, Kovacs, & Hollon, 1977), cognitive therapy has consistently outperformed various control conditions and at least equaled, if not exceeded, the performance of various alternate approaches to treatment, including tricyclic pharmacotherapy. There are even indications that cognitive therapy may provide stable skills that reduce the risk of relapse following treatment termination (Hollon, Tuason, Wiemer, DeRubeis, Evans, & Garvey, 1983; Kovacs, Rush, Beck, & Hollon, 1981). There is no indication of any negative interactions when combined with pharmacological treatment, and, perhaps, there is some evidence of superiority over either single modality alone (Beck, Hollon, Bedrosian, & Young, 1984; Blackburn *et al.,* 1981; Hollon *et al.,* 1983).

Clinical Depression

According to Beck (1967), clinical depression can be defined as a nosologic disorder consisting of *change* across five major areas of symptomatology including

1. *Negative Affect:* Typically sadness, unhappiness, and guilt, but, less often, irritability, profound boredom, or other negative affect
2. *Negative Cognitions:* Typically including a negative self-concept, pessimism, and a bleak view of one's surroundings
3. *Negative Motivations:* Including a loss of interest in typically preferred activities and suicidal ideation
4. *Behavioral Changes:* Typically including a reduction in typical rates of behavioral activities
5. *Vegetative Changes:* Typically including insomnia, reduced appetite, and loss of interest in sex

Lehmann (1959) has distinguished between depression defined as a *symptom,* a *syndrome,* and a *nosological disorder.* As a symptom, the term *depression* refers to the negative affective component described previously. Most people experience feeling sad or "blue" from time to time, but such affective states rarely last for any length of time. Thus, depression at the symptomatic level, is problematic only if very severe or very long lasting. Various mood adjective checklists, including Lubin's Depression Adjective Checklist (DACL) (Lubin, 1965) and Zuckerman's

Multiple Affect Adjective Checklist (MAACL) (Zuckerman & Lubin, 1965), probably represent instruments best suited for the assessment of depression at the single affective syumptom level.

Depression as a syndrome typically involves changes in most, if not all, of the five areas listed previously. Most standard rating scales, including Hamilton's Rating Scale for Depression (HRSD) (Hamilton, 1960) and the Raskin Depression Scale (RDS, Raskin, Schulterbrandt, Reating, & McKeon, 1970), and self-report measures, including the Beck Depression Inventory (BDI) (Beck, Ward, Mendelsohn, Mock, & Erbaugh, 1961) and the Zung Self-Rated Depression Scale (SDS) (Zung, 1965), are best suited for quantifying the degree to which the syndrome of depression is present in an individual.

Depression as a nosologic entity involves the presence of the syndrome of depression in the absence of other major types of psychopathologies (e.g., schizophrenia, organicity, substance abuse, etc.). The syndrome of depression is a common concomitant of a variety of other psychiatric disorders, a phenomenon sometimes referred to as secondary depression (Robins & Guze, 1969). As a primary nosologic disorder, depression is regarded to have a consistent syndromatic expression (actually several subsyndromes appear to be present), common course, common prognosis, common etiology (or several particular etiologies), and common treatment response (or several specific patterns of response). In general, depression as a primary nosologic disorder will have a good prognosis and will typically evidence an episodic, time-limited course even if left untreated. Depression secondary to other major types of psychopathologies typically proves either more chronic or, at least, more dependent on the successful resolution of those other problems for its own remission. A subset of primary depressed clients will evidence a somewhat more chronic course, with ongoing chronic dysphoria, typically of only moderate severity, apparent in 20 to 30% of all outpatients.

The differentiation of *depression* from *anxiety* may be particularly problematic. Many depressed clients evidence concomitant anxiety of panic attacks that subside as the depressive episode does. Other clients, particularly those with more chronic anxiety disorders, appear to have depressive episodes superimposed on top of ongoing neurotic disorders. For a number of clients, the early stages of an episode appear to be dominated by the experience of anxiety, with depression coming to the fore as the episode continues its course, with a return to predominant anxiety as the episode nears the end of its course.

The course of a typical episode appears to be about 3 to 6 months in outpatients and 6 to 9 months in inpatients (Beck, 1967). Estimates of the number of clients who will have subsequent episodes range from 50 to 80%, with the higher figures based on longer term follow-up studies that probably better reflect the true prevalence of relapse. A minority of clients will evidence psychotic depressions, defined by the presence of delusions, hallucinations, or stuporous condition. When delusions or hallucinations are present, they are typically mood congruent.

At least two distinctions within the primary nosologic depressions are important. First is the distinction between *bipolar* and *nonbipolar* depressions (Angst, 1966; Depue & Monroe, 1978; Leonhard, 1959; Perris, 1966; Winokur, 1970;

Winokur, Clayton, & Reich, 1969). Bipolar patients are those individuals who ever evidence a manic or hypomanic episode. Typically, such patients also evidence depressive episodes at some point in their lives. Nonbipolar patients (sometimes referred to as *unipolar*) are those patients who have only depressive episodes throughout their lives. At this time, there has been virtually no work done exploring the utility of cognitive therapy with bipolar depressed patients, even during their depressed phases.

The second distinction of note is that between *endogenous* versus *nonendogenous* (also known as reactive, neurotic, or exogenous) depression (Mendels & Cochrane, 1968). Although not so clearly established empirically as the bipolar-nonbipolar distinction, the endogenous-nonendogenous distinction has typically been presumed to have an important bearing on the selection of treatments. *Endogenous depressions* are those episodes evidencing a particular syndromal pattern dominated by vegetative signs and symptoms. The classic endogenous pattern typically involves a distinct quality of mood, profound anhedonia, early morning insomnia, appetite loss, loss of interest in sex, and psychomotor retardation. There is no clear nonendogenous pattern. Rather, *nonendogenicity* is most often defined simply as the absence of clear-cut endogenicity. It has typically been presumed that endogenous patients will respond better to pharmacotherapy, whereas nonendogenous patients will respond better to psychotherapy. Although endogenously depressed clients do typically respond better to drugs than do nonendogenous patients and although these differential predictions may well hold for the comparison of pharmacotherapy and most other types of psychotherapy, there is some evidence that endogenicity is not a differential predictor of response to cognitive therapy relative to pharmacotherapy (Blackburn *et al.*, 1981; Hollon *et al.*, 1983; Kovacs *et al.*, 1981).

Assessment of Depression

There are a plethora of useful assessment strategies for depression, all of which tend to converge on a common construct. The major error typically made is to ignore the distinction between symptom, syndrome, and nosologic disorder levels, selecting an assessment strategy appropriate at one level in an effort to establish the presence of the phenomenon at another.

The basic clinical interview is the mainstay of the appropriate assessment of depression. Unstructured interviews can, of course, be used, but the recent development of carefully structured diagnostic interviews, in particular the Schedule for Affective Disorders and Schizophrenia (SADS) (Spitzer, Endicott, & NIMH, 1978) or the Diagnostic Interview Schedule (DIS) (Robins, Helzer, Croughan, & Ratcliff, 1981) has greatly enhanced the reliability of diagnoses in this area. Such instruments facilitate the establishment of differential diagnoses, that is, the identification of primary affective disorder as opposed to secondary depression, and they represent the optimal strategy for identifying depression as a nosological entity distinct from other disorders.

The majority of the existing self-report and clinician-rated scales quantify depression as a syndrome rather than as a nosologic disorder. The sole exceptions to this statement may be the psychopathology batteries such as the Minnesota Multiphasic Personality Inventory (MMPI) (Hathaway & McKinley, 1951) or the Hopkins Symptoms Checklist, 90-item version (SCL-90) (Derogatis, Lipman, & Covi, 1973), which include syndrome depression subscales and numerous other subscales designed to assess other forms of psychopathologies. However, although the depression subscales of these instruments are serviceable measures of syndrome depression, efforts to make nosologic statements based on profile analyses remain problematic. For example, we have examined MMPIs on nearly 200 carefully diagnosed primary nonbipolar depressives as part of our ongoing treatment outcome studies. Although most of those patients evidence significant elevations (t scores $\geq$ 70) on the depression subscale (Scale 2), the modal primary outpatient depressive also evidences significant elevations on Scales 4 (psychopathic deviant), 7 (psychasthenia), and 8 (schizophrenia). Other profile patterns are also common in our samples. Most of the existing psychopathology batteries were normed against earlier, now outdated, diagnostic systems, making any reliance on such profile analyses for diagnostic purposes questionable.

We typically utilize at least one of the standard self-report instruments to assess the degree of depression at intake and to monitor changes in levels of depression across time. We tend to prefer the Beck Depression Inventory (BDI) (Beck *et al.*, 1961), a 21-item inventory that covers a range of symptoms present in the syndrome but recognize that there are a number of equally serviceable alternatives, for example, the Zung Self-Rating Depression Scale (Zung, 1965) or the Carroll Depression Scale (Carroll, Feinberg, Smouse, Rawson, & Greden, 1981). We typically ask our clients to complete a BDI at the beginning of each treatment session, providing a convenient check on the level, specific patterns, and changes in symptomatology. Whatever self-report measure is chosen, we strongly encourage its frequent utilization throughout the course of therapy.

As with the self-report syndrome measures, a plethora of clinician-rated measures also exist. Two of the more frequently utilized are the Hamilton Rating Scale for Depression (HRSD) (Hamilton, 1960) and the Raskin Depression Rating Scale (RDS) (Raskin *et al.*, 1970). Both require a brief interview targeted at specific signs and symptoms for completion. In our research and practice, we frequently complete clinician-rated measures (or preferably, have a colleague execute the clinical ratings) on our clients, although not so frequently as we have our clients complete self-report measures on themselves.

Our preferred battery would include the completion of a SADS diagnostic interview, leading to a DSM-III diagnosis, supplemented by an MMPI, BDI, and HRSD at intake. Self-report BDIs would be completed at each session (or weekly, when sessions become less frequent) and clinician-rated HRSDs would be completed monthly.

Finally, it is frequently useful to ascertain transient changes in mood, or depression at the symptom level. Although a variety of serviceable mood checklists exist, for example, the Lubin Depression Adjective Checklist (DACL) (Lubin, 1965) or the Multiple Affect Adjective Checklist (MAACL) (Zuckerman & Lubin,

1965), we prefer less cumbersome procedures. Typically, we ask our clients to rate their affect on a 0- to 100-point metric, in which 0 represents the "worst they've ever felt" and 100 represents the "best they've ever felt," or some such similar metric. Such an assessment system allows the quick, careful delineation of affective changes occurring during a session or at key points between sessions. As we shall describe in the sections to follow, this simple metric readily lends itself to the process of hypothesis testing that lies at the heart of cognitive therapy.

Description of Cognitive-Behavioral Therapy

Overview

Cognitive-behavioral therapy is *structured, collaborative, Socratic, empirical,* and *time limited.* The method focuses on the current situations and emphasizes the role of maladaptive beliefs, or cognitions. It is based on the premise that thoughts, feelings, and behaviors are related and that cognitive distortions are learned and can be unlearned. Each of these characteristics will be discussed in turn.

Structure

The individual session as well as the entire therapeutic process has a high degree of structure. Each time the client is seen, the Beck Depression Inventory (BDI) (Beck *et al.,* 1961) and the Automatic Thoughts Questionnaire (ATQ) (Hollon & Kendall, 1980) are administered. The interview may begin with a social exchange inquiring how the client has been doing in the past week and commenting on mundane life events. As the real business of the interview begins, the first order is setting an agenda. At this time, both client and therapist note items or situations that might be discussed. Priorities are set in the event that there is insufficient time to cover all items. The agenda is then covered, at the end of which the client is asked to summarize what was discussed, what became clearer, questions that remain or were not raised, and suggestions that they have as to their own focus in the next week. It is useful to ask the client at this time if the therapist did or said anything that was irritating or bothersome in some manner. As the therapeutic relationship develops, increasing trust and ease of communication, one may dispense with this query.

The course of therapy is structured to initially emphasize assessment, then move to a focus on behavior, and finally to cognitions, both automatic thoughts and underlying assumptions. The transition from one to another is neither abrupt nor discrete. There is further structure in that the client is expected to participate in the planning of various homework assignments to be done regularly between the interviews. Such self-help tasks reflect the emphasis on assessment initially, then on behavior, then on cognitions. These will be elaborated further in the discussion of specific techniques.

Collaborative

In cognitive therapy, the therapist and client are both active in assessing, planning, and evaluating. The therapist seeks to engage the client as an active participant in all phases of therapy, including agenda setting, *in vivo* self-monitoring, designing behavioral activation tasks, and cognitive hypothesis testing. Although the therapist is always prepared to take the lead in structuring the course of treatment, he or she typically attempts to involve the client in an active participation.

Socratic

This method emphasizes questioning, which leads the client to new revelations. The therapist refrains from verbalizing interpretations or assumptions about the meanings of clients' behavior or statements, preferring instead to lead the client through the process of guided discovery. Thus, the approach is typically "Socratic" in nature, with questioning, rather than argumentation, utilized to challenge existing beliefs.

Empirical

Training the client in the process of empirically testing the validity of his or her thoughts and beliefs is a primary goal of cognitive therapy. Frequently, the client is encouraged to utilize his or her own behaviors to test a belief. For example, the client who believes that he or she cannot accomplish anything is encouraged to engage in selected concrete tasks, using the consequences of those activities to test his or her belief. Thus, great emphasis is placed upon encouraging the client to engage in behaviors that actually put to the test his or her beliefs.

Time Limited

The course of cognitive-behavioral (C-B) therapy is generally 20 sessions in length. Typically, C-B begins with sessions twice weekly before shifting to sessions once weekly later in treatment. The therapist frequently points out that treatment is to be time limited as an impetus to working concretely on problems of major importance.

"Here and Now"

The focus is typically kept on current here-and-now concerns. This is not to say that attention to past events may not be helpful but simply that it is not necessary to do much historical reconstruction in order to teach the process. One may, at some point, wish to give attention to the past, for example, in an effort to demonstrate that the client's beliefs may once have had a reasonable basis but that is generally unnecessary to accomplish the goal of change in symptoms and development of skill in the empirical approach.

Focus on Cognition

In cognitive therapy, the greatest emphasis is placed on assessing and evaluating thoughts rather than on feelings. Although feelings and affects are typically of interest, they are treated as if they were dependent upon the antecedent beliefs. This is the aspect of C-B therapy that causes many therapists the greatest trouble and frequently elicits criticism. Rather than emphasizing support alone as the procedure for dealing with strong negative affect (e.g., sadness or anxiety), the cognitive therapist will attempt to help the client "distance" himself or herself from the belief and examine its validity. Although often misconstrued as being an insensitive approach, the optimal execution of cognitive therapy neither excludes empathetic support nor is limited to it.

Relationship between Thoughts and Feelings

The ABC model, which will be familiar to many from Rational Emotive Therapy, is used as a basis to teach clients the relationship between their thoughts and their feelings. *A* is the antecedent situation that precedes the thoughts; *B* is the thought or cognition, and *C* is the consequence of interest, typically either an affective state and/or behavior. Individuals generally focus on A and C and leave out B, tending to believe that certain situations cause a specific feeling (or compel a particular action) without recognizing the role played by their interpretation of the event. To illustrate, if you bring someone a gift and they think you were doing it out of friendship and affection for them, they will feel happy and affectionate toward you. On the other hand, if their thought is that you brought it with some ulterior motive and wish to manipulate, they will feel suspicious and wary. The event, of course, is the same in both instances. The cognitive processes and the subsequent feelings are, however, very different.

Cognitive Distortions Are Learned

In general, it is presumed that people develop certain patterns of thinking and believing as a result of previous experiences. Strictly speaking, of course, this need not be assumed. It is only necessary that content and/or process be malleable in therapy. A basic distinction is typically made between *automatic thoughts,* the contents of accessible conscious ruminations that seem to arise automatically, and *underlying assumptions,* attitudes presumably held by individuals even if rarely ever experienced in the client's stream of consciousness. Both are presumably acquired through experience, either actual or vicarious, and both are presumably modifiable through the process of empirical disconfirmation. Automatic thoughts are, however, more concrete and specific, and, presumably more readily modified.

Assessment Techniques and Tools

Depressed clients extensively distort the past, the present, and the future. It is important that the client and the therapist together get as accurate a picture as possible of the client's situation, his or her thoughts, feelings, and behaviors. There are at least five major tools and techniques that we like to use in this assessment phase and, in some cases, as ongoing assessment tools throughout therapy. These tools include a brief history, the Beck Depression Inventory, the Automatic Thoughts Questionnaire, the *Coping with Depression* pamphlet (Beck & Greenberg, 1974), and the Self-Monitoring Record or Daily Log.

History

The purpose of a brief history is not to enable the therapist or client to formulate some causative theory nor is it to delineate a core problem. It is, rather, to look at the client's cognitions and behaviors as these relate to the current depression and to anticipate possible problems in the course of therapy. Of interest is the client's description of his or her symptoms. It often is helpful to have the client rate the degree of depression he or she has experienced in the past on a scale from 1 to 10, with 10 being severe depression, and plotting the rises and falls in this metric over the course of the client's life. Eliciting a rating of what is usual for that client is useful, both for purposes of comparison and in order to establish more accurately the prior course of the client's affective experiences for prognostic purposes. Another important aspect is to explicate any theory the client may have as to the cause (or lack thereof) of his or her depression. Do they see themselves as being chronically depressed? If so, why? Has this been a lifelong affective state, an episodic affliction, or a new experience? Do they think that someone's action or lack of action has precipitated their depression? Such cognitions may indicate that the client sees the alleviation of his or her depression as beyond his or her means. One of the key aspects of cognitive therapy is to provide the client with an alternative formulation for his or her affective distress, one that stresses the role of dysfunctional attitudes in shaping the maladaptive behaviors (e.g., self-fulfilling prophecies; Darley & Fazio, 1980) that lead to objective failure and disappointments. Often, the depressed client can point to real disappointments in life. What he or she fails to recognize is the role his or her subject beliefs play in generating those disappointments.

Exploration of expectation and goals is also important. What symptom alleviation is hoped for? What degree of depression or lack thereof is expected at the end of therapy? What the client hopes to achieve in therapy may be quite different from what the therapist hopes to achieve. It is crucial that the therapist know and adjust to the client's expectations or assist the client in changing those expectations. For instance, on that 1 to 10 depression scale just described, some clients may be looking forward to a 5, whereas the therapist might assume that such a level would be intolerable. The therapist might then be very reluctant to allow termination of therapy, even once the client's goal was realized. A different situation would obtain with a chronically depressed client's seeking a depression level of 0 or 1, despite a history of lifelong dysphoria. In any case, it is important for the therapist and the client to have an accurate mutual understanding of the current situation and the goals.

Beck Depression Inventory

The Beck Depression Inventory (Beck *et al.*, 1961) (or a related self-report syndrome measure) should be administered at the beginning of each session as an indicator of the level of depression and progress of therapy. The numerical value of the circled items is totaled additively, taking only the *highest* circled item within each cluster. A score under 10 is considered normal and relatively nondepressed. Ten to 20 is considered marginally depressed, 20 to 30 is moderately depressed, 30 to 40 is moderately severe depression, and over 40 is severe depression. In general, the clinician can have less confidence in the discriminability of scores in the high 30s and up because severely neurotic outpatients will frequently report higher scores (high 40s and 50s) than obviously more severely depressed inpatients. Nonetheless, the guidelines provided can serve as a rough guide for the neophyte clinician. Additionally, the Beck Depression Inventory furnishes both the clinician and the client with information on the content of the depressive syndrome and some of the cognitive distortions.

Automatic Thoughts Questionnaire

The Automatic Thoughts Questionnaire (ATQ) (Hollon & Kendall, 1980) is a 30-item instrument designed to assess "depressotypic" cogntions at the level of automatic thoughts. The 30 items are each discrete thoughts such as, *"I'm a fail-ure"* or *"My future is bleak,"* each scored on a 1- to 5-point frequency scale. Total scores are derived by summing across the 30 items. The ATQ can be administered at the beginning of each interview and can serve a parallel function to the Beck Depression Inventory, indicating the extent to which the client is thinking nega-tively and providing a numerical indicator of the progress over time. It also fur-nishes the clinician and the client with cognitive content. Other cognitive assess-ment devices are also available, although few are as readily administrable or easily scored as the ATQ. These include the Dysfunctional Attitude Scale (DAS) (Weiss-man & Beck, 1978), a measure of "underlying assumptions"; the Attributional Styles Inventory (ASI) (Seligman, Abramson, Semmel, & von Baeyer, 1979), a mea-sure of depressotypic causal explanations; and the Cognitive Response Test (CRT) (Watkins & Rush, 1983), a free-response, sentence completion assessment device.

Coping with Depression *Pamphlet*

This pamphlet (Beck & Greenberg, 1974) presents illustrations of the ways in which people think negatively and various negative thoughts that are common. It further explains the emphasis of therapy and introduces the ABC model with rudi-mentary directions on how to assess thoughts. It is effective not only as an educa-tional device but also as an assessment tool. In the latter context, it can be given to the client at the first interview with directions that it be read before the second interview. We typically ask the client to underline portions that are either descrip-tive of him or her or that particularly do not apply or that seem unreasonable. Thus, the pamphlet serves as a good starting point for discussion, both about symp-toms and about treatment.

Self-Monitoring Record *(Daily Log, Activity Log)*

One standard assignment that we like to begin therapy with (at least for mod-erately depressed outpatients; more severely depressed, globally impaired patients are typically started on concrete activity schedules) is a simple self-monitoring task designed to assess events (and behaviors) and mood states outside of therapy. Fig-ure 1 presents a self-monitoring record completed by a client during the first 4 days of therapy. Typically, the client is asked to enter his or her major activity for each hour. Also noted for each hour is a mood rating, preferably on a scale from 0 to 100 (this client would only agree to use a 0 to 10 scale). This scale represents the client's range of actual experience, 0 being the worst the client has ever felt,

100 being the best. The third entry is an *M* (for "mastery") or *P* (for "pleasure") when appropriate. We prefer to define a mastery task as one that appears difficult before it is begun. For some clients (such as the client providing the record in Figure 1), even simple tasks such as getting out of bed in the morning is a mastery task. Pleasurable events are typically defined as any event that either leads the client to feel a little better or, at least, a little less badly.

This initial record revealed a real poverty of content. This client, an unem-

	TIME	Date: 1/18/85 Monday	Date: 1/19/85 Tuesday	Date: 1/20/85 Wednesday	Date: 1/21/85 Thursday
A.M.	9–10		Started to wake up	Got out of bed 3M	
	10–11		Got out of bed 3M	Sat on couch 3	
	11–12		Sat on couch, Listened to stereo 3	Slept	
P.M.	12–1		Went to apply for Welfare		
	1–2				
	2–3				
	3–4	In session 4	Sat on couch 2M	Turned on TV 3	In session 4 or 5
	4–5	Sat on couch 4	2		
	5–6	Listened to stereo/Ate 4	3		Watched News 3
	6–7	Listened to stereo	Watched TV 3		
	7–8	Watched simulcast 5	3		Gopher Basket-ball 5 4
	8–9	Read 5	3	4	
	9–10	Read 5	3	4	North Stars 5 4
	10–11	Read 5	3	4	
	11–12	Bed	Bed	4	

Figure 1. Client self-monitoring record.

ployed black male in his early 30s, evidenced few social contacts, minimal mastery experiences, virtually no pleasurable experiences, and virtually chronic dysphoria. It was apparent that reading and watching televised sporting events provided his primary sources of gratification. Following the second session, the client was asked to be more specific, to make some plans, and to predict his mood. This is reflected in the Thursday entries that specified he would watch the news, a basketball game, and a hockey game. Further, he predicted what his mood would be and circled the prediction so it could be compared with actual mood rating. These changes were made for several reasons. Increased attentiveness to the specifics of his immediate circumstances counteracted tendencies to ruminate and fantasize negatively and provided an opportunity for feeling better. Predicting mood for comparative purposes laid the foundation for the assessment and later discussion of expectations and other cognitions that regularly resulted in disappointment, discouragement, and increased avoidance of activity for this client. This client's expectation that both his teams would play well resulted, on that particular night, in his mood's being lower than he had expected. He stated that he had always enjoyed watching sports on television, but since becoming depressed, he no longer even enjoyed that. Further discussion revealed that previous to his depression, he had been far more resilient when his team did poorly because he would think differently about it.

Having begun with the very simple task of planning a specific television program to watch daily, a graduated planning approach was initiated that ended with this client's getting out for a walk every day. This was an activity that he had enjoyed earlier, prior to becoming depressed. Getting that activity back into his daily routine helped in lifting the worst of his depression.

When this assignment is given, it is important to ascertain whether or not it makes sense to the client and what difficulties are anticipated. The assignment is given to get an accurate picture of the client's life, to see if there is a relationship between what he or she is doing and how he or she is feeling. It further can serve as the basis for behavioral engineering, as in the example just provided, or as the basis for cognitive exploration and hypothesis testing, as will be discussed. It is, however, important to recall that depressed clients will often have problems in executing even simple assignments, such as self-monitoring. If difficulties are anticipated, the client can be helped to plan ways to solve those. Often clients anticipate forgetting to execute the self-monitoring. Placing the log in a conspicuous place, such as on the refrigerator or folded in a package of cigarettes, can often be helpful. Using the information gathered, the client can be engaged in problem solving with some very interesting and original results. Finally, it is good practice to invite the client to call before the next appointment if unforeseen difficulties are encountered.

Relationship of Mood and Activity Level

The point at which the client returns with the first record completed is the point at which he or she begins to see the blending of the ongoing assessment, behavioral activation strategies, and cognitive assessment and change that is the hallmark of cognitive therapy. In processing the first products of this self-monitoring process, it is helpful to ask the client to report what he or she experienced and whether or not he or she learned anything interesting in the process. The therapist might encourage the client to look at his or her general mood level and to notice whether this mood is stable or fluctuating. Clients who assumed that they were "in the pits" all of the time are often surprised to find that there is some alleviation or fluctuation in the course of their days. Any such variation can be explored for patterns. Are the moods different in the morning than in the evening? Are they different on the weekends than in the middle of the week? Does affect improve when the client is actively engaged in goal-directed behaviors? Any information gleaned from such variations can be used to guide behavioral activation strategies and as information for subsequent hypothesis testing.

It is particularly important to look at whether or not there is any relationship between what the client was doing and his or her mood. In essence, the client's own self-monitoring records can be used to examine the determinants of his or her moods. The therapist might ask the client to observe the times when his or her mood was the lowest and the times when his or her mood was the highest and ask that attention be paid to what he or she was doing at the time and what kinds of thoughts he or she was having. Was there any indication that the client felt better when he or she was engaged in activities that were pleasurable or when he or she was engaged in activities that were mastery tasks? Clients often note that they are surprised to see that they have done so little, that their lives are so boring, or that they are not having any fun. The therapist might ask the client if he or she believes there was any relationship between what he or she is doing and how he or she felt. Most often, clients will say "yes," they believe that there is, but often their thoughts about that relationship are misdirected. For instance, one young male client reported that he felt terrible when he was at work. However, when he submitted his activity log, it was discovered that his mood was somewhere between 40 and 65 on a 100-point scale when at work, ratings that tended to be higher than ratings when not at work. Occasionally, clients will report they do not believe there is any relationship between their moods and activities. At this point, they may engage in an experiment to see if that is true or not. We will return to a discussion of planning the testing of such predictions in the section that follows.

Behavioral Activation Strategies: Planning Activities and Testing Predictions

Beginning in the early sessions (anytime from the first session on), it is helpful to begin explicitly testing the client's predictions (again, for particularly behaviorally impaired clients, the early sessions might be devoted solely to behavioral activating strategies). At this point, it is helpful to discuss with the client what his or her mood and activity level was like previous to his or her current depression. The therapist may want to explore previously gratifying activities that have been discontinued and to determine *why* they have been discontinued. One major symptom of depression is that people often stop doing those things that used to make them feel good. Have any old interests been neglected? What new interests have been considered? What necessary tasks are not currently being performed? An example was the client (already discussed) who had always enjoyed going for regular walks but discontinued those walks after becoming depressed, sitting for hour upon hour in a darkened apartment. Another example was a client who had always wanted to go to some museums and art galleries but who believed that she could not do so alone. A third example was the client who no longer attempted even minimal housekeeping tasks and who felt worse as a result of living in domestic chaos.

The client may want to plan to execute one or two of these or related activities before the next interview. The therapist should exercise some caution and not allow the client to plan to try too much. Often, clients will become overzealous about taking on everything they have left undone for the last several months, setting themselves up for inevitable disappointment, triggering a whole litany of self-defeating thoughts. When they have chosen one or two activities, those behaviors can be entered as a plan in the daily log, marked in some way to designate these as preplanned activities. The therapist can anticipate problems, asking such questions as, (a) "If you don't accomplish this, what might keep you from accomplishing it?" (b) "Are you likely to make excuses at the last minute and, if so, what will those excuses be?" or, (c) "What sorts of life events could occur that would interfere with the accomplishment of this task?" Anticipating such problems will allow the client to make some plans for counteracting such eventualities or changing plans in such a way to increase the chances of success.

It is important to maximize the client's success in these efforts toward change. This can be done by breaking big tasks into their component steps, which can be attempted one by one ("chunking"), and/or by encouraging the client to engage in the simplest, most easily accomplished steps first ("success therapy"). Such assignments should always be approached so that they will be informative regardless of outcome rather than as tasks at which to "succeed" or "fail." Further, these behavioral activation strategies can be used to test the accuracy of the client's beliefs. The therapist might, for example, ask the client to predict his or her mood after he or she attempts the planned behavior. This prediction can be entered with a circle around it on the self-monitoring sheet to differentiate it from the actual reporting of mood at the time of doing the activity. The client, for example, might plan a walk and predict that his or her mood will not go up. The therapist can explore why he or she thinks the client's mood will not rise, paying particular attention to the cognitions the client reports, such as, "I used to enjoy doing this, but nothing seems to feel good anymore." The particular behavior can then be treated as an experiment designed to test the validity of that specific prediction, with the client's own mood ratings before and after the walk taken as the actual data, a truly empirical process. Typically, the client will experience greater pleasure than anticipated. This process assists him or her in beginning to make connections regularly between activities and moods as well as beginning the hypothesis-testing process.

When the client next returns, the therapist should continue to look at the general report of activity and mood as discussed before but should pay particular attention to those activities that were planned and the moods that were predicted. The therapist should discuss what activities were accomplished and how the individual felt when he or she accomplished them. If it was not accomplished, what kept that from happening? How accurate were the predictions? What were the cognitions regarding the accomplishment or nonaccomplishment of the activity? What are the current cognitions about the predictions? When planning tasks that are viewed as being necessary but not particularly pleasant (i.e., mastery tasks), clients will often predict a very low mood. One client planned to pick up some food for a party and predicted that that task would cause her mood to go down to 35, a very low mood for her. She anticipated that her mood would drop because she thought that this was going to be a very difficult task in which she would not be able to make the proper choice of party food and that it would take so long that it would keep her from doing other tasks that were equally important. With the assistance of her therapist, she planned her shopping trip so that when she actually engaged in the task it did not take her very long and her actual mood rating was much higher than she had predicted. She could see that by doing some planning in order to counteract her negative cognitions about the task, she was able to buttress her mood and disconfirm her cognitions.

The key point is that although cognitive therapy makes extensive use of a multitude of behavioral activation strategies, it does so in a fashion that allows the consequences of those interventions to serve as tests of the client's cognitions. Thus, although cognitive therapy typically begins by focusing on behavior change, it does so in a way that sets up the cognitive change strategies to be discussed in the sections to follow.

Eliciting Cognitions

Assisting the client in becoming aware of his or her thought processes is one of the most difficult aspects in the therapeutic process. Though clients typically find it relatively easy to understand the ABC model, they often find it difficult to actually report their ongoing cognitions. It is often helpful to describe what is meant by "automatic thoughts." In part, they are experienced as "automatic" because they become ingrained as a result of years of habit. Frequently, people become so habituated to their own thinking that their only awareness remains that of the situation and the subsequent feeling. Therefore, an important step in the therapeutic process is that of training the client to access his or her own beliefs, often by consistently focusing on examples of thoughts. The therapist can often facilitate this process by noticing and remembering examples from the client's conversation. For instance, one client reported at the first interview that one of the reasons for her depression was a weight gain of 23 pounds. As she talked about this, one of her statements was that "Sinequan makes you fat." This was an automatic thought that we later discussed, asking whether or not it was the pills that made her fat or whether it was what she ate that made her fat. Highlighting examples of thoughts from the client's conversation can facilitate his or her learning to recognize what is meant by an "automatic thought." In addition, such attention to careful labeling can be used to help highlight the difference between thoughts and feelings. Our culture is somewhat careless in this regard, often confusing the two and labeling thoughts as feelings. For example, an individual might say: "I *feel* that you don't understand what I am saying." This is, of course, not a statement of affect. Rather, it is a statement of a belief, albeit one accompanied by a feeling tone. It is important that the therapist educate himself or herself so as to better educate the client in this distinction.

As a method of further eliciting cognitions, the therapist might discuss with the client feelings and thoughts experienced just prior to the interview. Clients will often report much anticipatory anxiety that is catastrophic in nature. Asking what he or she thought about before coming in for the first session is often helpful. If the client is not able to provide any cognitions, the therapist can provide examples of things that are commonly reported by other clients. Some of the examples might be: (a) "I wonder what my therapist will be like"; (b) "I bet my therapist won't understand me"; (c) "I don't think anything is going to help"; (d) "I sure hope to get some answers about this"; (e) "What if my therapist tells me I'm crazy?" and (f) "What if I have to go to the hospital?"

A third way to assist the client in eliciting cognitions has been mentioned briefly before. That is, the daily activities log can be used to focus on high points and low points in mood. After eliciting a description of the activity associated with that mood state, it is frequently possible to reconstruct what the individual was thinking about at the time.

Once the client has gotten some basic instruction in the nature of cognitions and ways to sharpen his or her awareness of them, he or she can move to the use of a Dysfunctional Thought Record (DTR), as is illustrated in Figure 2.

It is useful for the client to begin the daily record of dysfunctional thoughts while he or she is still doing the activity log. The client can be instructed to regard any mood rating below a certain point, say 35, as a signal for cognitive introspection. The client is first asked to write the date and the situation, typically either an event or daydream. Initially, we ask the client to attempt to complete only the first four columns: the date, the situation (or A in the ABC model), the affect (or C in the model), and the belief (the B in the model), crossing out the columns for rational response and outcome. Initially, we are content to focus on assisting the client

DATE	SITUATION Describe: 1. Actual event leading to unpleasant emotion, or 2. Stream of thoughts, daydream, recollection leading to unpleasant emotion.	EMOTION(S) 1. Specify sad/ anxious/ angry, etc. 2. Rate degree of emotion, 1–100.	AUTOMATIC THOUGHTS 1. Write automatic thought(s) that preceded emotion(s). 2. Rate belief in automatic thought(s), 0–100%.	RATIONAL RESPONSE 1. Write rational response to automatic thought(s). 2. Rate belief in rational response, 0–100%.	OUTCOME 1. Rerate belief in automatic thought(s), 0–100. 2. Specify and rate subsequent emotions, 0–100.

Figure 2. Daily record of dysfunctional thoughts.

to become increasingly skilled in the recognizing of her or his own automatic thoughts. Our experience has been that clients easily become frustrated with the process, rapidly concluding that they cannot learn how to evaluate their beliefs if they are not carefully taught the process in discrete, manageable steps.

Let us give a brief example of what we might ask the client to generate. In Figure 3, the client reported an actual event leading to an unpleasant emotion. As can be seen, the cognition listed was closely congruent with both the negative affect noted and the triggering event. The neophyte therapist may find it useful to utilize his or her own capacity for affective empathy to determine whether he or she fully

	SITUATION	EMOTION(S)	AUTOMATIC THOUGHT(S)	RATIONAL RESPONSE	OUTCOME
DATE	Describe: 1. Actual event leading to unpleasant emotion, or 2. Stream of thoughts, daydream, or recollection, leading to unpleasant emotion.	1. Specify sad, anxious, angry, etc. 2. Rate degree of emotion, 1–100.	1. Write automatic thought(s) that preceded emotion(s). 2. Rate belief in automatic thought(s), 0–100%.	1. Write rational response to automatic thought(s). 2. Rate belief in rational response, 0–100%.	1. Rerate belief in automatic thought(s), 0–100%. 2. Specify and rate subsequent emotions, 0–100.
1/9	Jerry is two hours late.	Fear anger discouraged	He's not going to get here. He's doing something more important to him. What if he had an accident? He always does this to me. I'm the only one that has to work around here. I'm the one who has to take care of the kids. What if he's with someone else? I wonder if I should call the police?		

EXPLANATION: When you experience an unpleasant emotion, note the situation that seemed to stimulate the emotion. (If the emotion occurred while you were thinking, daydreaming, etc., please note this.) Then note the automatic thought associated with the emotion. Record the degree to which you believe this thought: 0% = not at all; 100% = completely. In rating degree of emotion, 1 = a trace; 100 = the most intense possible.

Figure 3. Partial sample record: Daily record of dysfunctional thoughts.

understands the client's idiosyncratic meaning system. If the therapist can readily understand both the client's affect and its degree, given the beliefs listed, then assessment has probably been adequate. If the therapist cannot image himself or herself experiencing either the type of affect listed or its magnitude, even if he or she believed what the client indicates he or she believed, then additional exploration of the client's idiosyncratic meaning system is required.

You will note the client has not rated the degree of emotion nor his or her belief in the automatic thought. This can be initiated immediately or left until later. Early on in the introduction of the Dysfunctional Thoughts Record DTR, we do not want clients to become confused or overwhelmed. Further, it is not important initially for the client to be very discriminating in terms of recording his or her emotions. Any variation on anxious, happy, sad, angry, and the like will do, with the finer nuances left for later. As the client becomes more adept at reporting automatic thoughts and emotions, he or she can enter ratings of both the degree of affect and the extent to which the cognitions are believed, thus increasing the level of sophistication.

Identifying Cognitive Errors

When the client is reasonably able to generate some automatic thoughts, it is time to move toward evaluating and correcting cognitions. A first helpful step is to give clients a list of cognitive errors commonly made by individuals. Table 1 provides a list that has been adapted from Burns's *Feeling Good: The New Mood Therapy* (Burns, 1980), which in turn was adapted from earlier work by Beck and colleagues (Beck, 1967; Beck *et al.*, 1979). It is not clear that these logical errors are necessarily unique to depressed individuals (e.g., similar processes have been noted in nondepressed normals under the rubric of *heuristics*; cf. Kahneman, Slovic, & Tversky, 1982; Nisbett & Ross, 1980), but it is clear that combined with the negative content of most depressives' beliefs, these logical errors serve to maintain erroneous beliefs and contribute to the maintenance of dysphoria (cf. Hollon & Garber, in press; Hollon & Kriss, 1984).

This list will acquaint the client in a beginning and basic way with some of the typical errors in logic frequently made by depressed clients. It is often useful to ask the client to write an example from his or her own life illustrating as many of the cognitive errors as he or she can. The therapist might ask the client to pay particular attention to the cognitive errors he or she "specializes" in and might urge that the examples be drawn from recent experience. Throughout the course of treatment, the therapist should be alert to instances of these and related logical errors, calling them to the client's attention as they occur.

Evaluating and Changing Cognitions

Three Questions: "Evidence," "Alternative Explanations," and "Implications"

The material that has been generated by the client on the cognitive error sheet and the Dysfunctional Thoughts Record furnishes material to work with in beginning to teach him or her how to evaluate the validity of such cognitions. There are at least three major questions that are useful in this process. The first is "What is the evidence?" The second is "Are there any other alternative explanations?" The third question is "What are the realistic implications?" We will discuss each in turn.

What Is the Evidence?

In asking this first question, it is important to define terms clearly, particularly labels such as *failure, dumb, stupid,* and *hopeless.* What kind of behavior, for instance, is subsumed under any particular label? Perhaps the term should be

Table 1. Cognitive Errors in Depression

1. ALL OR NOTHING THINKING: You see things as black or white; there is no gray or middle ground. Things are wonderful or awful, and if what you do isn't perfect, it is a total failure.
2. OVERGENERALIZATION: You see a single negative event as a never-ending pattern of defeat. If you have a misunderstanding with a person important to you, you think he or she doesn't understand you or care about you, never has, and never will. You think you will always be isolated and misunderstood.
3. MENTAL FILTER (SELECTIVE ABSTRACTION): You pick out a single negative detail and dwell on that until everything is affected by that negative. If you make a nice dinner but overcook the vegetable, then you think only of the ruined vegetable until you see the entire dinner as a disaster.
4. DISQUALIFYING THE POSITIVE: You "don't count" positive experiences for some reason or another and maintain a negative belief that is really not based on your everyday experience. You will not allow yourself to enjoy good feelings, for instance, because you will tell yourself that if you feel good, there must be bad feelings to follow, Thus, you even feel bad about feeling good.
5. JUMPING TO CONCLUSIONS (ARBITRARY INFERENCES): You see things as negative whether you have any facts or not.
   a. Mind Reading: You decide someone is responding negatively to you without checking it out. If an acquaintance meets you on the street and doesn't say hello, you assume she or he doesn't like you and doesn't want to speak to you. You don't ask to see if they were having other things on their mind and didn't notice you, or if something else was going on.
   b. Fortune Teller Error: You expect things to turn out badly and don't allow for the possibility they may be neutral or positive. You anticipate you will not have any fun at a party and in fact become so convinced of that, that you don't even go.
6. MAGNIFICATION AND/OR MINIMIZATION: You make an extra big deal about your own errors and an extra big deal about other people's success. On the other hand, you say that other people's errors don't really matter and that your successes and good qualities are really small and don't count for much.
7. EMOTIONAL REASONING: You assume that your negative feelings result from the fact that things are negative. If you feel bad, then that means the world situation is bad. You don't look around to see if it's actually true.
8. SHOULD STATEMENTS: You try to push yourself and improve yourself with *should's* and *shouldn't's, musts,* and *oughts.* "I should do more"; "I ought to have known better"; "I must have a good reason for saying no"; and "I shouldn't wish I didn't have any kids" are common examples. The emotional consequence is guilt, anger, and resentment. The phrase *I should* is often used when *I wish* or *I would like* is more accurate.
9. LABELING AND MISLABELING: This is major overgeneralizing. When you make a mistake, you say, "I'm a dope." When you don't get something you wanted, you say, "I'm a loser." When someone's behavior rubs you wrong, you say, "He's a louse." You refer to an event in emotionally loaded language. When labels are used, many characteristics that don't apply to the person are implied or included.
10. PERSONALIZATION: You see yourself as the cause of some external unfortunate or unpleasant event that you were not actually responsible for. An incest victim, for example, refuses to talk with her parents about the pain of the experience because she anticipates they will then feel hurt and that will be her fault.

looked up in the dictionary. What are the facts that support a belief such as "I can't handle this job anymore"? Perhaps it is important to acquire some actual information or to set up a test to see if the notion is correct. One client, for instance, who was working on a switchboard, was very depressed because so many of the calls that she received were abusive. She concluded that she had to quit her job. What she decided to do was to keep a running record of the calls that were neutral, those that were abusive, and all of the calls that were tolerable or even pleasant. What she discovered was that less than 2% of the calls were abusive and more than 60% of the calls were either tolerable or pleasant. It was not necessary for her to go any further in assessing that thought. Had she discovered the opposite was true, however, that many of the calls were really abusive, she could have gone on to the third question (described later) that asks: "Given that this is true, what are the real implications and consequences?"

A recently widowed client who believed that she could no longer continue life without her husband exhibited dysphoria that continued long past what would be expected for a typical grief reaction. What proved important for her in evaluating the evidence regarding her belief was to think back to whether or not there had ever been a time in her life when she had been happy without her husband or whether there had been times in her life when he was still living that she had found solace or pleasure in activities that did not include him. By recognizing she had experienced both such experiences, she was able to begin to entertain the possibility that life was not totally bleak without her husband.

Thus, the "evidence" question can be addressed either by collecting new evidence (typically the consequences of the client's own hypothesis-testing behaviors) or by reviewing existing information in a dispassionate manner. It is typical that both steps are helpful. The key is that the therapist assist the client in conducting an unbiased search or review. In most instances, clients will tend to search for information in a manner likely to confirm their existing beliefs—a phenomenon known as "confirmatory bias" (Snyder, 1981). For example, if the switchboard operator in the earlier example had recorded only the occurrence of abusive calls, not the full range of calls, she might very well have continued to overestimate their frequency of occurrence.

Are There Any Other Alternative Explanations?

This second major question asks the client to entertain other possible explanations for observed events than those initially inferred. There are three major ways to evaluate beliefs in terms of this question. One is to re-review the responsibility for what is going on. Persons who are depressed paradoxically think of themselves as worthless and unimportant, but at the same time, as being at the center of the universe in terms of their impact on others (Abramson & Sackheim, 1977). They will regularly take responsibility for events that they have little or nothing to do with and frequently fail to understand that there are situations in which no one is particularly at fault, or particularly responsible.

Second, depressed persons are often reluctant to look for other interpretations for unpleasant events beyond ascribing the responsibility to themselves. They will assume that someone does not relate to them because there is something wrong with them, neglecting to assess whether or not, for example, that other individual shows a capacity for warmth and close relationships with others. It is frequently helpful to encourage the client to generate a number of possible interpretations for various situations if only as a prelude to returning to the "evidence" question in order to choose between the competing explanations.

Third, the client can be encouraged to remain open to various possible outcomes or points of view. In interpersonal relationships, for example, individuals will often say, "I didn't say anything to him because I knew how he would react." It can often be helpful to elicit thoughts about how the client would view someone else in exactly the same situation he or she is in. What kind of advice would they give to that friend? Would they be quick to blame someone else who did as they did? Role reversal often seems to stimulate depressed clients to apply different, less harsh, sets of rules, similar to what they apply to others, to evaluate the extent of their own responsibility (Garber & Hollon, 1980; Hollon & Garber, in press).

What Are the Realistic Implications?

This third major question encourages the client to explore the *realistic* consequences or implications of a belief that might have some element of truth to it. First, the client is asked to think about what it would mean to him or her or what it would mean about him or her if a given belief were true. (One may end up back at Question 1, "What is the evidence?", in this manner.) The client is encouraged to think about what will happen next, what will happen after that, and so forth. It is important to assess whether or not this is indeed catastrophic, or whether it really will not make much difference. If the conclusion is that the likely consequences would indeed be important and undesirable, the therapist's task becomes one of helping the client consider how the consequence can be coped with. For example, one client indicated, "I am going to lose my house. I'm going to lose everything." We first defined what she meant by "everything" (Question 1) and then encouraged her to list the things that were important to her in her life that she would not risk losing even if she did lose the house. Next, we moved to the "implications" question by means of evaluating the actual probability of losing her house. She estimated that the probability was about 70% that she was going to lose her house. We talked about what would happen if, indeed, she lost the house. Contrary to her original thought that this would be catastrophic, she concluded that it would be a serious setback but one from which she could recover and, indeed, find a few small positives. Though her home was very important to her, its importance paled in comparison to her child and her health. Although this was not an attempt to minimize the impact of the loss of her home, her perspective changed sufficiently so that she no longer thought it catastrophic and life threatening.

Completing the Dysfunctional Thought Record

Returning to the "Dysfunctional Thoughts Record," the evaluations that are generated to response in one or more of the three questions are written in the fifth column, the "rational response" column. Following that, the client is asked to rerate his or her belief in his or her initial automatic thoughts and to then specify and rerate his or her subsequent emotions. Figure 4 illustrates an example of these last two steps on the DTR.

It is important for the client to generate responses to the three questions that make real sense to him or her. It is not sufficient for clients to simply substitute some "rational" or "positive thinking" and expect that to influence their moods. All of us have learned the platitudes of positive thinking and know that looking for the "silver lining" in the cloud does not always work. The substitution of "positive platitudes" for real empirical inquiry is one of the problems most often encountered in the practice of this method. The rated degree of belief in the "rational

DATE	SITUATION Describe: 1. Actual event leading to unpleasant emotion, or 2. Stream of thoughts, daydream, or recollection, leading to unpleasant emotion.	EMOTION(S) 1. Specify sad, anxious, angry, etc. 2. Rate degree of emotion, 1–100.	AUTOMATIC THOUGHT(S) 1. Write automatic thought(s) that preceded emotion(s). 2. Rate belief in automatic thought(s), 0–100%.	RATIONAL RESPONSE 1. Write rational response to automatic thought(s). 2. Rate belief in rational response, 0–100%.	OUTCOME 1. Rerate belief in automatic thought(s), 0–100%. 2. Specify and rate subsequent emotions, 0–100.
8/4	I haven't rented my house and can't make the mortgage payment.	Anxious 100%	I'm going to lose my house. I'm going to lose everything. I can't go on. It's all hopeless. 100%	There is about a 70% chance I will lose the house. Losing my house is not the same as losing everything. There are other things that are important to me. My job is important and I'm not going to lose that. My child is important and I'm not going to lose her. I do have my apartment in Arizona which is an adequate place for us to live. If I lose the house, that means I don't have all the worry about rental and upkeep. Even though I will hate to see the house go, I will have the basic important things left in my life. 90%	Belief 15% relief 90% sad 50%

EXPLANATION: When you experience an unpleasant emotion, note the situation that seemed to stimulate the emotion. (If the emotion occurred while you were thinking, daydreaming, etc., please note this.) Then note the automatic thought associated with the emotion. Record the degree to which you believe this thought: 0% = not at all; 100% = completely. In rating degree of emotion: 1 = a trace; 100 = the most intense possible.

Figure 4. Complete sample record: Daily record of dysfunctional thoughts.

responses" in the sixth column of the DTR can serve as a useful guide in this regard.

A second problem clue that is sometimes encountered involves the client's saying, "My head tells me one thing, but my 'gut' or 'heart' tells me another." The "head" and the "heart" are always congruent. More accurately, the client is likely believing two different, relatively incompatible, things, each with their associated affects, but paying attention to one belief while monitoring the affect associated with the other. One client was puzzled by her response to her husband's mistress, stating, "Rationally I know that she didn't kidnap him against his will, but I am consumed by rage toward her." As shown in Figure 5, this could be conceptualized in the following fashion.

The client was attentive to the thoughts on Track 1, for those were the ones she found more acceptable, given her preferences for her own behavior. She rejected as undesirable the thoughts on Track 2, yet she still, in part, believed them. Hence, she was puzzled by the intensity with which she felt the emotion of rage attendant on the second track of cognition. What she experienced seemed to her to be an incongruence between thought and feeling, but it really reflected an unwillingness on her part to acknowledge beliefs she would have preferred to have thought herself above believing.

Uncovering "Underlying Assumptions"

The final step in cognitive therapy typically involves uncovering "underlying assumptions." In this approach, such generalized attitudes are typically inferred only after observing the client's specific reactions to multiple situations. For example, the therapist might begin to suspect that a client has an underlying assumption that he or she must be "approved of by everyone at all times" if that client is observed reacting with distress whenever others do not appear to accept his or her actions. Ideally, underlying assumptions are identified inductively, presented tentatively, and subjected, as best as can be done, to potential disconfirmation.

Typically, these larger organizing principles can be traced to important experiences earlier in life, one of the few times when historical reconstruction is utilized in cognitive therapy. For example, one recent client appeared to operate as if she believed that she must always be on her guard in social interactions lest she do or

	TRACK 1	TRACK 2
THOUGHTS:	These are two adults, and they share the responsibility equally. My husband has more responsibility to consider my feelings than she does.	She knew he was married. Women should have more consideration. She is the more responsible. She took the most important thing in my life away from me.
FEELINGS:	Sad, hurt	Rage

Figure 5. Two "tracks" of thinking.

say something to offend the other party. As a consequence, she felt excessive tension and stress in even the most casual interpersonal interactions. As a child, this client had had a history of being dominated by a mercurial, cyclothymic father who frequently went into unpredictable rages that could only be resolved if the client and her mother engaged in protracted bouts of abject apologies for their unknown transgressions. Identification of both the client's underlying assumption regarding interpersonal vigilance and the sense of perspective that grew out of tracing its childhood antecedents facilitated the process of both cognitive and behavioral change.

A Clinical Case Study

Ellen was a 57-year-old woman, the mother of six children, separated from her husband for more than 15 years. She came into therapy for the first time in her life experiencing what she considered to be her second major depressive episode. She was placed on imipramine and began a course of cognitive behavioral therapy. She complained of sadness, tearfulness, and chronic fatigue that she feared would jeopardize her professional career.

She was living alone; all of her five children were grown. Most were married and lived out of town, though she had one married daughter in the city and a son in college near home. She was very much involved with this daughter and her grandchildren. She was also heavily involved in seeing to her elderly mother who was in a nursing home. Her husband, an invalid since before their divorce, also was in a nursing home, and she would go to see him on a somewhat regular basis.

Her focus of concern was on her perception of herself as a failure in what she considered to be the two most important areas of life: as a wife and as a mother. She was wondering if she should "go back" to her husband who had been partially paralyzed and invalided for the past 32 years. She expressed much guilt at having finally given up on that marriage, though she continued to say that she had gotten nothing from him since shortly after the illness that paralyzed him.

The first several sessions were involved with providing a basic treatment rationale, teaching her the ABC model and testing to see if it fit with her experiences, training her in self-monitoring and behavioral activation skills, and introducing her to initial cognitive assessment and cognitive hypothesis-testing skills, including the use of the Dysfunctional Thoughts Record. At the sixth session, she came in with some writing she had begun on the Dysfunctional Thoughts Record and then elaborated.

T: How has your week been?
C: It's been bad. I've done a lot of crying. In fact, just on Sunday I cried for about 4 hours.
T: What brought that on? That's unusual for you.
C: I began writing all about my marriage and my life. I wrote till I was crying so hard I couldn't write anymore. It was very painful.
T: Would you be willing to read aloud what you wrote?
C: Okay, but I kind of hate to start to go over it again. Here goes. "When I met him I

remember how handsome he was. He was in his uniform, and oh, I loved him so much. We spent a lot of time together and were very close. He wanted me to have sex with him, and I resisted him for so long, but finally gave in. It was very good, but I have always felt guilty that I did that before we were married. I got pregnant, and then we got married. We were very happy for a few years; we had three babies, one, two, three, that fast. We didn't have much money and it was hard with all those little ones, but still nice until he got sick. Then we were all in quarantine, and everyone was so frightened by this illness that for a long time no one, not even any of my family, would come and see us. I thought he was going to die, but he finally came home. He couldn't do much for himself, and I had to go to work to support the family. We had three more children, and as much as I love them all, things got really tough. I know that that's when the kids began to resent me so much."

T: How do you know that?

C: My husband always told me that all the kids were very resentful of me.

T: Did the kids ever tell you that they were resentful?

C: No, but they showed it.

T: How did they do that?

C: By not doing the things that I told them to do.

T: Can you give an example?

C: Yes, I remember one very clearly. I worked from four to midnight so that my husband would be home with the kids at night. I would be home to get them off to school in the morning and make meals for the day. I had left word that my son was to do up all the dishes, but when I got home at nearly one in the morning, the kitchen was an absolute mess, and none of the dishes were done. They had all eaten their suppers and just left everything.

T: And what did that mean to you or about you.

C: That meant that they resented me, that I couldn't make them do what a mother should be able to make her kids do. I mean, it was a hard go around that place. I had a lot of responsibility, and when I said something had to be done, it had to be done and right now or the whole place would fall apart.

T: Were you then, or are you now aware of other families who have teenagers who did not do what their parents told them to do?

C: [Laughing] Oh, yes. That happens in all families; I know that now. Back then I didn't have much to compare it with, but I've had a lot more experience since.

T: Even with that experience, you are still thinking that this incident is illustrative of your children's resentment of you, and your failure, as you've described it before, as a mother?

C: Yes. Not just that incident, but a lot of things like it and the fact that my husband always made such a point of telling me that the kids resented me.

T: When you see kids in other families who are not doing all the things their parents tell them to, do you conclude that they are resentful of their parents?

C: Oh, no. There are lots of reasons for that. That's just kids.

T: Somehow you don't conclude that about your children, is that right?

C: I think the difference is that my husband made such a point of it.

T: Is there any possibility that your children did not resent you?

C: I guess there's a possibility.

T: How could you find out?

C: I guess I could ask them.

T: What do you think about doing that?

C: I guess I could. I've never thought about it. I guess I could call one of them.

T: Or all of them?

C: Well, yes. Except I don't think some of them would know what to say.

T: Why wouldn't they know what to say?

C: Well, except for my one daughter, we've just never talked about such things, so I think they would be surprised and wonder what is going on.

T: How could you best handle their surprise and questions about what is going on?

C: I think maybe I could write each of them a letter and tell them what is happening. A few of them know that I have been depressed and have gone to get some help. Then I could ask them if they resented me.

T: "Is there anthing else you would like to know while you're at it?"

C: [*Long pause*] Yes. I'd like to know how they saw my relationship with their father and if they think I did the right thing to leave.

T: Anything else?

C: [*After a very long pause*] Yes. I'd like to know if they have any pleasant memories of me.

The client wrote the letters to her children in order to collect evidence regarding whether her beliefs about her functioning as a mother were accurate or not. She received replies from four of the five children to whom she wrote. She had previously said that these four were the ones whose opinions most counted to her. What she was told was that she had been a tough taskmaster and that as the children grew up they had, indeed, resented her discipline. However, they had many pleasant memories of her and had never doubted her love and affection for them. As they grew into adulthood, they recognized that she had managed a tremendously difficult situation very well, and they had patterned many of their actions as parents after hers. Further, they had long felt sad about the little support and comfort their father had been to her, for the most part, through no fault of his own. They had understood when she left and thought it a sound decision.

When Ellen had begun therapy, she had scored 23 on the Beck Depression Inventory. As she began dealing with initial issues such as whether or not she was performing adequately at work, her Beck score dropped to 17. When she received replies from her children, there was a precipitous drop to a score of 7 accompanied by a totally changed set of cognitions around her performance as a mother. Her perceptions of herself as a wife also changed as she received confirmation that her children thought that she had "gone the last mile" in a difficult marital situation. In the last 3 weeks of therapy she made a final decision not to return to her husband, and her Beck scores remained under 5.

Problems Encountered, Assessing Efficacy, and Follow-Up

Problems Encountered in Treatment

There are numerous difficulties that one encounters in executing this approach to therapy. Learning to practice cognitive therapy is much like acquiring any other set of skills: modeling and symbolic instruction can prepare the potential practitioner, but there is no substitute for the acquisition of experience. Typically, this experience involves "trial and error." Not infrequently, the neophyte cognitive therapist finds himself or herself performing strategic maneuvers in what seems to be a "clumsy," uncomfortable fashion. This perception (and the reality behind it) often changes with experience.

Perhaps the most common problem encountered involves the client's inability to execute the various behavioral and cognitive change strategies outlined by the therapist. Such "noncompliance" is frequently interpreted by the therapist as an indication that the client is "sabotaging" the therapeutic process, motivated by an unconscious "need to fail." However, it would be unreasonable to expect a depressed client to be any more able to execute therapeutic assignments than to deal with any of the other life situations that have brought him or her into treatment.

Typically, such noncompliance can be dealt with as a "technical" problem. Most of these problems can be overcome through careful attention to the interplay between how the "homeworks" are presented and the client's cognitions about that homework and that client's behavioral capacities. In fact, the problems encountered in doing "homeworks" are so often similar to the problems encountered by the client in real-life events that their occurrence can be "diagnostic." Further, the process of working through these issues can serve as a model for the kinds of steps necessary to follow to solve major life problems. Thus, rather than being problems in therapy that force the adoption of dynamic, motivational explanatory models, the occurrence of such noncompliance with assignments can often be turned to therapeutic advantages by staying within a cognitive-behavioral model (Hollon, 1983).

This is far from the only type of problem encountered. Such issues as dealing with "realistic depressions," passivity in the client, overwhelming pessimism, suicidity, and the like are all important, but they are beyond the scope of the present discussion. The interested reader is referred to Beck and colleagues' comprehensive treatment manual (Beck *et al.*, 1979).

Assessing Efficacy

The same self-report and clinician-rated procedures that we have been emphasizing for use before and during treatment are ideal for assessing the efficacy of treatment. The main point that needs to be emphasized is that such assessment is an integral part of the change process and should be integrated into therapy from the very beginning. Thus, behavioral engineering in the first few sessions can be directly assessed against short-term mood ratings, and, with lesser confidence, against session-by-session changes in self-reported syndrome measures.

Because pessimism is such a pervasive aspect of depression, recourse to short-term "experimentation," in which therapeutic efforts are carefully evaluated against objective mood or syndromal measures, is particularly useful. The neophyte therapist should be careful not to fall prey to (or allow the client to fall prey to) "all-or-none" thinking. Particularly early in therapy, very small indications of change are all that can be expected and, if they occur, are indications that therapy is proceeding appropriately.

Typically, 20 sessions over 12 weeks is a sufficient period of time within which to expect full clinical remission. About 70% of primary depressed outpatients can be expected to evidence full remission within that period. In fact, our experience has been that nearly 90% of that change will be evident within the first 6 to 8 weeks, with the remainder of the treatment period being devoted to working on uncovering underlying assumptions and developing relapse prevention strategies. Nonetheless, individual response rates can be quite variable. Some clients evidence slow, gradual change, with few dramatic "drops," but with few sudden increases either. Others evidence far greater affective lability. Whatever the case, we prefer encouraging the client to keep careful charts and graphs of levels of symptomatology, and we frequently use these data as adjuncts to the hypothesis-testing process. Knowing the client's prior history can also be important because such knowledge will color our expectations for remission. Clients with associated personality problems or with histories of chronic depression are less likely to evidence a full remission within this 12-week interval. For such clients, it may be wise to anticipate a longer course of therapy from the outset (Hollon, 1984).

Follow-Up

Most clients who have been depressed are at risk for subsequent episodes. Although any of several interventions are effective in the resolution of the acute episode, any approach that reduces the probability of relapse would be particularly welcome. We stress preparing the client for termination throughout the course of treatment, emphasizing the skills acquisition nature of the therapy and our own desire to make ourselves obsolete. More than in many other therapies, we attempt to explicate the process we utilize to understand the client's difficulties and to achieve change in an effort to enhance the client's capacity to deal with his or her own depression. For example, reductions from twice weekly to once weekly sessions are presented as "experiments" to assess how well the client can function when treatment contact is reduced, a prelude to later termination. Not infrequently, we suggest planning a "relapse" during treatment, just to establish that improvement is linked to what the client does, not simply to spontaneous remission or external factors. Finally, we role play with the client what he or she will do if a relapse begins to occur. We make very sure to communicate that such an occurrence does not mean that treatment failed; rather, such an insipient relapse should signal the client to reinitiate therapeutic self-management activities. We like to use an analogy to taking showers. Taking a shower may get you clean, but it will not necessarily keep you from getting "dirty" again. However, if you do, it is a relatively simple matter to shower again. In short, we emphasize regarding therapy as an opportunity to learn skills that may well help prevent or retard relapses, without implying that relapses will not occur. Further, we try to prepare clients to think of relapses, if they occur, as a time to practice therapeutic self-management skills. We do not expect relapse-free follow-ups (although we do expect a reduction in vulnerability), but we do strive to create a climate in which clients can utilize such occurrences to improve their capacity to deal with their own depressions. As such, our relapse prevention model is quite similar to that utilized in the "controlled drinking" models for alcoholism (Marlatt & Gordon, in press).

Booster sessions are frequently useful during the follow-up period, but extended courses are rarely necessary, unless relapse occurs. Typically, treatment during a relapse proceeds more rapidly and efficiently than the initial course of treatment. Our clinical experience has been that the typical course of *successful* treatment involves one or two brief courses of treatment during the follow-up period, usually lasting only a half-dozen sessions or so, and often occurring anywhere from months to years after the initial treatment course.

Summary

Clinical depression can be defined as a symptom, syndrome, or nosological entity. Assessment efforts need to be carefully tailored to the level of the disorder specified. Several useful assessment instruments are available at each level of conceptualization.

Cognitive therapy is a time-limited, active therapeutic intervention that utilizes an integrated combination of cognitive and behavioral change techniques to alter the passivity, dysfunctional cognitive processes, and negative beliefs associated with depression. The process is one of *collaborative empiricism,* in which the client is encouraged to treat his or her beliefs as hypotheses to be tested, relying heavily on the consequences of his or her own behaviors to provide the necessary evidence. Thus, the client's own experience (influenced by the consequences of behavioral engineering) are used to test his or her beliefs, rather than relying solely on didactic persuasion.

Finally, the whole approach is structured as a skills-training model, with the goal of helping the client develop skills useful long after formal therapy has ended. Given the recurring, episodic nature of most depressions, any truly effective intervention should be able to address the long-term course of the disorder, not just the acute episode. The initial outcome studies have suggested that the time spent in cognitive therapy preparing the client to deal adaptively with future relapses is time well spent.

ACKNOWLEDGMENTS

The authors wish to express their appreciation to V. B. Tuason, Head, Department of Psychiatry, St. Paul-Ramsey Medical Center, for his support and to Mary K. Jones for her secretarial assistance.

References

Abramson, L. Y., & Sackheim, H. A. (1977). A paradox in depression: Uncontrollability and self-blame. *Psychological Bulletin, 84,* 838–851.

Angst, J. (1966). *Zur atiologic and nosologic endoener depressiver Psychosen.* Berlin: Springer, 1966.

Beck, A. T. (1967). *Depression: Clinical, experimental, and theoretical aspects.* New York: Hoeber.

Beck, A. T. (1970). Cognitive therapy: Nature and relation to behavior therapy. *Behavior Therapy, 1,* 184–200.

Beck, A. T., & Greenberg, R. L. (1974). *Coping with depression.* New York: Institute for Rational Living.

Beck, A. T., Ward, C. H., Mendelson, M., Mock, J. E., & Erbaugh, J. K. (1961). An inventory for measuring depression. *Archives of General Psychiatry, 4,* 561–571.

Beck, A. T., Rush, A. J., Shaw, B. F., & Emery, G. (1979). *Cognitive therapy of depression: A treatment manual.* New York: Guilford Press.

Beck, A. T., Hollon, S. D., Bedrosian, R. C., & Young, J. (in press). Treatment of depression with cognitive therapy and amitriptyline. *Archives of General Psychiatry.*

Blackburn, I. M., Bishop, S., Glen, A. I. M., Whalley, L. J., & Christie, J. E. (1981). The efficacy of cognitive therapy in depression: A treatment trial using cognitive therapy and pharmacotherapy, each alone and in combination. *British Journal of Psychiatry, 139,* 181–189.

Burns, D. (1980). *Feeling good: The new mood therapy.* New York: Morrow.

Carroll, B. J., Feinberg, M., Greden, J. F., Tarika, J., Albala, A. A., Haskett, R. F., James, N. McI., Kronfol, Z., Lohr, N., Steiner, M., de Vigne, J. P., & Young, E. (1981). A specific laboratory test for the diagnosis of melancholia. *Archives of General Psychiatry, 38,* 15–22.

Carroll, B. J., Feinberg, M., Smouse, P. E., Rawson, S. G., & Greden, J. F. (1981). The Carroll Rating Scale for Depression: Vol. I. Development, reliability and validation. *British Journal of Psychiatry, 138,* 194–200.

Darley, J. M., & Fazio, R. (1980). Expectancy confirmation processes arising in the social interaction sequence. *American Psychologist, 35,* 867–881.

Depue, R. A., & Monroe, S. M. (1978). The unipolar-bipolar distinction in the depressive disorders. *Psychological Bulletin, 85,* 1001–1029.

Derogatis, L. R., Lipman, R. S., & Covi, L. (1973). The SCL-90: An outpatient psychiatric rating scale. *Psychopharmacology Bulletin, 9,* 13–128.

Ellis, A. (1962). *Reason and emotion in psychotherapy.* New York: Lyle Stuart.

Garber, J., & Hollon, S. D. (1980). Universal versus personal helplessness in depression: Belief in uncontrollability or incompetence? *Journal of Abnormal Psychology, 89,* 56–66.

Hamilton, M. (1960). A rating scale for depression. *Journal of Neurology, Neurosurgery, and Psychiatry, 23,* 56–61.

Hathaway, S. R., & McKinley, J. C. (1951). *The Minnesota Multiphasic Personality Inventory Manual.* New York: Psychological Corporation.

Hersen, M., Eisler, D., Alford, G., & Agras, W. S. (1973). Effects of token economy on neurotic depression: An experimental analysis. *Behavior Therapy, 1973, 4,* 392–397.

Hollon, S. D. Resistance and noncompliance in cognitive behavior therapy for depression. (1983, December). In N. S. Jacobson (Chair), *Resistance and noncompliance in cognitive behavior therapy.* Washington, DC: Institute conducted at the annual convention of the Association for the Advancement of Behavior Therapy.

Hollon, S. D. (1984). Cognitive therapy for depression: Translating research into practice. *The Behavior Therapist, 7,* 125–127.

Hollon, S. D., & Beck, A. T. (1979). Cognitive therapy of depression. In P. C. Kendall & S. D. Hollon (Eds.), *Cognitive-behavioral interventions: Theory, research, and procedures* (pp. 153–204). New York: Academic Press.

Hollon, S. D., & Garber, J. (in press). Cognitive therapy: A social cognitive perspective. In L. Y. Abramson (Ed.), *Social-personal inferences in clinical psychology.* New York: Guilford Press.

Hollon, S. D., & Kendall, P. C. (1980). Cognitive self-statemetns in depression: Development of an automatic thoughts questionnaire. *Cognitive Therapy and Research, 4,* 383–395.

Hollon, S. D., & Kriss, M. R. (1984). Cognitive factors in clinical research and practice. *Clinical Psychology Review, 4,* 38–78.

Hollon, S. D., Tuason, V. B., Wiemer, M. J., DeRubeis, R. J., Evans, M. D., & Garvey, M. J. (1983). *Combined cognitive-pharmacotherapy versus cognitive therapy alone and pharmacotherapy alone in the treatment of depressed outpatients: Differential treatment outcome in the CPT project.* Unpublished manuscript, University of Minnesota/St. Paul-Ramsey Medical Center, Minneapolis-St. Paul.

Kahneman, D., Slovic, P., & Tversky, A. (Eds.). (1982). *Judgment under uncertainty: Heuristics and biases.* Cambridge, England: Cambridge University Press.

Kovacs, M., Rush, A. T., Beck, A. T., & Hollon, S. D. (1981). Depressed outpatients treated with cognitive therapy or pharmacotherapy: A one-year follow-up. *Archives of General Psychiatry, 38,* 33–39.

Lehmann, H. E. (1959). Psychiatric concepts of depression: Nomenclature and classification. *Canadian Psychiatric Association Journal Supplement, 4,* 51–512.

Leonhard, K. (1959). *Aufteilung der endogenen Psychosen.* Berlin: Akademie Verlag.

Lewinsohn, P. M. (1974). Clinical and theoretical aspects of depression. In K. S. Calhoun, H. E. Adams, & K. M. Mitchell (Eds.), *Innovative treatment methods in psychopathology.* New York: Wiley.

Lewinsohn, P. M., Biglan, A., & Zeiss, A. M. (1976). Behavioral treatment of depression. In P. O. Davidson (Ed.), *The behavioral management of anxiety, depression, and pain.* New York: Brunner/Mazel, 1976.

Lewinsohn, P. M., Munoz, R. F., Youngren, M. A., & Zeiss, A. M. (1978). *Control your depression.* Englewood Cliffs, NJ: Prentice-Hall.

Lubin, B. (1965). Adjective checklists for measurement of depression. *Archives of General Psychiatry, 12,* 57–62.

Marlatt, G. A., & Gordon, J. R. (in press). *Relapse prevention: Maintenance strategies for addictive behavior change.* New York: Guilford Press.

Mendels, J., & Cochrane, C. (1968). The nosology of depression: The endogenous-reactive concept. *American Journal of Psychiatry, 124* (Suppl. 11), 1–11.

Murphy, G. E., Simons, A. D., Wetzel, R. D., & Lustman, P. J. (1984). Cognitive therapy and pharmacotherapy, singly and together, in the treatment of depression. *Archives of General Psychiatry, 44,* 33–41.

Nisbett, R. E., & Ross, L. (1980). *Human inference: Strategies and shortcomings of social judgment.* Englewood Cliffs, NJ: Prentice-Hall.

Perris, C. (1966). A study of bipolar (manic-depressive) and unipolar recurrent depressive psychoses. *Acta Psychiatrica Scandinavia, 42* (Suppl. 194), 1–189.

Raskin, A., Schulterbrandt, J. C., Reating, N., & McKeon, J. J. (1970). Differential response to chlorpromazine, imipramine, and placebo: A study of hospitalized depressed patients. *Archives of General Psychiatry, 23,* 164–174.

Rehm, L. P. (1977). A self-control model of depression. *Behavior Therapy, 8,* 787–804.

Robins, E., & Guze, S. B. (1969). Classification of affective disorders: The primary-secondary, the endogenous-reactive, and the neurotic-psychotic concepts. In T. A. Williams *et al.* (Eds.), *Recent advances in the psychobiology of the depressive illnesses.* Chevy Chase, MD: U.S. Department of Health, Education, and Welfare.

Robins, L. N., Helzer, J. E., Croughan, J., & Ratcliff, K. S. (1981). National Institute of Mental Health Diagnostic Interview Schedule: Its history, characteristics, and validity. *Archives of General Psychiatry, 38,* 381–389.

Rush, A. J., Beck, A. T., Kovacs, M., & Hollon, S. D. (1977). Comparative efficacy of cognitive therapy versus pharmacotherapy in outpatient depressives. *Cognitive Therapy and Research, 1,* 17–37.

Seligman, M. E. P., Abramson, L. Y., Semmel, A., & von Baeyer, C. (1979). Depressive attributional style. *Journal of Abnormal Psychology, 88,* 242–247.

Shaw, B. F. (1977). Comparison of cognitive therapy and behavior therapy in the treatment of depression. *Journal of Consulting and Clinical Psychology, 45,* 543–551.

Snyder, M. (1981). Seek and ye shall find: Testing hypotheses about other people. In E. T. Higgins, C. P. Herman, & M. P. Zanna (Eds.), *Social cognition: The Ontario Symposium* ((pp. 277–304). Hillsdale, NJ: Erlbaum.

Spitzer, R. L., Endicott, J., and the NIMH Clinical Research Branch Collaborative Program on the Psychobiology of Depression. (1978). *Schedule for Affective Disorders and Schizophrenia-Lifetime Version* (3rd ed.). New York: Psychiatric Institute, Biometrics Research Division.

Spitzer, R. L., Endicott, J., & Robins, E. (1972). Research diagnostic criteria: Rationale and reliability. *Archives of General Psychiatry, 35,* 773–782.

Taylor, F. G., & Marshall, W. L. (1977). Experimental analysis of a cognitive-behavioral therapy for depression. *Cognitive Therapy and Research, 1977, 1,* 59–72.

Watkins, J. J., & Rush, A. J. (1983). Cognitive response test. *Cognitive Therapy and Research, 7,* 425–436.

Weissman, A., & Beck, A. T. (1978, November). *The Dysfunctional Attitudes Scale: A validation study.* Paper presented at the annual meeting of the Associate for the Advancement of Behavior Therapy, Chicago.

Winokur, G. (1970). Genetic findings and methodological considerations in manic-depressive disease. *British Journal of Psychiatry, 117,* 267–274.

Winokur, G., Clayton, P. J., & Reich, T. (1969). *Manic-depressive illness.* St. Louis: C. V. Mosby.

Zuckerman, M., & Lubin, B. (1965). *Manual for the Multiple Affect Adjective Check List.* San Diego, CA: Education and Industrial Testing Service.

Zung, W. W. K. (1965). A self-rating depression scale. *Archives of General Psychiatry, 12,* 63–70.

Social Skills Training Approaches

ROBERT E. BECKER AND RICHARD G. HEIMBERG

Introduction

In this chapter we outline the application of social skills training approaches to the treatment of nonpsychotic unipolar depressive disorder. *Social skills training* is a collection of techniques including instructions, modeling, behavior rehearsal, corrective feedback, social reinforcement, and selected cognitive restructuring techniques that have been effectively utilized to modify the social behavior of clients with a broad range of interpersonal difficulties. Social skills training has been applied to the treatment of persons suffering from major depressive episodes, and preliminary results suggests that it may be as effective in remediating depressive symptoms as some pharmacologically based treatment approaches (Bellack, Hersen, & Himmelhoch, 1983; Hersen, Bellack, Himmelhoch, & Thase, 1984). At the Mood Disorders Clinic of Albany Medical College, we are currently engaged in a study of the effectiveness of social skills training and antidepressant medication for the treatment of chronic intermittent depressive disorder. In addition to cognitive therapy (see Chapter 7, this volume), social skills training may represent a viable alternative to drug treatment for some depressed individuals.

We begin the chapter with a brief discussion of the diagnosis of depressive disorder, a description of the various subtypes of depressive disorder, and an overview of methods for the measurement of the severity of depressive symptoms. In the remainder of the chapter, we focus our efforts on a description of the strategies

ROBERT E. BECKER • Behavior Therapy Unit, Department of Psychiatry, Medical College of Pennsylvania at EPPI, 3200 Henry Avenue, Philadelphia, Pennsylvania 19129. RICHARD G. HEIMBERG • Center for Stress and Anxiety Disorders, State University of New York at Albany, 1535 Western Avenue, Albany, New York 12203. Preparation of this manuscript was supported in part by grant No. RO1 MH35.9901 TDAA awarded to the authors by the National Institute of Mental Health.

employed at the Mood Disorders Clinic to assess social behavior and the techniques involved in the application of social skills training to the treatment of chronically depressed individuals.

Diagnosis and Subtypes of Depressive Disorder

The first task for any therapist who treats depressed individuals is to assess the client's affective state and determine if he or she is, in fact, depressed. This task first involves the identification of a series of specific symptoms that define the class of affective disorders as specified by the American Psychiatric Association (1980) in the *Diagnostic and Statistical Manual of Mental Disorders* (DSM-III). The clinician must also attempt to specify which type of affective disorder is present and further attempt to rule out the possibility that whatever depressive symptoms are demonstrated by the client are a secondary result of some other medical or emotional disorder. Although full explication of the clinical procedures utilized in the processes of diagnosis and differential diagnosis is well beyond the scope of this chapter, a brief discussion is warranted. In this discussion, we will concentrate only on those procedures and devices in use at the Mood Disorders Clinic.

The primary device utilized in the process of structured clinical diagnosis is the Schedule for Affective Disorders and Schizophrenia (SADS) (Endicott & Spitzer, 1978). The SADS is a structured interview guide that allows an experienced interviewer to collect necessary diagnostic information in an efficient manner. By asking questions about the presence or absence of essential symptoms, it surveys the range of affective disorders, schizophrenia, and several competing diagnostic categories (e.g., the anxiety disorders) in 60 to 90 minutes. Data collected during a SADS interview may be compared against specific criteria for each disorder as described in the manual for the Research Diagnostic Criteria (RDC) (Spitzer, Endicott, & Robins, 1978). A diagnosis of major depressive disorder may be applied if the following criteria are met (American Psychiatric Association, 1980, pp. 213–215):

1. Dysphoric mood or loss of interest or pleasure in all or almost all usual activities and pastimes.
2. Four or more of the following must be present nearly every day for a period of at least two weeks: poor appetite/significant weight loss or increased appetite/significant weight gain; insomnia or hypersomnia; psychomotor agitation or retardation; loss of interest or pleasure in usual activities or decrease in sex drive; loss of energy, fatigue; feelings of worthlessness, self-reproach, or excessive guilt; diminished ability to think or concentrate; recurrent thoughts of suicide or death.
3. Symptoms do not appear to be a result of Schizophrenia, Organic Mental Disorder or Uncomplicated Bereavement.
4. The patient has no history of manic episodes.

Other types of affective disorder listed in the *Diagnostic and Statistical Manual of Mental Disorders* (DSM-III) include bipolar disorder, cyclothymic disorder, dysthymic disorder, adjustment disorder with depressed mood, and atypical affective disorder. Dysthymic disorder (or intermittent depressive disorder as it is called in the RDC), the diagnostic group under study at the Mood Disorders Clinic, is defined in DSM-III (1980, pp. 222–223) as follows:

1. During the past two years the individual has been bothered by symptoms characteristic of the depressive syndrome but that are not of sufficient severity and duration to meet the criteria for a major depressive episode.
2. Depressive mood may be relatively persistent or separated by periods of normal mood lasting a few days to a few weeks, but no more than a few months at a time.
3. During depressive periods, a prominent depressed mood or marked loss of interest in almost all usual activities and pastimes.
4. At least three of the following must be present during depressive periods: insomnia or hypersomnia; low energy level or chronic tiredness; feelings of inadequacy; decreased effectiveness or productivity at school, work, or home; decreased ability to concentrate; social withdrawal; loss of interest in pleasurable activities; irritability or excessive anger; inability to respond with pleasure to praise or rewards; less active or talkative than usual; pessimistic attitude toward the future, brooding about the past, or feeling sorry for oneself; tearfulness or crying; recurrent thoughts of death or suicide.
5. Absence of psychotic features.

Measurement of the Severity of Depression

After a client has been suitably diagnosed and any issues of differential diagnosis have been resolved, the degree of depressive impairment must be assessed. This is a necessary step in outcome evaluation because it is the severity of the symptoms at pretreatment with which the client will be most concerned and that will later provide the basis for evaluating the effectiveness of treatment interventions. Next we describe the measures employed at the Mood Disorders Clinic for the assessment of the severity of depression. It should be kept in mind, however, that although these measures are a necessary part of clinical and outcome evaluation, they provide little information about the client that will be specifically useful in the formulation of a social skills training program. These measures are described in a later section.

Self-Report Measures

Self-report scales attempt to assess those subjective feelings, attitudes, and mood states that make up a central component of the depressive experience. As such, they ask the client to report on those experiences to which only he or she has access. Although this assessment is critical, the clinician should always keep in mind that self-report measures not only assess depressive symptoms but are themselves affected by these symptons. Depressed individuals may have difficulty concentrating or following directions. They may believe that the clinician is not really interested in them. Furthermore, they may have a severe tendency to see things as worse than they really are. Several laboratory studies (e.g., DeMonbreun & Craighead, 1977) support the view that depressed persons selectively recall negative events, whereas others (e.g., Jacobson & Anderson, 1982) suggest that they emit a high number of negative self-referent statements. These propensities may affect the quality and accuracy of the information provided on self-report scales. Nevertheless, these scales provide important information about the client's perceived state.

Several self-report scales are available to the clinician interested in the assessment of depression, including the MMPI-D30 (Comrey, 1957), the Zung Self-Rating Depression Scale (Zung, 1965), the Depression Adjective Checklist (Lubin, 1965), the Center for Epidemiologic Studies Depression Scale (Radloff, 1977), and the depression factor of the Hopkins Symptom Checklist (Derogatis, Lipman, Rickels, Uhlenhuth, & Covi, 1974). Probably the most widely used self-report measure of depression (and the one in use at the Mood Disorders Clinic) is the Beck Depression Inventory (BDI) (Beck, Ward, Mendelson, Mock, & Erbaugh, 1961). The BDI includes 21 items, each with four response alternatives that receive scores of 0 to 3 depending on the severity of depression implied by the response. It is scored simply by summing the scores for each item. Although items sample the range of depressive symptoms, they draw somewhat more heavily from the cognitive than the behavioral or somatic domains. A split-half reliability of .93 has been reported by Beck *et al.* (1961). The BDI relates well to independent clinical judgment of depression (Beck *et al.,* 1961; Metcalfe & Goldman, 1965) and to behavioral measures of depression and the Hamilton Rating Scale for Depression Scores (Williams, Barlow, & Agras, 1972). Readers interested in further information about self-report measurement of depression are referred to papers by Bellack and Hersen (1977) and Hammen (1981).

Clinical Rating Scales

A number of rating scales that are completed at the end of a clinical interview are available for the assessment of depressive symptoms and are currently employed at the Mood Disorders Clinic. These scales include the Hamilton Rating Scale for Depression (Hamilton, 1960), the Raskin Global Severity of Depression Scale (Raskin, Schulterbrandt, Reatig, & Rice, 1967), and the Schedule for Affective Disorders and Schizophrenia, Change version (SADS-C) (Spitzer & Endicott, 1977). The Global Assessment Scale (Endicott, Spitzer, Fleiss, & Cohen, 1976), a measure of the degree of impairment in social, occupational, and family functioning, is also employed at the Mood Disorders Clinic.

The original Hamilton scale consists of 17 items sampling subjective, behavioral, and somatic/vegetative symptoms of depression. Twenty-one and 24-item versions of the scale are also available, including a recent version developed for the National Institute of Mental Health collaborative study evaluating cognitive therapy, interpersonal therapy, and imipramine hydrochloride as treatments for major depressive disorder. Depending on the specific version, items are scored on 0–3 or 1–4 scales. The Hamilton scale was originally developed for use by trained clinical interviewers, but a study by O'Hara and Rehm (1983) demonstrates that acceptable levels of interrater agreement can be achieved by doctoral students in psychology. Similarly, at the Mood Disorders Clinic, agreement of 85 to 90% has been achieved between the ratings of a psychiatrist and psychiatric nurses.

The Raskin scale is also completed after a detailed clinical interview, based on the client's self-report, observation of client behavior, and identification of secondary symptoms of depression. Each of three items is rated on a 1–5 scale, and a score of 7 to 9 of a possible 15 is interpreted as an indication of moderate depression. Preliminary data from the NIMH collaborative study on the long-term preventive treatment of recurrent affective disorder suggest that Raskin scores were predictive of recurrence of depressive symptoms (Prien, personal communication, 1983). In this study, patients whose scores declined to 3 and remained at that level for three successive weekly assessments experienced fewer recurrences than patients with higher scores.

The SADS-C is a device similar to the SADS but employed specifically to measure posttreatment change. It contains 65 items divided into several subscales including Depressive Syndrome, Endogenous Features, Manic Syndrome, Anxiety, Delusions and Disorganization, and Miscellaneous Psychopathology. The Global Assessment Scale is included, and a Hamilton scale score may be derived from SADS-C items.

Assessment of Social Skills

The determination of the type and severity of depression is a necessary step in the evaluation of treatment interventions. However, by themselves, these data provide little direction to the clinician in his or her attempt to formulate a plan for psychotherapeutic treatment. Such formulations will ultimately be derived from the clinician's theoretical notions about the factors that precipitate and maintain depressive experience. The clinician who chooses to implement a social skills training program with a depressed patient assumes, explicitly or implicitly, that depressive behavior is in some way related to inadequate interpersonal functioning. At the Mood Disorders Clinic, our social skills training program for chronically depressed patients is based on the following assumptions:

1. Depression is a result of an inadequate schedule of positive reinforcement contingent on the person's nondepressed behavior.
2. A meaningful portion of the most salient positive reinforcers in the adult world are interpersonal in nature.
3. A meaningful portion of the noninterpersonal rewards in adult life may be received or denied, contingent on the person's interpersonal behavior.
4. Therefore, any set of treatment techniques that helps the depressed patient increase the quality of his or her interpersonal behavior should act to increase the amount of response-contingent positive reinforcement and thereby decrease depressive affect and increase the rate of "nondepressed behavior."

5. Inadequate interpersonal behavior may arise from any number of sources including, but not restricted to, the following:
    a. Insufficient exposure to interpersonally skilled models at key developmental periods.
    b. Insufficient opportunity to practice important interpersonal routines at key developmental periods.
    c. Learning of inappropriate or maladaptive interpersonal behaviors at key developmental periods.
    d. Failure to "discard" old behaviors and adopt new ones during periods of transition, that is entry into adolescence or adulthood.
    e. Decaying of specific behavioral skills due to disuse, as in the case of a newly divorced individual who must now enter the singles' world.
    f. Failure to recognize the appropriate or inappropriate times for the execution of specific behavioral routines.
    g. Nonexecution of a potentially adaptive behavior because of a belief in the inevitable failure of the behavior to produce the desired result or one's belief that he or she cannot perform the required behavior adequately.

Background Literature

The assumptions listed before are based on a large body of literature on the behavioral analysis of depression, the interpersonal behavior of depressed and nondepressed persons, and the cognitive processes of depressed and nondepressed persons. Because we have reviewed these literatures in two previous papers (Becker & Heimberg, 1984; Becker, Heimberg, & Tassinari, in press), we will not attempt a lengthy review here. However, a brief examination of these literatures will be undertaken.

Charles Ferster (1965, 1973), the first behavioral psychologist to devote his attention to the study of depression, defined *depression* as a low rate of operant behavior emitted by the individual. The low rate of behavior was said to result from a disruption in the person's ongoing system of positive reinforcement as might occur when a person sees a long-term relationship come to an end, loses his or her job, or faces restricted physical activity as a result of injury or advancing age. Previously reinforced behavior was placed on extinction, returned to its operant level, and nothing moved in to "replace" it. Ferster's formulations initiated the behavioral study of depression but were not adequate to explain differences among people in their tendencies to react to events such as those first described with depression. Peter Lewinsohn expanded on Ferster's work by stressing the importance of *response-contingent* positive reinforcement. The amount of response-contingent positive reinforcement was said to be a function of (a) the number of activities that the person may find potentially rewarding; (b) the availability of those events in the person's immediate environment; and (c) *the skillfulness and rate of emission of interpersonal behaviors that elicit a maximum of positive reinforcement and a minimum of punishment for the individual,* that is, social skill. According to Lewinsohn (1975), depression-prone individuals are lacking in this important area. As a result, when they find their lives disrupted for any number of reasons, they may be less able than other persons to develop alternative sources of personal gratification.

Several studies demonstrate the poor quality of the interpersonal behavior of depressed individuals. Although these studies do not indicate the specific reasons for deficits in social behavior (i.e., they do not demonstrate that depressed persons lack behavioral knowledge; they simply demonstrate that effective behaviors are not forthcoming from depressed persons in social situations), they provide support for many of Lewinsohn's contentions and are clearly supportive of the broad-based approach to social skills training to be described in a later section of this chapter.

Coyne (1976) asked nondepressed persons to spend time engaged in conversations with persons who were depressed. At the end of these conversations, the nondepressed persons reported a large drop in their own mood. They found the conversations to be quite unpleasant and expressed a desire to avoid the other (depressed) person in the future. In another study (Jacobson & Anderson, 1982) depressed and nondepressed persons were again placed in dyads. Although the two groups of subjects were similar on most counts, depressed subjects made more negative self-referent statements. They also emitted more self-disclosing statements, presumably of the same negative tone, without being questioned by the other person. We might speculate that this tendency toward unsolicited negative self-disclosure was what Coyne's nondepressed subjects found so unpleasant!

Studies by the Lewinsohn group have examined the performance of depressed persons in a group situation. In a study by Libet and Lewinsohn (1973), depressed subjects exhibited several deficits in social behavior including a slower response time, less frequent attempts to initiate conversation with others, and a lower probability of responding positively to the initiations of others. Youngren and Lewinsohn (1980) report that clinically depressed psychiatric patients were less involved than other persons in social interactions and found them less rewarding. Finally, in an intriguing study by Sanchez and Lewinsohn (1980), depressed outpatients were asked to monitor their mood and the frequency with which they behaved assertively over a period of several weeks. Assertive behavior and mood were negatively correlated. Assertive behavior was found to significantly predict the next day's mood, whereas mood did not predict the next day's assertive behavior.

Our social skills training package also relies upon the literature examining the role of cognitive factors in depression and/or social behavior. Components of treatment are based upon Morrison and Bellack's (1981) concern that social skills training include specific attention to the interpretation of others' communications and to the analysis of the effect of social mores on the probability that specific behaviors will result in positive outcomes, a realm they have labeled *social perception.* We also rely on the work of Rehm (1977) relating depression to deficits in self-monitoring, self-evaluation, and self-reinforcement.

Assessment: Goals and Procedures

With the preceding review as background, we may now address the goals and procedures involved in the assessment of interpersonal behavior. At the Mood Disorders Clinic, an extensive assessment battery consisting of clinical interviews, self-report questionnaires, and behavioral roleplays is utilized to fulfill several goals:

1. to provide an initial evaluation of the client's social behavior and, therefore, the potential appropriateness of various components of social skills training;
2. to determine the specific content of social skills training sessions;
3. to monitor clients' progress across sessions especially in reference to specific situations addressed in treatment:
4. to establish whether or not the client's social behavior has changed in a positive direction by the end of treatment and during a 1-year follow-up period;
5. to determine if change in a client's social behavior relates to changes in the client's affective state; and
6. to evaluate whether social skills training has produced a change in social behavior and related cognitive processes when compared with other treatment conditions.

These goals, of course, are inextricably bound together, and most assessment modalities contribute toward multiple goals. However, in the interest of brevity, we will concentrate only on the use of clinical interviews and behavioral roleplays in the assessment process. Those readers interested in pursuing the use of self-report measures of social skills are referred to J. G. Beck and Heimberg (1983). Those interested in cognitive assessment are referred to volumes on that topic by Kendall and Hollon (1981) and Merluzzi, Glass, and Genest (1981).

The Clinical Interview

Although the initial goal of the clinical interview is the determination of a SADS-RDC diagnosis, the bulk of interview time routinely is devoted to a discussion of the client's life circumstances. During this screening interview and extending into the first one or two therapy sessions, the patient is specifically queried about interpersonal difficulties he or she may experience in several different settings—work or school, family relationships, sexual or intimate emotional relationships, friendships, casual social encounters, and interactions with strangers. As we have noted elsewhere (Becker, Heimberg, & Tassinari, in press), we attempt to identify those *behavior settings* and *interaction partners* that have a strong functional relationship to the client's mood—when interactions with these partners in these settings turn out well, the client feels better; when they go badly, the client feels worse. Similarly, we attempt to identify situations that a client must be able to handle competently before a desired goal might be accomplished. A client must be able to present himself or herself well in a stressful job interview before he or she may obtain that desired position; and he or she must be able to initiate casual conversations with the opposite sex before he or she is likely to be successful in requesting a date.

In the discussion of each interaction partner and behavior setting, it is necessary to obtain very detailed descriptions of the partner and his or her likely response to the situation at hand (as perceived by the client) so that this material may be used in later therapy sessions to construct scenarios for social skills training. The interviewer may wish to inquire about any of the partner's behavioral habits, including gestures, facial expressions, postures, or favorite sayings. It is often helpful to ask the client to roleplay the interaction partner's likely response to the situation in as much detail as possible. It is also important to realize the limitations of this source of information. It is less likely to reflect objective reality than it is to represent the client's worst fears. In fact, the client may have no objective information to rely on because these fears may have inhibited any attempt to resolve the situation at all. One of our female clients, for example, when asked to demonstrate her husband's likely response to her desire to obtain employment outside the home, roleplayed her husband's response liberally spiced with shouts, obscene gestures, and descriptions of the client's probable ancestry. However, the client had never voiced her desire for fear that her husband would respond in precisely that way. Later in treatment, the client was encouraged to discuss the situation with her husband, and he was thrilled that she would now contribute to the family's troubled finances! Although the client's initial perceptions may have been inaccurate, it was useful to obtain them and to train her to be prepared for what she saw as the worst possible outcome. As she approached her husband, she felt she could respond competently to anything he might have said because she was prepared for the worst.

Not only must the interviewer assess the relevant interaction partners and behavior settings, he or she must also assess the adequacy of the client's performance of several types of behavioral skills. Our training program focuses on three specific behavioral repertoires that are of potential significance to our depressed clients—negative assertion, positive assertion, and conversational skills—in addition to specialized repertoires that may be of significance to smaller numbers of clients (e.g., job interviewing or dating skills).

Negative assertion involves those behaviors that allow a person to stand up for himself or herself and act in his or her own best interest when the needs and desires of people conflict. Negative assertion skills that are addressed in our program include refusal of requests or demands that the client deems unreasonable, requesting that other persons change their behavior when it infringes on the client in some important way, negotiating a solution to conflict, and reaching a compromise.

Positive assertion and *conversational skills* involve the performance of behaviors that should make the client more socially attractive to other people. When we address positive assertion skills, we focus on expressing affection to others, giving compliments, expressing praise, approval, or appreciation, and giving appropriate apologies. From the complex area of conversational skills, we devote specific attention to the skills of initiating conversations, asking questions, providing appropriate information about oneself, being socially reinforcing to the conversational efforts of others, and ending conversations gracefully. Each of these three general repertoires appears to be of special importance to depressed patients.

Self-monitored and self-reported negative assertion has been shown to be inversely related to depression levels (Lea & Pacquin, 1981; Sanchez & Lewinsohn, 1980). Positive assertion and conversational skills derive their importance from the studies reviewed previously, demonstrating the problematic interpersonal behavior of depressed persons in dyads and groups.

To teach the general categories of skills noted before, it is necessary to analyze them one step further. Each skill area must be broken down into its component behaviors before social skills training may be effectively applied. In addition to *speech content,* the interviewer should also pay attention to *paralinguistic aspects of speech* such as volume, pitch, or tone, *nonverbal behaviors* such as eye contact, facial expression, posture, or gestures, and the *timing* of the delivery of a response. All aspects of a response must be delivered in an integrated fashion, or the desired effect may be lost, as in the case of a person who attempts to deliver a negative assertive response in a whiny voice. In order to obtain this information about the client's performance in the situations of concern, the interviewer should roleplay the target situations with the client during therapy sessions and carefully observe the client's performance of all relevant aspects of the response. The interviewer may also wish to avail himself or herself of the results of a standardized roleplay test, such as the one to be described next.

The Behavioral Roleplay Test

Although roleplaying in the clinical interview provides much information necessary for the proper conduct of social skills training, assessment of the effects of social skills training on clients' social behavior requires different measurement strategies. It would be most useful if we could collect samples of social behavior in the specific situations that each client finds problematic as these situations occur in real life. However, these situations occur at irregular and unpredictable intervals and are often of such a private and sensitive nature that observation would be not only cumbersome but unethical. As a result, most researchers in the area of social skills training employ standardized roleplay tests. In the prototypical roleplay assessment, a narrator reads a brief description of the situation to be roleplayed, an assistant gives the client a prompt (i.e., roleplays the opening line of the interaction), and the subject responds. This brief interaction is recorded on (video)tape and several measures of speech content and nonverbal behavior are derived from the taped records. Standard roleplay tests like the Behavioral Assertiveness Test-Revised (Eisler, Hersen, Miller, & Blanchard, 1975) include many situations from different behavioral domains (e.g., positive and negative assertion) in order to obtain a representative sample of the client's response style. Although roleplay tests have been employed as a regular part of almost all studies of social skills training conducted since 1970, the last few years have witnessed an increased concern over the external validity of roleplay assessment data. Several recent studies (reviewed by Bellack, 1981) suggest that roleplay scores may not relate to independent criteria of social performance in a systematic manner, and the results of studies utilizing roleplay tests have been called into question. It is possible, however, that the relatively poor showing of roleplay assessments is a function of inattention to several subtle but important aspects of their administration. For instance, the rapid-fire sequence of narration/prompt/response/narration/prompt/response may prevent the client from "getting into role" appropriately, or the standardized nature of the roleplay stimuli may reduce their salience to the client. As a result, the client may become anxious or confused or remain uninvolved in the entire assessment process (Bellack, 1983). To test this last assertion, a study of the impact of standardized roleplay scenarios versus scenarios constucted on the basis of data provided by clients about personally relevant real-life situations ("personalized" roleplays) is being conducted at the Mood Disorders Clinic. Personalized roleplays are constructed during the initial diagnostic interview and appended to the standardized roleplay test that is administered to all clients. Clients provide ratings of the relevance of each personalized and standard scenario and the amount of discomfort they experience during each. Roleplays are recorded on videotape for later behavioral observation. Relevance and discomfort ratings have now been collected for 20 clients. Preliminary analyses indicate that clients rate the personalized roleplays as significantly more relevant and as leading to significantly more discomfort. In line with Bellack's (1983) formulations, these findings suggest that personalized roleplay scenes may produce greater involvement on the part of clients. If so, a personalized approach to roleplay assessment, in which all scenes are similarly formatted but scenes are selected to represent individually meaningful situations, may lead to a more accurate appraisal of clients' social competence.

The roleplay procedure utilized at the Mood Disorders Clinic owes much to the writings and consultation of our colleague Alan Bellack. Twelve standard dual-response roleplay scenarios are administered to each client in addition to two personalized scenarios. The 12 standard scenes are equally divided into 6 positive and 6 negative assertion scenes, 2 each with family members, friends, and co-workers. Prior to the administration of the roleplay scenes, the client is provided with a typewritten sheet that contains the scene descriptions with blanks where the names of the interpersonal partner should go. Clients are instructed to select that person from real life who most accurately fulfills the proper role, and his or her name is inserted in the scene description. When role playing is initiated, it is the client who actually reads the scene description (which is written in the first person). A roleplay assistant then provides the required prompt, the client responds, the assistant gives another prompt, and the client responds again. The client then gives his or her ratings of relevance and discomfort, and the next scene is introduced. In this way, we attempt to maximize client involvement in the entire roleplay procedure.

In addition to the ratings provided by the client, a number of measures are derived from videotapes of the roleplayed interactions. Included in this list are measures of overall response quality, speech fluency, latency to respond, duration of response, loudness, affect, eye contact, and body orientation. Several of these measures are operationalized in the form of *bidirectional* rating scales. Extremely high levels of a behavior *and* extemely low levels of a behavior both receive low ratings, whereas more moderate performances receive high scores. For example, someone who shouts receives a rating similar to someone who speaks barely loud enough to be heard, whereas someone who maintians a conversational volume is more positively rated. As noted by Bellack (1983), this type of scoring procedure assures that high scores represent a greater degree of social competence. Simple duration or frequency scores are unidirectional and cannot take such complexities into account.

Cognitive-Behavioral Social Skills Training: Procedures

The treatment offered at the Mood Disorders Clinic draws heavily on a package developed by Bellack, Hersen, and Himmelhoch (1981; Hersen, Bellack, & Himmelhoch, 1982) at the University of Pittsburgh. It includes training on both expressive and receptive communication skills and an emphasis on cognitive factors such as social perception, self-evaluation, and self-reinforcement. The package contains segments on *direct behavior training, practice and generalization, social perception training,* and *self-evaluation and self-reinforcement training.* In the interest of clarity, we present each technique separately, but in the actual delivery of treatment, they are applied in an *integrated manner.* Each set of techniques is applied on an individualized basis to the treatment of specific performance problems in specific behavior settings until a minimally acceptable level of skill is attained. Direct behavior training and practices usually receive the greatest attention early in treatment, whereas cognitive strategies are increasingly invoked as treatment moves along.

Direct Behavior Training

At the point that training actually begins, the therapist and client will already have spent two to three sessions together (including the initial diagnostic interview), and a list of problematic interpersonal situations related to the client's depression will have been developed. The client should already have been exposed to the rationale for treatment, and a general outline of what should occur during treatment should have been presented. Direct behavior training begins with the selection of a specific situation for attention, preferably one that has a number of desirable characteristics—it is important to the client; it has relevance to the client's present life; it does not represent a "crisis"; and it does not hold potentially disastrous consequences for the client. Although clients desire most often to attack the most pressing issues, these situations inevitably provide a poor environment for the training of varied and flexible social skills. A less intense, less emotionally loaded situation will provide a better vehicle for instruction on the specific behavioral skills isolated during the clinical interview and behavioral roleplay test.

During all cognitive behavioral social skills training procedures, the clinician adopts an educational stance and provides detailed and specific instructions about behaviors targeted for change. Behaviors are focused upon one at a time, and the clinician instructs the client both in the specifics of behavioral performance and in the reasons that the target behavior is important. Instructions should be *brief* and focus on what the client *should do.* After the client has been carefully instructed, several roleplay rehearsals of the problematic situation are conducted. Typically, rehearsals progress through the following steps:

1. An initial brief roleplay in which the client makes an attempt to produce the desired behavior.

2. Further instructions along with demonstration of the target behavior by the therapist in the form of a *modeling display.* Therapist modeling of new behavior occurs during roleplays in which the client assumes the role of the other person. Some additional benefits may attend this procedure. First, the clinician will gain additional information about the other person's behavior that may be incorporated into later rehearsals. Second, the client may be placed in a position to experience some of the thoughts and feelings of the prospective interaction partner. Because of the latter effects, this procedure has been labeled *role reversal.*

3. A second roleplay is conducted in which the client resumes his or her original role but attempts to incorporate new content gleaned from instructions and modeling displays.

4. Upon completion of the second roleplay, the clinician provides *response-specific feedback.* Praise is given for attempts or approximations to desired behavior, and clear, concrete instructions for change in future rehearsals are given.

5. Further roleplays follow this format until the therapist believes the behavior has been mastered. Additional behaviors are incorporated until an integrated response is achieved.

6. When all targets of training have been improved to minimally acceptable levels, roleplaying takes a slightly different turn. The therapist varies his or her response to the client so as to be less agreeable (more angry, self-righteous, hostile, etc.) in order to develop flexibility in the client's response style. This step may also serve another purpose in that the response is actually overtrained. Overtrained responses may be experienced by the client as more "natural" and may be more likely to compete with and replace less functional habits.

7. Upon completion of flexibility training, the in-session treatment of the specific situation is temporarily completed.

Practice and Generalization

When flexibility training has been accomplished, the clinician should be prepared to make homework assignments so that newly acquired skills may be put into practice in everyday life. Homework serves to provide practice for newly learned responses and to promote generalization or transfer of the new skills into the client's natural environment. The following guidelines should be followed when making homework assignments:

1. The assignment should be worked out with and agreed upon by the client.

2. The instructions for homework assignments must be detailed. For example,

rather than simply requesting that a client notice and compliment his or her spouse's positive behaviors, the assignment might specify the kinds of behaviors that should be praised, the possible types of compliments that might be given, and a specification of the setting where a compliment might be offered. The assignment should be recorded in the chart and a copy provided to the client. Additionally, the client should maintain a written record of attempts to carry out assignments.

3. The assignment should have a high probability of success. Therefore, assignments should be made if and only if the client can reasonably execute a good response and the recipient of that response is likely to react in the manner predicted in treatment. Early in treatment, unsuccessful homework assignments may result in a justifiable hesitation to attempt future behaviors. Successes may greatly enhance clients' motivation and investment in treatment. Definition of what constitutes a successful outcome is a thorny issue to be addressed further in a later section.

Social Perception Training

This series of techniques focues on the *where*'s and *when*'s of adaptive responding rather than the *how*'s. Morrison and Bellack (1981) have labeled these skills *social perception.* In our treatment package social perception training is introduced during the flexibility portion of direct behavior training, after basic behavioral skills have been mastered. Information is provided about the social and environmental context in which a response occurs. Particular attention is paid to appropriate times, places, and reasons for a response. Additionally, attention is paid to the historical context of a situation, the possible impact of recent interactions between the client and the other person, and how these factors may influence the timing and selection of a response. The client is encouraged to adopt a reflective posture in social situations and to avoid impulsive responding. However, didactic training alone is often insufficient and is followed by the utilization of roleplay rehearsals to demonstrate the points outlined before. Social perception training is typically integrated into flexibility training roleplays. The therapist varies his or her behavior to communicate various mood states on the part of the interaction partner. The client is asked to identify a mood state, assess its implications, and respond accordingly. For example,

> A woman who wanted her boyfriend to visit her more often decided she would do something about it. However, her strategy was to wait until he told her of plans to go off with friends before she raised the issue. When she did so, she was impulsive, angry, and whiny. He responded defensively, and a serious argument ensued. She reported to the therapist that her boyfriend was unreasonable and never listened to her. When asked what she wanted to do, she finally admitted that she would simply like to have more private time with him. Roleplays commenced, and a more reasoned behavioral response was soon evident. However, the client indicated that she would still wait until her boyfriend next told her of a social plan that excluded her. The therapist suggested that she seek a better time. Upon questioning, she reported that he would sometimes accept her own independently initiated invitation to spend time together, especially if

the invitations were paired with expressions of affection for him, occurred at times when he was relaxed, and if he had not previously announced other plans. Rehearsals of this situation were initiated, and a high level of behavioral skill was immediately demonstrated. Repetitions involved roleplays in which the therapist portrayed differing amounts of relaxation, made references to plans or not, etc. Further rehearsals concerned discussion of the general issue of time spent together, initiated when they were alone together and relaxed.

Self-Evaluation and Self-Reinforcement Training

Evidence is abundant that depressed individuals tend to make inappropriately negative evaluations of themselves and their behavior and that they reward themselves for positive behavior very sparingly. They may also tend to perceive objective successes as failures and to overlook positive events when they do occur. These distortions may serve not only to maintain or prolong depressed affect but may also lead clients to devalue or overlook positive strides made in treatment and to negatively evaluate their homework performances. This potential negative impact requires that active strides be taken to overcome it.

Soon after clients have become comfortable and familiar with social perception training, self-evaluation and self-reinforcement training is implemented. After each roleplay response, clients assign a letter grade (A–F) to their performance. They are also instructed to engage in verbal statements of their accomplishments after A or B grades. Clients typically begin this procedure by assigning "failing" grades. They are then questioned in detail about the standards employed to grade their response. Perfectionistic standards are common; frequently, the client can specify no way in which the response could meet the standard because the standard itself is so extreme. To aid clients in modifying these standards, they are asked, (a) What could make the response acceptable? (b) Is this modification realistically attainable? and (c) What standard might be more adaptive? Adaptive evaluative criteria are modeled by the therapist. Self-evaluative and self-reinforcing operations are also applied to homework responses. In these situations, evaluative criteria for success are determined in advance by clients and therapists to decrease the opportunity for perfectionistic standards to come into play. For example, a client who had been assigned to call someone up for a date when he had initiated no social activity for the previous 6 months might require that the woman actually accept the date before he would allow himself a passing grade. However, by prior attention to evaluative criteria, the therapist would help the client understand that simply placing the call is a large step in the right direction and that further positive steps should result in even greater judgments of success. His success is not diminished if he makes a good effort and the woman declines. In general, clients have little actual control over the behavior of others. As a result, it is wiser to set grading criteria on the basis of *the client's own behavior.*

Limitations of Social Skills Training as a Treatment for Depression

The approach outlined before may be a potentially powerful treatment for nonpsychotic unipolar depression. However, depression is a complex, multifaceted disorder that may arise as the result of a multitude of interpersonal, intrapersonal, biological, or environmental events. We do not believe that social skills training procedures, even those including the cognitive components outlined herein, are the appropriate treatment for all occurrences of unipolar depression. On the basis of outcome research (including our own preliminary studies), we can state that these are promising procedures, but research to determine which clients might benefit most remains to be conducted. We may, however, offer the following speculations:

1. For clients lacking in generalized or situational social *skills* (as opposed to simply giving a poor performance), skills training would appear to be a necessary component of a treatment program. Other therapy procedures or pharmacologic interventions may also be necessary, but by themselves, would seem insufficient.

2. Social skills training would seem beneficial to clients whose depression is related to unassertiveness or anxiety related to interpersonal behavior, regardless of whether the problem results from insufficient skills. The repetitive nature of skills training may have anxiety-reducing effects.

3. Social skills training may be appropriate for depressions that, at first blush, appear to lack an interpersonal basis. We recently completed an analysis of the relevance of these procedures for persons whose depression is related to chronic illness or handicap (Becker, Heimberg, & Tassinari, in press). For instance, depression in a spinal-cord-injury patient, while multiply determined, may rest in part on difficulties in interpersonal interaction (e.g., heterosexual) precipitated by the injury. These issues can be confronted easily within the confines of social skills training.

4. For persons who possess quite reasonable social skills, the modular aspect of treatment may allow the utilization of roleplaying for purposes other than direct behavior training, and treatment may then take a more cognitive turn.

5. Unfortunate events in any area of life may have reduced impact if other areas of life are in good shape. Social skills training may therefore have effects on noninterpersonal areas by virtue of this "spillover" mechanism.

Social skills training, in our experience, *does not* work effectively with a number of clients—those who do not accept the rationale, those who do not acknowledge their role in modifying unsatisfactory life circumstances, those who are too afraid of negative consequences to risk trying anything, those who wish to control the flow of therapy, those who steadfastly refuse to roleplay, those who do not attempt homework assignments or do so in a half-hearted fashion, and those who react to daily events as if they were monumental crises. Clients who experience severe psychomotor retardation may have initial problems finding the energy to become involved in treatment. Some of these problems will be detailed in a later section. First, however, we turn to the following case example to demonstrate the integrated application of cognitive-behavioral social skills training to the treatment of depression.

In this section, we describe the application of social skills training to the treatment of a depressed client. Joyce, a 43-year-old unmarried Caucasian female was self-referred to the Mood Disorders Clinic after an unremitting depression of several years' duration. At the initial intake she appeared composed, pleasant, and alert, but quickly became tearful when questioned about her current job situation and her (virtually nonexistent) social life. She reported a variety of depressive symptoms, including prolonged sadness, low energy, poor concentration on household and occupational tasks, sleep-onset insomnia, and obsessive overconcern with her worth as a person. Joyce reported a moderately active but unsatisfying social life during college, but since that time, she has removed herself from the dating scene. She spends almost all of her nonwork hours in solitary pursuits, and although she endorses traditional desires for marriage and family, she has never had an intimate relationship. She characterizes herself as lonely and alone and spends considerable time berating herself for this state of affairs. In the absence of meaningful relationships, she has devoted herself almost entirely to her job, as an office manager for a local business executive. She works long hours at the job and is generally acknowledged as top-notch. She is also thought of as cold and unfeeling. Nevertheless, her relationships with her boss and co-workers represent the totality of her social network. The referral was precipitated by the client's recent declining mood pursuant to increasing conflict with her boss, who (according to Joyce) fails to provide her with adequate direction and then blows up at her when jobs are completed late or incorrectly. Further discussion revealed that Joyce reacts to these interactions by becoming angry and depressed and aimlessly struggling to do better. At the time of referral, she had begun to miss work for fear of being criticized by her boss. Additional discussion highlighted the client's need to develop a diversified social network. On the basis of SADS-RDC criteria, Joyce received a diagnosis of intermittent depressive disorder, and pursuant to pretest assessment and physical examination, was accepted for treatment. Pretest score on the (24-item) Hamilton was 17; her BDI score was 23.

Social Skills Training

Sessions 1 and 2 were devoted to further specification of the client's interactions with her boss and co-workers and her need to develop an adequate social system. During these sessions, social skills training and the theory on which it is based were further explained to the client, and the functional link between the outcomes of social events and her depression was demonstrated. A treatment plan was laid out specifying which situations were to be addressed first, second, and so forth. Although the therapist believed that the development of a social network was critical for ameliorating the client's depression, it was agreed that work should begin on specific problems on the job—situations for which an intervention might demonstrate an effect relatively quickly. Furthermore, job situations appeared to represent an area of relatively higher functioning for the client, and progress might therefore occur more quickly. The first situation to be confronted in the job area (and the one to be described in this segment) involved a behavior on the part of the boss that was extremely problematic. Specifically, he would assign multiple tasks to the client but provide no information on relative importance, priority, or dates for completion of the various tasks. Training on this situation, described next, began in Session 3. However, some preliminary assessment data were already available because this situation had been included in the set of personalized role-plays. In response to her roleplayed boss, Joyce displayed distressed affect and several behaviors that made self-expression a difficult issue. She bowed her head, avoided eye contact, stuttered, took a long time to "get it out," and then simply gave a lame excuse. Examination of other negative assertion situations in the standard roleplay battery revealed a similar but less extreme pattern. Discussion with the client suggested that this was a fairly typical response.

In Session 3, direct behavior training was initiated on the situation described previously. The client reported that she usually apologized to her boss for not doing his work as he wanted it and rushed off to get it done. She felt that she always ended up looking bad, even though the problem was not really hers. The first rehearsal of the situation assessed her typical response. On the basis of description provided by the client, the therapist (T) acted the part of the boss. The client (C) portrayed herself.

T: Joyce, where's that memo I asked you to do? I need it now!
C: I'll h . . . have it d . . . done in 10 minutes [*looking away, stuttering*]. I just didn't know you needed it so soon. I'm so, so sorry!
T: Joyce, you *never* seem to be on top of things. Hurry it up, will you!
C: Right away [*feeling angry and depressed*].

At this point the therapist stopped the roleplay. A brief discussion of the adequacy of the therapist's portrayal of the boss was conducted, and the strong and weak points of Joyce's response were addressed. Joyce was given instructions to focus on particular behaviors and how they should be changed. However, before the situation was rehearsed again, the therapist provided a modeling display.

T: [*Giving instructions to Joyce*] Let's try a different kind of response to your boss. In fact, let's try to prevent this situation from happening by informing your boss about the problem before it actually happens. What we want to do here is (a) to get his undivided attention; (b) point out the problem specifically; (c) suggest a solution to the problem; and (d) do so in a way that does not embarrass you publicly [*therapist actually sketches these out on a chalkboard*]. Let's try it with you acting the part of your boss, and I'll be you so I can show you what I mean. I'll model a response for you to try.
C: [*Acting as the boss*] Joyce, where's that memo I asked you to do? I need it now!
T: [*Modeling a response*] I'm sorry, Mr. Jones, but you never told me it was a priority so I've been working on what I thought was first priority. I know we can't talk about it now, but this problem happens a lot, and it *can* be solved. As soon as I've done this memo, can we talk about this in your office?
C: Well, OK, but let's get this memo out quickly.

Now the therapist asks the client to try this new response and provides further instruction about how to behave. He specifically calls attention to critical aspects of his verbal and nonverbal responses, in this case, his eye contact, voice quality, and specificity of content.

T: Now, I'll be your boss, and you try to respond just as I did a minute ago. Remember to look at him as you're talking, keep your voice steady, and be specific. Ready, let's try it. Joyce, where's that memo I asked you to do? I need it now!
C: I'm sorry, Mr. Jones. I'll have it ready in 10 minutes [*hesitates and looks down*]. This happens a lot, and it might help if we talk about it. Can I see you later in your office?
T: [*Responding positively to a good first attempt*] Oh, OK, I'm glad you brought it up. I'll see you as soon as this memo is done.

Consistent with out earlier descriptions, the therapist should point out the positive aspects of the response first and then suggest constructive areas of improvement. In this case, the therapist provided feedback.

T: That's quite an improvement over your original response. You pointed out the problem clearly and did ask for a private meeting to talk about the problem. You spoke clearly, loud enough, and without a quiver in your voice. Now let's try it again. Try to point out the problem in more detail than before and remember to keep looking at my face as we talk.

Rehearsals continued until the therapist felt that a minimally adequate response was attained, in this case, less hesitation, direct specification of the problem area, good eye contact, and a request for a specific meeting time. The homework assignment from this session set the stage for social perception training to come. The client was asked to monitor her boss's mood to see if it varied in any systematic way in order to pick a good time to speak with him. She was also asked to watch her co-workers to see how they handled their bosses in similar situations.

Session 4 began with a review of homework and revealed that the client's coworkers handled their own bosses in the way recommended by the therapist; however, the client expressed concern that her boss would be harder because he rarely seemed to be in a good mood. More roleplays were conducted until two consecutive adequate-quality responses were achieved. At this point, the therapist began flexibility training by varying the boss's response.

T: Where's that memo I asked you to do? I need it now.
C: I'm sorry, Mr. Jones, but I was working on the transistor project which I thought was first priority. This problem has come up before, and I think it could be settled if we handled it differently. After I finish this memo I'll come in to your office so we can discuss it.
T: Joyce, not now, just do the memo quickly.
C: [*Hesitating*] Ah, I'll check with you later.

During this stage the client mastered the first part of the response and, in fact, was overtrained to some degree. The second response was not the expected one, and, even though the therapist had given the client sufficient warning, she was not prepared for the response. Variations of this nature were included in rehearsals until minimally adequate responses were consistently demonstrated. During this phase, rehearsals became extended so as to better accommodate variations. At the completion of this session, the client was assigned the homework of trying this new response with her boss during the week.

Session 5 once again began with a review of homework, a process that took on added importance because it represented the client's first try of a new response outside the confines of the consulting room. Her report revealed that she had attempted the new response the day after the last therapy session and had obtained a reasonable response from her boss. Yet she was not entirely pleased by her performance and the outcome that she obtained. After a brief discussion, the therapist asked her to roleplay the interaction in order to better assess her performance.

T: Joyce, where's that memo that I asked you to do a while ago? I need it now!
C: I'm sorry, Mr. Jones, but I was working on the reports for the new electrical insulators which you told me were so important. This problem has come up before, and I think it can be cleared up by you and I meeting briefly in the morning to set priorities. I'll do the memo now and bring it to you. Then can we talk about changing the way we handle priorities?
T: [*Responding as the boss did during the homework assignment*] What? . . . I can't do it now, but how about 11:30?
C: OK, I'll be there.

The discussion at 11:30 did not resolve the issue, but her boss agreed to talk to her about it again next week. She felt that her boss was putting her off and that she should just forget the idea, even though the first request was received better than expected. She also believed that her co-workers did not have to go through "this ordeal" and that their bosses would have corrected the problem without extended discussion. Social perception training was initiated at this point, utilizing role reversals as the vehicle for discussion about the client's predictions of the boss's behavior.

T: Let's try another roleplay, but you play the part of your boss and I'll be you. I want you to try to think and feel like your boss as much as possible. Remember that your administrative assistant rarely suggests things to you about ways to run the office, but is always busy and cooperative. Now you start.
C: Joyce, where's that memo that I asked you about? I need it now!
T: [*As Joyce*] "I'm sorry, Mr. Jones, but I've been busy on that report on the new electrical insulators that I thought was first priority. This problem has come up before, and I think the way to solve it is for you and I to meet briefly in the morning and set priorities for the day. I'll do your memo now and bring it in to your office, and then we can talk about starting this.
C: [*Surprised by the difference in his assistant's response and not sure what to do*] Ah, OK, but I can't really talk about it seriously until next week.

The purpose of this roleplay was for the client to experience some of the emotions that the boss may have felt and to question the negative motives she ascribed to his delaying behavior. That response could have resulted from surprise at the new behavior of his assistant or from realizing that she was right and that he had not been doing his job correctly. He may have wanted some time to think. Clarification of the boss's motives made it much easier for Joyce to accept his response and to follow through with what she had started.

At this point, self-evaluation and self-reinforcement training was also initiated. The grading procedure was explained to Joyce, and she received some practice by grading the therapist's responses from the previous roleplay. She was then asked to grade her homework performance and assigned herself a D. The therapist gave that same performance an A. Discussion revealed that Joyce felt that her performance was poor because she did not get an immediate resolution of the situation. Joyce felt, however, that she had executed "a technically competent response." The therapist pointed out the many good qualities of Joyce's response and asked her to grade her performance again, this time ignoring the response of her boss. When this comparison was made, the two grades coincided at A. The therapist also replayed a tape recording of the first roleplay that Joyce had done and asked her to compare her two performances. Again, Joyce saw the improvement in her performance. Further discussion revolved around the observations Joyce had of the other bosses, specifically whether or not they had delayed things at times. Indeed they had, so her boss was not that much different. She also remembered that her boss usually mellows with time and is easier to handle after he has thought about an issue for a day or so. With that in mind, another set of roleplays was undertaken with the purpose of reminding Mr. Jones that they should talk about the problem of priority setting and probably the sooner the better. Several roleplays produced an adequate response and a judgment by Joyce that she had done well. The session ended with a homework assignment for her to make this new request of her boss before the next session.

Session 6 began with a review of homework. Joyce had made her additional request and received quite a favorable response. The new system they set up was working well, and Joyce felt more on top of her work and more recognized for her performances because things were not late anymore. She felt better about her boss, and he seemed to be treating her more reasonably. Her scores on the BDI and the Hamilton were 11 and 6, respectively. At this point, training moved to a different skill area of making conversation and increasing her social contacts.

Problems in Treatment

Although the course of social skills training treatments for depression is frequently smooth, a number of problems may arise that impede client progress or, in some cases, lead to a negative treatment outcome. Several of these problems were briefly mentioned in an earlier section. Although it is not possible to entertain all potential treatment complications, we highlight four major classes of difficulties: (a) noncompliance with therapeutic procedures; (b) control of the content of therapeutic sessions; (c) information transfer between therapist and client; and (d) inappropriate goal selection.

Clients may often be hesitant to engage in roleplay rehearsals during skills training sessions and may be similarly disinclined to implement therapeutic homework assignments. The idea of roleplaying may be rejected because the client does not accept the theoretical rationale for social skills training, because the client fears that he or she would be embarrassed by a poor acting performance, because the client is suffering from a loss of energy as a part of the depressive syndrome, or because the client feels hopeless about the chances of a successful recovery. In the first case, the client may be induced to participate in roleplays for a trial period; the therapist may then be able to demonstrate to the client that his or her roleplay performance, if duplicated in real life, may produce unanticipated negative consequences. This trial period may lead to a reevaluation of the treatment rationale and also provide time for the therapeutic relationship to gain importance for the client. However, if the client's evaluation of treatment or expectations for treatment outcome remain low, referral, termination, or reformulation of the treatment plan may be the most appropriate course.

If the client expresses a desire to avoid roleplays on the basis of depressive pessimism, inertia, or anxiety, the therapist may typically move the client along with a firm but tender hand. Again, the client may be induced to roleplay if the therapist is appropriately supportive but, at the same time, indicates that continuation of sessions without roleplaying is not an available option. Initial roleplays should be brief, highly structured, and deal with relatively benign topics until the client becomes comfortable with the general procedure. Even if the client's roleplayed performance is woefully inadequate, a strong initial focus on positive feedback is required.

Like roleplaying, failure or refusal to initiate homework assignments may occur for any of the preceding reasons and may be reasonably handled with analogous procedures. However, if the problem persists despite the client's expressed intent to comply or if it arises in the middle of treatment after a series of successfully completed assignments, a cognitive-behavioral analysis of the client's performance is required. Homework failure may often occur as a result of the client's fear of severe negative consequences or because the client's significant others are not supportive of his or her efforts at behavior change. In either case, the completion of a homework assignment may be treated as any other problematic situation—it may be roleplayed, possible variations may be confronted in flexibility training and social perception training, and reasonable goals may be established via self-reinforcement procedures.

Control of the Content of Therapeutic Sessions

Social skills training attempts to teach an integrated set of cognitive and behavioral skills and, like any other educational endeavor, requires careful attention to the "student's" experience. The therapist must design the session to maximize the opportunity for skill acquisition and may emphasize repeated rehearsal and practice of skills to be applied in future situations. However, clients' lives are often turbulent and filled with situations that they feel are critical and in need of immediate attention. If, for example, a heterosexual relationship goes sour, the client may desire that therapy be directed toward salvaging it. The therapist may believe that the "crisis" deserves some attention but that the client would be better served if he or she were to develop skills for meeting other potential partners, for behaving more assertively in intimate relationships, or for negotiating the conflicts that are inevitable between partners. Attention to the immediate situation may take away from the therapist's ability to teach the necessary skills and hamper the client's ultimate path toward progress. The situation is compounded for the not-infrequent client who experiences a different crisis almost every week. Attention to each crisis as it arises prevents the establishment of a coherent treatment flow, produces a series of patchwork solutions to problems, and impedes skill acquisition. It also ignores the very real possibility that the tendency for the client to bring in crises arises from an overestimation of the likelihood of negative consequences, a lack of the behavioral skills necessary to prevent situations from assuming crisis proportions, or inappropriate reinforcement of the part of the therapist. The judgment of whether a particular situation requires immediate attention or should be shelved in favor of other priorities is one of the most difficult to confront the social skills therapist, but failure to make this judgment correctly will result in a waste of valuable session time. The therapist should always keep in mind, however, that the client's concerns should be treated with the utmost respect and empathy and that efforts at skill learning should be related to future efforts to handle similar crises.

Information Transfer between Therapist and Client

Most of our information about specific problematic situations in clients' everyday lives necessarily comes from their verbal reports. Although the therapist may rely on the various other assessment devices described earlier or conduct a series of collateral interviews, the client's report will be the primary source of information about the specific situations or the behavior of the other persons involved. Two problems may arise as a result of this situation. First, the client may provide a poor or inadequate description of the other person's behavior or motivation. As a result, the therapist may provide an inaccurate portrayal of the other person, provide inappropriate behavioral strategies, or actually train the client for improbable variations of the situation. However, most of these problems can usually be avoided by repeated questioning of the client, especially in reference to the adequacy of the therapist's portrayals. Second, the client may avoid the disclosure of information that fundamentally alters the nature of the problematic situation.

Consider the case of the young woman who recently sought treatment for her depression at the Mood Disorders Clinic. She complained that her husband was inattentive to her, and after some discussion, she was trained in the skills of positive assertion for intimate relationships. It was later revealed, however, that our client had engaged in several extramarital affairs, and her husband's discovery of this fact coincided with the beginning of treatment. Although the skills she learned were still relevant, treatment has obviously taken a less-than-productive course.

Not infrequently, a client is confronted with a relationship partner or family member who appears to be acting in an unreasonable way. After a seemingly productive series of rehearsals and attempts by the client to resolve an interpersonal conflict, the other person's behavior remains difficult, and the situation remains unchanged. Clients often react to this state of affairs with feelings of despair and hopelessness and evaluations of themselves as incompetent and worthy of punishment. But the problem here may not be the client's performance but rather his or her expectations about the outcome of behavior change efforts. Stated otherwise, a problem in goal setting exists. The definition of a successful outcome has been tied to the behavior of a person other than the client, and, as a result, remains forever beyond the control of the client. The social skills trainer must pay careful attention to goal setting (an integral part of self-evaluation and self-reinforcement training) and define successful outcomes in terms of the client's behavioral performance. The client must learn to behave as competently as possible, to persist in that effort until a satisfactory outcome occurs or it appears realistically futile, and then to be satisfied with a job well done. Any other goal can never be consistently related to the client's own effort.

Summary

The cognitive behavioral approach to social skills training outlined in this chapter appears to be a viable method for the treatment of many depressed individuals. It focuses on a number of areas of known difficulty among depressed patients and allows the social skills therapist to tailor the treatment to the specific deficits of the individual patients. Evidence exists for its effectiveness with major depressive disorder (Hersen *et al.*, 1984), and preliminary data about its effectiveness with dysthymic disorder is encouraging. However, much work remains to be done. Future research efforts might reasonably be directed toward

1. further investigation of the effectiveness of skills training with different types of affective disorder;
2. isolation of the necessary and effective components of social skills training in order to further increase the effectiveness of the procedures;
3. comparison of the package with other psychotherapeutic approaches such as Beck's Cognitive Therapy;
4. comparison of the package to the range of pharmacological and somatic procedures for the treatment of depression; and
5. specification of client characteristics that might suggest a successful treatment outcome for social skills training.

With this knowledge, social skills training may assume an even greater role in the treatment of depressed clients.

American Psychiatric Association. (1980). *Diagnostic and statistical manual of mental disorders* (3rd ed.). Washington, DC: Author.

Beck, A. T., Ward, C. H., Mendelson, M., Mock, J., & Erbaugh, J. (1961). An inventory for measuring depression. *Archives of General Psychiatry, 4,* 561–571.

Beck, J. G., & Heimberg, R. G. (1983). Self-report assessment of assertive behavior: A critical analysis. *Behavior Modification, 7,* 451–487.

Becker, R. E., & Heimberg, R. G. (1984). Cognitive-behavioral treatments for depression: A review of controlled clinical research. In A. Dean (Ed.), *Depression in multidisciplinary perspective.* New York: Brunner/Mazel.

Becker, R. E., Heimberg, R. G., & Tassinari, R. (in press). Social skills training for depression among chronically ill or injured patients. In D. Schubert (Ed.), *Depression in the medical patient.* New York: Plenum Press.

Bellack, A. S., (1981). A critical appraisal of strategies for assessing social skills. *Behavioral Assessment, 1,* 157–176.

Bellack, A. S. (1983). Recurrent problems in the behavioral assessment of social skill. *Behaviour Research and Therapy, 21,* 29–41.

Bellack, A. S., & Hersen, M. (1977). Self report inventories in behavioral assessment. In J. Cone & R. Hawkins (Eds.), *Behavioral assessment: New directions in clinical psychology* (pp. 52–76). New York: Brunner/Mazel.

Bellack, A. S., Hersen, M., & Himmelhoch, J. M. (1981). Social skills training compared with pharmacotherapy and psychotherapy in the treatment of unipolar depression. *American Journal of Psychiatry, 138,* 1562–1567.

Bellack, A. S., Hersen, M., & Himmelhoch, J. M. (1983). A comparison of social skills training, pharmacotherapy and psychotherapy for depression. *Behaviour Research and Therapy, 21,* 101–107.

Comrey, A. (1957). A factor analysis of items on the MMPI depression scale. *Educational and Psychological Measurement, 17,* 578–585.

Coyne, J. C. (1976). Depression and the response of others. *Journal of Abnormal Psychology, 85,* 186–193.

DeMonbreun, B. G., & Craighead, W. E. (1977). Distortion of perception and recall of positive and neutral feedback in depression. *Cognitive Therapy and Research, 1,* 311–329.

Derogatis, L. R., Lipman, R. S., Rickels, K., Uhlenhuth, E. H., & Covi, L. (1974). The Hopkins Symptoms Checklist (HSCL): A self-report symptom inventory. *Behavioral Science, 19,* 1–15.

Eisler, R., Hersen, M., Miller, P., & Blanchard, E. (1975). Situational determinants of assertive behavior. *Journal of Consulting and Clinical Psychology, 43,* 330–340.

Endicott, J., & Spitzer, R. (1978). A diagnostic interview: The Schedule for Affective Disorders and Schizophrenia. *Archives of General Psychiatry, 35,* 837–844.

Endicott, J., Spitzer, R. L., Fleiss, J. L., & Cohen, J. (1976). The Global Assessment Scale: A procedure for measuring overall severity of psychiatric disturbance. *Archives of General Psychiatry, 33,* 766–771.

Ferster, C. B. (1965). Classification of behavioral pathology. In L. Krasner & L. P. Ullmann (Eds.), *Research in behavior modification: New developments and implications* (pp. 6–26). New York: Holt, Rinehart & Winston.

Ferster, C. B. (1973). A functional analysis of depression. *American Psychologist, 28,* 857–870.

Hamilton, M. (1960). A rating scale for depression. *Journal of Neurology, Neurosurgery, and Psychiatry, 23,* 56–62.

Hammen, C. L. (1981). Assessment: A clinical and cognitive emphasis. In L. P. Rehm (Ed.), *Behavior therapy for depression: Present status and future directions* (pp. 255–274). New York: Academic Press.

Hersen, M., Bellack, A. S., & Himmelhoch, J. M. (1982). Skills training with unipolar depressed women. In J. P. Curran & P. M. Monti (Eds.), *Social skills training: A practical handbook for assessment and treatment* (pp. 159–183). New York: Guilford Press.

Hersen, M., Bellack, A. S., Himmelhoch, J. M., & Thase, M. E. (1984). Effects of social skills training, amitriptyline, and psychotherapy in unipolar depressed women. *Behavior Therapy, 15,* 21–40.

Jacobsen, N. S., & Anderson, E. A. (1982). Interpersonal skill and depression in college students: An analysis of the timing of self-disclosures. *Behavior Therapy, 13,* 271–282.

Lea, G., & Paquin, M. (1981). Assertiveness and clinical depression. *The Behavior Therapist, 4,* 9–10.

Lewinsohn, P. M. (1975). The behavioral study and treatment of depression. In M. Hersen, R. M. Eisler, & P. M. Miller (Eds.), *Progress in behavior modification* (Vol. 1). New York: Academic Press.

Libet, J., & Lewinsohn, P. M. (1973). The concept of social skill with special reference to the behavior of depressed persons. *Journal of Consulting and Clinical Psychology, 40,* 304–312.

Lubin, B. (1965). Adjective checklists for measurement of depression. *Archives of General Psychiatry, 12,* 57–62.

Metcalfe, M., & Goldman, E. (1965). Validation of an inventory for measuring depression. *British Journal of Psychiatry, 111,* 240–242.

Morrison, R. L.. & Bellack, A. S. (1981). The role of social perception in social skill. *Behavior Therapy, 12,* 69–80.

O'Hara, M. W., & Rehm, L. P. (1983). Hamilton Rating Scale for Depression: Reliability and validity of judgments of novice raters. *Journal of Consulting and Clinical Psychology, 51,* 318–319.

Radloff, L. S. (1977). The CES-D Scale: A self-report depression scale for research in the general population. *Applied Psychological Measurement, 1,* 385–401.

Raskin, A., Schulterbrandt, J., Reatig, N., & Rice, C. E. (1967). Factors of psychopathology in interview, ward-behavior, and self-report ratings of hospitalized depressives. *Journal of Consulting Psychology, 31,* 270–278.

Rehm, L. P. (1977). A self control model of depression. *Behavior Therapy, 8,* 787–804.

Sanchez, V., & Lewinsohn, P. M. (1980). Assertive behavior and depression. *Journal of Consulting and Clinical Psychology, 48,* 119–120.

Spitzer, R., & Endicott. J. (1977). *The Sads-Change Interview.* (Available from [Research Assessment and Training Unit, New York State Psychiatric Institute, 722 West 168th Street, New York, New York 10032])

Spitzer, R., Endicott, J., & Robins, E. (1978). Research diagnostic criteria: Rationale and reliability. *Archives of General Psychiatry, 34,* 773–782.

Williams, J. G., Barlow, D. H., & Agras, W. S. (1972). Behavioral measurement of severe depression. *Archives of General Psychiatry, 27,* 330–333.

Youngren, M. A., & Lewinsohn, P. M. (1980). The functional relationship between depression and problematic interpersonal behavior. *Journal of Abnormal Psychology, 89,* 333–341.

Zung, W. (1965). A self-rating depression scale. *Archives of General Psychiatry, 12,* 63–70.

Behavioral Medicine

IV

A Problem-Solving Approach to the Treatment of Obesity

LINDA WILCOXON CRAIGHEAD

Introduction

The treatment of obesity presents a rather unique challenge to today's professionals. Obesity has been considered both a medical problem, because of its biological consequences, and a psychological problem, because of its social/personal consequences. Thus, professionals from many health fields have been involved in efforts to understand the causes of obesity and to work toward more effective ways to treat it or at least minimize its negative consequences. This chapter is designed to organize currently available information in a way that will be most useful to the professional who must make treatment and/or referral decisions regarding a disorder that is still poorly understood. The decision-making perspective that is being suggested offers a flexible framework within which the professional and the client can make more realistic, rational, and humane decisions. The ambiguous and contradictory research findings, the presence of pervasive cultural stereotypes and individual beliefs, and the commercial marketing of "miracle" cures and fad diets make rational choices nearly impossible for the client (consumer). Thus, the client must be educated in the decision-making process and become an active participant in treatment decisions.

Adopting a decision-making perspective rests on three assumptions. The first assumption is that it is reasonable to ask the question "Should this person lose

LINDA WILCOXON CRAIGHEAD • Division of Counseling and Educational Psychology, The Pennsylvania State University, University Park, Pennsylvania 16802.

weight?" This assumption is based on compelling evidence in three areas (Bennett & Gurin 1982; Polivy & Herman 1983).

1. The negative consequences of obesity may be more variable than were initially hypothesized and appear to depend on a number of individual characteristics such as type of fat deposits, sex, family medical history, and presence of other risk factors. The risks associated with gross obesity are also much clearer than those associated with mild (under 30%) obesity. However, weight reduction is clearly associated with changes in various health indexes such as blood pressure and cholesterol, so even some mildy overweight people may be able to influence their individual risk. Thus, for one individual weight loss may, in fact, result in substantial health benefits, whereas for another they may be minimal.

2. Although there is a clear social bias against obesity, the negative psychological consequences of certain weight loss strategies and/or certain weight maintenance strategies (e.g., constant restraint) may, at least in some individuals, be more severe than the psychological consequences of remaining overweight. Thus, some individuals may benefit substantially from treatment on psychological criteria, whereas others may not, and some individuals may even deteriorate.

3. Initial assumptions that weight loss/maintenance is an achieveable goal for almost every person are now being questioned. Preliminary evidence suggests that there may be individuals for whom substantial weight loss is nearly impossible due to unknown regulatory disorders and others for whom it could be achieved only through extreme measures that may well not be worthwhile in terms of the benefits that are accrued.

The second assumption is that it is possible to ask the question, "What weight loss strategy is best for this person at this time?" This assumption depends on the availability of several distinctively different treatment options and evidence that these options have different advantages and disadvantages; these options are detailed in the treatment section.

The third assumption is that a particular individual's treatment must be approached in a trial-and-error fashion. An initial treatment decision can be made, but it must be followed by a series of critical redecision points. The client must be actively involved in this decision making, which is a continuous reevaluation of whether the benefits of the current strategy are worth the costs. Essentially, the client is asking himself or herself, "At what personal cost am I willing to lose (or maintain) weight?" This assumption is based on the fact that very few predictors of treatment response have been identified. The professional can give the client initial guidance based on average (typical) responses to various strategies, but subsequent redecisions must be based on the individual's response.

The professional can give the client only rough estimates of the amount of weight he or she is likely to lose with a particular strategy and whether such a loss, if achieved, will actually produce physical or psychological benefits. However, based on the client's personal response to treatment, the second and subsequent decision points may lead to an optimal strategy that maximizes the benefits and minimizes the costs for that individual. One individual may eventually decide not to diet and to work toward being more comfortable with his or her overweight status. Another may decide dieting extracted too high a personal cost but that increased exercise provided sufficient payoff to be continued. This person might also need help in becoming more comfortable with a less stringent personal goal weight. Some people may realize they can maintain their "personal goal weight" but only through continuous self-regulation and/or a rigorous exercise program. Of those, some may decide the benefits are worth the costs, whereas others may choose to be satisfied with a higher weight. The professional's role is to stick with the client through the trial-and-error process until an acceptable strategy for coping with the client's obesity is found.

Weight loss is only one of several acceptable solutions for a client's obesity problem. Within the decision-making framework, a client may come to an entirely different but satisfactory resolution of the problem. Deciding that a certain weight loss is not a viable alternative or that the personal costs are higher than the personal benefits is, at least psychologically, an entirely different outcome than concluding one is a failure at yet another weight loss effort. In a sense, the only unacceptable solution to an obesity problem is for the client to decide that he or she cannot or chooses not to do what it takes to lose weight but that he or she will continue to be miserable about being overweight and will continue to subject himself or herself to repeated failures with whatever fad diet comes out next.

The essence of a decision-making approach is fairly simple and straightforward. The basic steps are those that have been described elsewhere (Golfried & Davidson 1976; Horan 1979), but the procedure takes on special significance when utilized as a framework for obesity treatment. The success of obesity treatment depends largely on the client's willingness to make life-style changes and his or her ability to maintain these changes. Thus, the decision-making model is used initially to focus attention on the need for the client to make an active decision to lose weight and to do so via certain specific strategies. Polivy and Herman (1983) put it this way:

> If people have chosen dieting, know the risks, but still have confidence that losing weight will help some aspect of their lives, they may be willing to control their eating cognitively and try to ignore or overcome the "side effects" of dieting. It is the person who has been dieting without really thinking about it or making a choice who is most likely to feel compelled and uncomfortable. If such people add up the costs and the benefits dieting has produced thus far in their lives, they might decide that losing weight is not after all, the answer for them. (pp. 187–188)

The decision-making approach is not used to persuade an individual either to diet or not to diet but to help the individual initially to make a more informed treatment decision and to help the individual revise his or her decision based on his or her own experiences. Many individuals will initially choose fairly short-term diet approaches, but if not successful they may eventually adopt alternative, long-term-oriented strategies.

Step 1: Define the Problem

During the initial stages of assessment, which is described in a later section, the professional helps the client more clearly define the problem.

Step 2: Generate Alternative Strategies

The professional plays a major role at this point. He or she elicits information about strategies the client has used before or is currently using. The professional then provides information about other types of strategies that are available. The following types of strategies may be considered (see treatment section): cognitive/behavior therapy techniques, modest calorie restriction, severe calorie restriction, pharmacotherapy, exercise, "undiet," psychotherapy for related psychological difficulties, and/or psychotherapy focused on accepting self, decision not to diet, and possible negative reactions of others.

Step 3: Evaluate Alternatives

The professional's role at this point is to alert the client to the typical advantages and disadvantages of each strategy insofar as current research has been able to delineate them. The professional also makes it clear that response to these strategies is highly variable and that the individual client may or may not respond like the "average person." The professional clarifies how the client's subsequent experiences will be used to modify and/or add to this initial decision-making matrix. It is explained that clients will need to come back to this step at several points as they get more information about how their own body responds to various procedures and as their sensitivity to their own values and priorities increases.

Step 4: Rank Order Alternatives and Implement

The client takes the major role in ranking the alternatives and deciding to implement a strategy. Three important decisions must be made. Several of the alternatives can be combined, whereas others are fairly incompatible. Many clients will initially choose a combination program (e.g., behavioral techniques, diet, and exercise) because these have the best average success rates. However, other clients may wish to start with a single strategy, such as behavioral techniques, but rank order others as acceptable alternatives. Then, at a future redecision point, the client may decide either to add a second procedure or to switch to a second procedure.

A decision must be made regarding when to implement the procedure. It is helpful for a client to assess whether now is the most appropriate time to start a particular program because many programs necessitate a considerable investment in time and energy. The client's life need not be free from stress or other problems in order to begin treatment, but these additional variables should be explicitly assessed at this time. The client may be best advised to postpone his or her efforts until he or she can make this personal concern a high priority.

Because obesity occurs in a gradual manner and typically represents a constant, low-level (not crisis) personal issue, individuals typically have been dealing with it in one of two ways. One way is to ignore the problem most of the time and then make periodic, frantic, short-term efforts such as crash diets. The second way is to make very modest continual efforts (always dieting), which do not amount to much. Within this framework, if a client does choose one of the potentially more effective weight loss strategies (e.g., behavioral techniques and exercise), he or she is asked to make a very different kind of commitment. The commitment is to a fairly long-term period of sustained effort. A person overweight by 20 pounds must think in terms of a 6-month commitment, and a 40-pound loss typically means a 1-year commitment.

Once a decision regarding the general strategy has been made, a decision must be made regarding the treatment modality that is preferred. For example, the client choosing behavioral techniques may have a choice of bibliotherapy, individual or group professional therapy, self-help (lay) groups, and the like. The person choosing exercise must decide on the type and whether to exercise alone or with others. If this framework is being used within an already predetermined program, this is simply the time to insure that the client understands the program. Some clients may need to be counseled out of a group program at this point if it is not at least close to what they want.

Step 5: Monitor Progress and Reevaluate

This reevaluation step is the most critical part of the model. The client continues with the chosen strategy as long as progress is satisfactory. At any point when progress appears to have stopped or when the client becomes discouraged over a slower than expected rate of loss or other difficulties, going back through the decision-making steps is the best way either to reconfirm and restore the client's commitment to the particular strategy or to reevaluate the pros and cons based on the new experiential evidence. In many treatment programs, a client who does not do well either concludes the program is not for him or her or that he or she is once again a failure. In either case, they typically drop out and continue their search for yet another "cure." A client who has been given a decision-making framework is more likely to see lack of progress as a cue to reevaluate and to seek help from the professional regarding how to modify his or her strategies. In a sense, lack of progress or feeling discouraged is reconstrued for clients as important new information about themselves and their bodies rather than something terrible and awful. Thus, clients may begin to cope with their weight problem more rationally and may be more likely to ultimately find a satisfactory resolution. Hopefully, this resolution will include at least some weight loss because for most people there are associated physical and mental health benefits. However, even if it does not, clients are less likely to add further psychological complications to whatever negative consequences are already associated with their obesity.

Assessment

Current State of Obesity

Assessment of the client's current state of obesity is relatively straightforward. The clinician will be interested first in determining how much the client would like to weigh. Then, a simple measure of actual body weight provides the initial assessment of level of obesity. Using the recently revised 1983 Metropolitan height–weight charts the clinician can determine the general weight range that would be considered appropriate for that client and compare this to the client's stated goal weight. The clinician can then make some initial determination regarding the general category of obesity. At some point, the client's specific personal goal may need to be challenged, but this can easily be done later within the decision-making framework. If the client's weight is already within the normal range, it is important to assess more carefully the client's stated personal goal to understand what perceptions and information base have been used to arrive at this goal weight. This goal would need to be challenged at this point if the client were already near or below the lowest recommended weight for his or her height and wished to lose more. Such clients may have excessive concern over potential weight gain, a previous history of anorexia, or bulimic episodes, and they need to be treated differently than clients who actually need to lose weight.

The possibility of bulimia or anorectic episodes should always be assessed because the client, especially if currently overweight, may not bring these up initially. Bulimic clients who are not overweight need to be treated differently (see Boskind-White & White, 1983, and Hawkins, Fremouw, & Clement, 1984). Bulimic clients who are overweight may need a combination of procedures relevant to obesity and bulimia. Depending on the severity of the binging and/or purging, a decision may be made regarding where to start with that client. The presence of binging by itself does not preclude behavioral treatment. Dubbert and Wilson (1983) reported no correlation between binge scores and weight loss. Currently overweight clients with a history of anorexia or anorectic episodes will need to be treated with special care because attempts to lose weight may exacerbate their problems. The professional may elicit information regarding these issues as the weight history is taken or use one of the standardized questionnaires that are available (Garner, Olmstead, & Polivy, 1982; Hawkins & Clement, 1980).

Simple assessments of body weight and percentage overweight are recommended even though they are clearly not synonymous with measures of actual body fat because they are reasonably highly correlated (except in fairly extreme cases). Body fat measures are important for research purposes; preliminary evidence suggests that body fat may be a more critical determinant of health risk than percentage overweight. However, because the majority of clients are losing weight primarily for cosmetic reasons, body weight alone is typically adequate. The most precise measures of body fat are expensive and impractical. Skinfold calipering, however, is a viable option and may be useful in some cases. Skinfold calipering involves measuring subcutaneous fat by taking a pinch of skin at several different sites around the body and measuring the width of the fold very precisely with a caliper. A trained technician is needed to obtain a reliable and valid measurement, but such assessments are readily available and are not very expensive. Several different formulas are available to calculate percentage body fat (see recommendations by Rogers, Mahoney, Mahoney, Straw, & Kenigsberg, 1980), and norms for various populations are available. A body fat measure may be important information for a mildly overweight person to consider in the decision of whether to lose weight or when to stop. Because muscle weighs more than fat, a very fit person may need to pay more attention to body fat and worry less about reaching a particular weight. Persons who decide to focus on exercise or incorporate exercise into their weight loss efforts may need feedback regarding improvement in body fat as their actual weight change may not be as dramatic as they anticipate.

Weight History

Several guidelines are available for obtaining information about a client's weight history (Ferguson, 1975), success or failure of previous attempts to lose and/or maintain weight, family weight history, and medical conditions. However, few of these variables have been demonstrated to accurately predict response to treatment. Gormally, Rardin, and Black (1980) presented data indicating that success in losing weight on previous diets was the best predictor of weight loss in a behavioral program (18% of the variance accounted for). Initial amount of overweight was not a significant predictor. Their data identified certain clients that fit a pattern of chronic dieting and weight regain, and they found that a majority of these clients also demonstrated weight regain after the behavioral program. Thus, clients so identified may need special emphasis on relapse prevention procedures and continued support during the first year of maintenance.

Other data from a weight history may be useful at various redecision points. For example, a client reports a fairly stable weight of 140 over a period of 10 years that she has maintained without much difficulty. In a program, she is highly motivated and loses 20 pounds but finds that maintenance is difficult and she must constantly focus on her diet to stay at 120. The previous stable weight may suggest that her "natural weight" is closer to 140. Thus, at a redecision point she may want to reevaluate her personal weight goal or to focus on increasing exercise as a potentially more viable strategy than constant restraint.

Current Energy Balance

An initial assessment of daily caloric intake and activity levels is important to clearly define the client's obesity problem. Self-monitoring for a period of 1 to 2 weeks before any treatment is started is frequently suggested. In fact, given the critical role of self-monitoring during treatment, many professionals recommend using such a requirement as an initial screening device. Clients who are not willing to monitor initially are poor risks.

The client's records will help establish whether the problem is primarily overeating or an underactive life-style, although it is most typically some combination of the two. Katahn (1982) suggests the following guidelines: average daily intake of approximately 2,000 calories for a 128-pound woman and 2700 calories for a 154-pound man are considered "normal" eating levels. Intake over these amounts suggests an "overeating" problem, but intake at or below these levels suggests that lack of adequate exercise may have upset the natural energy balance. An active woman of 128 will stay slim eating at those levels, whereas an inactive woman of

200 will remain obese. Exercise is a very slow way to *lose* weight, and modest calorie reduction is usually required initially, but adequate exercise may be a more effective and more palatable alternative for maintenance than continued restriction.

Physiological Functioning

Because obese patients typically state they are losing weight for cosmetic and/or social reasons (Dubbert & Wilson, 1983), assessment of physiological functioning may not be warranted in all cases. However, when a client has been referred by a physician and/or states that improving his or her health is a primary motivation, physiological assessment may be quite useful. Changes in various indexes such as blood pressure and cholesterol levels may be more important feedback than weight change. Decreased need for insulin injections or blood pressure medication can be very powerful factors in a client's "redecision" to continue weight control efforts. Whatever factor is relevant for the individual client can be assessed through self-monitoring and/or periodic physical assessments. Data collection is important because the client's own improvement is a far more salient piece of information to plug into a redecision evaluation than a general statement such as weight loss is likely to decrease blood pressure.

Similarly, measures of physical fitness are perhaps most useful in terms of sustaining adherence to exercise. Although the more sophisticated measures of fitness (e.g., stress tests) may not be very practical, clients can monitor exercise and recovery pulse rates, chart distances or times, and carry out other assessments such as the 12-minute walk/run. A client who sees clear evidence of improved physical fitness may choose to continue this strategy (for its own health benefits) even though he or she may not have lost significant weight.

Psychological/Social Functioning

The relationship between psychological functioning and weight reduction has not been extensively evaluated despite the fact that the majority of clients seek treatment because they expect that weight loss will make them feel better about themselves and improve their interpersonal relationships. Several research studies have demonstrated improvements in depression, self-esteem, marital relationships, and the like associated with weight loss achieved through behavior therapy (Wilson & Brownell, 1980). However, Stunkard and Rush (1974) have noted that depression and anxiety have also resulted from some dieting efforts.

For the practicing clinician, assessment of psychological functioning might include measures of depression, anxiety, daily mood, general psychopathology, self-esteem, marital adjustment, social interaction, and body image. Because these measures have not been shown to predict differential treatment response, however, they would only be useful in the following ways. Clinicians doing treatment in groups might choose to exclude certain clients as they may be disruptive to the group. Evidence of pathology, severe depression, or marital discord may be important information to consider in initial or subsequent treatment decisions. These problems may need to be resolved before the client can benefit from participation in an educationally oriented, structured weight-loss program.

Assessment of mood on a daily or weekly basis may be useful as an indicator of client response. If clients can see that their mood clearly improves as they exercise or control their eating, this is again powerful information to utilize at subsequent decision points. In the absence of clearly recorded data, clients may not be aware of small changes, and if a relapse occurs they may find it difficult to remember how they were feeling before. On the other hand, if clients' moods deteriorate, this may be evidence that they need to reevaluate the method of weight loss they have chosen or at least take some measures to counteract the negative emotional effects that may accompany dieting efforts.

Eating Habits and Thoughts

Several self-report measures have been developed to assess client eating habits and thoughts related to eating. At this point, they have been used primarily as research tools rather than treatment guides because the measures correlate only modestly with weight loss during treatment and have not predicted differential response to treatments.

Two scales (Herman, 1978; Stunkard, 1981) are available that measure the degree of conscious restraint (habitual dieting) a person typically exhibits. People with high scores on restraint are those who are keeping their weight below a level that is easy to maintain, but they may or may not be "overweight." Blum and Craighead (1982) did find reported restraint increased as a result of participating in a behavioral program. Although there is currently no validation, these data would suggest that low-restraining obese clients might particularly benefit from a behavioral program in which they learn strategies for effective self-control (restraint). Highly restraining obese clients may benefit from learning more effective restraint techniques; however, it may be that these clients are the ones who have a higher "natural weight." If so, the degree of restraint necessary for them to lose and/or maintain a "normal" weight may be excessive. They might do better with exercise and "undieting."

The Master Questionnaire (Straw, Straw, Mahoney, Rogers, Mahoney, Craighead, & Stunkard, 1984) is a self-report measure with several scales that has been used primarily for research. It has been shown to register change following cognitive-behavioral treatment. The stimulus control scale assesses problematic eating habits, and three cognitive scales assess problematic thinking patterns (hopelessness, physical attribution, lack of motivation). From a clinical perspective, it may be useful to the extent that it provides a quick initial assessment of eating habits and cognitions that may suggest where intervention is needed. However, careful self-monitoring of actual eating patterns and idiosyncratic negative thoughts will be needed to implement relevant interventions.

Physiology and Obesity

One of the most important functions of the clinician treating obesity is to educate the client about the "biological facts" as best as we currently know them.

Although the current picture is still quite cloudy (cf. Brownell, 1981, 1982), there are several points that may be useful in helping clients understand some of the biological implications of obesity. This understanding may allow them to more critically evaluate their own responses, although care must be taken that such information is not used inappropriately to "rationalize" failure to lose weight.

Types of Obesity

Many obese clients might be happy to find a biological explanation for their obesity, but unfortunately, at this time only a very few, relatively rare, obesity syndromes have been identified (Callaway & Greenwood, 1983). Except for these few exceptions, most obese are lumped into the "exogenous" category and are thus treated as essentially similar. Callaway and Greenwood suggest that obesity is likely to be a heterogeneous condition that might result from any number of pathophysiologic mechanisms. Continuing to lump all obese individuals together makes it difficult to identify any specific mechanism. Failure to distinguish subtypes would also help explain current treatment failure rates.

Greenwood and Brunzell (1982) have suggested a regulatory scheme that, if validated, would help clinicians match people to appropriate treatments. Three possible types of deficits are hypothesized. Type C (cognitive) regulatory deficits would involve not paying attention to appropriate internal cues; Type C people would be likely to respond positively to a behavioral approach. Type S (short-term, metabolic, meal-to-meal) regulatory deficits would involve problems in the persons' "satiety" signals. Cognitive regulation (i.e., behavioral treatment) might help such people compensate for their disordered signals, but they would need to be constantly on the alert because they could never depend on their internal cues. Type L (long-term regulatory) disorders would involve problems in the body's signals regarding fat storage. This type of inborn error would not respond well to cognitive regulation as the body would always attempt to compensate in some way. Although such types cannot currently be identified, it may be useful to clients to understand this notion as it may help explain why some people may lose and maintain relatively easily; others must feel constantly deprived if they are to be successful; and still others appear to fail completely. Appropriate causal attributions might relieve some of the sense of failure and/or self-blame.

Set Point or "Natural Weight"

Set point theories suggest that each person has an ideal biological weight (which may be higher then cultural weight norms) and that the body will utilize physiological mechanisms, such as appetite, to defend this weight against efforts to modify it. The data supporting these theories are quite strong as far as animals are concerned, but they are far more controversial for humans (see Bennett & Gurin, 1982). If there is a "natural weight" in humans, it is more flexible than in animals. Clearly, there is a range within which a person's weight can be altered intentionally (in either direction). However, as one would approach either extreme of this range, greater conscious effort would be needed to compensate for biological counter-responses. At the present time, there is no clear way to determine what this range might be for a given individual. Weight at about age 21, if the person had not been dieting, would be the closest approximation. Gradual weight gain due to a sedentary life-style, metabolic decreases associated with aging, and dieting efforts make inferences more difficult at later stages. Biological processes appear to resist weight loss somewhat more strongly than weight gain, even though the theory would suggest that both would be resisted. Such a mechanism would have been adaptive for prehistoric man, but it is not now.

Response to Dieting

Whether or not there is a "natural weight" that is being defended, there is clear evidence that whenever caloric intake is restricted the body responds physiologically by becoming metabolically more efficient, attempting to minimize further loss. Initial biological responses have been noted within the first 48 hours and decreases in basal metabolic rate as high as 20% have been noted within the first 2 weeks of restriction (Bray, 1969). Alternating short periods of modest and more severe caloric restriction may be a way to minimize this effect (Clausen, Silfen, Coombs, Ayers, & Altshul, 1980). Evidence from animal research suggests that repeated caloric restriction may have long-term effects. Metabolic reduction may occur more and more quickly with each restriction, and it may fail to return to prerestriction levels when the restriction is lifted (Wooley, Wooley, & Oyrenforth, 1979). Thus, there appear to be physiological limits on the possible rate of loss that can be achieved. There is concern that with constant dieting, persons might, in essence, train themselves to maintain their weight on even fewer calories than they ate previously. There is, in fact, little evidence that the overweight eat more than normals, although this is partly accounted for by lower activity levels. Physiological responses might also help explain plateaus and daily weight fluctuations. The relationship between calorie intake and weight gain or loss appears to be rather complex; it is mediated by many variables that we do not clearly understand. Thus, clients must be trained to look at trends in weight over a period of a week or two rather than focusing on a given day's weight.

Dietary Factors

Evidence from animal research strongly suggests that the content of a diet can influence the biological regulatory system. Rats given a "supermarket" diet (high in sweetness and fat and a variety of food choices) will gain large amounts of weight quite quickly, even though they had previously remained at normal weight when given free access to laboratory chow (Sclafoni & Springer, 1976). Evidence also suggests that the effect may only be partially reversible (Scalfoni, 1980), probably because biological processes are set to favor weight gain. The high-fat content appears to be the most critical aspect of the diet. Drewnowski and Greenwood's (1983) research on obese and normal taste preferences indicates that the obese prefer higher fat content then normals but not higher sweetness, and this preference does not change even if the obese successfully lose weight. Although it has not been clearly demonstrated in human research, the inference is that a low-fat, low-variety diet may in itself influence physiological processes and perhaps lower a person's current "set point" (Bennett & Gurin, 1982).

Fat Cells

Fat-cell size and number may ultimately help explain the notion of "natural weight." Adults with juvenile-onset obesity typically have more than the normal number of fat cells, whereas those with later onset typically have a normal number but larger fat cells. Fat-cell number, however, does not decrease with weight loss, only fat-cell size. Bjorntorp (1975) has presented evidence that weight loss typically stops once fat-cell size reaches normal, regardless of whether the person is still "overweight." Sjostrom (1980) reported that 80% of the variance in weight reduction could be accounted for by pretreatment measures of fat-cell number and metabolic rate. However, age of onset has not been a notable predictor in treatment studies, and people with juvenile-onset obesity have been quite successful in treatment (Dubbert & Wilson, 1983). It may be that such people were still at the point of reducing cell size so they had not yet encountered biological limitations. Currently, assessment of fat-cell number is expensive and fairly painful, but further work may ultimately allow these data to be helpful in a client's decisions regarding appropriate goal weight.

Fat cells may also effect weight in another way. It takes fewer calories to sustain fat tissue than lean body tissue (Katch & McArdle, 1977). Thus, a person with a higher percentage of body fat will maintain his or her weight on fewer calories then a person with more muscle tissue.

Cognitive-Behavioral Therapy[1]

Although there are many variations of what is frequently referred to as a standard behavioral program, considerable agreement exists about the major components or techniques that are involved. A number of manuals or texts are available that describe the clinical application of these techniques in greater detail (Ferguson, 1975; Jeffrey & Katz, 1977; Johnson & Stalonas, 1981; Jordan, Levitz, & Kimbrell, 1976; Katahn, 1982; Mahoney & Mahoney, 1976; Stuart, 1977; Stuart & Davis, 1972).

Comprehensive reviews, including data from over 100 controlled studies, have carefully documented the effectiveness of behavioral programs (Brownell, Heckerman, & Westlake, 1979; Foreyt, Goodrick, & Gotto, 1981; Jeffery, Vender, &

[1]From *Behavior Modification* (2nd ed.) (pp. 286–312) by W. E. Craighead, A. E. Kazdin, and M. J. Mahoney, 1981, Boston: Houghton Mifflin. Copyright 1981 by Houghton Mifflin Company. Reprinted by permission.

Wing, 1978; Lebow, 1981; Wilson & Brownell, 1980; Wing & Jeffery, 1979). These studies support the following conclusions:

1. Behavioral treatment programs are designed for slow weight loss, an average of ½ to 2 pounds per week. Most of the programs are 10 to 12 weeks with an average loss of 11 pounds reported. The most effective programs are longer (16 to 25 weeks) and report larger average losses, from 17 to 24 pounds. The range of response is quite variable, from slight gains to over 80-pound losses. Concurrent improvement in psychological functioning has also been noted.

2. Weight loss is very similar across programs that vary widely in terms of location, types of clients (volunteers vs. medical referrals), treatment fees, level of therapist training, and client demographics. Self-help bibliotherapy with minimal contact is a cost-efficient alternative for the mildly overweight (Craighead, McNamara, & Horan, 1984).

3. Few clients, perhaps 25%, continue to lose after treatment is terminated, but weight already lost is typically well maintained. The average loss reported at 1-year follow-up is 10 pounds; however, higher losses have been reported in the most effective, longer programs (e.g., average 20-pound loss at 1 year in Craighead, Stunkard, & O'Brien, 1981). Variability of response increases the longer the period of follow-up.

The following elements, each of which consists of several specific techniques, currently characterize standard behavioral programs: self-control model, analyzing and modifying eating behaviors, stimulus control, and cognitive restructuring. The individual contribution of any particular technique, or even of each element, is still in question. No one technique (except self-monitoring) seems indispensable, nor does any one technique appear to account for a significant proportion of the variance. McReynolds, Lutz, Paulsen, and Kohrs (1976) reported a small but significant difference at follow-up in favor of a simple stimulus-control program compared to a more comprehensive, complex self-control program. Stalonas, Johnson, and Christ (1978), however, reported a small difference at follow-up in favor of a program including very specific self-reinforcement procedures compared to a program that did not include the contingency component. The addition of a strong component of problem solving and cognitive restructuring (Mahoney, Rogers, Straw, & Mahoney, 1977) did not enhance weight loss compared to more traditional, less cognitively oriented programs.

The relationship between adherence (applying the techniques) and weight loss is also not clear (Brownell & Stunkard, 1978; Lansky, 1981). Some data suggest that compliance accounts for only a small part of the variance (Bellack, Rozensky, & Schwartz, 1974; Jeffrey *et al.*, 1978; Stalonas, Johnson, & Christ, 1978). However, these self-reports generally indicate a high level of adherence, which may be inaccurate. That so many variations work and that researchers cannot yet explain how or why the techniques work suggests that more general or nonspecific factors may be largely responsible for the success of the behavioral programs. However, behavior therapy has clearly been more effective than a number of placebo or comparison therapies. Stalonas *et al.* (1978) suggested the following hypothesis. Most behavioral programs demand an extremely large amount of out-of-therapy time (for example, to record, graph, monitor) compared to other weight-reduction regimens. Thus, the procedures may be effective because they continuously prompt the client's (and other's) attention to weight loss.

Self-Control Model

Self-control is seen as a complex process in which the individual learns to manage his or her own behavior. The three basic steps involved are self-monitoring, self-evaluation, and self-reinforcement. Studies have indicated that external reinforcement (e.g., earning back money deposited with the therapist) is effective during treatment, but the results are not maintained as well (Jeffrey, 1974). Reinforcement by a significant other, however, appears to be more effective (Israel & Saccone, 1979). Thus, current programs rely primarily on self-reinforcement but may include contracting with significant others.

Self-monitoring appears to be the most indispensable component of behavioral programs, even though it is not sufficient by itself in the long run. Two studies reported on very brief, 4-week programs, but during that time daily self-recording of weight and caloric intake was as effective as a behavior management program or a combined approach (Romanczyk, 1974; Romanczyk, Tracey, Wilson, & Thorpe, 1973). Evidence suggests that premonitoring (recording immediately before eating) is slightly more effective than postmonitoring (after eating) (Bellack, Rozensky & Schwartz, 1974) and that self-monitoring of caloric intake is more effective than monitoring eating habits (Green 1978).

The second step, self-evaluation, is often considered an implicit part of the self-reinforcement procedure, although recent research points out its critical role. Assessment of general self-evaluative style on nonweight-related tasks indicated that subjects who were more likely to evaluate themselves positively (self-reinforce) lost more weight and responded particularly well to self-control programs compared to therapist-controlled programs (Bellack, Glanz, & Simon, 1976; Carroll, Yates, & Gray, 1980; Rozensky & Bellack 1976).

Specific self-reward procedures appear to enhance self-monitoring. There seems to be little difference whether money or more symbolic rewards are used or whether subjects self-reinforce or self-punish (Bellack 1976; Mahoney 1974; Mahoney, Moura, & Wade, 1973). Castro and Rachlin (1980) suggest that any procedure that serves as feedback to the person who wants to lose weight is sufficient, although money may make the feedback more salient for some. Evidence indicates that self-reinforcement based on eating habit change is more effective than if based on weight loss (Israel & Saccone, 1979; Mahoney, 1974).

Analyzing and Modifying Eating Behaviors

The following procedures are utilized to modify undesirable eating patterns so that the overweight person develops an appropriate, controlled eating style.

There is conflicting evidence regarding whether an "obese" eating style is truly characteristic of overweight persons and to what extent this causes their weight problem. Nonetheless, most programs have assumed this to be the case, and there is a wealth of clinical evidence that clients find such procedures useful.

Pace of Eating

The purpose is to slow down the rate of eating so the person will eat less. The extra time allows the person to sense the feeling of fullness and to stop before feeling stuffed. In addition, the person avoids the temptation to nibble while waiting for others to finish. Clients are instructed to put down their forks completely between each bite. They stretch out the mealtime by introducing short (2 minute) delays, in which they just socialize. Including foods with high bulk or that take a long time to eat (for example, salads, artichokes) is also helpful.

Timing of Eating

Clients are instructed to avoid skipping meals and subsequently eating when starved, when they are more likely to eat too fast and too much before they will feel full. Regular, planned meals and snacks promote controlled eating.

Focusing on Internal Cues

Clients deliberately practice leaving a small amount of food on their plate to overcome the habit of automatically eating whatever is in front of them. The purpose is to get clients to attend to internal cues to regulate their eating rather than to external cues. In addition, clients practice asking themselves, "Am I really hungry?" whenever they feel an urge to eat impulsively. They learn to discriminate externally cued impulses and to eat only in response to internal cues.

Altering Behavioral Chains

Once clients have learned to discriminate environmentally cued eating, they practice substituting alternative, competing (noneating) responses when this occurs. Clients make lists of activities (for example, dusting, taking a walk, taking a bubble bath) that will get them out of the situation or distract them until the urge subsides. Another method is to set a timer for 10 minutes to introduce a delay; frequently, the urge subsides during this period. As clients become more sophisticated in their abilities to look for and analyze behavioral patterns (antecedents, behaviors, consequences), they learn to intervene early in a chain of behaviors to avoid situations that are particularly likely to lead to eating. It is far easier to substitute early in a chain than to wait until the urge actually occurs.

Typical problem behavior chains involve eating when tired (a better alternative is a 15-minute nap), bored, depressed, or anxious. It is a widely held assumption that obese people are more likely to eat in response to negative emotional states; however, the experimental evidence relating anxiety or boredom to eating is ambiguous (see Abraham & Stinson, 1977; Reznick & Balch, 1977). Leon and Chamberlain (1973 a,b) found that 25% of both obese and normal subjects report eating when lonely or bored. Eating in response to negative emotional states may be more of a problem for the obese even if it is not initially causally related to their being overweight. Clients who find themselves eating in response to negative emotions can be encouraged to deal with them more directly by figuring out what the problem is and doing something about it (e.g., relaxation training, assertive training, interpersonal problem solving, etc.). Meditation, imagery, or other experiential techniques can be used to help clients tolerate negative affect without relying on eating. Because behavioral interventions for obesity are usually conducted in groups within an educational framework, clients with serious or recurring emotional problems are typically referred to other professionals to deal with those issues.

Refusing Food Offers

Clients often feel uncomfortable refusing food in social situations. Behavior rehearsal is used to teach clients to refuse food assertively. Clients are asked to eat only food that they have specifically requested because they must learn to control their intake based on internal cues rather than letting other people or situational cues control their eating.

Stimulus-Control Modification

Stimulus control refers to modifying environmental cues so that a particular, desirable response will be more likely to occur. Used in a self-control framework, it refers to something that a person does ahead of time to alter the probability of subsequent events. The use of these procedures in controlling obesity is based on the still-controversial assumption that the obese person is overly responsive to environmental cues. The procedures are designed to eliminate cues for impulsive, uncontrolled eating and to introduce new cues that will promote controlled eating. Clients learn to monitor and self-reinforce for making these self-controlling responses.

Eliminate Extraneous Visual Food Cues

Clients do not have tempting foods available. All food is stored away in opaque containers. Extra food is put away before starting to eat and is not left on the table.

Narrow the Range of Cues Associated with Eating

Clients are asked to designate specific places to eat and to eat only in these approved places (not all over the house). Clients are not allowed to pair other activities (such as TV) with eating because those activities are frequently discriminative stimuli for eating.

Minimize Contact with Food

Clients eliminate any unnecessary exposure to food (for example extensive baking/cooking). Other people may be enlisted to prepare food and/or clean up. Leftover food or tempting food gifts are immediately thrown out or given away. Clients are encouraged to shop and to prepare foods ahead of time (when they are not feeling hungry).

Clients use graphs, signs, and other cues to remind themselves to use new eating habits. A special placemat or set of dishes can serve as new cues; small dishes may also make small portions appear larger.

Preplan

Clients are asked to plan their meals and snacks and to write down their plan so they will be more likely to stick with it. Planning is done the day before; clients then monitor their actual intake, writing down any changes when they do not adhere to it. The continuous feedback for planning enhances the client's control over his or her intake. It is particularly useful in handling parties, dinners out, or other special occasions, when a person is more likely to overeat if not committed ahead of time to a particular plan. Frequently, clients not only preplan but also preprepare snacks in specified amounts to decrease the probability of eating more than was planned.

Cognitive Restructuring

Cognitive-restructuring techniques, widely used in many areas of behavioral treatment (Goldfried & Davidson, 1976), have been specifically adapted to the treatment of obesity. Clinical reports indicate that overweight clients think about food a great deal, and their subsequent internal monologues are frequently maladaptive because they do not reliably lead to controlled eating. Little data are available to suggest that cognitive factors are causally related to obesity, but evidence suggests that adaptive cognitions are related to success in treatment (Sjoberg & Person, 1979; Straw *et. al.,* 1984). Mahoney and Mahoney (1976) have identified five general categories of problematic thoughts: rigid, unrealistic goals; negative evaluations of personal capability to lose weight; justifications (excuses) for eating; inability to distract from food thoughts; and impatience with slow rates of loss. Clients self-monitor their thoughts and replace the negative self-defeating thoughts with more adaptive, encouraging self-talk.

Modest Calorie Restriction

Nutrition education is part of almost all behavioral treatment packages. The major focus of traditional behavioral programs is to modify eating habits so clients will eat smaller amounts and will more often choose low-calorie foods. However, the value of a nutritionally sound diet is always upheld. Clients are strongly advised not to skip meals, not to exclude any food groups, and not to rely on faddish, atypical eating habits. The message is to cut down not out and to substitute low for high-calorie foods. Many programs do not include any specific diet plan because clients are to focus more generally on changing eating style and habits. However, many of the more effective behavioral programs have included a flexible, exchange-type diet as a guide. These diets typically recommend 1,000 calories/day as an absolute minimum and up to 1,500 or 2,000, depending on age, sex, and initial weight. The specific contribution of nutrition/diet information cannot be isolated from the overall effectiveness of these programs. However, one study (Jeffrey & Wing, 1979) found that self-reported calorie intake was the best predictor of weight loss. For our purposes, modest calorie restriction is considered a strategy that is typically used in conjunction with behavioral techniques. Ample data indicate that the effectiveness of simply providing diet information is so poor that this strategy would rarely be used alone.

Research suggests that the specific content, timing, or calories recommended in a diet may make little difference, at least in the long run. Wing and Epstein (1981) demonstrated no differences in initial or subsequent weight loss whether clients were asked to reduce their caloric intake by small, moderate, or large amounts during the first 5 weeks of a behavioral program. Wing, Epstein, and Shapiro (1982) found no differences in weight loss during the first 2 weeks in a behavioral program between subjects who were instructed to follow a specific-content diet (Scarsdale Medical Diet) and those who were given a daily calorie goal. When only those subjects who completed the subsequent 8 weeks of treatment and were available at follow-up were considered, those in the Scarsdale condition had lost more weight during those first 2 weeks on the diet; these initial differences were no longer significant at end of treatment or follow-up. Thus, even for those who are successful in initially losing a little faster due to a particular diet, there seems to be little long-term advantage.

Severe Calorie Restriction

Fairly recently, a number of specific, severe-calorie-restriction diets have been evaluated in conjunction with behaviorally oriented programs. The use of such diet strategies alone will not be considered in this chapter because there does not appear to be any situation in which such a strategy would be advantageous to a client. The problem of relapse after such efforts has been well documented (Wadden, Stunkard, & Brownell, 1983). Careful medical screening and supervision is critical with any such program to reduce the potential for physical problems.

Musante (1976) reported on 229 clinically obese clients who were treated in an outpatient program in which all meals were provided in a supervised dining area. A very restricted, standardized 700-calorie diet was provided in conjunction with an intensive behavioral program. Treatment was individualized and of varying lengths, which makes comparisons to other studies difficult, but substantial weight losses were reported. Over half the patients lost more than 20 pounds and a quarter lost more then 40 pounds. No follow-up data were reported.

A report by Wadden, Stunkard, Brownell, and Day (1984) provides the strongest evidence to date that substantial weight loss achieved through severe calorie restriction might be maintained. Seventeen clinically obese subjects (averaging 85% overweight) lost an average of 20.5 kg (45 pounds) during a 6-month treatment program combining a very low calorie diet with behavior modification. During the initial month, behavioral techniques were taught, and clients followed typical modest calorie-restriction (1,000 to 1,200 calorie) diets. During the second and third months, clients followed a severe calorie-restriction diet (400 to 600 calories) under careful medical supervision. There was no difference between the use of a prescription powdered protein-formula diet or a diet of lean meat, fish, and fowl. Clients then returned to the balanced diet of conventional foods and spent the remaining 3 months learning behavioral techniques designed specifically for relapse prevention. Clients continued to lose (at a much slower rate) during this final treatment period but, most importantly, regained an average of only 2.1 kg (4.6 lb) over the subsequent 1-year follow-up. Psychological effects were also monitored and results indicated that clients did not experience increased depression or anxiety even while on the very low calorie diet. Preliminary evidence suggested that clients who were initially fairly depressed did not lose as well as initially nondepressed clients while on the very low calorie diet but they were able to lose as well while on modest calorie restriction. Results from a subsequent, larger controlled trial (Wadden & Stunkard, 1984) replicated the weight loss previously achieved (average 41 pound loss), however, maintenance was not quite as good (average 31 pounds loss).

Pharmacotherapy

Pharmacological treatments for obesity typically are not recommended due to their short-lived weight losses and the abuse potential of many of the drugs that have been used. Recent efforts to utilize such interventions to produce initially more rapid weight loss in combination with behavioral interventions to produce long-term adherence to modified eating and activity patterns have not been particularly successful. Results from an initial investigation (Craighead *et al.*, 1981) found that adding fenfluramine (a mild appetite suppressant with sedative rather than stimulant properties) did enhance the initial effectiveness of a behavioral program by an average of 8 pounds (total loss 31 pounds). However, during the 1-year follow-up, the behavioral treatment alone demonstrated excellent maintenance, whereas subjects in combined treatment regained substantial weight. The final weight losses were not statistically different due to increased variability but favored the behavioral treatment alone (average 20-pound loss) over the combined treatment (average 12-pound loss).

The failure of behavioral treatment to insure long-term maintenance of the initial losses was both surprising and disappointing. Most clients had initially responded extremely positively to the use of medication. Morale and enthusiasm, as reported by the group leaders, was much higher in the combined treatment groups. Even though the additional weight loss averaged only 8 pounds, this seemed to be clinically significant in terms of preventing discouragement and enhancing continued compliance over what was a fairly long treatment period (6 months).

A second study (Craighead, 1984) was designed to evaluate alternative ways to combine these two strategies that might utilize their strengths more effectively. In one group, the behavioral program was continued for 2 months after the medication was terminated. This sequence was effective in preventing relapse as long as the clients remained in the supportive group treatment, but slow weight regain was still observed over the subsequent 1-year follow-up. A second group in this study consisted of behavior therapy alone followed by a period of combined medication and therapy to provide a boost at the point that weight loss typically slows and clients become discouraged. Medication was substantially more effective when used this way, as these subjects continued to lose at a modest but steady rate. However, the superior weight loss in this group was not maintained during follow-up, probably due to the fact that both medication and therapy were terminated at the same time. Further work is needed to determine if this relapse can be prevented by a period of intensive relapse prevention training after medication is terminated.

Post hoc analyses were used in the second study to identify clients who were good responders at 8 weeks (at least 8 pounds lost in 8 weeks) or poor responders (less than 8 pounds) to behavior therapy alone. Subsequent provision of medication enhanced weight loss in both groups, but it was particularly effective with the poor responders. All six initially poor responders who subsequently took medication lost at least 8 pounds in the next 8 weeks, whereas none of the six poor responders who continued with behavior therapy alone were able to do so. Thus, medication may be worth considering if clients do not initially respond to behavioral techniques. It may or may not be that these are the same people who, for whatever reasons (e.g., naturally high "set points"), are not able to maintain weight loss, but the possibility deserves further investigation.

Exercise

The appropriateness of increasing energy expenditure as well as decreasing caloric intake in order to balance the energy equation has long been acknowledged. The notion of changing both eating and activity patterns is inherent in the behavioral model of treating obesity, however, the relative emphasis put on these two strategies varies considerably among programs. For our purposes, it is useful to consider exercise programming as a separate strategy from behavioral techniques to change eating habits. Initial assessment of the client may indicate the extent to which their obesity problem appears to be due to low activity levels rather than to overeating. Client willingness and ability to exercise, at least initially, vary so widely that it is useful to think of exercise as a separate decision the client must make. Making a separate decision helps the client better understand what exercise can and cannot do in coping with an obesity problem. There are four major reasons why a client might choose to exercise: modest effects on initial weight loss, fairly strong effects on weight maintenance, improved physical health and appearance, and improved psychological functioning.

Exercise has often been relegated to a secondary position in weight loss efforts due to the popular notion that it takes an inordinate amount of exercise to burn off any substantial amount of calories. To a certain extent, this perception is correct. Charts detailing the number of calories needed for various types and lengths of exercise are apt to be more discouraging than encouraging. In fact, controlled studies have shown that combined behavior modification and exercise programs produce only slightly greater initial weight loss than behavior modification alone (Dahlkoetter, Callahan, & Linton, 1979; Stalonas, Johnson, & Christ, 1978). In addition, Jeffrey and Wing (1979) found that self-report of exercise was not significantly related to weight loss (self-reported calorie intake was). However, most of the more effective behavioral programs reported in the literature (e.g., Craighead *et al.*, 1981; Dubbert & Wilson, in press; Katahn, Pleas, Thackery, & Wallston, 1982) have included a strong exercise component.

The mechanisms mediating the effect of exercise on weight loss are not clearly understood, but there is preliminary evidence for the following possibilities. In normally sedentary people, a substantial increase in energy expediture appears to be tolerated before the person begins to compensate by increasing intake. In fact, increased activity may decrease appetite (Bjorntorp, 1978). There is little evidence that increased exercise produces greater appetite except at high levels. Although some clients may report being very hungry after even modest exercise, this is probably due more to what they are saying to themselves (e.g., "I exercised so hard, I deserve a treat") or to social conditioning (e.g., going out for pizza after volleyball practice) than to physiological hunger. Cognitive restructuring and reeducation about exercise may be helpful in those cases. Second, evidence suggests that periods of sustained exercise alter metabolic functioning for a period of several hours after the exercise is stopped. Thus, current notions of the caloric "value" of exercise probably underestimate the true effect (Brownell, 1982). Third, several researchers (Bennett & Gurin, 1982) have argued that vigorous, regular exercise may lower, or "reset," a person's "natural weight." Fourth, a greater percentage of fat rather than lean body tissue is lost when diet and exercise are combined (Bray 1976). Fifth, exercise may serve as an alternative response to snacking (Epstein & Wing, 1980).

Until recently, behavioral treatment programs addressed the need to increase activity in two ways. First, the person's life-style was analyzed, and suggestions were made to increase "routine" exercise such as using stairs instead of elevators, walking to work or at least parking a few blocks away, and the like. This approach may be the most viable since it requires only minor life-style changes. Initial evidence suggests clients are more likely to adhere to such a program (Epstein, Wing, Koeske, Onip, & Beck, 1982). However, the payoff from such efforts in terms of weight loss and fitness is likely to be fairly modest.

The second approach has been to devise a specified, gradually increasing, individualized exercise program. Once agreed upon, a written contract is usually signed, and the client keeps self-monitoring records that are reviewed by the group leader. A specific self-reinforcement plan may or may not be added to the contract. This type of system allows the client to choose the type and amount of exercise that is most acceptable and can be most easily fit into his or her life-style, hopefully facilitating long-term compliance. Unfortunately, it is very difficult to monitor adherence to such programs and difficult to insure that sufficiently vigorous and sustained effort is put out to obtain maximum benefits. Some clients, particularly the more severely obese, are not willing or able to do strenuous activities, and some would need to be closely monitored if they should decide to try vigorous activities. Thus, for fairly obese clients, a gradual walking program is most often recommended.

Katahn (1982) has provided an excellent and detailed example of the type of exercise program that can be recommended even for the severely overweight. Katahn also makes a very significant point that needs to be highlighted within the decision-making approach. The value of exercise is directly related to the frequency, duration, and intensity of the effort. Occasional or sporadic attempts are probably not even worth the effort, at least from a weight-loss perspective. It is Katahn's contention that one must make a serious commitment to a life-style change due to the amount of exercise needed to have a serious impact on an obesity problem. He suggests that clients must plan to expend at least 200 calories a day on exercise; this translates into walking an extra 3 miles a day which takes approximately 45 minutes.

Blum and Craighead (1982) suggest that initial use of a formal, supervised group exercise program may be more effective than relying on individual efforts. In this study, subjects assigned to participate in a supervised exercise group (a graduated walk/run program) three times a week for 10 weeks (in addition to the regular behavior therapy meeting) lost only slightly more weight during treatment than subjects who contracted to expend the same amount of time in exercise of their choice on their own (a standard exercise contract). During the 1-year follow-up, all subjects were asked to continue their exercise programs on their own. At the final assessment, the subjects who had initially been supervised maintained a significantly greater average weight loss than those in the exercise contract group. Thus, even if clients eventually find it more convenient to exercise on their own, the initial structure, supervision, and/or group support may be important in facilitating a life-style change that will be successfully maintained.

Effect on Weight Maintenance

Evidence for a fairly strong long-term effect of exercise on weight maintenance is accumulating. In several experimental studies (Dahlkoetter *et al.,* 1979; Stalonas *et al.,* 1978), the initially small difference favoring exercise over no-exercise conditions increased from posttreatment to follow-up. In addition, post hoc evidence suggests that those who do adopt an exercise life-style change maintain better than those who do not. At 1-year follow-up, Katahn, Pleas, Thackrey, and Wallston (1982) found that 39% of subjects reported they continued to exercise at the recommended level. These subjects maintained all their (approximately 30 pound) losses, whereas the nonexercising subjects regained an average of 11.3 pounds. Gormally *et al.* (1980) reported that six of the seven successful maintainers in their study were rated as still engaging in much or extensive exercise according to interview data at follow-up.

The major problem with exercise programs has been poor adherence. Reviews of the exercise adherence literature (Martin & Dubbert, 1982) suggest that in all populations fewer than half of all people who begin an exercise program, whether on their own or in a structured program, will still be exercising after 3 to 6 months; obese subjects are even more likely than others to drop out despite the fact that exercise would be especially useful for them. Gwinup (1975) illustrated substantial weight loss (22 lb) among 11 obese women who continued to exercise 1 hour a day for 1½ years, but only one-third of those who had initially enrolled were still in the program. Martin and Dubbert (1982) highlight a number of factors that may facilitate exercise adherence; however, it is difficult to arrange for clients to have a "perfect" program. Group-based obesity programs might do best to consider an integrated exercise program (e.g., Katahn *et al.*, 1982) that includes some group-based and some individual exercise.

Effect on Physiological and Psychological Functioning

Although the primary effect of exercise on weight appears to be in long-term maintenance, there are several additional payoffs that may be evident much more quickly. Focusing client attention on these factors may be helpful in establishing and maintaining regular exercise behavior. Considerable research is available to document the physiological changes associated with weight loss and the accompanying improvements in cardiovascular risk (see Brownell, 1982). Improved physical appearance may result from improvements in body composition (lean to fat ratio); this may be particularly important for those who are losing considerable weight, but some changes can be noted even with little weight loss.

Evidence is also rapidly accumulating that exercise is associated with general improvements in psychological functioning in both normal and clinical populations (Folkins & Sime, 1981; Fremont & Craighead, 1984). Fremont and Craighead found that positive changes in mood occurred rather quickly (within 3 to 5 weeks). Strong, positive changes were evident across a variety of mood scales (e.g., less anxious, less depressed), and positive changes were evident both in mildly depressed "normals" as well as the more severely depressed. Mood changes did not correlate with physiological improvements, suggesting that high levels of conditioning are not necessary. The extent to which the effects were due to nonspecifics rather than physiological effects of exercise is unclear, but the effects persisted over a period of several months. Thus, they do not appear simply to be transient effects due to starting some new activity.

Psychological improvements are clearly worthwhile even if the client does not lose weight, but they may serve an important indirect function in weight loss. Polivy and Herman (1983) have noted that continual efforts to diet appear to be quite stressful and may increase emotionality. Furthermore, stress tends to disinhibit cognitive restraint, disrupting diet efforts. Foreyt, Goodrick, and Gotto (1981) have suggested that exercise may reduce stress (whether from dieting or other sources) and thus may allow many people to comply with weight loss programs more effectively. This may be particularly critical for clients identified as "emotional" eaters.

Undiet

Polivy and Herman (1983) have provided a "natural weight undiet" program as a rather dramatic alternative to other approaches to obesity. At the present time, there are no experimental studies evaluating this program or its relative effectiveness compared to other approaches. The theoretical premise of such an approach is based on the still controversial hypothesis that people have a "natural weight" and that deprivation (dieting) sufficient to alter this natural weight can be accomplished only by learning to ignore normal hunger cues. Chronic dieters eventually lose their ability to regulate weight naturally and may, in fact, end up at weights even higher than their initial "natural weight." The undiet program is designed to reinstate normal regulatory processes and allow the person to assume his or her natural weight. The authors contend that many people will be pleasantly surprised to find they lose weight despite the fact that they may well never reach their hypothetical "ideal."

The seven major recommendations of the undiet program as proposed by Polivy and Herman (1983) can be outlined as follows. The "undiet" is not incompatible with behavioral techniques, exercise, and even nutrition education, although it has a different emphasis; these procedures can be used to aid resumption of "normal" eating habits, but they must not be used to set up a feeling of "deprivation."

1. Learn to distinguish between hunger (the physiological cue for food), appetite (the psychological desire for a particular taste or sensation), and stomach sensations (feeling satisfied versus feeling full or even bloated).
2. Recondition hunger signals so they occur at normal meal times by initially forcing oneself to eat three or four times a day on a fairly regular schedule.
3. Redefine *satiety* as absence of hunger, not stomach feeling full; learn to stop eating when hunger has been satisfied, that is before a stomach feels any discomfort.
4. Put food in the proper perspective in one's life instead of making it a central concern. Learn to identify the other, psychological functions that food has been fulfilling and find alternative ways to fill those needs (e.g., other, less destructive self-indulgences or ways of celebrating).
5. Make an effort to deliberately counteract the magical (addictive) power of food. Toilet binges are recommended for bingers; bingers are to buy the food for a binge and crumble it into the toilet to help make the point that

this is food that is in excess of what is truly needed by the body and is just being wasted anyway (i.e., stored as fat or perhaps even purged).

6. The person is to eat any food he or she wishes but only when hunger has been identified, and they are to stop when the hunger is satisfied. Thus, one eats as much as one *needs*, not as much as one *wants*. There are no forbidden foods, and the undieter may incorporate occasional splurges without guilt as they are not to make themselves feel "deprived."

7. Learn to cope with social pressures to eat and unhelpful interference by significant others by brief explanations of the basic principle and/or assertive counterresponses.

From a decision-making perspective, this alternative is worth cautious consideration as we await further validation. It may be useful as a first choice in situations when clients decide it is not a good time to put the time and resources into a demanding program. For others, it may be useful as a secondary strategy. Their initial experiences with other techniques may tell them they are not willing to pay the personal price of constant deprivation. The undiet is an alternative to giving up, and it is distinctly different from saying, "I just don't care, and I'll eat all I want." The person choosing the undiet is working to restore natural biological and psychological functioning so that his or her weight reflects his or her biological needs rather than his or her psychological needs. Thus, even if the person's natural weight is higher than what is socially desirable, he or she may be better able to accept this weight and avoid some of the negative psychological consequences of feeling like a failure. As noted earlier, "overeating" not "overweight" may turn out to be the more serious culprit in terms of negative biological consequences. Evidence is also accumulating that rapid weight gain and large weight fluctuations may be more stressful to the body than overweight itself (Wooley, Wooley, & Dyrenforth, 1979). Thus, a program focusing on natural regulation that will lead to a more stable weight may have fewer medical risks than the up-and-down pattern characteristic of many "chronic dieters."

Typical Problems

Attrition

Attrition in traditional medical treatment of obesity and in self-help groups has been quite high (Stunkard, 1975; Stunkard & Brownell, 1979). One of the strengths of behavioral programs has been lower attrition, typically not more than 20% (Wilson & Brownell, 1980). The use of a refundable deposit is typically associated with even lower rates (Hagen, Foreyt, & Durham, 1976), and this is now recommended as standard procedure. In an analysis of treatment dropouts, Dubbert and Wilson (1983) found that none of their subject variables predicted retention except that fewer men than women dropped out. Weight loss during the first month did not predict dropping out; most of their dropouts had lost at least 5 pounds before they left.

Failure to Lose during Treatment

Reviews of research on predictors of treatment response indicate that subject variables account for a relatively small portion of the variance (Cooke & Meyers, 1980), although specific weight variables appear to be more directly relevant. Analyzing the available research on treatment predictors plus data from their own treatment program, Dubbert and Wilson (1983) identified five indicators that are fairly stongly related to failure to reduce. Clients exhibiting such characteristics, however, should not be simply eliminated as a significant number of such clients are successful. Dubbert and Wilson recommend a careful reassessment of such clients after the first month of treatment to reappraise their progress; this can easily be accomplished within a decision-making framework.

The following indicators were associated with failure to reduce:

1. High (45% or greater) percentage body fat; this accounted for even more variance than actual body weight or percentage overweight.
2. Older (over 50) age; this effect appeared to be largely related to the higher percentage body fat among the older group.
3. High pretreatment marital satisfaction scores and/or an obese spouse; this may be a result of less pressure to lose weight and/or less support in weight loss efforts.
4. Minimal (less than 2 pounds) weight loss during the first 3 weeks of treatment; note, however, that 20% of ultimately successful losers did have such a slow start.
5. Failure to self-monitor calories for at least a week during the first month of treatment.

Dubbert and Wilson (1983) concluded that failure to respond to treatment, whether in a behavioral or nonbehavioral program, does not appear to be highly related to success in subsequent efforts. The number of previous unsuccessful efforts was not correlated with weight loss during their behaviorally oriented program. Other authors, including Katahn *et al.* (1982), have reported that success in maintenance was associated with joining another weight group. These results seem to support Schachter's (1982) conclusions that looking at a single attempt to lose weight may be misleading. According to retrospective personal weight history interviews, 62.5% of those sampled who had at some point been obese could be considered successful (no longer obese). These people reported using a variety of techniques and several different attempts before they were ultimately successful.

Failure to Reach Goal Weight

Even in the most successful behavioral programs, only a small proportion of clients reach their goal weight. Very few of those who still need to lose more weight are able to continue weight loss on their own even if they do maintain what they have lost. It has frequently been suggested that longer treatment, that is, until goal weight is reached, is the obvious solution, but there have been no direct tests, of this hypothesis. The better average losses achieved in longer programs suggest this may be at least a partial solution, but practical problems and cost-efficiency indexes must also be carefully considered. Combining more rapid initial weight loss techniques with behaviorally oriented maintenance strategies is another promising alternative that might increase the percentage who actually reach the goal weight. The typically slowed rate of loss over time suggests that physiological aspects of weight loss must also be considered. Once a clear plateau has been reached, the focus may need to shift to techniques designed to counteract biological responses to dieting and/or biological limitations of "natural weight."

Failure to Maintain Weight Loss

Behavioral programs have demonstrated by far the best maintenance, but successful maintenance varies considerably across individuals, and researchers are just beginning to understand some of the reasons for relapse. Reviews of the effect of periodic booster sessions have revealed inconsistent results (Foreyt *et al.*, 1981; Wilson & Brownell, 1980), and clearly their contribution, if any, is quite modest and inadequate. A significant problem in the literature has been a failure to differentiate between those who have lost significant amounts and have relapsed and those who were never very successful. Intervention appears to be needed very early in the relapse process to help clients cope with their own reactions to a "slip" and to restore their disrupted self-regulation. At this point, the best clinical suggestion that can be made is to teach clients relapse prevention strategies *before* treatment is terminated and then provide immediate access to assistance as needed. Scheduling frequent checkups on clients may even be needed because some reports show that clients frequently are reluctant to initiate contact once they "slip," even when access is made available.

The relapse prevention model developed by Marlatt (1982) is the most fully articulated specific maintenance strategy that is available. It was initially developed as a general model to use with a variety of addictive behaviors. Empirical evaluation of its effectiveness as a specific maintenance strategy for obesity, however, is still in the preliminary stages. Wadden *et al.* (1984) successfully used relapse prevention techniques as a way to prevent the substantial weight regain that typically occurs following a very low-calorie diet. Also, a direct comparison between a "standard" and a "relapse prevention" program (Sternberg, 1985) found a small (5 pound) but significant difference in favor of relapse prevention at the 3-month follow-up, whereas there had been no differences at the end of treatment. Twice as many of the subjects in the standard group had regained at least some weight. A subsequent effort to replicate (Collins, Wilson, & Rothblum, 1980) found only a smaller, nonsignificant difference; however, the length of the follow-up was longer (7 and 12 months). Perri, Shapiro, Ludwig, Twentyman, and McAdoo (1984) found superior long-term maintenance with relapse prevention but only when it was combined with extensive posttreatment contact by telephone and mail.

Research on the correlates of maintenance has provided some support for the potential utility of many of the techniques suggested by the model. Although the effect may not be as large as one would like, the relative ineffectiveness of other strategies suggests this is currently the most promising alternative. The following factors have been identified as important in weight maintenance (or lack thereof):

1. Exercise
2. Continued self-monitoring of progress (either body weight or eating habits); mentally self-monitoring not sufficient
3. Setting a specific weight regain (3 to 5 pounds) as a cue to reinstate self-regulatory strategies
4. Continued use of specific strategies that had been identified as being useful during weight loss
5. Spouse support in weight loss efforts
6. Making more general, life-style changes
7. Absence of disruptive life events and/or ability to cope effectively with emotional states

The data suggesting a link between relapse and emotional states seem particularly compelling given the frequency of clinical reports of emotionally related eating and the relative lack of emphasis on emotions characteristic of traditional behavioral programs. Retrospective client reports indicate that unsuccessful maintainers are more likely to say they eat in response to emotional states (depression, stress) (Gormally *et al.*, 1980; Leon & Chamberlain, 1973). Unexpected, unpredictable stressful life events also appear to be associated with relapse (Dubbert & Wilson, 1983; Gormally *et al.*, 1980). A detailed analysis of reported initial dieting "slips" during the first 2 months after treatment (Rosenthal *et al.*, 1980) highlights the role of emotions. Intrapersonal (reactions within the person to nonpersonal environmental states) and interpersonal (reactions to situations involving other persons) determinants were approximately equally likely to be responsible for these "slips." Responding to negative emotional and/or physical states (e.g., bereavement) accounted for most of the intrapersonal slips (31% of the total slips), whereas positive emotional states (e.g., enjoying a vacation) accounted for most of the interpersonal slips (36% of the total slips). Data from Dubbert and Wilson (1983) regarding stated reasons for relapse were amazingly similar. The authors also noted that none of those who had relapsed had resumed calorie recording after their slips despite the fact that the program had very explicitly set a 5-pound regain as a salient cue to resume self-regulation strategies. Thus, more attention must be paid to developing strategies to deal with negative emotional states and to help people find alternative ways to socialize and celebrate special events in nonfood-centered ways.

Relapse Prevention Techniques

Identifying High-Risk Situations

The client first learns to identify situations that are likely to be a problem. Situational descriptions involve both a specific environmental situation (such as being at a party) and an emotional state (such as anxiety). Self-monitoring is the most useful technique because the situations are typically quite idiosyncratic. If clients are currently eating appropriately, it may be useful for them to review their initial eating records to draw up a list of high-frequency problem situations. Clients can also monitor current urges or impulses to identify temptation situations. Relapse fantasies can be used to help clients become more aware of possible relapse situations. Clients then learn to respond to these high-risk situational (danger) cues as discriminative stimuli. They signal clients to avoid or to leave the situation if possible or, if not, to institute specific coping responses to "get through" the situation. The notion is that the earlier clients can identify potential trouble and prepare for it, the more successful they will be. Once clients find themselves already "in the act," it is more difficult to stop.

Coping Skills for High-Risk Situations

In some cases, the client's usual coping skills are being blocked by fear or other emotional reactions. In such cases, anxiety-reduction techniques are needed. In other cases, the client lacks the necessary skills. General problem-solving skills (e.g., Goldfried & Davison, 1976) plus specific response skills (a combination of instruction, modeling, rehearsal, coaching, feedback, and self-instructions) are taught so the client will have numerous alternative responses for problem situations. For example, a person facing free doughnuts being provided every morning at coffee break might develop the following alternative coping skills: taking an orange to eat instead, walking around the block or meditating instead of eating, assertively refusing the doughnuts, contracting to limit doughnuts to once a week and so forth. Cognitive decision-making techniques are also used to help clients overcome the tendency to focus only on the pleasant short-term effects of the indulgent behavior. Marlatt has labeled this the *problem of immediate gratification,* or the *PIG phenomenon.* Clients are taught to use a decision matrix to force themselves to look at the total picture. If clients become aware that they will tend to exaggerate the positive aspects, especially if they have been avoiding something for some time, they will be less likely to give in to their perceived need for immediate indulgence. For example, the person who has avoided the doughnuts for a month may begin to focus on how great one would taste, and this builds up until he or she feels he or she just must have one. The person can remind himself or herself that the doughnut probably will taste good but probably will not live up to his or her exaggerated expectations; plus the 2 minutes of pleasure may not be worth the long-term weight problem.

Marlatt recommends the use of a "programmed relapse" in which the client who feels compelled to resume an old habit agrees to come in and have the first cigarette or drink under the direct supervision of a therapist. The client who resumes the habit as a response to stressful conditions is likely to attribute the ability to cope to the substance and be more likely to turn to it again when under stress. Also, the client who resumes the habit under particularly pleasant circumstances (a birthday celebration) is likely to exaggerate his or her own positive response (the ice cream tastes absolutely wonderful), which will make subsequent abstinence more difficult. Clients need to experience the behavior apart from its usual negative (or positive) circumstances so they can more objectively evaluate their own response. For example, a person who has been avoiding chocolate bars may sit down under neutral conditions and very carefully note his or her reactions as he or she slowly eats a candy bar. Often, he or she can begin to identify that the real pleasure is in the first few bites and that it rapidly diminishes. In many cases, even the initial taste is not quite as wonderful as the person had been anticipating. Such experiences may help clients avoid unrealistic expectations about the effects of food, encourage them to eat moderate amounts rather than binge and help them understand how strongly the social context effects their pleasure with food.

As is evident here, the abstinence model must be adapted to some degree for eating problems because total abstinence from eating is not a possibility. However, many clients do tend to think about certain "problem" foods in an abstinence-oriented manner. The psychological consequences of this type of dichotomous thinking are part of the reason that in most behaviorally oriented programs abstinence from specific "problem" foods is not advised. Carefully structured, limited eating of forbidden foods can reduce the power that certain foods appear to have and will promote moderated, or controlled, eating. These skills are critical during maintenance as the client is likely to feel it is safe to indulge to some degree. If clients have not learned to limit amounts, initially small indulgences may well trigger a binge or lead to gradual weight gain.

A slip or lapse in the relapse prevention model is typically defined as the first cigarette or the first drink after a period of abstinence. For eating problems, the model must be modified. For some people a true binge or a party weekend may serve as a clear cue. The first doughnut, cookie, or second helping, however, is not likely to be a salient cue. A slow, almost imperceptible, gradual increase in amounts eaten may not trigger off the appropriate relapse prevention mechanisms. Thus, it may be critical to set up a specific early warning signal that will serve to define an initial "lapse." Data from Stuart and Guire (1978) indicated that successful maintainers weighed themselves weekly and set an upper limit of a 3-pound gain, at which time they reinstated certain procedures.

Coping with an Initial Lapse

Once the client has identified that a lapse has occurred, behavioral and cognitive techniques are applied to prevent a full-blown relapse. A behavioral contract is typically set up ahead of time to limit the extent of use should a lapse occur. Clients are prepared to cope with the negative emotional reactions they are likely to experience. Marlatt and his colleagues have described a phenomenon called the *abstinence violation effect* (AVE), a combination of cognitive dissonance (conflict and guilt) and personal attribution (blaming self), which is frequently sufficient to trigger a relapse. To the extent that a person holds a dichotomous view that he or she is either in control or out of control, any perceived violation is likely to result in a shift to a period of indulgence during which it is difficult to restore a sense of control.

Cognitive techniques are used to teach the client to reconceptualize a violation as a single, independent event that can be corrected rather than a sign of failure.

Clients will tend to *overgeneralize,* to make the slip more catastrophic than it really is. An external-type attribution explaining the slip in terms of an interaction of a high-risk situation and lack of coping responses is more adaptive than an internal-type attribution of lack of will power or control. The lapse is viewed as a potential learning experience. The client is not to punish himself or herself but to analyze the situation to figure out what happened and what he or she needs to learn in order to handle such a situation better in the future. Clients are also taught that conflict/guilt feelings are to be expected and that this negative affect will tend to trigger additional eating. Clients are reassured that such feelings will subside over time if they do not give in to them (reinforce them by eating) but simply wait them out. Meditation is often used as a technique to tolerate or detach oneself from the negative affect until it passes. Clients may even carry a small reminder card with their AVE instructions including the appropriate self-statements, a list of "what to do next" generated from their relapse contract to limit use, and possibly a person or "hot line" number to call if more assistance is needed.

Promoting a Balanced Life-Style

Research by Marlatt and his colleagues suggests that an unbalanced life-style, one characterized largely by *shoulds* (activities perceived as external demands) rather than *wants* (activities for pleasure or self-fulfillment), tends to set the stage for a relapse. The more a person feels deprived, the greater the desire for self-indulgence and immediate gratification and the more easily it can be justified or rationalized. Frequently, the person manages to get himself or herself into a high-risk situation and feels overwhelmed. The person then feels he or she just could not help himself or herself: "It just happened." The goal of response prevention is to help clients become aware of life-style problems and the way very early decisions (apparently irrelevant decisions) contribute to putting themselves in temptation situations that they are not able to resist. Life-style changes must be quite individualized but may focus on rescheduling to avoid the stress of a constant, hectic pace, setting aside some type of individual time, modifying interactions with significant others, or making changes in type of employment or even living situations. A more generally positive life-style appears to reduce the desire for self-indulgence; the client learns to substitute other, more adaptive forms of self-indulgence, that is, "positive addictions" (Glasser, 1976).

Case Study

The following case study is used to illustrate the three typically critical redecision points within the problem-solving approach to treatment of obesity. Mary is an excellent example of the "typical" obese client who has been described by Wilson and Brownell (1980) as follows: female, 40 years old, 200 lb (approximately 50% overweight).

Mary's initial assessment indicated she weighed 200 lb (49% overweight). Her initial goal was to weigh 140 lb. She was currently 30 years old, happily married, and had a 4-year-old son. She worked part-time as a file clerk. Her husband was not overweight; he encouraged her efforts to control her weight but was not critical of it. She had been mildly overweight since high school but had gained considerable weight after she was married and again during her pregnancy. During and since her pregnancy, she had moderately high blood pressure that was being monitored, although no medication had been prescribed. Her physician had strongly recommended weight loss, but her weight had remained stable over the past 2 years despite her efforts to follow the diet recommendations. She was concerned about this health issue but also stated she was particularly motivated at this time as she was anticipating her husband's graduation from college and induction as an officer in the armed services the next spring, or in 1 year. She was anticipating a large family celebration and wanted to weigh what she had when she had gotten married. She was also thinking of having another child at some point and felt she must get her weight under control first.

In discussing initial treatment alternatives, Mary easily identified cognitive-behavioral therapy plus modest calorie restriction as her preferred option. She was willing to make a long-term commitment to slow, steady weight loss and did not feel under any pressure to lose weight rapidly. She wanted an approach that would be least disruptive to her family's eating habits and their life-style. She did not feel she had the time and interest at this point to exercise. Assessment of Mary's initial 2 weeks of self-monitoring records confirmed that this would be an appropriate initial decision. She was, in fact, "overeating," not consistently but a few days each week and had developed some maladaptive eating patterns (e.g., hiding or sneaking food in to eat alone, moderate binges if certain foods were left in the house, and eating in response to boredom). She had little physical activity other than housework and looking after her son, but she was reluctant to change this. A decision was made to reconsider this issue at a later point because she was likely to lose some initial weight even without increasing her activity level. Mary felt she needed more support than would be available with bibliotherapy and did not feel a self-help group would be sufficient either. She was willing to take either group or individual therapy. Our group programs were not scheduled to start for several months, so she chose to continue to work with the individual therapist (a master's-level counselor in training) who was doing the initial assessment and decision making.

Mary received a student manual (Ferguson, 1975) that outlined the procedures that would be taught and contained the forms that were used for self-monitoring. The first 10 weeks focused primarily on the more traditional behavioral procedures (the self-control model, altering eating style and stimulus control). Mary was very conscientious about recording and following the procedures and lost at a slow but steady pace (15 pounds). During the next 2 weeks Mary experienced a plateau, which is typical at this point in such a program. Many programs are, in fact, only set up for 8 to 12 weeks, but this is a serious mistake. Only the mildy overweight will be near their goal, and few people continue to lose on their own. As in Mary's case, external reassurance and intervention is needed to sustain client efforts. Mary reevaluated her initial decision but decided to renew her efforts and give this strategy another 2 weeks before considering a switch to another strategy. Mary and the therapist identified a few of the techniques that had been the most helpful before and focused on reinstating them. In addition, the therapist introduced cognitive restructuring to help Mary counteract negative statements of discouragement.

Mary had several other plateaus over the course of the year as would be expected in long-term treatment for the more severely obese. At one point, she was able to make a commitment to a walking program that she was not willing to do before. At another point, she focused specifically on learning to be more assertive in refusing food offers, especially on visits home to family and in-laws. Relapse prevention techniques were also introduced after the first 6 months and proved quite helpful in coping with her occasional binges. Mary was able to make some life-style changes to alleviate some of the boredom she experienced. She became willing to leave her son at the baby-sitter's for longer periods of time so she had some time for herself outside of work and began a crafts class and an exercise class. She started some initial career exploration with the counselor to develop a plan for when her husband finished school and she would be free to get further training or consider other jobs. She practiced a technique we label *sitting with feelings.* When she felt bored and wanted to eat, she would sit down and really pay attention to her feelings, often writing down *what* she was feeling. She began to realize that she did not need to always escape from negative feelings by eating (or doing something else) but that she could tolerate them; they would not overwhelm her, and eventually they would subside. As she put it,

> It wasn't a pleasant experience, but afterwards I would feel pretty good because at least I hadn't eaten. In the past I would feel bad and eat and then feel even worse because I had eaten. It started to make sense to me to face the feelings instead of compounding the problem by eating.

Frequently, it was these reflective periods that gave her ideas about other changes she wanted to make in her life.

Once Mary reached her goal weight, 60 lb lost in 48 weeks, the decision-making framework was utilized to decide on an explicit maintenance strategy because clients tend to go "off" programs and revert to old patterns. Mary's strategy included continuing her exercise class, an abbreviated self-monitoring form and weekly weighing with a 5-lb gain set as the "danger" cue.

Many clients, including Mary, maintain quite well, but others encounter difficulties once treatment is terminated. Again, the explicit decision-making framework gives the client a new way to conceptualize and cope with weight regain. Maintenance difficulty is seen as important new information about the self that must be added into the decision-making matrix. The client knows now he or she can lose weight at a certain personal "cost." Thus, the question is reframed as "At what cost am I willing to maintain my weight?" Many clients who were willing to "pay a high price" (e.g., cognitive restraint, exercise, curtail certain social functions, etc.) to lose weight are unpleasantly surprised to find that, for them, the price of maintaining their new weight is also quite high, higher than they had anticipated.

Most people, even if they know they will have to "watch it," expect to resume more "normal" eating habits and to be less consistent in their efforts once the goal weight is reached. This does seem to be true for some, but for others it is not sufficient. Thus, a reevaluation is necessary. The client may decide continued efforts are worth it, may decide new strategies are needed, or may decide to modify his or her goal weight to some degree to one that is more easily maintained. For example, two clients who successfully lost to target weight came back in 2 months perplexed and unhappy over weight regain. One client was able to identify strong feelings of resentment over the fact that even though now at "normal weight" she could not eat the same way as her husband or other normal weight friends. Continued stringent restraint for the rest of her life seemed a harsh sentence. Although she had already begun a modest exercise program, she decided to try a quite rigorous one as she felt that would be a more positive alternative that might allow her to eat more normally yet maintain her weight. The second client chose to resume fairly stringent restraint. She concluded she had initially chosen what was for her an unrealistic maintenance strategy. She had felt that she deserved a break after all her hard work and could take it easy for a while but now she knew what she had to do and was willing to do it. She decided to come in for a few individual sessions of cognitive restructuring to help her rethink some of her expectations, such as "I should be able to maintain my weight as easily as other people, and it's terribly unfair if I have to work harder at it."

Summary

A problem-solving approach to the treatment of obesity has been presented as a flexible framework within which professionals and clients can make more realistic, rational, and humane treatment decisions regarding a disorder that is still poorly understood. The initial assessment is used to clarify the client's obesity problem and to educate him or her about the important role that physiology may play in weight regulation. Because many people do lose weight fairly easily and maintain with modest effort, the notion persists that obesity is a fairly simple matter of eating too much and/or exercising too little. Lack of knowledge concerning physiological factors may, however, lead to maladaptive dieting patterns. Dieters want weight loss to be fast, steady, easy, and permanent when, in fact, it is more likely to be slow, inconsistent, costly in terms of time and personal effort, temporary, and perhaps nearly impossible for certain individuals. Thus, the person with a weight problem typically continues to seek out new, promising methods but terminates them when they do not show quick results or when it becomes clear they require effort. Or, if they do lose weight, they regain it fairly quickly, setting up a yo-yo pattern of feast or famine. It usually takes many such unsuccessful efforts before dieters are willing to revise their beliefs and accept the notion of slow, effortful weight loss plus continued life-style change to insure maintenance.

In the problem-solving model, the professional helps the client evaluate available treatment alternatives and make an initial decision but makes it clear that subsequent reevaluations will be based on the client's personal response. The goal is to stick with the client through a trial-and-error process until an optimal strategy can be found that maximizes the benefits and minimizes the costs for that individual.

Initial treatment recommendations reflect the state of the art and currently may be summarized as follows (Stunkard, 1983). For the mild to moderately (less than 40%) overweight, which includes 90.5% of obese women, cognitive-behavior therapy plus exercise and moderate calorie restriction is clearly the treatment of choice. Weight loss for such clients may be primarily a cosmetic matter as medical consequences are quite variable and uncertain. Self-help groups or bibliotherapy with minimal therapist contact are the most cost-efficient alternatives and should be considered particularly by those who are only mildly overweight. Short-term structured group programs led by professionals are a viable option for those who do not want or have not been successful with self-help approaches. Those who have more than 30 pounds to lose may best consider an intensive, professionally led behavioral program that is of sufficient length that it might be likely that they could reach the goal weight. Individual therapy may be needed if an appropriate group program is not available. Clients should be informed that only a small proportion are able to continue to lose once they terminate treatment. It is appropriate to encourage clients to try a new behavioral program even if they have previously not been successful with other behavioral (or nonbehavioral) programs, especially if they indicate that they are in some way motivated differently this time. For unknown reasons, past efforts do not reliably predict success in subsequent efforts.

Recommendations for the moderately to severely obese (40 to 100% overweight), which includes 9% of obese women, are more complex. There is a greater likelihood of medical complications to consider and greater possibility of pathological physiology that might limit weight loss. Many such individuals have done well in long-term, comprehensive behavioral treatment programs, and this is still the best recommendation if clients are willing to persevere in a long-term commitment. A combination of severe calorie restriction (under medical supervision) plus behavioral treatment plus exercise may, however, be a more realistic alternative in that a large weight loss can be achieved in a more reasonable period of time. Preliminary evidence suggests that maintenance may be adequate, but the possibility of relapse suggests caution and careful attention to follow-up. Exercise must be very gradually increased, and consultation with medical and/or exercise specialists may be necessary to prevent or reduce risk. An extensive life-style change is likely to be critical in terms of maintaining new exercise and eating habits.

The very severely (over 100% overweight) obese constitute only a very small proportion (approximately .5%) of the obese, but their treatment is by far the most problematic. Severe medical complications are almost always present, and pathological physiology is a likely hypothesis. Clients who do not respond positively to the most effective combination of behavior treatment and severe calorie restriction may, for medical reasons, need to consider the possibility of surgical measures, but this alternative has not been discussed in this chapter.

In the decision-making approach difficulty in either weight loss or weight maintenance is reconstrued as important new information about one's body and one's values and priorities. Thus, in reevaluating their efforts, clients may eliminate or incorporate additional techniques. Clients who are not successful and who have no additional compelling medical reasons to lose weight may need to reevaluate their goals. Some clients may need to focus on exercise or "undieting" rather than emphasizing restraint to such a degree. In a sense, the only unacceptable solution to an obesity problem is for the client to decide that he or she cannot, or chooses not to do what it takes to maintain a weight that is acceptable but that he or she will continue to be miserable about being overweight and will continue to subject himself or herself to repeated failure with whatever fad diet comes out next.

References

Abramson, E. E., & Stinson, S. G. (1977). Boredom and eating in non-obese individuals. *Addictive Behaviors, 2,* 181–185.

Bellack, A. S. (1976). A comparison of self-reinforcement and self-monitoring in a weight reduction program. *Behavior Therapy, 7,* 68–75.

Bellack, A. S., Glanz, L., & Simon, R. (1976). Self-reinforcement style and covert imagery in the treatment of obesity. *Journal of Consulting and Clinical Psychology, 44,* 490–491.

Bellack, A. S., Rozensy, R., & Schwartz, J. (1974). A comparison of two forms of self-monitoring in a weight reduction program. *Behavior Therapy, 5,* 523–530.

Bennett, W., & Gurin, J. (1982). *The dieter's dilemma: Eating less and weighing more.* New York: Basic Books.

Bjorntorp, P. (1975). Effect of an energy-reduced dietary regimen in relation to adipose tissue cellularity in obese women. *American Journal of Clinical Nutrition, 28,* 445–452.

Bjorntorp, P. (1975). Effect of an energy-reduced dietary regimen in relation to adipose tissue cellularity in obese women. *American Journal of Clinical Nutrition, 28,* 445–452.

Bjorntorp, P. (1978). Exercise and obesity. *Psychiatric Clinics of North America, 1,* 691–696.

Blum, M., & Craighead, L. W. (1982, November). *Evaluation of a supervised exercise component in behavioral treatment of obesity.* Paper presented at the meetings of the Association for the Advancement of Behavior Therapy. Los Angeles.

Boskind-White, M., & White, W. C. (1983). *Bulimarexia: The binge/purge cycle.* New York: Norton.

Bray, G. A. (1969). Effect of caloric restriction on energy expenditure in obese patients. *Lancet, 2,* 397–398.

Bray, G. A. (1976). *The obese patient.* Philadelphia: Saunders.

Brownell, K. D. (1981). Assessment of eating disorders. In D. Barlow (Ed.), *Behavioral assessment of adult disorders* (pp. 329–404). New York: Guilford Press.

Brownell, K. D. (1982). Obesity: Understanding and treating a serious, prevalent and refractory disorder. *Journal of Consulting and Clinical Psychology, 50,* 820–840.

Brownell, K. D., Hecerman, C. L., & Westlake, R. J. (1979). The behavioral control of obesity: A descriptive analysis of a large scale program. *Journal of Clinical Psychology, 35,* 864–869.

Brownell, K. D., & Stunkard, A. J. (1978). Behavior therapy and behavior change: Uncertainties in programs for weight control. *Behaviour Research and Therapy, 16,* 301.

Callaway, C. W., & Greenwood, M. R. C. (1983). Progress in characterizing human obesities. *Nutrition News, 46* (3), 9.

Carroll, L. J., Yates, B. T., & Gray, J. J. (1980). Predicting obesity reduction in behavioral and nonbehavioral therapy from client characteristics: The self-evaluation measure. *Behavior Therapy, 11,* 189–197.

Castro, L., & Rachlin, H. (1980). Self-reward, self-monitoring, and self-punishment as feedback in weight control. *Behavior Therapy, 11,* 38–48.

Clausen, J. D., Silfen, M., Coombs, J., Ayers, W., & Altschul, A. M. (1980). Relationship of dietary regimens to success, efficiency, and cost of weight loss. *Journal of the American Dietetic Association, 77,* 249–256.

Collins, R. L., Wilson, G. T., & Rothblum, E. (1980, November). *The comparative efficacy of cognitive and behavioral approaches in weight reduction.* Paper presented at the annual meeting of the Association for Advancement of Behavior Therapy, New York.

Cooke, C. J., & Meyers, A. (1980). The role of predictor variables in the behavioral treatment of obesity. *Behavioral Assessment, 2,* 59–69.

Craighead, L. W. (1984). Sequencing of behavior therapy and pharmacotherapy for obesity. *Journal of Consulting and Clinical Psychology, 52,* 190–199.

Craighead, L. W., McNamara, K., & Horan J. J. (1984). Perspectives on self-help and bibliotherapy: You are what you read. In S. D. Brown & A. W. Lent (Eds.), *Handbook of counseling psychology* (pp. 730–769). New York: Wiley.

Craighead, L. W., Stunkard, A. J., & O'Brien, R. (1981). Behavior therapy and pharmacotherapy of obesity. *Archives of General Psychiatry, 38,* 763–768.

Dahlkoetter, J., Callahan, E. J., & Linton, J. (1979). Obesity and the unbalanced energy equation: Exercise versus eating habit change. *Journal of Consulting and Clinical Psychology, 47,* 898–905.

Drewnowski, A., & Greenwood, M. R. C. (1983). Cream and sugar: Human preferences for high-fat foods. *Physiology & Behavior, 30,* 629–633.

Dubbert, P. M., & Wilson, T. (1983). Treatment failures in behavior therapy for obesity: Causes, correlates, and consequences. In E. Foa & P. M. G. Emmelkamp (Eds.), *Treatment failures in behavior therapy* (pp. 263–288). New York: Wiley.

Dubbert, P., Wilson, G. T., Augusto, F., Langenbucher, J., & McGee, D. (1981, November). *Cooperative behavior of involved and non-involved spouses of weight control program participants.* Paper presented at the annual convention of the Association for Advancement of Behavior Therapy, Toronto.

Epstein, L. H., & Wing, R. R. (1980). Aerobic exercise and weight. *Addictive Behaviors, 5,* 371–388.

Epstein, L. H., Wing, R. R., Koeske, R., Ossip, D., & Beck, S. (1982). A comparison of lifestyle change and programmed aerobic exercise on weight and fitness changes in obese children. *Behavior Therapy, 13,* 651–665.

Ferguson, J. M. (1975). *Learning to eat: Behavior modification for weight control.* Palo Alto, CA: Ball.

Folkins, C. H., & Sime, W. E. (1981). Physical fitness training and mental health. *American Psychologist, 36,* 373–389.

Foreyt, J. P., Goodrick, G. K., & Gotto, A. M. (1981). Limitations of behavioral treatment of obesity: Review and analysis. *Journal of Behavioral Medicine, 4,* 159–174.

Fremont, J., & Craighead, L. W. (1984, November). *Aerobic exercise in the treatment of mild to moderate depression.* Paper presented at the meetings of the Association for the Advancement of Behavior Therapy. Philadelphia.

Garner, D. M., Olmsted, M. P., & Polivy, J. (1982). Development and validation of a multidimensional eating disorder inventory for anorexia nervosa and bulimia. *International Journal of Eating Disorders, 2,* 15–34.

Glasser, W. (1976). *Positive addiction.* New York: Harper & Row.

Goldfried, M. R., & Davidson, G. C. (1976). *Clinical behavior therapy.* New York: Holt, Rinehart & Winston.

Gormally, J., Rardin, D., & Black, S. (1980). Correlates of successful response to a behavioral weight control clinic. *Journal of Counseling Psychology, 27,* 179–191.

Green, L. (1978). Temporal and stimulus factors in self-monitoring by obese persons. *Behavior Therapy, 9,* 328–341.

Greenwood, M. R. C., & Brunzell, J. D. (1982). *A classification of human obesity based on a regulatory model.* Manuscript submitted for publication.

Gwinup, G. (1975). Effect of exercise alone on the weight of obese women. *Archives of Internal Medicine, 135,* 676–680.

Hagen, R. L., Foreyt, J. P., & Durham, T. W. (1976). The dropout problem: Reducing attrition in obesity research. *Behavior Therapy, 7,* 463–471.

Hawkins, R. C., & Clement, P. F. (1980). Development and construct validation of a self-report measure of binge eating tendencies. *Addictive Behavior, 5,* 219–226.

Hawkins, R. C., Fremouw, W. F., & Clement, P. F. (1984). *Binge eating: Theory, research, and treatment.* New York: Springer.

Herman, C. P. (1978). Restrained eating. *Psychiatric Clinics of North America, 1,* 593–607.

Horan, J. J. (1979). *Counseling for effective decision making.* North Scituate, MA: Duxbury Press.

Israel, A. C., & Saccone, A. J. (1979). Follow-up effects of choice of mediator and target of reinforcement on weight loss. *Behavior Therapy, 10,* 260–265.

Katahn, M. (1982). *The 200 calorie solution.* New York: Norton.

Katahn, M., Pleas, J., Thackrey, M., & Wallston, K. A. (1982). Relationship of eating and activity self-reports to follow-up maintenance in the massively obese. *Behavior Therapy, 13,* 521–528.

Katch, F. I., & McArdle, W. D. (1977). *Nutrition weight control and exercise.* Boston: Houghton Mifflin.

Jeffrey, D. B. (1974). A comparison of the effects of external control and self control on the modification and maintenance of weight. *Journal of Abnormal Psychology, 83,* 404–410.

Jeffrey, D. B., & Katz, R. C. (1977). *Take it off and keep it off.* Englewood Cliffs, NJ: Prentice-Hall.

Jeffrey, R. W., Vender, M., & Wing, R. R. (1978). Weight loss and behavior change one year after behavioral treatment for obesity. *Journal of Consulting and Clinical Psychology, 46,* 368–369.

Jeffrey, R. W., & Wing, R. R. (1979). Frequency of therapist contact in the treatment of obesity. *Behavior Therapy, 10,* 186–192.

Johnson, W. G., & Stalonas, P. M. (1981). *Weight no longer.* Gretna, LA: Pelican Publishing Co.

Jordan, H. A., Levitz, L. S., & Kimbrell, G. M. (1976). *Eating is okay!* New York: Rawson, Wade Publishers.

Lansky, D. (1981). A methodological analysis of research on adherence and weight loss: Reply to Brownell and Stunkard. *Behavior Therapy, 12,* 144–149.

Lebow, M. D. (1981). *Weight control. The behavioral strategies.* New York: Wiley.

Leon, G. R., & Chamberlain, K. (1973a). Comparison of daily eating habits and emotional states of overweight persons successful or unsuccessful in maintaining a weight loss.
Journal of Consulting and Clinical Psychology, 41, 108–115.

Leon, G. R., & Chamberlain, K. (1973a). Comparison of daily eating habits and emotional states of overweight persons successful or unsuccessful in maintaining a weight loss. *Journal of Consulting and Clinical Psychology, 41,* 108–115.

Mahoney, K., Rogers, T., Straw, M., & Mahoney, M. J. (1977, December). *Results and implications of a problem-solving treatment for obesity.* Paper presented at the 11th Annual Convention of the Association for Advancement of Behavior Therapy, Atlanta.

Mahoney, M. J. (1974). Self-reward and self-monitoring techniques for weight control. *Behavior Therapy, 5,* 48–57.

Mahoney, M. J., & Mahoney, K. (1976). *Permanent weight loss.* New York: Norton.

Mahoney, M. J., Moura, N. G., & Wade, T. C. (1973). Relative efficacy of self-reward, self-punishment, and self-monitoring techniques for weight loss. *Journal of Consulting and Clinical Psychology, 40,* 404–407.

Marlatt, G. A. (1982). Relapse prevention: A self-control program for the treatment of addictive behaviors. In R. B. Stuart (Ed.), *Adherence, compliance and generalization in behavioral medicine* (pp. 329–378). New York: Brunner/Mazel

Martin, J. E., & Dubbert, P. M. (1982). Exercise applications and promotion in behavioral medicine: Current status and future directions. *Journal of Consulting and Clinical Psychology, 50* 1004–1017.

McReynolds, W. T., Lutz, R. N., Paulsen, B. K., & Kohrs, M. B. (1976). Weight loss resulting from two behavior modification procedures with nutritionists as therapists. *Behavior Therapy, 7,* 283–291.

Metropolitan height and weight tables for men and women. (1983). *Statistical Bulletin, 1,* 2–9.

Musante, G. J. (1976). The dietary rehabilitation clinic: Evaluative report of a behavioral and dietary treatment of obesity. *Behavior Therapy, 7,* 198–204.

Perri, M. G., Shapiro, R. M., Ludwig, W. W., Twentyman, C. T., & McAdoo, W. G. (1984). Maintenance strategies for the treatment of obesity: An evaluation of relapse prevention training and posttreatment contact by mail and telephone. *Journal of Consulting and Clinical Psychology, 52,* 404–413.

Polivy, J., & Herman, C. P. (1983). *Breaking the diet habit.* New York: Basic Books.

Resnick, H, & Balch, P. (1977). The effects of anxiety and response cost manipulation on the eating behavior of obese and normal-weight subjects. *Addictive Behaviors, 2,* 219–255.

Rogers, R., Mahoney, M. J., Mahoney, B. K., Straw, M. K., & Kenigsberg, M. I. (1980). Clinical assessment of obesity: An empirical evaluation of diverse techniques. *Behavioral Assessment, 2,* 161–181.

Romanczyk, R. G. (1974). Self-monitoring in the treatment of obesity: Parameters of reactivity. *Behavior Therapy, 5,* 531–540.

Romanczyk, R. G., Tracey, D. A., Wilson, G. T., & Thorpe, G. L. (1973). Behavioral techniques in the treatment of obesity: A comparative analysis. *Behavior Research and Therapy, 11,* 629–640.

Rosenthal, B., Allen, G. J., & Winter, C. (1980). Husband involvement in the behavioral treatment of overweight women: Initial effects and long term follow-up. *International Journal of Obesity, 4,* 165–173.

Rozensky, R. H., & Bellack, A. S. (1976). Individual differences in self-reinforcement style and performance in self- and therapist-controlled weight reduction programs. *Behavior Therapy, 14,* 357–364.

Schachter, S. (1982, August). Don't sell habit-breakers short. *Psychology Today*, 27–33.

Sclafani, A. (1980). Dietary obesity. In A. J. Stunkard (Ed.), *Obesity* (pp. 166–181). Philadelphia: Saunders.

Sclafani, A., & Springer, D. (1976). Dietary obesity in adult rats: Similarities to hypothalamic and human obesity syndromes. *Physiology and Behavior, 17,* 461–471.

Sjoberg, L., & Person, L. (1979). A study of attempts by obese patients to regulate eating. *Addictive Behaviors, 4,* 349–359.

Sjostrom, L. (1980). Fat cells and body weight. In A. J. Stunkard (Ed.), *Obesity* (pp. 72–100). Philadelphia: Saunders.

Stalonas, P. M., Johnson, W. G., & Christ, M. (1978). Behavior modification for obesity: The evaluation of exercise, contingency management, and program adherence. *Journal of Consulting and Clinical Psychology, 46,* 463–469.

Sternberg, B. (1985). Relapse in weight control: Definitions, processes, and prevention strategies. In G. A. Marlatt & J. R. Gordon (Eds.), *Relapse prevention: Maintenance strategies in the treatment of addictive behaviors* (pp. 521–545). New York: Guilford Press.

Straw, M. K., Straw, R. B., Mahoney, M. J., Rogers, T., Mahoney, B. K., Craighead, L. W., & Stunkard A. J. (1984). The Master Questionnaire: Preliminary reports of an obesity assessment device. *Addictive Behavior, 9,* 1–100.

Stuart, R. B. (1977). *Act thin, stay thin.* New York: Norton.

Stuart, R. B., & Davis, B. (1972). *Slim chance in a fat world.* Champaign, IL: Research Press Company.

Stuart, R. B., & Guire, K. (1978). Some correlates of the maintenance of weight loss through behavior modification. *International Journal of Obesity, 2,* 225–235.

Stunkard, A. J. (1975). From explanation to action in psychosomatic medicine: The care of obesity. *Psychosomatic Medicine, 37,* 195–236.

Stunkard, A. J. (1981). Restrained eating: What it is and a new scale to measure it. In L.A. Cioffi, W. P. T. Jones, & L. T. Van Kellie (Eds.), *The body weight regulatory system: Normal and disturbed mechanisms* (pp. 243–251). New York: Raven Press.

Stunkard, A. J. (1983). The current status of treatment for obesity in adults. *Psychiatric Annals, 13,* 862–867.

Stunkard, A. J., & Brownell, K. D. (1979). Behavior therapy and self-help programs for obesity. In J. F. Munno (Ed.), *Treatment of obesity* (pp. 199–230). Lancaster, England: MTP Press.

Stunkard, A. J., & Rush, J. (1974). Dieting and depression reexamined. *Annals of Internal Medicine, 81,* 526–533.

Wadden, T. A. & Stunkard, A. J. (1984, November). A controlled trial of the effectiveness of very low calorie diet and behavior modification in the treatment of moderate obesity. Paper presented at the meeting of the Association for the Advancement of Behavior Therapy, Philadelphia.

Wadden, T. A., Stunkard, A. J., & Brownell, K. D. (1983). Very low calorie diets: Their efficacy, safety and future. *Annals of Internal Medicine, 5,* 675–684.

Wadden, T. A., Stunkard, A. J., Brownell, K. D., & Day, S. C. (1984). Treatment of obesity by behavior therapy and very-low-calorie diet: A pilot investigation. *Journal of Consulting and Clinical Psychology, 52,* 692–694.

Wilson, G. T., & Brownell, K. D. (1980). Behavior therapy for obesity: An evaluation of treatment outcome. *Advances in Behavior Research and Therapy, 3,* 49–86.

Wing, R. R., & Epstein, L. H. (1981). Prescribed level of caloric restriction in behavioral weight loss programs. *Addictive Behaviors, 6,* 139–144.

Wing, R. R., & Jeffrey, R. W. (1979). Outpatient treatments of obesity: A comparison of methodology and clinical results. *International Journal of Obesity, 3,* 261–279.

Wing, R. R., Epstein, L. H., & Shapiro, B. (1982). The effect of increasing initial weight loss with the Scarsdale diet on subsequent weight loss in a behavioral treatment program. *Journal of Consulting and Clinical Psychology, 50,* 446–447.

Wooley, S. C., Wooley, O. W., & Dyrenforth, S. R. (1979). Theoretical, practical, and social issues in behavioral treatments of obesity. *Journal of Applied Behavior Analysis, 12,* 3–25.

Anorexia Nervosa

Francis C. Harris and Carolyn F. Phelps

Introduction

Over the past 20 years, an increasing interest in eating disorders such as anorexia nervosa and bulimia can be evidenced by examining the proliferation of professional publications on these topics, the formulation of special interest groups, and the creation of journals devoted exclusively to eating disorders. Since Richard Morton (1694) first described anorexia nervosa, the literature has become rich with clinical descriptions of a variety of therapeutic modalities employed in the treatment of eating disorders. Although most of these treatments appear to be adequate in short-term restoration of weight and normal eating behavior, reports of long-term maintenance and generalization of treatment effects seldom appear in the literature (Bemis, 1978; Garfinkel & Garner, 1982; Schwartz & Thompson, 1981).

The *Diagnostic and Statistical Manual of Mental Disorders* (DSM-III) outlines the cardinal features of anorexia as (a) loss of 25% of original body weight (adjusted for growth if under the age of 18); (b) distorted body image; (c) intense fear of becoming obese; (d) refusal to maintain normal body weight; (e) no known physical illness that would account for the weight loss (American Psychiatric Association, 1980). In addition, research diagnostic criteria (RDC) indicate that onset of the disorder must occur prior to 25 years of age and patients must exhibit a loss of appetite (Feighner, Robins, Guze, Woodruff, Winokur, & Munoz, 1972). However, many have noted the onset of primary anorexia nervosa to occur in patients over 15 years old, and the presence of true "anorexia" either occurs late in the course of the disorder or is completely absent (Garfinkel, 1974; Hsu, 1983). Hence, these

FRANCIS C. HARRIS • Western Psychiatric Institute and Clinic, University of Pittsburgh School of Medicine, Pittsburgh, Pennsylvania 15213.   CAROLYN F. PHELPS • Department of Psychology, University of Pittsburgh, Pittsburgh, Pennsylvania 15260.

criteria may be too strict by excluding many individuals who have the essential features of the disorder. Rollins and Piazza (1978) underscored this when they reported only 23% of their clinically diagnosed anorexic patients would meet the criteria Feighner proposed (Feighner *et al.*, 1972).

Anorexia occurs predominately in females (85 to 95%) and during adolescence or young adulthood (American Psychiatric Association, 1980; Bemis, 1978). Although precise statistics regarding the incidence of anorexia are not available due to inconsistent diagnostic criteria and inadequate records, there are data suggesting that the prevalence of the disorder is increasing (Duddle, 1973; Jones, Fox, Babign, & Hutton, 1980). Particularly, investigators have noted a sharp rise in the number of cases reported in the last 10 years of study. For example, Jones *et al.* (1980) discovered that the number of diagnosed cases of anorexia nervosa increased from .35/100,000 in 1960–1969 to .64/100,000 in 1970–1976. Unfortunately, it is not clear how much of this increase is simply due to an increase in professional and public knowledge of the disorder. Although methodologically adequate investigations regarding the prevalence of anorexia are lacking, other estimates suggest 1 in every 250 females develops the disorder, with girls 12 to 18 years of age at particular risk (American Psychiatric Association, 1980; Crisp, Palmer, & Kalucy, 1976). Previous reports have enumerated the psychological and physical correlates of the disorder (Bemis, 1978; Bruch, 1973; Crisp, Hsu, Harding, & Hartshorn, 1980; Morgan & Russell, 1975). A cluster of psychological and social characteristics that typify the anorexic are (a) intense fear of eating in the presence of others; (b) idiosyncratic and monotonous diets (particularly prevalent is the avoidance of carbohydrates and fats); (c) preoccupation with food; (d) binging; (e) vomiting; (f) laxative abuse; (g) hyperactivity; (h) stealing; and (i) lying. So much time is devoted to engaging in anorectic behavior that positive interpersonal interactions begin decreasing until relationships have virtually deteriorated. Social interactions appear to become aversive and often consist of battles over food and weight-related issues. Thus, the anorexic's environment appears to contain problematic situations consisting of stressful interpersonal interactions. It is not surprising, then, that she exhibits poor social adjustment and has been characterized as withdrawn, isolated, introverted, stubborn, selfish, and perfectionistic. Clinically, the anorexic often is highly manipulative and incessantly denies the existence of eating problems (Bemis, 1978; Garfinkel & Garner, 1982).

Seven prospective and retrospective studies utilizing self-report and archival data have described anorexia nervosa as a heterogeneous disorder (Beumont, 1977; Beumont, George, & Smart, 1976; Casper, Eckert, Halmi, Goldberg, & Davis, 1980: Crisp, Hsu, Harding, & Hartshorn, 1980; Garfinkel & Garner, 1982; Janet, 1919; Russell, 1979). Subtypes of obsessional and hysterical forms of anorexia were originally described by Janet (1929). More recent attempts to identify subtypes of anorexia have focused on the consummatory patterns of the individual, dividing anorexia into (a) "restricters" or "abstainers"—those who control weight by rigorous caloric restriction; and (b) "bulimics"—those whose weight loss is a function of vomiting and/or laxative and diuretic abuse. It is estimated that 40% of anorexic patients also meet the diagnostic criteria for bulimia (Crisp *et al.*, 1980; Garfinkel & Garner, 1982). These studies reveal a subgroup of bulimic-anorexics who differ significantly from restricter anorexics on clinical and psycho-social variables as well as weight loss methods. All of the investigations concluded that "bulimic-anorexics" were more psychologically disturbed than their "restrict-ing" counterparts. Specifically, bulimic-anorexics were reported to exhibit (a) increased levels of depressive features such as decreased ability to concentrate, recurrent suicidal ideation, subjective feelings of gloom, and marked irritability that resulted in impaired social relationships (Casper et al., 1980; Crisp et al., 1980; Russell, 1979); (b) increased impulsivity as exhibited by a higher rate of heavy drinking, stealing, mood lability, and suicidal ideation (Casper et al., 1980; Crisp et al., 1980; Garfinkel & Garner, 1982); (c) increased levels of anxiety (Casper et al., 1980; Crisp et al., 1980); (d) increased levels of sexual activity (Beumont, 1977; Beumont et al., 1976; Casper et al., 1980; Crisp et al., 1980; Garfinkel & Garner, 1982; Russell, 1979); and (e) higher rates of histrionic behavior (Beumont, 1977; Beumont et al., 1976). However, it is unclear whether or not these psychological correlates predate the anorexia.

Although bulimic-anorexics were found to be more sociable than restricting anorexics (Casper et al., 1980; Crisp et al., 1980; Garfinkel & Garner, 1982), much greater sociability appears to be an artifact of their ability to form new relation-ships. That is, although bulimic-anorexics were able to initiate social contacts more frequently than restricting anorexics, they reported being dissatisfied with their relationships, including bulimic-anorexics, who are unable to maintain positive social interactions over sustained periods of time.

It is clear, then, that bulimic patients with anorexia can be differentiated from abstaining anorexics (Garfinkel & Garner, 1982; Garner & Garfinkel 1980; Russell, 1979). Palmer (1979) coined the phrase *dietary chaos syndrome* to describe bulimic behavior that may or may not be accompanied by anorexia nervosa. He describes the essential features of this pattern as:

1. Preoccupation with eating food and weight that often overrides other thoughts
2. An aberrant eating pattern that includes abstinence, binging, vomiting, and/or purging via laxatives or diuretics
3. Rapid fluctuations in body weight occurring as a result of abrupt intake and output

Representing a combination of Russell's (1979) and Palmer's (1979) diagnostic cri-teria, DSM-III defines bulimia as (a) recurrent episodes of binge eating that result in fasting, vomiting, or purging to negate the effects of caloric intake; (b) awareness that the eating pattern is abnormal, accompanied with feelings of loss of control; and (c) depressed mood and self-deprecating thoughts following a binge (American Psychiatric Association, 1980).

Two recent epidemiological studies have documented the existence of bulimia as a distinct disorder. Halmi, Falk, and Schwartz (1981) surveyed 355 college stu-dents by assessing weight over the past year, history of lowest and highest weight, use of diet aids and medication, behavioral aspects of bulimia according to DSM-III criteria, and a number of demographic variables. Results indicated that 13% (n = 46) fulfilled DSM-III criteria for bulimia. Importantly, no significant relationships were found between bulimic behavior and a history of abnormally low weight. Fairburn and Cooper (1982) assessed the degree of bulimia nervosa in a sample ($n = 669$) of women who admitted to using self-induced vomiting as a weight control mechanism. Those who had stopped engaging in bulimic behavior prior to completing the questionnaire ($n = 49$) and those who fulfilled diagnostic criteria for anorexia ($n = 19$ or 3.1%) were excluded from the analyses. Four hundred and forty-nine of the remaining 601 respondents fulfilled diagnostic criteria for bulimia. Of those, it is most remarkable that less than half had ever been of low enough body weight to be diagnosed with primary anorexia. Unfortunately, precise statistics regarding the prevalence of anorexia in this sample were not available. However, there remained a large number of individuals who were bulimic but never had been anorexic, lending further empirical support to the existence of bulimia as a separate entity.

Treatment

Based primarily on the theoretical perspective of the clinician and the presumed etiology of the disorder, many interventions for anorexia and bulimia have been proposed. These interventions may be classified as either biological, family systems, psychodynamic, or behavioral approaches to the conceptualization and treatment of eating-disordered patients.

Biological Approaches

A variety of drug therapies have been utilized in the treatment of anorexia nervosa. The use of psychoactive medication has involved three generic categories of pharmacological agents: phenothiazines, tricyclic antidepressants, and serotonin antagonists. Each of these is used to treat a specific feature of the disorder (Johanson & Knorr, 1977).

On the assumption that the sedating effects of a major tranquilizer would (a) decrease the patient's anxiety; and (b) increase the patient's compliance to a prescribed lowered activity level, phenothiazines have been advocated as an intervention for anorexia nervosa (Garfinkel & Garner, 1982). Three investigations have reported that chlorpromazine is effective in restoring weight in anorexic patients (Crisp, 1965; Dally & Sargant, 1960, 1966). However, severe side effects stemming from the use of phenothiazines with anorexics may further endanger the patient's health (Dally & Sargant, 1966, 1969; Garfinkel & Garner, 1982).

Due to their appetite-stimulating effect and the belief held by some that anorexia nervosa is a variant of affective disorder (Cantwell, Sturzenberger, Burroughs, Salkin, & Green, 1977), medications used in the treatment of affective disorders have been employed in the treatment of anorexia nervosa. Seven studies have examined the effectiveness of tricyclic antidepressants as a primary intervention for anorexia (Katz & Walsh, 1978; Kendler, 1978; Mills, 1976; Moore, 1977; Needleman & Waber, 1976, 1977; White & Schnaultz, 1977).

Six investigations described a total of nine anorexic patients whose weight increased following the administration of amitriptyline (Katz & Walsh, 1978; Kendler, 1978; Moore, 1977; Needleman & Waber, 1976, 1977; White & Schnaultz, 1977). Although there was no systematic evaluation of the medication, all of the investigators attributed the weight gains to the drug. Furthermore, Needleman and Waber (1976, 1977) contend that their data are supportive of tricyclic antidepressants as an effective treatment for anorexia nervosa. However, methodological problems in the extant literature cast doubt on the validity of these conclusions. Mills (1976) reports that Needleman and Waber (1976, 1977) have overstated the effectiveness of amitriptyline and notes that success with this drug is highly variable. Additionally, two of the studies (Katz & Walsh, 1978; White & Schnaultz, 1977) reported that increased weight was coupled with hypomania in the former case and obesity in the latter. These results can hardly be deemed favorable. More serious are the cardiotoxic properties with which tricyclic antidepressants have been credited. These side effects would strongly contraindicate the use of tricyclic medication in many cases (Mitchell & Gillum, 1980).

Results from investigations evaluating the effectiveness of lithium carbonate in the treatment of anorexia nervosa also are equivocal (Barcai, 1977; Hsu, Crisp, & Harding, 1979). Moreover, the use of lithium salts with anorexics may be contraindicated because these patients would be at significant risk for lithium poisoning due to their chaotic dietary patterns (Barcia, 1977; Garfinkel & Garner, 1982).

Cyproheptadine, a serotonin antagonist and appetite-stimulating medication, also has been employed in an effort to increase the caloric intake of anorexic patients. Two well-designed investigations of cyproheptadine report conflicting results, suggesting further research is needed prior to judging its utility as an effective treatment for anorexia nervosa (Goldberg, Halmi, Eckert, Casper, & Davis, 1979; Vigersky & Loriaux, 1977). There appear to be numerous methodological problems with studies evaluating the effectiveness of various drugs in the treatment of anorexia nervosa. Examples of problems in the extant literature are (a) failure to include double-blind procedures; (b) inadequate follow-up periods; and (c) outcome criteria that are based solely on weight. In addition, it appears that psychoactive medication may not adequately address all aspects of anorexia nervosa. Moore (1977) suggested that effectiveness of drugs in the treatment of anorexia nervosa was restricted to the instigation of food consumption and that other features of the disorder (e.g., weight phobia) must be remedied by psychotherapy. Additionally, Garfinkel and Garner (1982) emphasized that regardless of a drug's ability to increase weight, it does little to alter maladaptive cognitions. Thus, it appears that pharmacological interventions may do little to increase the anorexic's ability to respond effectively in a variety of problematic situations.

Family Systems Approach

Because the onset of anorexia nervosa usually occurs during adolescence when the patient is living at home, the role of the family both as an etiological factor and a target for intervention has often been examined. Although Crisp and his colleagues (Crisp, Harding, & McGuinness, 1974) stated family psychopathology was nonspecific, both the Minuchin group (Minuchin, Rosman, & Baker, 1978) and Palazzoli (1978) have expanded the role of family psychopathology in anorexic patients by adopting a model that emphasizes the interdependence and circularity of each component of the system (i.e., individuals within a family). According to this model, the behavior of one is simultaneously caused and causative (Minuchin *et al.*, 1978).

It is from the systems formulation that Minuchin contends anorexia nervosa is an interpersonal problem that is best treated by restructuring the dysfunctional family (Minuchin *et al.*, 1978). Diagnosis and intervention with anorexic patients and their families is carried out during the "family therapy lunch session." This method of assessment gives the therapist direct observational data, allowing the formulation of specific treatment strategies designed to correct faulty communication patterns occurring in the dysfunctional system.

Unfortunately, no controlled investigations of the effectivenss of the lunch session itself or structural family therapy in general have been conducted. However, anecdotal accounts suggest family therapy may be a useful and appropriate intervention for treating some (e.g., early to middle adolescence) patients. One limitation of family therapy is that it continues to involve an already enmeshed family in the patient's problem. In contrast, individual therapy may serve as a model of separation/individuation for both the patient and her family.

Behavior Therapy

Many investigators have described the implementation of behavior therapy in the treatment of anorexia nervosa. Although operant conditioning procedures have been employed most frequently, other behavioral interventions have included systematic desensitization, social skills training, and a variety of cognitive-behavioral strategies. Each of these procedures has focused on a particular factor, such as weight loss, weight phobia, poor social interactions, or maladaptive cognitions.

Operant conditioning procedures have been aimed at rapid weight restoration by manipulating the patient's environment. With one exception (McGlynn, 1980), all of these investigations describe the treatment of hospitalized patients where the environment can be controlled easily. In seven studies, positive reinforcement, either social or material, was contingent upon appropriate eating behavior (Azzerad & Stafford, 1969; Bachrach, Erwin, & Mohr, 1965; Bhanji & Thomson, 1974; Fichter & Kessler, 1980; Kehrer, 1975; Neumann & Gaoni, 1975, Stumphauzer, 1969). In contrast, 25 investigations, implementing operant conditioning techniques, utilized weight gain as the criterion for positive reinforcement (Agras & Werne, 1977; Agras & Werne, 1978; Bianco 1972; Blinder, Freeman, & Stunkard, 1980; Blue, 1979; Brady & Rieger, 1972; Eckert, Goldberg, Halmi, Casper, & Davis, 1979; Elkin, Hersen, Eisler, & Williams, 1973; Garfinkel, Kline, & Stancer, 1973; Garfinkel, Moldofsky, & Garner, 1977; Geller, 1975; Halmi, Powers, & Cunningham, 1975; Hauserman & Lavin, 1977; Leitenberg, Agras, & Thomson, 1968; Lobb & Schaefer, 1972; McGlynn, 1980; Parker, Blazer, & Wyrick, 1977; Pertschuk, 1977; Pertschuk, Edwards, & Pomerleau, 1978; Poole & Sanson, 1978; Rosen, 1980; Rosman, Minuchin, Liebman, & Baker, 1976; Vandereyeken & Pieters, 1978; Werry & Bull, 1975; Wulliemier, 1978). Twelve of the 33 investigations examining the efficacy of operant conditioning procedures in the treatment of anorexia were single-subject studies, whereas 21 were multiple-subject investigations that with two exceptions (Eckert *et al.*, 1979; Wulliemier, 1978) employed single-subject methodology.

Methodological problems were common in these studies and include inadequate diagnostic criteria, inadequate experimental designs, inadequate follow-up methods in terms of variables assessed, method of assessment, and duration of follow-up periods. Only 5 investigations employed the appropriate control procedures such that treatment outcome genuinely appeared to be the result of the application of an operant conditioning program (Eckert *et al.*, 1979; Garfinkel *et al.*, 1977; Pertschuk, 1977; Vandereyeken & Pieters, 1978; Wulliemier, 1978).

Despite the methodological problems, all of the investigations reported *short-term* improvements in weight that were achieved quickly. Unfortunately, psychosocial competence was assessed in only 13 studies (Agras & Werne, 1978; Blinder *et al.*, 1970; Blue, 1979; Brady & Rieger, 1972; Fichter & Kessler, 1980; Garfinkel *et al.*, 1977; Geller, 1975; Halmi *et al.*, 1975; Kehrer, 1977; Neumann & Gaoni, 1975; Pertschuk, 1977; Rosman *et al.*, 1976). These assessments consisted of clinician's global ratings (i.e., poor, fair, good) based on information that was often obtained (a) by telephone and (b) from someone other than the patient. Thus, in the 14 studies assessing psychosocial competence, competence never was defined adequately. Moreover, 9 of these investigations reported no improvements in, or a deterioration (e.g., suicide) of, psychosocial functioning (Agras & Werne, 1978; Blinder *et al.*, 1970; Brady & Rieger, 1972; Fichter & Kessler, 1980; Garfinkel *et al.*, 1977; Halmi *et al.*, 1975; Pertschuk, 1977; Rosman, Minuchin, Baker, & Liebman, 1976).

Thus, it appears that positive reinforcement for appropriate eating behavior or weight gain yields rapid weight restoration in the treatment of hospitalized anorexic patients. However, the use of operant conditioning procedures in the treatment of anorexia nervosa has two major limitations. First, an increase in weight is less likely to occur when the patient's environment cannot be controlled easily. Thus, similar results may be difficult to achieve when treating anorexics in an outpatient setting. Furthermore, weight gain achieved during hospitalization may be difficult to maintain once the anorexic is discharged from the hospital because the variables controlling the behavior may not be present in the natural environment. Second, operant conditioning procedures do not address related issues such as interpersonal competence, problem-solving skill, maladaptive cognitions, or other factors that might exacerbate eating problems.

As a result of these limitations, several investigators (Bianco, 1972; Blinder *et al.*, 1970; Garfinkel *et al.*, 1977; Geller, 1977; Hauserman & Lavin, 1977) emphasized that weight restoration should be viewed as the *initial* phase of treatment for anorexic patients. Therefore, it is reasonable to assume that a more broadly based application of behavior therapy in which interventions were aimed at decreasing the patient's fear of maintaining a normal body weight, restructuring maladaptive cognitions, and increasing problem-solving skills would result in a more long-term, successful outcome both in terms of weight and psychosocial functioning.

Focusing on the weight phobia found in anorexic patients, four studies have examined the effectiveness of *systematic desensitization* in the treatment of anorexia nervosa (Hallsten, 1965; Lang, 1965; Ollendick, 1979; Schnurer, Rubin, & Roy, 1973). The rationale for this behavioral intervention is twofold. First, dieting behavior is viewed as a learned anxiety reduction response that has continued to be used by the patient, long after it has ceased to be effective. Second, weight phobia is seen as the primary maintaining factor in anorexia nervosa (Schnurer *et al.*, 1973). As with other behavioral interventions, systematic desensitization has been effective in promoting short-term improvements in weight (Hallsten, 1965; Lang, 1965; Ollendick, 1979; Schnurer *et al.*, 1973). Ollendick's (1979) combination of cognitive restructuring and systematic desensitization produced results indicating that cognitive restructuring may be more effective than systematic desensitization alone in producing long-term maintenance of weight gain. Unfortunately, none of the investigations provided data on psychosocial adjustment either pretreatment, posttreatment, or in follow-up reports. The primary limitation of systematic desensitization is that it only addresses one feature of the disorder. That is, systematic desensitization is sufficient in decreasing anxiety related to weight gain. However, it does not provide alternative coping strategies in many situations that result in subjective feelings of anxiety and elicit a food-refusal response.

Clinical Assessment

Kanfer and Saslow (1969) provided an excellent outline of topics that should be covered in a comprehensive behavioral assessment of any clinical problem. Our basic assessment plan is based on their outline with other areas evaluated and certain areas emphasized rather heavily based on our clinical experiences and relevant research. The specific questions to be answered during the assessment have been described elsewhere (Harris, Hsu, & Phelps, 1983; Kanfer & Saslow 1969).

Following is an abbreviated summary of the areas typically assessed:

I. Presenting problem
   A. Frequency, duration, intensity, and antecedents of urges to restrict intake or binge and purge, including specific stressors and moods
   B. Specific features of food consumption, including the type and quantity of food consumed, and temporal, ecological antecedents of consumption during binge *and* nonbinge consumption
   C. Pattern, frequency, and methods of purging
   D. Knowledge of basic nutrition information
   E. Current weight and history of the patient's actual or attempted weight changes
   F. Specific fears associated with weight gain.
II. Biological functioning including metabolic status, renal and thyroid functioning, and menstrual cycle

Assessment Methods

An interview focusing on the areas described previously is the typical starting point for the assessment process. After the first interview, the patient is asked to begin a diary in which she records her actual consumption and purging behaviors as well as their antecedents. The Eating Attitudes Test (Garner & Garfinkel 1979) and Beck Depression Inventory (Beck, Ward, Mendelson, Mock, & Erbaugh, 1961) also are administered to each patient.

More specialized assessments of particular areas of functioning that are related to the eating disorder often are undertaken based upon information obtained during the interview. These areas might include anxiety problems, depression, anger control, jealousy, social skills deficits, marital dysfunction, or alcohol abuse. Comprehensive behavioral assessment plans for each of these areas have been described elsewhere in great detail (Barlow, 1981; Ciminero, Calhoun, & Adams, 1977).

Case Study

Background Information

Laura is a 22-year-old, white, single, female who was voluntarily admitted to the Adolescent and Young Adult Module at Western Psychiatric Institute and Clinic (WPIC) with a primary diagnosis of anorexia nervosa. Prior to entering the hospital she had been working as a field representative for a sales organization.

Presenting Problem

Upon presentation, Laura weighed 72 pounds and stood 60 inches tall. During the initial evaluation, Laura stated that she was seeking treatment "because the anorexia is interfering with my social life." She reported being terrified of becoming fat and feeling bloated despite her low body weight. In addition to caloric restriction, she reported engaging in excessive exercising (400 sit-ups per day) and one to six instances of binging and vomiting daily for the previous several months. Additionally, she noted that onset of amenorrhea occurred 4 years prior to admission when her weight fell below 95 pounds. She denied any use of laxatives, diuretics, or diet pills.

Upon admission the patient's affect was controlled but appropriate, and she denied any suicidal thoughts. No psychotic features were present. Laura also denied any alcohol or drug use. She described three previous unsuccessful attempts to seek treatment for anorexia nervosa that included individual psychotherapy, family therapy, and religious counseling. No history of psychopathology in other family members was noted either by the patient or her parents.

History of the Problem

Laura reports having begun dieting at the age of 17 when her boyfriend challenged her to lose weight. She described herself as "a bit chunky then" (125 pounds, 5 feet). She achieved her target weight of 105 pounds through caloric restriction, by eliminating "junk food" and carbohydrates from her diet, and by exercising. Her weight remained stable for 1 year.

The second significant weight loss occurred when Laura was approximately 18, 1 year later. At this time she had traveled abroad to study for 3 months. This was to be the patient's first extended period of time away from home. However, she returned home 2 weeks after her departure complaining of "homesickness." She was extremely embarrassed by this failure. Shortly after her return, she began to experience problems with her boyfriend who expressed an interest in dating other people. Laura was "very depressed" and "unable to eat" during this time such that a 10- to 15-pound weight loss ensued. Subsequent to this weight loss, many people commented on "how skinny I was" and "that made me feel better." Her weight remained stable at 90 to 95 pounds for the next 3.5 years.

The onset of amenorrhea and binge vomiting occurred during that 3.5-year period. She had learned of binge-vomiting through a magazine article and described it as "the perfect solution" because it enabled her to eat without gaining weight. Her first vomiting episode occurred after overeating in a restaurant. She reported having felt "terribly guilty for wasting the food" afterward. For the next 6 months, episodes were infrequent, occurring approximately once per month.

Laura reported that her episodes increased to once a week after beginning college. She would binge alone at home on ice cream and "other junk food." The patient stated that her distress increased as she continued to binge and vomit. In an attempt to alleviate her discomfort, she confided in some friends "about this terrible thing I was doing." Although she reports they were supportive, her weekly episodes did not decrease.

The third significant weight loss began 6 months after she was transferred to a city approximately 100 miles from her home and 8 months prior to hospitalization. Although she reported performing well in her job, Laura stated that she was overwhelmed by the amount of responsibility it entailed. She began leaving work early to go home to binge. At that time the frequency of her binge episodes increased to 4 days per week. On "binge days," she stated that she binged twice a day. Binges consisted of ½ gallon of ice cream and a bag of approximately 40 to 50 cookies. Laura also reported ritualizing her binges "to make them perfect." Prior to the binge, she would carefully break up the cookies into crumbs. She stated this would take approximately 45 minutes, during which time she was careful not to eat anything. It was also during this time that the patient began to feel as if the binging "was controlling my life," noting that as her binging increased, she became more socially isolated. Six months prior to her admission to the WPIC, she began dieting more rigorously, decreasing her weight by 20 pounds to 72 pounds. Three months prior to admission, Laura's request for a transfer back to her hometown was granted, and she moved in with her family. She reported eating 500 to 600 calories on nonbinge days (approximately two per week). She continued her pattern of binging and vomiting twice daily on "binge days."

Family and Social History

Laura is the oldest of three children who was raised in an intact family. She is followed by two brothers who are 4 and 11 years younger than she. Laura's parents described her as a perfectionistic, independent child who got along well with her siblings and who had many friends. They reported no prenatal problems or developmental delays. Additionally, both parents noted that she "became an adult when she was still a child." This is highlighted by the fact that at 11 years of age she assumed all household and child-care responsibilities of her siblings when her mother began working.

Socially, Laura reports having had many male and female friends while growing up. She reported that she began casual dating in high school and described having had one significant, long-term (3 years) relationship that ended during her junior year in college. She noted a marked decrease in the frequency of her social contacts 6 months prior to hospitalization. This coincided with the onset of her third significant weight loss.

Academic Performance and Intellectual Functioning

Academically, Laura has performed well throughout grade school and high school, graduating from high school early. Following high school, she attended a small liberal arts college where she also graduated early with a bachelor's degree in fine arts. At that time, Laura entered a sales management training program.

Neuropsychological Assessment

Performance on all tests of neuropsychological functioning, including attention, memory, visuoconstructive skills, visual-perceptual skills, language, and motor skills revealed no deficits. No evidence of neuropsychological deficits either as a function of current psychological problems or a central nervous system (CNS) dysfunction secondary to the weight loss were present.

Medical Evaluation

A medical evaluation showed normal awake EEG pattern and normal thyroid functioning. Physiological correlates of anorexia nervosa secondary to the weight loss were bradycardia and amenorrhea.

Additional Assessment Information

The Eating Attitudes Test (EAT) also was administered. The EAT is a 40-item, forced choice, self-report questionnaire that quantifies features commonly associated with anorexia nervosa. A higher score is indicative of a more severe eating disturbance, with a score above 30 in the "anorexic range." Upon admission, Laura's total EAT score was 48.

Treatment Plan

The assessment information suggested several areas to be addressed in a broad spectrum behavior therapy framework. These areas were

1. Laura's unstable and chaotic eating patterns
2. Her low body weight
3. Laura's difficulty in becoming independent from her parents
4. Her binging and vomiting in response to stressful situations
5. Laura's diminished peer social contacts and social support

Laura's low weight and problematic eating patterns were designated to be treated in the context of an operant/response prevention program, whereas the independence and social contacts were addressed in a rational restructuring (D'Zurilla & Goldfried, 1971) process. These programs are described next in detail.

Course of Inpatient Treatment

Laura was hospitalized for 9 weeks. In addition to the treatment program described next, she participated in twice-weekly psychotherapy process groups, a unitwide token economy program, and weekly family sessions that included her mother and father.

Her individual inpatient treatment consisted of dietary advice, an operant program to restore normal weight and eating patterns as safely and rapidly as possible, and cognitive-behavioral problem-solving training. She met with her primary therapist 3 to 5 times per week for approximately 30 minutes each session.

Dietary Advice

During the first week of the hospitalization a registered dietician met with Laura to review and discuss basic nutrition information. In addition, she was taught to use a calorie exchange system (Stuart & Davis, 1972) to record her intake. She also used this exchange system to order meals from the hospital cafeteria. Throughout the hospitalization she met with the dietician to compare intake and weight gain. During the 2 weeks after the target weight was reached, these meetings concentrated on selecting the general calorie level required for her to maintain the target weight.

Laura participated in the general milieu treatment of the Adolescent Unit, which is a Token Economy Program (Privilege Level Economy) in which patients earn points for meeting various expectations, lose points for violating unit rules, and spend points to gain access to various privileges. Laura also participated in an individual operant/response prevention program that focused on weight and eating related factors.

The goals of the program were to

1. Increase Laura's weight from 72 pounds to 105 pounds
2. Establish a throughout-the-day eating pattern
3. Prevent her from vomiting after eating
4. Enable Laura to assume "self-control" of the program after discharge

Until her target weight (105 lb) was reached the program included the following:

1. Laura was weighed daily before breakfast.
2. She received 3,000 calories daily divided into four "meals" and two snacks. She selected items from a prepared checklist 1 day in advance.
3. She was observed constantly by a staff member during each meal and snack and for the 45-minute period thereafter.
4. She earned token economy points for eating meals.
5. She lost points for concealing food, leaving the table without permission, or having "nonhospital food."
6. She had access to all unit privileges such as the telephone, game room, TV room, and visitors on days when her weight was at least 0.50 lb greater than her previous highest weight during the hospitalization.
7. An increase of 0.25 lb entitled her to privileges for 8 hours during the day.
8. A gain of less than 0.25 lb, remaining the same, or a weight loss resulted in no access to privileges for the day.
9. Laura graphed her weight daily.

After the target weight was reached, the following generalization and maintenance program was implemented:

1. Laura weighed herself daily with random, frequent "reliability checks" made by a member of the nursing staff.
2. She planned her meals a day in advance, ate them in the hospital cafeteria, and selected her own food.
3. She recorded and graphed her daily calorie consumption and adjusted her intake to maintain a weight of 105 to 110 lb.
4. She was not observed constantly while eating. She was asked on a daily basis whether she experienced urges to binge and vomit.
5. She was permitted to participate in a 1-hour daily exercise group activity.

Problem Solving/Self-Instruction Training

This component of the treatment proceeded in three consecutive phases. The purpose of the first phase was to provide Laura with a set of self-statements to use when she experienced urges to restrict her scheduled intake, binge, or vomit. The self-statements were structured according to the problem-solving model as presented by D'Zurilla and Goldfried (1971). Specifically, Laura was trained to go through the following steps cognitively whenever she experienced an urge to binge or eat less than the planned amount.

1. Identify the Problem Situation and Likely Antecedents
   "It is 7:00 P.M., and I feel like binging and vomiting, and it probably is a function of being home alone; not having eaten breakfast or supper; and my actual weight being 10 lb less than my target weight."
2. List Possible Alternative
   a. "Binge and vomit as I feel like doing."
   b. "Go alone to a restaurant and order a meal."
   c. "Stay at home and try to resist the urges as best as I can."
   d. "Call a friend."
3. Evaluate the Likely Short-Term and Long-Term Consequence of Each Alternative in Terms of Short- and Long-Term Goals
   a. "If I binge and vomit, I'll occupy myself for a while, while I enjoy the food, but I know I will feel guilty later. I might get a stomachache, and it certainly won't help me get over my eating problems in the long run."
   b. "If I go alone to a restaurant, I will be able to avoid vomiting if I can manage to stay out of my house for at least an hour, but this has never worked in the past, and I've ended up eating a big meal, hurrying home and vomiting."
   c. "If I stay at home alone I know I will binge, vomit, and go to bed."
   d. "If I call a friend to talk, she might not be home, and then I would have to call someone else who I don't really want to talk with, but this has been my most effective strategy in the past."
4. Select a Course of Action
   "All things considered, calling a friend probably would be the best course of action right now. It probably would be even more effective in the future if I would eat my meals on schedule and plan my evening activities in advance."

During this review, Laura described each urge experienced in the past day and the self-talk she had employed to counteract it. The problem-solving/self-instruction procedure continued throughout the hospitalization.

The remainder of each session for the next 3 weeks was devoted to work in two of the areas previously targeted for intervention. These target areas were (a) an ongoing comparison of the pros and cons of maintaining her eating disorder; and (b) her irrational beliefs regarding the immediacy and "permanence" of substantial weight gain as the result of consuming a relatively small amount of food. In each session during this period, the therapist engaged the patient in a review of previous eating behavior and urges to vomit or restrict intake. This was followed by a discussion of the pros and cons of maintaining her eating problem. The most compelling *pro* was the opportunity for keeping her dependence on others, including her family and mental health professionals. The *cons* were the physical health risks, pain, and guilt she experienced. During these discussions the therapist emphasized the notion that Laura must "pay a price" for giving up her eating disorder and that one part of the "price" was the temporary discomfort associated with increasing her calorie intake and body weight. Specific areas of discomfort were approached in a rational restructuring format (Goldfried & Davison, 1976), which challenged her experiences of discomfort and problematic assumptions. In addition, Laura was encouraged to look at the likely consequences of maintaining her problematic assumptions.

During the final 2 to 3 weeks of the hospitalization, the structure of the session remained the same, but the problem-solving discussions focused on problems especially likely to be encountered after discharged. These problem areas were (a) Laura's diminished social contacts with male and female peers; and (b) the establishment of an independent living arrangement.

Because Laura previously had enjoyed a relatively full social life, social skills training, *per se,* was not indicated. However, it was necessary to develop a list of potential social activities and set specific goals regarding the frequency of her social contacts. Laura agreed to initiate and follow through on at least two "outings" (e.g., moving, weekend lunch, play, etc.) per week after discharge. After several problem-solving discussions, Laura decided to return to work full-time with her previous employer and to move in with two female friends on a temporary basis. This living arrangement was viewed as a compromise between living with her parents and establishing an independent residence.

Laura complied with all aspects of the program, ate virtually all meals and snacks, and made no attempts to vomit throughout the hospitalization. She reached her target weight of 105 lb by the end of the seventh week. She kept her weight above 105 lb for the next 2 weeks as she selected her own meals in the hospital cafeteria.

Outpatient Follow-Up

Outpatient work was intended to maintain and generalize the improvements she had made during the inpatient stay. Sessions were held twice weekly immediately after discharge, and their frequency was faded gradually to brief "check-ins" at 6-month intervals. At this writing, 20 months have passed since Laura's discharge from the hospital. The session format and general topics were identical to those used during the last week of the hospitalization. After being weighed, Laura reviewed her self-recorded eating behavior, vomiting, social activities with family and peers, and her use of problem solving/self-instructions since the last visit.

During the first week of follow-up outpatient work, the following specific goals were formulated: (a) 2,000 to 2,400 calories daily; (b) maintain body weight at 100 to 105 lb; (c) establish an independent residence within 3 months; (d) schedule at least two social events per week to occur on weekends or after 5:00 P.M. weekdays; and (e) no vomiting.

The time period since the last meeting was reviewed in terms of these goals. Specific problems in meeting any of the goals were addressed in the same cognitive/behavioral style that was established during the inpatient stay.

Laura has been successful in terms of her establishment of an independent living situation. Indeed, she moved in with friends for 2 months after being discharged, rented an apartment by herself 4 months later, and 1 year later purchased a small house that she occupies alone. In addition, she has developed several friendships with other women and has become active in various church social groups and activities. She also has dated four different men for brief periods during this time.

Table 1 shows the frequency of Laura's binge-vomit episodes and her weight over the 20 month follow-up period. Although there were periods when she vomited as much as twice per week, these instances were not nearly as intense as her pretreatment episodes during which she often would spend an entire day binging and vomiting. For the most part she maintained her weight within the target range, and at no time did her weight fall below 94 pounds.

This is an excerpt of Laura's most recent follow-up interview, during which she appeared to demonstrate a relatively thorough understanding of the application of the problem-solving model to problem situations in her life.

THERAPIST: So there was a 1-week period where you did it for three times and that's the only time for the past 5 months.

LAURA: Yes.

THERAPIST: Well, what happened during that week?

LAURA: We've had a new manager which has been since August of last year, and I had never spoken with the man. I decided I was just going to have to talk to him because I was seeing myself start to hate the job, and I wanted to feel that if I was going to be working

Table 1. *Weight, Binging, and Vomiting since Discharge*

Months since discharge	Average weekly binge–vomit frequency since last meeting	Average weight[a]
1	1.75	103.75
2	0.25	100.50
3	1.50	96.50
4	1.50	96.00
5	2.75	95.50
6	2.25	95.50
7	2.25	99.75
8	1.50	102.50
9	1.00	103.50
10	1.00	103.50
11	0.50	101.75
12	0.00	103.00
14	0.25	100.00
20	0.00	104.00

[a]Target range: 100 to 105 lb.

as hard as I was, like only taking a half-hour lunch and coming in an hour early and things like that, then I was going to be appreciated. So I just went in and said, "I deserve to be promoted." I want to know that my work is appreciated now but that I would have to wait until my fourth anniversary with the company. They've been telling me all along that they feel I deserve a promotion. Well, they started telling me this in September, and my anniversary's next June. I guess this might have been about a month ago that this happened. I said I don't want to hear that, I want to know that you're going to do something as soon as possible because I deserve it, not because my anniversary's coming. Supposedly they're going to promote me, and it's going to happen January 1. I haven't been told that for sure, but that's what they told me back in November. So anyway, I just felt better that I had done something about talking to somebody and letting them know how I felt.

THERAPIST: Sure.

LAURA: I mean, that was like a real springboard for me to talk to the manager and confront him because I always felt you had to have a promotion bestowed upon you, not that you knocked on the door and said, "Look, I deserve it." And anyways, I think that had a lot to do with why I went home and binged because I just really, really felt frustrated.

THERAPIST: You went home and binged after you confronted him?

LAURA: No, prior.

THERAPIST: Oh, I see.

LAURA: Prior to and that's when I . . . I mean, I think the fact that I was driven to that point of despair made me realize that I had to do something, take an active change . . . I mean, do something out of my normal routine.

THERAPIST: What made you decide to do that?

LAURA: Just thinking that I consciously did not want to see myself become so frustrated that I would start hating the job. I really liked the job, and I wanted to keep it that way until I had to sit back and think well, what can I do to keep it this way?

THERAPIST: It seems different than what you would have done a couple years ago.

LAURA: Oh, yeah. Well, I think that going home and binging was like the automatic reaction of what to do with something that I was frustrated about. I thought there was nothing easy I could do. Not that talking to somebody is difficult, but motivating myself to get up the nerve to talk to this person is difficult.

THERAPIST: Right. Well, it was just that probably in the past you would have went home and binged and vomited and that would have been it.

LAURA: Right, right.

THERAPIST: Well, what do you think is different? Instead of just keeping on binging and vomiting, you decided to go and talk to the boss about it, get your point across, and in fact get what you wanted in the end.

LAURA: Just the recognition of similar circumstances in the past. Where it led or what it accomplished was nothing insofar as dealing with what was bugging me. I mean really, I mean I don't think there was any like magic factor or anything. It's just that I felt like I've come this far, look where I am as far as my job and where I'm living, and I didn't want to jeopardize any of that. I've really consciously thought about what are my priorities; just not in that instance but in a lot of other things too. How can I put it? There were two different things that I wanted at the same time, but one had to take precedence over the other, so I'd have to make a sacrifice as far as . . . I mean, just little things like, taking the bus or driving to work. Well it would be a lot less wear and tear on my car etc., etc., if I take the bus. I'd like to save the mileage, you know, not put the miles on my car but my job's really important to me and I want to get there when I want to get there. If I want to get there an hour early it's OK or I want to leave a little late, OK.

THERAPIST: So you took control of things basically. Set your priorities and your objectives.

LAURA: Yeah. I mean, things aren't real "hunky-dory" or anything, but those are just things I see that I'm consciously decisive with. I mean, I still feel real shitty sometimes. I hate being by myself and I really resent that. You know, and friends telling me that uh . . . you know, married friends saying, "Look, it's just different when you're married and you can't understand what I'm going through." I don't really need to hear something like that when I'm particularly down. But I just leave then if I don't want to be in the house alone or have somebody come over.

THERAPIST: Sounds basically like you're sizing up the situations a little bit better, maybe evaluating the things in the way we've talked about evaluating them; potential courses of action and the likely outcomes of them. Making some decisions based on that. At least it sounds like that.

LAURA: Yeah, I think. I still dread coming home by myself and I frequently make up lists, like seven or eight things to do in a particular evening and actually check them off and that just keeps me busy but it's necessary for me to do that.

THERAPIST: OK, so it's a way to get by, right? You can cope planning your activities. You take control rather than waiting for the eating problem or whatever else it is to swoop down and take control of you. That seems to be what you're doing. How are things with your family?

LAURA: Well, OK. Now I think my mom depends on me more than I do on the family, more like she wants me to come over, I usually spend 1 day of the weekend there.

THERAPIST: How about your social life?

LAURA: I had all the people from work over for a party. I spent the day Saturday getting ready for that and had all the fun planning for it and I was a nervous wreck because I was going to be entertaining these people but . . . I just . . . that was natural and I felt really good that I had done it and I've had other people from the neighborhood over and people from the church and things like that.

THERAPIST: You were just moving into your new place the last time we met. How do you like it?

LAURA: I like it. I've been getting to know the neighbors. I visit some of them. We just had a neighborhood block party. I mean it's just mundane stuff, but it's OK. I'm too tired when I come home from work to do anything that takes a lot of thought.

THERAPIST: It's not unlike many, many, many people who aren't coming in for therapy. It's a positive sign to me that you're able to keep the "eating disorder" under control and still muddle through life pretty well in spite of the fact that earth-shaking and wonderful things aren't happening left and right for you.

LAURA: I think I still spend a lot of time making an issue of what I'm eating or what I'm not eating. I mean I still . . . make it a point that there are just certain things that I avoid. I mean, I just try and eat the healthy, good stuff. If I go out to eat I get something like the seafood and salad bar and I don't eat a lot of fried stuff.

THERAPIST: You're not allowed to eat any?

LAURA: I'll allow myself a little but not a whole fried meal. It would maybe be the broiled seafood and french fries or something. When I pack my lunch it will just be a salad, and tuna, and then maybe a bag of potato chips with that but it won't be just a bunch of fried, starchy things.

THERAPIST: How about sweets?

LAURA: No, I just stay away from them. I'm still scared of them, I guess.

THERAPIST: So you can't have ice cream?

LAURA: I haven't for a while now.

THERAPIST: How long?

LAURA: Ever since my last binge.

THERAPIST: Cookies? Doughnuts?

LAURA: Nothing. No.

THERAPIST: OK. So that's the only thing that you cut out considerably, almost totally?

LAURA: Yeah. I never have dessert.

THERAPIST: You basically cut out sweets, then. Sounds like your diet is pretty healthy.

LAURA: I think it is. I'm keeping my weight up. I'm real glad about that because I really feel like my clothes still fit, not that I was shrinking but I felt like maybe I weighed a little bit more because some stuff is snug, but I wasn't sure, and that kinda confirms it. So, I feel good. And I have been keeping track of how many calories I've been eating. I kinda roughly eat the same amount for breakfast, lunch, and dinner.

THERAPIST: Fruits and vegetables? Are you eating those?

LAURA: Oh, yeah.

THERAPIST: In that area; eating a balanced diet to keep your weight up and controlling your binging and vomiting, it sounds to me like you're doing real well. Would you agree with that assessment?

LAURA: Yeah.

THERAPIST: The social end of your life . . . although it's not as spectacular as you may like, you're doing some things, and you're relatively happy with those?

LAURA: I go through my *ups* and *downs*. Sometimes I'm just content with things and sometimes not. You know, there's bad things, but it could be worse, it really could. I've got a house, I was 23 years old and I bought my very own house and I can decorate however I want and I've got real nice parents and I've got a good job and I like my friends and I feel like I'm pretty accepted at work and I feel I'm competent in what I'm doing there. I feel confident at what I'm doing at my house. My house has just done wonders for my self-confidence. I put up my very own curtain rods. Nobody helped me. And I picked out my very own furniture and the other night I took a double bed and I lifted up the box springs and the mattress and I put them on the bedframe all by myself and there was nobody helping me. My electricity went out the other night and I didn't call anybody. Like my first thought was, "Oh, my God! I've got to empty the freezer and go to my parents and spend the night there so I make sure I get up in time." And I thought, "No that's not really a good idea because you know how would I feel if my parents' electricity went off and they came running up to my house?"

THERAPIST: Mhhmhh.

LAURA: You know, this is my house and they would stay in their house and cope, and everybody else in the entire community; their electricity is out and they're not running up to their parents. So, if I'm late for work I'll just tell them my electricity went out. There's nothing I can do about it and if everything melts in my freezer, I'll buy more, you know. And I mean I felt real good.

Summary

This case study describes the assessment and apparently successful treatment of a severe case of anorexia nervosa. Prior to treatment Laura weighed 72 lb and had been binging and vomiting several times per day such that her social life and job performance were restricted severely. Inpatient treatment consisted of an operant/response prevention program, dietary advice, and problem-solving/self-instruction training. Her weight was above 105 lb for the last 2 weeks of the hospitalization, and she did not vomit while hospitalized. Follow-up outpatient treatment was conducted for 20 months during which Laura kept her weight within the target range for the last 12 months and reduced her rate of self-induced vomiting to zero for the last 6 months. In addition she has developed and maintained various interpersonal relationships and established an independent residence.

References

Agras, S., Barlow, D. H., Chapin, H. N., Abel, G., & Leitenberg, H. (1974). Behavior modification of anorexia nervosa. *Archives of General Psychiatry, 30,* 279–286.

Agras, S., & Werne, J. (1978). Behavior therapy in anorexia nervosa, a data-based approach to the question. In J. P. Brady & H. K. H. Brodie (Eds.), *Controversy in psychiatry.* Philadelphia: Saunders.

American Psychiatric Association. (1980). *Diagnostic and statistical manual of mental disorders* (3rd ed.).) Washington, DC: Author.

Azzerad, J., & Stafford, R. L. (1969). Restoration of eating behavior in anorexia nervosa through operant conditioning and environmental manipulation. *Behaviour Research and Therapy, 7,* 165–171.

Bachrach, A. H., Erwin, W. S., & Mohr, J. P. (1965). The control of eating behavior in an anorexic by operant conditioning techniques. In L. P. Ullmann & Krasner (Eds.), *Case studies in behavior modification.* New York: Holt, Rinehart & Winston.

Barcai, A. (1977). Lithium in anorexia nervosa: A pilot report on two patients. *Acta Psychiatrica Scandinavica, 55,* 97–101.

Barlow, D. H. (1981). *Behavioral assessment of adult disorders.* New York: Guilford.

Beck, A. T., Ward, C. H., Mendelson, M., Mock, J. E., & Erbaugh, J. K. (1961). An inventory for measuring depression. *Archives of General Psychiatry, 4,* 561–571.

Bemis, K. M. (1978). Current approaches to the etiology and treatment of anorexia nervosa. *Psychological Bulletin, 85,* 593–617.

Beumont, P. J. V. (1977). Former categorization of patients with anorexia nervosa. *Australian and New England Journal of Psychiatry, 11,* 223–226.

Beumont, P. J. V., George, G. C. W., & Smart, D. E. (1976). "Dieters" and "vomiters and purgers" in anorexia nervosa. *Psychological Medicine, 6,* 617–622.

Bhanji, S., & Thompson, J. (1974). Operant conditioning in the treatment of anorexia nervosa: A review and retrospective study of eleven cases. *British Journal of Psychiatry, 124,* 166–172.

Bianco, F. J. (1972). Rapid treatment of two cases of anorexia nervosa. *Journal of Behavior Therapy and Experimental Psychiatry, 3,* 223–224.

Blinder, B. J., Freeman, D. M. A., & Stunkard, A. J. (1970). Behavior therapy of anorexia nervosa: Effectiveness of activity as a reinforcer of weight gain. *American Journal of Psychiatry, 126*(8), 72–82.

Blue, R. (1979). Use of punishment in the treatment of anorexia nervosa. *Psychological Reports, 44,* 743–746.

Brady, J. P., & Rieger, W. (1972). Behavioral treatment of anorexia nervosa. In T. Thompson & W. S. Dockens, III (Eds.), *Proceedings of the International Symposium on Behavior Modification.* New York: Appleton-Century-Crofts.

Bruch, H. (1973). *Eating disorders: Obesity, anorexia nervosa and the person within.* New York: Basic Books.

Cantwell, D. P., Sturzenberger, S., Burroughs, J., Salkin, B., & Green, J. K. (1977). Anorexia nervosa: An affective disorder? *Archives of General Psychiatry, 34,* 1087–1093.

Casper, R. C., Eckert, E. D., Halmi, K. A., Goldberg, S. C., & Davis, J. M. (1980). Bulimia: Its incidence and clinical importance in patients with anorexia nervosa. *Archives of General Psychiatry, 37,* 1030–1034.

Ciminero, A. R., Calhoun, K. S., & Adams, H. E. (1977). *Handbook of behavioral assessment.* New York: Wiley.

Crisp, A. H. (1965). Clinical and therapeutic aspects of anorexia nervosa—A study of thirty cases. *Journal of Psychosomatic Research, 9,* 67–68.

Crisp, A. H., Harding, B., & McGuinness, B. (1974). Anorexia nervosa. Psychosomatic characteristics of parents: Relationship to prognosis. A quantitative study. *Journal of Psychosomatic Research, 18,* 167–173.

Crisp, A. H., Palmer, R. L., & Kalucy, R. S. (1976). How common is anorexia nervosa? A prevalence study. *British Journal of Psychiatry, 128,* 542–554.

Crisp, A. H., Hsu, L. K. G., Harding, J., & Hartshorn, J. (1980). Clinical features of anorexia nervosa. *Journal of Psychosomatic Research, 24,* 179–191.

Dally, P. J., & Sargant, W. (1960). A new treatment for anorexia nervosa. *British Medical Journal, 1,* 1770–1773.

Dally, P. J., & Sargant, W. (1966). Treatment and outcome of anorexia nervosa. *British Medical Journal, 2,* 793–795.

D'Zurilla, T. J., & Goldfried, M. R. (1971). Problem-solving and behavior modification. *Journal of Abnormal Psychology, 78,* 107–126.

Duddle, M. (1973). An increase of anorexia nervosa in a university population. *British Journal of Psychiatry, 123,* 711.

Eckert, E. D., Goldberg, S. C., Halmi, K. A., Casper, R. C., & Davis, J. M. (1979). Behavior therapy in anorexia nervosa. *British Journal of Psychiatry, 134,* 55–59.

Elkin, T. E., Hersen, M., Eisler, R. M., & Williams, J. G. (1973). Modification of caloric intake in anorexia nervosa: An experimental analysis. *Psychological Reports, 11,* 707–711.

Fairburn, C. G., & Cooper, P. J. (1982). Self-induced vomiting and bulimia nervosa: An undetected problem. *British Medical Journal, 284,* 1153–1155.

Feighner, J. P., Robins, E., Guze, S. B., Woodruff, R. A., Jr., Winokur, G., & Munoz, R. (1972). Diagnostic criteria for use in psychiatric research. *Archives of General Psychiatry, 26,* 57–63.

Fichter, M. M., & Kessler, W. (1980). Behavioral treatment of an anorexic male: Experimental analysis of generalization. *Behavioral Analysis of Medicine, 4,* 152–168.

Garfinkel, P. E. (1974). Perception of hunger and satiety in anorexia nervosa. *Psychological Medicine, 4,* 309–315.

Garfinkel, P. E., & Garner, D. M. (1982). *Anorexia nervosa: A multidimensional perspective.* New York: Brunner/Mazel.

Garfinkel, P. E., Kline, S. A., & Stancer, H. C. (1973). Treatment of anorexia nervosa using operant conditioning techniques. *Journal of Nervous and Mental Disease, 157,* 428–433.

Garfinkel, P. E., Moldofsky, H., & Garner, D. M. (1977). The role of behavior modification in the treatment of anorexia nervosa. *Journal of Pediatric Psychology, 2,* 113–121.

Garner, D. M., & Garfinkel, P. E. (1979). The eating attitudes test: An index of the symptoms of anorexia nervosa. *Psychological Medicine, 9,* 273–279.

Garner, D. M., & Garfinkel, P. E. (1980). Socio-cultural factors in the development of anorexia nervosa. *Psychological Medicine, 10,* 647–656.

Geller, J. L. (1975). Treatment of anorexia nervosa by the integration of behavior therapy and psychotherapy. *Psychotherapy and Psychosomatics, 26,* 167–177.

Goldberg, S. C., Halmi, K. A., Eckert, E. D., Casper, R. C., & Davis, J. M. (1979). Cyproheptadine in anorexia nervosa. *British Journal of Psychiatry, 134,* 67–70.

Goldfried, M. R., & Davison, G. C. (1976). *Clinical behavior therapy.* New York: Holt, Rinehart & Winston.

Hallsten, E. A. (1965). Adolescent anorexia treated by desensitization. *Behaviour Research and Therapy, 3,* 87–91.

Halmi, K. A., Falk, J. R., & Schwartz, E. (1981). Binge-eating and vomiting: A survey of a college population. *Psychological Medicine, 11,* 697–706.

Halmi, K. A., Powers, P., & Cunningham, S. (1975). Treatment of anorexia nervosa with behavior modification. *Archives of General Psychiatry, 32,* 93–96.

Halmi, K. A., Goldberg, S. C., Eckert, E., Casper, R., & Davis, J. M. (1977). Pretreatment evaluation in anorexia nervosa. In R. A. Vigersky (Ed.), *Anorexia nervosa.* New York: Raven Press.

Harris, F. C., Hsu, L. K. G., & Phelps, C. F. (1983). Problems in adolescence: Assessment and treatment of bulimia nervosa. In M. Hersen (Ed.), *Outpatient behavior therapy: A clinical guide.* New York: Grune & Stratton.

Hauserman, N., & Lavin, P. (1977). Post-hospitalization continuation treatment of anorexia nervosa. *Journal of Behavior Therapy and Experimental Psychiatry, 8,* 309–313.

Hsu, L. K. G. (1983). The etiology of anorexia nervosa. *Psychological Medicine, 13,* 231–238.

Hsu, L. K. G., Crisp, A. H., & Harding, B. (1979). *Outcome of anorexia nervosa. Lancet, 1,* 61–65.

Janet, P. (1929). *The major symptoms of hysteria.* New York: Macmillan.

Johannson, A. J., & Knorr, N. J. (1977). L-dopa as treatment for anorexia nervosa. In R. A. Vigersky (Ed.), *Anorexia nervosa.* New York: Raven Press.

Jones, D. F., Fox, M. M., Babigan, H. H., & Hutton, H. E. (1980). Epidemiology of anorexia nervosa in Monroe County, New York: 1960–1976. *Psychosomatic Medicine, 42,* 551–568.

Kanfer, F. H., & Saslow, G. (1969). Behavioral diagnosis. In C. M. Franks (Ed.), *Behavior therapy: Appraisal and status.* New York: McGraw-Hill.

Katz, J. L., & Walsh, B. T. (1978). Depression in anorexia nervosa. *American Journal of Psychiatry, 135,* 507.

Kehrer, H. E. (1977). Behandlug der Anorexia nervosa mit Verhaltens-Therapie. *Medizinische Klinik, 70,* 427–432.

Kendler, K. S. (1978). Amitriptyline-induced obesity in anorexia nervosa: A case report. *American Journal of Psychiatry, 135,* 1107–1108.

Lang, P. J. (1965). Behavior therapy with a case of anorexia nervosa. In L. P. Ullmann & L. Kranser (Eds.), *Case studies in behavior modification.* New York: Holt, Rinehart & Winston.

Leitenberg, H., Agras, W. S., & Thompson, L. E. (1968). Sequential analysis of the effect of selective positive reinforcement in modifying anorexia nervosa. *Behaviour Research and Therapy, 6,* 211–218.

Lobb, L. G., & Schaefer, H. H. (1972). Successful treatment of anorexia nervosa through isolation. *Psychological Reports, 30,* 245–246.

McGlynn, F. D. (1980). Successful treatment of anorexia nervosa with self-monitoring and long distance praise. *Journal of Behavior Therapy and Experimental Psychiatry, 11,* 283–286.

Mills, H. (1976). Amitriptyline therapy in anorexia nervosa. *Lancet, 2,* 687.

Minuchin, S., Rosman, B. L., & Baker, L. (1978). *Psychosomatic families: Anorexia nervosa in context.* Cambridge, MA: Harvard University Press.

Mitchell, J. E., & Gillum, R. (1980). Weight-dependent arrhythmia in a patient with anorexia nervosa. *American Journal of Psychiatry, 137,* 377–378.

Moore, D. C. (1977). Amitriptyline therapy in anorexia nervosa. *American Journal of Psychiatry, 134,* 1303–1304.

Morgan, H. G., & Russell, G. F. M. (1975). Values of family background and clinical features as predictors of long term outcome in anorexia nervosa: Four year follow-up of 41 patients. *Psychological Medicine, 5,* 355–371.

Morton, R. (1689). *Phthisiologica: Or a treatise of consumptions.* London: S. Smith & B. Walford.

Needleman, H. L., & Waber, D. (1976). The use of amitriptyline in anorexia nervosa. *Lancet, 2,* 580.

Needleman, H. L., & Waber, D. (1977). The use of amitriptyline in anorexia nervosa. In R. A. Vigersky (Ed.), *Anorexia nervosa.* New York: Raven Press.

Neumann, M., & Gaoni, B. (1975). Preferred food as the reinforcing agent in a case of anorexia nervosa. *Journal of Behavior Therapy and Experimental Psychiatry, 6,* 331–333.

Ollendick, T. H. (1979). Behavioral treatment of anorexia nervosa: A five year study. *Behavior Modification, 3,* 124–135.

Palazzoli, M. S. (1978). *Self-starvation.* New York: International Universities Press.

Palmer, R. L. (1979). The dietary chaos syndrome: A useful new term? *British Journal of Medical Psychology, 52,* 187–190.

Parker, J. B., Jr., Blazer, D., & Wyrick, L. (1977). Anorexia nervosa: A combined therapeutic approach. *Southern Medical Journal, 70,* 448–452.

Pertschuk, M. J. (1977). Behavior therapy: Extended follow-up. In R. A. Vigersky (Ed.), *Anorexia nervosa.* New York: Raven Press.

Pertschuk, M. J., Edwards, N., & Pomerleau, O. F. (1978). A multiple-base-line approach to behavioral intervention in anorexia nervosa. *British Journal of Psychiatry, 139,* 553–539.

Poole, A. D., & Sanson, R. W. (1978). A behavioral program for the management of anorexia nervosa. *Australian and New England Journal of Psychiatry, 12,* 49–53.

Rollins, N., & Piazza, E. (1978). Diagnosis of anorexia nervosa: A critical reappraisal. *Journal of the American Academy of Child Psychiatry, 17,* 126–137.

Rosen, L. W. (1980). Modification of secretive or ritualized eating behavior in anorexia nervosa. *Journal of Behavior Therapy and Experimental Psychiatry, 11,* 101–104.

Rosman, B. L., Minuchin, S., Liebman, R., & Baker, L. (1976). Input and outcome of family therapy in anorexia nervosa. In J. L. Claghorn (Ed.), *Successful psychotherapy.* New York: Brunner/Mazel.

Russell, G. F. M. (1979). Bulimia nervosa: An ominous variant of anorexia nervosa. *Psychological Medicine, 9,* 429–448.

Schnurer, A. T., Rubin, R. R., Roy, A. (1973). Systematic desensitization of anorexia nervosa as a weight phobia. *Journal of Behavior Therapy and Experimental Psychiatry, 4,* 149–153.

Schwartz, D. M., & Thompson, M. G. (1981). Do anoretics get well? Current research and future needs. *American Journal of Psychiatry, 138*(3), 319–323.

Stuart, R. B. & Davis, B. (1972). *Slim chance in a fat world: Behavioral control of obesity.* Champaign, IL: Research Press.

Stumphauzer, J. S. (1969). Application of reinforcement contingencies with a 23 year old anorexic patient. *Psychological Reports, 24,* 109–110.

Vandereyeken, W., & Pieters, G., (1978). Short-term weight restoration in anorexia nervosa through operant conditioning. *Scandinavian Journal of Behaviour Therapy, 7*(4), 221–236.

Vigersky, R. A., & Loriaux, D. L. (1977). The effect of cyproheptadine in anorexia nervosa: A double-blind trial. In R. A. Vigersky (Ed.), *Anorexia nervosa.* New York: Raven Press.

Werry, K. S., & Bull, D. (1975). Anorexia nervosa: A case study using behavior therapy. *Journal of the American Academy of Child Psychiatry, 14,* 567–568.

White, J. H., & Schnaultz, N. L. (1977). Successful treatment of anorexia nervosa with imipramine. *Diseases of the Nervous System, 38,* 567–568.

Wulliemier, F. (1978). Anorexia nervosa: Gauging treatment effectiveness. *Psychosomatics, 19,* 497–499.

Alcohol and Drug Abuse

David M. Lawson and Henry M. Boudin

Introduction

The use of alcohol and other drugs is a pervasive and widely accepted part of our society. Unfortunately, the abuse of these substances is also increasingly widespread. In the United States alone, it has been recently estimated that between 9 to 13 million people suffer the direct effects of alcohol abuse and dependence and that as many as 45 million others are indirectly affected (Brandsma, Maultsby, & Welsh, 1980). Moreover, it has been estimated that between 3 to 7% of the American workforce uses illicit drugs on a daily basis (Quale, 1983). Altogether, the financial cost to the nation of alcohol and drug abuse in terms of health care utilization, property damage, and diminished productivity is estimated at 70 billion annually (Quayle, 1983). The cost in terms of human pain and suffering is incalculable.

The adverse personal consequences arising from the excessive use of alcohol and other drugs are often used to distinguish two clinical conditions (American Psychiatric Association, 1980). In the first, *substance abuse,* alcohol and/or drug ingestion persists despite the individual's efforts to reduce or discontinue usage and despite significant impairment in the areas of physical, occupational, and social functioning. Some abusers, for example, feel unable to function adequately without daily ingestion of their substance(s) of abuse. Many sustain injuries in accidents and assaults and suffer the effects of acute intoxication such as alcohol blackouts and opioid overdosages. Reduced productivity and increased absenteeism associ-

DAVID M. LAWSON • Division of Psychology, Shaughnessy Hospital, 4500 Oak Street, Vancouver, British Columbia V6H 3N1 and Department of Psychology, University of British Columbia, 2136 West Mall, Vancouver, British Columbia V6T 1Y7, Canada.   HENRY M. BOUDIN • Center for Psychological Services, Suite 310, Chin Hills Building, 3915 Talbot Road South, Renton, Washington 98055.

ated with substance abuse often result in repeated job loss and financial difficulties. Marital and other social relationships suffer, often irreparably, and legal entanglements may arise from possession, purchase, or sale of illicit drugs or from the criminal activities often necessary to support an expensive habit.

The second condition associated with excessive use of alcohol or other drugs is *substance dependence.* This condition is almost always accompanied by the impairments associated with substance abuse and is characterized by the presence of either or both of two additional clinical phenomena: tolerance and withdrawal. Tolerance refers to the diminished effect of a fixed dosage after repeated usage or to the substantially increased dosages necessary to attain the same effect that was originally produced by a small amount of the substance. Withdrawal refers to a substance-specific syndrome that occurs when ingestion of the substance is reduced or discontinued. The extent to which tolerance and withdrawal occur varies in proportion to the frequency, dosage, and chronicity of ingestion and depends largely upon the nature of the substance ingested.

Three generally defined classes of substances are typically associated with abuse and/or dependence. The depressants, including alcohol, opiate analgesics (heroine, morphine, methadone, and codeine), barbiturates, and tranquilizers, all act to reduce arousal in the central nervous system (CNS). Chronic, excessive use of many of these substances produces tolerance and a wide range of withdrawal symptoms, including psychomotor tremor, profuse sweating, muscle cramps, seizures, and hallucinations. The stimulants, including amphetamines and cocaine, act on the central nervous system to increase arousal. Like many of the depressants, amphetamines are associated with dependence because tolerance can develop, and withdrawal symptoms, such as depressed mood, fatigue, disturbed sleep, and increased dreaming may also occur. Cocaine, however, is classified only as a substance of abuse because the signs of physical dependency, tolerance, and withdrawal have not been demonstrated following its use. The third general class of substances, the hallucinogens, include lysergic acid diethylamide (LSD), psilocybin, mescaline, cannabis (marijuana), phencyclidine (PCP), and a variety of other organic and synthetic compounds. Although all of these substances distort perception and consciousness, the pharmacological mechanism by which they produce their effects is poorly understood. With the exception of cannabis, which may produce tolerance, the hallucinogens are generally classified as substances of abuse. Nevertheless, the deleterious effects of the hallucinogens, including panic reactions, depersonalization, psychosis, and "flashbacks" may be extreme. Substances such as nicotine and caffeine warrant separate attention and will, therefore, not be considered in this chapter.

In recent years, behavioral approaches to substance abuse and dependence have generated an increasing amount of research and have led to the development of numerous assessment and treatment techniques. These developments are predicated on a general behavioral model according to which substance abuse and dependence are viewed as learned, socially acquired patterns of behavior that develop and are maintained by a wide range of antecedent cues and consequent events (Marlatt & Donovan, 1981). Initial formulations of the behavioral model emphasized the role of learning and of the pharmacological effects of alcohol and other drugs. These substances were conceptualized as positive reinforcers to the extent that they produced euphoria or other positive subjective experiences and negative reinforcers to the extent that they provided either relief from aversive states such as tension, anxiety, and depression, or avoidance of the anticipated effects of withdrawal. In addition, the fellowship provided by the abuser's peer group and the attention provided by concerned family and friends were conceptualized as positive social reinforcements. Relevant antecedent events include both environmental cues previously associated with the use of drugs or the occurrence of withdrawal and negative mood states such as boredom and loneliness, all of which have been conceptualized as discriminative stimuli that may precipitate resumption or continuation of drug ingestion.

More recent formulations of the behavioral model recognize, in addition, the role of cognitive variables and social skills deficits (Marlatt & Donovan, 1981). In particular, the abuser's expectations and beliefs concerning the effects of alcohol and other drugs appear to contribute importantly to the maintenance of substance abuse and dependence (Brown, Goldman, Inn, & Anderson, 1980; Southwick, Steele, Marlatt, & Lindell, 1981). Despite the fact that increased or continued alcohol or drug usage typically intensify negative affect among chronic users, many persist in taking these substances in anticipation of beneficial effects. Similarly, the belief among alcoholics that consumption of a small amount of alcohol will trigger a physiological mechanism compelling them to continue to drink appears to be an important determinant of the loss-of-control phenomenon. Moreover, the widespread belief that alcohol or drug ingestion will enhance interpersonal effectiveness or self-esteem has particular significance for socially unskilled or self-deprecating abusers. To the extent that the abuser's behavioral repertoire is deficient in alternative, nonpharmacological coping responses, it is likely that drug or alcohol usage will recur. Not surprisingly, the circumstances most likely to reveal social skills deficits among alcohol abusers appear to be those that call for a proffered drink to be declined (Twentyman, Greenwald, Greenwald, Kloss, Kovaleski, & Zibung-Hoffman, 1982).

It is evident from the preceding introduction that abuse of, or dependence on, alcohol or other drugs produces pervasive and devastating consequences both for the individual and for society. It is equally evident that with the accumulation of clinical and research data, the behavioral model of these disorders has become increasingly refined and complex. It is our conviction that such reformulation on the basis of empirical findings is essential for the continuing development and increased efficacy of interventions intended for a problem of such magnitude. Our objective in writing this chapter, therefore, is to acquaint the reader with assessment and treatment techniques derived from a behavioral model of alcohol and drug abuse.

Clinical Assessment

The behavioral model of substance abuse and dependence has several important implications for clinical assessment, which will be briefly reviewed before specific assessment procedures are described. The first implication is that alcohol and drug ingestion are viewed as continuous rather than dichotomous variables, and it is, therefore, not sufficient simply to diagnose the presence or absence of these conditions. Rather, the clinician must determine the extent or degree of abuse or dependence.

Second, although the possibility of genetic predisposition is recognized, the behavioral model does not assume any exclusive physiological basis for substance abuse and dependence. Rather, alcohol and drug ingestion are presumed to be functionally related to a variety of internal and external factors, all of which have to be assessed. Internal factors include not only physiological states such as intoxication and withdrawal, but also mood, covert self-statements, and beliefs and expectations regarding drug and alcohol effects. External factors include social and environmental cues, such as the presence of drug dealers or drinking companions, arguments with a spouse or employers, reexposure to the physical setting in which drugs or alcohol had been consumed, or merely the sight of a liquor advertisement or of the paraphernalia for injecting drugs. Consequently, it is not only essential to investigate in detail the antecedents and consequences of drug ingestion, it is also appropriate to assess the client's social skills, marital adjustment mood, and problem-solving skills. Procedures for the assessment of these latter areas of functioning are detailed in other chapters of this volume and in Hersen and Bellack (1981).

A third implication of the behavioral model is that the factors associated with the initial development of substance abuse or dependence are not necessarily the same as those that maintain it. A case in point is an alcohol abuser who attributed his abusive drinking habits to a major disruption of his social and family life and his forced isolation with abusive drinkers. He had, in fact, been separated from his family and friends during World War II and had been transferred to a geographically remote aircraft refueling station where he had worked in close quarters with a crew who, when alcohol was in short supply, mixed cocktails with airplane antifreeze. At the time of the assessment, however, he had been reunited with his family and friends and had been residing in Montreal for more than 20 years! Thus, although history taking remains an important part of behavioral assessment, an examination of the patient's *present* life circumstances is usually essential in identifying factors that are functionally related to the maintenance of abuse or dependence.

Another implication of the behavioral model concerns the client's motivation for treatment. Just as alcohol and drug ingestion are influenced by a variety of factors, so too is the client's commitment to the objectives of treatment. Because the factors that predispose a client to seek treatment vary in terms of the duration of their influence, it is important to identify them. In cases of illicit drug abuse or dependence, the client may have been charged with a criminal offense, and the act of seeking treatment may be little more than a gesture intended to impress the court. The same may apply to the alcohol abuser charged with driving while intoxicated. In other cases, the client's reasons for entering treatment may not be time limited to the same extent. Continuation of employment, marital, or other social relationships, for example, may have been made contingent upon actual behavior change. Thus, although the patient's motivation for treatment may be enhanced during therapeutic contact (W. R. Miller, 1983a), it is nevertheless important to determine the extent to which it may also be sustained by extratherapeutic influences.

Finally, the behavioral model emphasizes the importance of objectivity of assessment. This, however, must not be construed as an exclusive reliance upon direct observation or any other single modality of assessment. It is recognized by behavioral clinicians (Hay & Nathan, 1982) that every modality of assessment has inherent limitations and that the optimal degree of objectivity is achieved by multimodal assessment, including self-report, behavioral, and physiological measures. In the section that follows, practical examples of each of these different types of measures will be briefly described.

Assessment Methods

The Drinking Profile developed by Marlatt (1976) is probably the single most widely used structured interview for the assessment of alcohol abuse and dependence. It is equally applicable to inpatients and outpatients and includes 14 pages of open- and closed-ended questions regarding employment and drinking histories, physical, social, and psychological consequences of drinking, treatment motivation, and expectations regarding treatment outcome. The Drinking Profile also elicits detailed information regarding current drinking practices, including beverage preferences, drinking settings and companions, and the cognitive and affective antecedents and consequences associated with drinking episodes. It takes approximately 1 hour to administer, and it can be easily and reliably scored using a manual specifically developed for this purpose. A matching follow-up questionnaire is also available to facilitate the evaluation of treatment outcome.

Unfortunately, no corresponding structured interview for the assessment of drug abuse and dependence has been published. As a result, many drug abuse treatment programs utilize standardized interview formats specifically developed for their own clientele. One such unpublished instrument is the G-DATS (Gainsville Drug Abuse Treatment Services) described by Boudin *et al.* (1977). Although this structured interview is similar in many respects to the Drinking Profile, it provides less information relevant to a functional analysis of drug self-administration but more detailed information on criminal activities, other substances of abuse, current income and expenses, and life goals. The G-DATS was developed for use in an outpatient setting, and although it is unpublished, it is available from the second author.

Over the years many scales have been developed to assess abuse and dependence on drugs, particularly alcohol (P. M. Miller, 1976). Most of these instruments, however, were based on assumptions that are inconsistent with a behavioral model and are, therefore, of limited usefulness to behaviorally oriented clinicians. A noteworthy exception, however, is the Alcohol Use Inventory (AUI) (Wanberg & Horn, 1983), which is probably the most valuable psychometric instrument for the assessment of alcohol abuse. The AUI is based on a multidimensional model of alcoholism and a series of factor-analytic studies. It includes 147 forced-choice items that are divided into 22 empirically derived scales that focus on the circumstances of drinking, the anticipated effects of drinking, drinking topography, and the cognitive, social, physical, and behavioral consequences. The AUI scales are, therefore, especially useful in the identification and quantification of factors that are functionally related to alcohol consumption. Moreover, the standardization sample, predictive validity, internal consistency, and test–retest reliability of the AUI scales are impressive, and norms are available for inpatients of both sexes and for a number of subgroups of alcohol abusers. Unfortunately, there is no comparable psychometric instrument for the assessment of abuse or dependence on drugs other than alcohol (Siegel, 1976).

Two screening tests for alcohol and drug abuse are also worthy of mention. The Michigan Alcoholism Screen Test (MAST) is a very widely used instrument that includes 25 forced-choice items relating to the social, medical, and interpersonal problems typically associated with excessive drinking (Selzer, 1971). It can be self-administered or used as a structured interview and usually takes less than 10 minutes to complete. Recent studies of its psychometric properties indicate that it is both reliable and valid for use in clinical settings (Skinner, 1979; Zung, 1979). The Drug Abuse Screening Test (DAST) is a more recently developed instrument that was closely modeled after the MAST (Skinner, 1982). It shares with its prototype a comparable level of psychometric sophistication, brevity, and ease of administration, and it yields a quantitative measure of a wide range of problems arising from drug abuse.

The structured interviews and psychometric instruments just described, like all direct self-report measures, are subject to distortion as a result of deliberate faking, inaccurate recall, and failure to observe relevant events. None of these instruments, therefore, should be administered to patients while they are intoxicated or undergoing withdrawal; all should be used in conjunction with other types of measures; and consideration should be given to the possibility that sanctions imposed by the court or by the treatment program may militate against valid self-report. For further discussion of the validity of self-report among alcohol and drug abusers, the interested reader is referred to Polich (1982), Callahan and Rawson (1980), and Brownell (1982).

Self-monitoring is a widely used strategy for the assessment of both alcohol and drug abuse or dependence. Following the intake interview, patients are trained to define and record their drinking or drug ingestion using as units of measurement the number of ounces of liquor or the absolute ethanol content of beverages consumed (Miller & Muñoz, 1976); the number of "tokes" or inhalations of marijuana (Boudin & Valentine, 1972); or the weight in milligrams of other substances. In addition, the client is usually instructed to record the date and time of ingestion, the setting in which it occurred, including the identity of any companions, and any thoughts, feelings, or behaviors that preceded or followed alcohol or drug ingestion. If self-administration of alcohol or drugs is infrequent, clinically useful information may also be obtained by instructing patients to monitor subjective urges to engage in this behavior.

Self-monitoring data are usually obtained throughout treatment and not only serve as a basis for clinical decision making and an objective index of improvement but also aid in the functional analysis of alcohol and drug ingestion. In the program developed by Boudin and his colleagues (Boudin, Valentine, Ingram, Brantley, Ruiz, Smith, Katlin, & Regan, 1977), clients were also instructed to monitor factors such as anxiety, depression, and school or work attendance that, on the basis of structured interviews, were suspected of being functionally related to drug ingestion. These additional data, which were monitored on wrist counters and relayed to the paraprofessional staff during regularly scheduled daily telephone calls, were subsequently used as a basis for predicting impending drug use and scheduling emergency interventions.

Self-monitoring as an assessment procedure is subject to all the limitations previously described in relation to self-report measures. In addition, as Callahan and Rawson (1980) noted, less well-educated clients may have difficulty acquiring self-observational skills, especially if they are not carefully trained by skilled clinical staff. It also is essential to review periodically with clients the operational definitions used in self-monitoring to ensure consistency of the data.

Although direct observations of alcohol and drug self-administration have been reported in the research literature (Barbor, Meyer, Mirin, McNamee, & Davies, 1976; Mirin, Meyer, & McNamee, 1976; Nathan & O'Brein, 1971; Rosenbluth, Nathan, & Lawson, 1978), they are seldom practical or appropriate in clinical settings. As a result, two indirect observational strategies are often implemented. The first, which is widely used in the assessment of alcohol abuse, is to obtain observational data from collaterals such as the client's friends, relatives, or co-workers. Admission to many alcohol abuse treatment programs, in fact, is contingent upon the client's providing the name of at least one person who is likely to be aware of the client's drinking, should it occur. It is noteworthy, however, that self- and collateral reports of drinking are seldom in perfect agreement, and correlations between them can range between .06 and .92 (Miller, Crawford, & Taylor, 1979).

In the second indirect observational strategy, alcohol or drug ingestion can be confirmed or disconfirmed on the basis of direct observation of the ingestion of antagonists, which block the effect of the substance of abuse. A narcotic abuser who takes Naltrexone daily, for example, will not experience a "rush" following the injection of heroin. Therefore, as long as the client is observed to be taking Naltrexone regularly, concurrent self-administration of heroin is unlikely. Similarly, a drug used in the treatment of alcohol abuse, disulfiram (Antabuse), reacts with alcohol to produce an aversive physical reaction characterized by nausea, vomiting, and a variety of other symptoms (Kwentus & Major, 1979). When it can be confirmed by direct observation that an alcohol abuser is ingesting disulfiram daily, it can be reasonably assumed that alcoholic beverages will be avoided. Needless to say, the presence of acute withdrawal symptoms or physical signs such as fresh needle tracks may also be used with a moderately high degree of confidence to infer alcohol or drug ingestion.

Biochemical measures are generally regarded as the most objective indices of alcohol and drug use. Breath-testing instruments permit a precise estimate of blood alcohol concentration that, in turn, is highly correlated with the amount consumed. Urinalyses can detect the presence of a wide range of other drugs. These measures are commonly used at the initial intake for diagnostic purposes and on a continuing basis thereafter as an indicator of treatment efficacy. Contrary to popular belief, however, both assessment procedures have serious limitations that should not be overlooked.

The major limitation shared by both procedures is that their validity depends largely upon random scheduling of assessment. Because alcohol and other drugs are present in the body only for a limited time following ingestion, a client could evade detection by refraining from alcohol or drug use prior to anticipated sampling periods. Thus, to obtain optimally valid measures would necessitate virtually constant monitoring of the client's whereabouts as well as sufficient personnel to conduct assessments throughout the day and night, 7 days a week.

Urinalysis also has several other limitations. Unlike breath testing for alcohol consumption, data from urinalyses are qualitative rather than quantitative, and there is typically a delay of a week or longer before the results are available from an independent laboratory. By contrast, inexpensive portable breath-testing devices are available that provide relatively accurate estimates of blood-alcohol concentration immediately after testing (Sobell & Sobell, 1975). An additional problem with urinalysis is that strict sample collection procedures have to be implemented to ensure that the sample is authentic. Clients have been known to conceal a "clean" sample in ballons or prophylactics on their person or in the bathroom and to present it for analysis. Needless to add, direct observation of the client while urinating raises a host of ethical and legal problems that must be seriously addressed by the clinician.

Archival records may also provide a potentially valuable source of assessment data. It is, of course, necessary to obtain the patient's consent before requesting information from outside sources regarding employment status, absenteeism (especially following weekends and paydays), arrests, driving charges, and hospitalizations. Some archival records, however, such as paycheck stubs, rental agreements, and prescription records can be provided by clients themselves. Like all assessment procedures described previously, however, archival information may also be misleading. It is often difficult, for example, to ensure that a client who submits a prescription record is not obtaining additional prescriptions from other sources.

Treatment Techniques

The behavioral model has three important implications for the treatment of alcohol and drug abuse, which will be briefly discussed before treatment techniques are described. The first implication can be drawn from the assumption that substance abuse and dependence are complex behavioral disorders that are functionally related to a variety of cognitive, affective, social, and environmental influences. It follows from this assumption that there is no single best treatment and that treatment should be individually tailored on the basis of a detailed and objective assessment. Accordingly, in the section to follow, a wide range of techniques will be presented.

Second, the behavioral model has important implications for the locus of treatment. To the extent that abuse and dependence occur as a function of the relationship between the client and the surrounding environment, a clinician cannot reasonably expect therapeutic changes produced in inpatient settings to generalize to the natural environment (Lawson, Wilson, Briddell, & Ives, 1976). Consistent with this view, recent surveys of hospital facilities for the treatment of substance abuse reveal a decline in the availability of inpatient services and an increase in outpatient services (Knowles, 1983).

Unquestionably, the most controversial implication of the behavioral model of alcohol and drug abuse concerns treatment goals. Substance ingestion is conceptualized in this model as a continuum extending from abstinence and nonproblematic ingestion at one end to abusive, problematic patterns of ingestion at the other. Stated simply, the objective of treatment according to this model is to reduce consumption patterns to a nonproblematic level. In the case of alcohol abuse, abstinence and controlled drinking are considered equally legitimate treatment goals. Adherents of the traditional model, by contrast, view alcoholism as a progressive and irreversible disease manifested by an irresistible compulsion to drink and an inability to discontinue drinking. By definition, abstinence is the only appropriate treatment goal according to this model.

It is perhaps not surprising that such a fundamental difference between these models would be the focus of controversy. It is, however, lamentable that the debate, which has continued for more than 20 years, shows little sign of waning despite the accumulation of an impressive body of research that supports the appropriateness of controlled drinking as a treatment goal for selected alcohol abusers. More specifically, it has been consistently demonstrated that controlled drinking is an attainable goal for many younger (less than 40 years) problem drinkers who are not physically dependent on alcohol and who report less than 10 years of problem drinking (Miller & Hester, 1980). In addition, those who succeed in moderating their drinking tend not to subscribe to the traditional disease model of alcoholism nor to consider themselves to be "alcoholics." For further discussion of the issues related to controlled drinking, the interested reader may refer to Brownell (1984), Marlatt (1983), and W. R. Miller (1983b).

The selection of goals in the treatment of drug abuse has been much less controversial. It is noteworthy, however, that treatment approaches for heroin dependence have historically fallen into one of two categories: (a) those in which clients strive to become totally abstinent from opiates; and (b) those in which clients have limited and supervised access to opiates such as methadone. Unlike the literature on alcohol abuse, little empirical data exist for the differential assignment of clients to abstinence-oriented or drug substitution treatment programs. Consequently, the goal of treatment for narcotic dependence depends largely on the orientation of the treatment program. As in the case of alcohol abuse, however, both treatment goals are consistent with the behavioral model to the extent that they reduce problems associated with drug use.

Behavioral treatment programs for alcohol and drug abuse usually consist of combinations of techniques, many of which are described next. Although there is growing empirical support for many such programs (Miller & Hester, 1980; Stitzer, Bigelow, & McCaul, 1983), relatively few studies have assessed the efficacy of the individual treatment components. Because all of the treatment techniques also have some methodological limitations that restrict their applicability, descriptions of both the procedures and their shortcomings are provided.

Aversive Conditioning

One of the earliest behavioral approaches to the treatment of alcohol and drug abuse, aversion therapy, is based on a classical conditioning model. According to this model, the repeated association of an aversive event with stimuli related to alcohol or drug ingestion will eventually result in an avoidance of these substances. Typically, the sight, smell, taste, or thoughts of these substances or stimuli previously associated with their use, such as the paraphernalia used to prepare an injection, are paired with a noxious stimulus. Although a variety of different types of noxious stimuli have been used, the most popular have been nausea-producing drugs, electric shock, and imaginal events.

During the past 10 years, the use of chemical aversion has become increasingly widespread in the treatment of alcoholism (Wiens & Menustik, 1983). Clients are admitted to hospital for approximately 14 days during which time five aversion conditioning sessions are scheduled. During each 30-minute session, the client is administered an intramuscular injection of emetine hydrochloride and, shortly before the onset of nausea and vomiting, is invited to drink an alcoholic beverage. After discharge, "booster" sessions are typically scheduled at various intervals according to the needs of the client. Only two reports of the use of chemical aversion with emetic drugs were included in a recent, exhaustive review of the behavioral literature on the treatment of drug abuse (Stitzer *et al.,* 1983). Both of these reports described similar treatment procedures, which were also administered on an inpatient basis.

Chemical aversion in the treatment of alcohol as well as drug abuse is yet to be adequately evaluated. From a practical viewpoint, it has several serious limitations; it requires medical screening and supervision, and it is expensive, highly unpleasant, and often unacceptable to clients.

Electric shock has numerous technical advantages over drug-induced nausea as a unconditioned stimulus (UCS) in aversion conditioning. Its onset, intensity, and duration can be precisely controlled, and it can be repeatedly paired with alcohol- or drug-related stimuli during a single treatment session. The use of electrical aversion as a component in the treatment of alcoholism has been the subject of considerable outcome research. The results of this research indicate that electrical aversion is associated with a high degree of attrition and is relatively ineffective. As a result, there is a growing concensus that its use in the treatment of alcoholism can no longer be justified (Nathan & Briddell, 1977; Nathan & Lipscomb, 1979; Wilson, 1978).

In contrast to the literature on alcoholism, there are very few reports of electrical aversion in the treatment of drug abuse, and many are uncontrolled case reports. An exception, however, is the report by Copemann (1976) in which 37 heroin abusers were administered electrical aversion therapy in a 6-month residential treatment program. At follow-up 2 years after treatment termination, 80% of those who completed treatment were, on the basis of detailed assessment including urinalysis, judged to be abstinent. Although data from such a multicomponent treatment program are inconclusive, they are promising and consistent with our own clinical experience.

In the drug project in Gainesville, Florida (Boudin *et al.* 1977), electric aversion was occasionally used during the initial stages of treatment to reduce the frequency of drug urges. The procedure consisted of a simulated, intravenous heroin injection that was immediately preceded by a strong electric shock delivered to the injection site by a portable shocker. In one case, daily treatment sessions for 3 weeks were followed by a complete suppression of drug urges, which was maintained for 7 weeks.

Electric aversion shares some of the same limitations that characterize chemical aversion. It is an unpleasant form of treatment, which increases the rate of attrition during treatment, and, although it may result in conditioned aversion responses in some clients, it does not contribute directly to the development of alternative, prosocial coping responses.

In covert sensitization, clients are first instructed to relax and then to imagine as vividly as possible a scene in which they are about to consume either alcohol or drugs. Detailed information is obtained beforehand about the typical antecedents of drinking or drug use, and they are incorporated into the imagined scene to make it as realistic as possible. Immediately after the consummatory response, a detailed and disgusting description is given of the onset of nausea and vomiting. This includes images of foul-tasting vomitus being regurgitated and expelled through the mouth and nose and contaminating the remaining alcoholic beverage or bag of heroin. The scene may end with the suggestion that the client will experience relief of these symptoms on leaving the setting and on deciding to refrain from alcohol or drug use in the future.

Although controlled research on the efficacy of covert sensitization is limited, it has been suggested that it is as effective in the treatment of alcoholism as chemical aversion (W. R. Miller, 1982). Certainly, it is far less intrusive and presumably much more acceptable than either chemical or electrical aversion. Covert sensitization, however, may not be appropriate for psychologically unsophisticated clients who have difficulty producing vivid images (Callahan & Rawson, 1980).

Extinction Techniques

Like aversion therapy, most extinction techniques used in the treatment of alcohol and drug abuse are based on a classical conditioning model (Siegel, 1979; Wikler, 1965). Rather than attempting to develop a conditioned aversion to alcohol- and drug-related stimuli, however, these techniques are intended to extinguish previously developed conditioned anticipatory responses, such as increased subjective craving, tremulousness, sweating, and pulse rate. Extinction of classically conditioned responses is achieved through repeated presentations of the conditioned stimuli and has been conducted in several different ways. Rankin, Hodgson, and Stockwell (1983), for example, have employed *in vivo* cue exposure and response prevention in an 8-week inpatient treatment program. During each of six 45-minute sessions, clients were first "primed" with two drinks of their perferred alcoholic beverage and then instructed to resist drinking a third. During successive 3-minute intervals, it was placed on a table in front of the client, held by the client at arm's length, and finally held near the mouth and sniffed. The results obtained on analog-drinking measures and on subjective ratings of craving following 18 such *in vivo* cue exposure trials together with the impressive effect of these procedures in the treatment of obsessive-compulsive disorders indicate that the procedure is worthy of further development and evaluation.

Classical conditioning procedures have also been implemented in the treatment of drug abuse and dependence. Narcotic abusers, for example, have been encouraged to engage repeatedly in the drug injection ritual using an inert substance (O'Brien, Greenstein, Ternes, McLellan, & Grabowski, 1980) or to imagine themselves engaging in the self-injection ritual using drugs but without experiencing any "rush" or euphoria (Götestam & Melin, 1974). These extinction procedures appear to hold greater therapeutic promise than the paradigm in which the subjective effects of actual drug injection are blocked by the prior administration of a narcotic antagonist. The difficulty with this latter procedure is that the administration of the antagonist appears to eliminate the conditioned anticipatory responses that must occur and go unreinforced before they can be extinguished.

Although it is based on a cognitive/behavioral rather than on a classical conditioning model, Marlatt's (1978) relapse prevention program also includes a component that may be classified as an extinction technique. More specifically, Marlatt recommends that abusive drinkers rehearse a relapse episode, either in imagination or overtly without actually drinking, in order to extinguish their self-defeating expectations that an initial "slip" will inevitably lead to a complete relapse. In extreme cases he recommends that the clinician schedule and supervise a "programmed relapse" during which the client actually consumes a drink. Procedurally, this technique resembles closely the cue exposure and response prevention technique developed by Rankin *et al.* (1983) except that it is specifically scheduled at the end of treatment and may occur outside the treatment setting. Presumably, these differences would enhance the generalizability of the extinction effect.

Controlled-Drinking Skills Training

Although reports of controlled drinking outcomes following abstinence-oriented treatment for alcoholism began to appear more than 20 years ago, it has only been in the last decade that serious consideration has been given to the development of techniques specifically intended to teach moderate drinking. Not surprisingly, there is no corresponding development to foster moderation in the use of illicit drugs, although the approach may have merit for the treatment of prescription drug abusers. Methadone and heroin maintenance are probably the most closely related developments in the treatment of drug abuse, but they do not incorporate training in the controlled use of these substances because they are already strictly controlled by legal authority.

The most widely used controlled-drinking program is behavioral self-control training (BSCT), developed by Miller and Muñoz (1976). BSCT is a comprehensive program that includes training in each of the following skills: (a) self-monitoring of alcohol consumption; (b) specification of appropriate limits for alcohol consumption; (c) drinking-rate reduction strategies; (d) self-reinforcement; (e) stimulus control procedures; and (f) alternative coping strategies. For example, a 35-year-old union negotiator in treatment with the first author was provided with wallet-sized cards on which he recorded the time, date, location, and amount of each drink. After a baseline rate of consumption was obtained, he was then provided with reading material that included information on the behavioral and physiological effects of alcohol and charts for estimating blood-alcohol concentration following the consumption of variable amounts of alcohol. Upper limits of three drinks per hour and four drinks per session were then agreed upon to ensure that his blood-alcohol concentration always remained well within the legal limit for driving. Rate reduction strategies such as alternating alcoholic and nonalcoholic beverages and ordering regular drinks rather than "doubles" were proposed as were stimulus control strategies such as drinking with moderate rather than with excessive drinkers and in locations where he was least likely to exceed his self-imposed limits. Several pleasurable activities that were assumed to function as reinforcers of his behavior were identified and made contingent upon goal attainment. Weekly consumption rates were also plotted on a graph at each session.

All of these self-control procedures were implemented within a 2-week period during which the client's self-monitored drinking rate fell from a weekly average of 64 drinks during baseline to a total of 23 drinks during the third week of treatment. Later in treatment, three sessions were devoted to heterosocial skills training and one to self-management of depression. Further treatment gains had been achieved by the time of a 3 month follow-up, and an unsolicited report from the client's wife 1½ years after treatment indicated that he had continued to drink in a nonproblematic manner. It is also noteworthy that the positive treatment outcome in this case is consistent with the available empirical evidence for the efficacy of BSCT (Miller, 1983b).

As noted previously in this chapter, controlled drinking is an appropriate treatment goal only for a selected minority of problem drinkers. Candidates for BSCT, therefore, must be carefully screened not only by a behaviorally oriented clinician, but preferably also by a physician.

Alternative Coping Skills Training

Recent analyses of relapse episodes among alcohol abusers and opiate addicts reveals that a majority of relapses occur in response to negative emotional states, including anger and frustration stemming from interpersonal conflict and direct social pressure to resume drinking and drug taking (Chaney, Roszell, & Cummings, 1982; Marlatt & Gordon, 1980). This research has given further impetus to the implementation of training programs that develop social and other skills that will serve as alternative responses to predictable antecedents of substance abuse.

Assertiveness training is probably the most widely implemented example of this approach in the treatment of alcohol and drug abuse. *Assertiveness* generally refers to the direct and appropriate expression of both positive and negative thoughts and feelings and includes a wide variety of verbal and nonverbal behaviors. In their functional analysis of the drinking episodes of a 34-year-old client following his promotion from night clerk to motel manager, Eisler, Hersen, and Miller (1974) identified three antecedent situations, all of which demanded assertive responses: (a) requesting housekeeping staff to clean the motel rooms more thoroughly; (b) refusing salesmen who insisted that he purchase items he did not need; and (c) handling unreasonable complaints made by motel patrons. After he had acquired the requisite assertive skills, the client coped more effectively with the demands of his new job, experienced less frustration and anger, and abstained from alcohol.

Although similar reports of the use of assertiveness training as a treatment component also appear in the literature on drug abuse (Callner & Ross, 1978; Hollonds, Oei, & Turecek, 1980), specific training in resisting social pressure has only been reported with alcoholics (Foy, Miller, Eisler, & O'Toole, 1976). In drink refusal training, therapists or, in the case of group treatment, other alcohol abusers, assume the roles of "friends" or relatives who repeatedly insist that the client drink with them. The client is taught to resist their efforts by (a) requesting that they stop insisting that he or she drink; (b) by suggesting an alternative activity to drinking; (c) by redirecting conversation to a topic unrelated to alcohol; (d) by maintaining eye contact while speaking to his or her companion; and (e) by using gestures, facial expressions, and voice qualities to communicate his or her resolve not to drink.

Dealing with feelings of anger and frustration and with social pressure to drink are two of the situations specifically addressed by a problem-solving skills training program developed by Chaney, O'Leary, and Marlatt (1978). Unlike assertiveness and drink refusal training, however, problem-solving training provides a more general coping skill applicable to a wider variety of problematic situations including negative emotional states such as loneliness, boredom, and depression and apparently spontaneous urges to drink. In an initial treatment outcome study, problem-solving training has been shown to reduce significantly the duration and severity of relapse episodes during the first year after treatment (Chaney *et al.*, 1978).

Training in job placement skills has been included in treatment programs for both alcohol and drug abusers. Such programs typically include training in the preparation of resumes, completion of job application forms, relaxation techniques for use before job interviews, and shaping of appropriate verbal and nonverbal behavior during roleplayed interviews. Particular attention is often given to the client's responses to questions regarding previous criminal activity and alcohol or drug abuse. The greatest shortcoming of job placement skills training and, for that matter, of all the alternative coping skills training approaches is one of generalization. Not only must the targeted skills be acquired, but they must also occur in the natural environment if they are to be of any benefit.

Contingency Management

During the last 20 years, numerous studies conducted in residential laboratories and hospital research wards have demonstrated the potent effect of environmental contingencies on the self-administration of alcohol and other drugs by substance abusers. More recently, clinical researchers have developed procedures for implementing therapeutic contingencies in the natural environment.

One of the most widely used of these procedures is the behavioral contract. Essentially, a behavioral contract is a formal written agreement between the client and the clinician that specifies the target behaviors that are to be the focus of treatment and the consequences if they occur. Behavioral contracts typically include reinforcing contingencies for the occurrence of desired behaviors, such as self-monitoring and work performance, and punishing consequences for maladaptive behaviors, such as failing to keep appointments or the use of drugs. A detailed example of a behavioral contract used in the treatment of a heroin abuser follows in a later section of this chapter.

The literature on alcohol and drug abuse includes numerous examples of contingency management in outpatient settings. In one study, 10 chronic public drunkenness offenders who ordinarily had noncontingent access to meals, cigarettes, clothing, and accommodation at a Salvation Army shelter forfeited them for a period of 5 days if they were judged by agency personnel to be grossly intoxicated or if their blood-alcohol concentration exceeded 10 mg/% at randomly scheduled breath tests (Miller, 1975). In the treatment of clients with alcohol and heroin dependence, Liebson, Tommasello, and Bigelow (1978) made methadone consumption contingent upon prior consumption of disulfiram. Because disulfiram reacts with alcohol to produce a variety of aversive physical reactions including nausea and vomiting, the contingent administration of methadone for the treatment of heroin dependence also ensured continued sobriety. To reduce multiple illicit drug use among other methadone maintenance clients, Glosser (1983) made the acquisition of methadone contingent upon drug-free urinalyses. A final example is the comprehensive community reinforcement program developed by Azrin and his colleagues (Azrin, 1976; Azrin, Sisson, Meyers, & Godley, 1982; Hunt & Azrin, 1973). After ensuring access to multiple social reinforcers in the community, including employment, recreational activities at a social club for abstainers, and reestablished marital and family relationships, behavioral contracts were prepared that made these reinforcers contingent upon taking disulfiram, attending therapy sessions, providing daily activity reports, and meeting with a peer adviser. The treatment outcome in this program, as in all these examples provided with contingency management procedures, was impressive.

Detecting the occurrence and verifying the nonoccurrence of target behaviors is probably the greatest limitation to the implementation of contingency contracting on an outpatient basis. In addition to the technical limitations inherent in the assessment procedures themselves, considerable resources, including treatment personnel, laboratory, and communication equipment are often required for extended periods of time to maintain the necessary degree of client surveillance (Boudin, 1980). Although utilization of collaterals such as the friends, relatives, and employers of clients may reduce these costs, contingency management programs are often expensive to operate and, consequently, are subject to the threat of discontinued or reduced funding. Gaining access to potent reinforcers and ensuring that the treatment is acceptable to potential clients may also pose problems. Despite the stringent behavioral control in some outpatient contingency management programs, they are in many respects no more restrictive than inpatient or residential treatment programs.

Case Study

Miss W. L., a 25-year-old secretary, referred herself to the Drug Project in Gainesville, Florida, for treatment of heroin dependence. She reported that she could not continue to be absent from work without losing her job and that she was feeling depressed and "losing hold of reality." She had begun using heroin intermittently while in another state 2 years earlier; during the year prior to her referral she was using one to three bags (60 to 80 mg) daily.

Miss W. L. was the oldest of three children and the daughter of a self-employed building contractor who had a history of alcoholism that began after his return from active duty overseas. She recalled episodes when he became angry and depressed and left the house for hours at a time. She also recalled having been unfavorably treated by her parents who doted on her younger sister. Her feelings of anger and rejection at this time appeared to contribute to a general sense of low self-esteem and persistent anxiety and depression that, during her later teens, were alleviated by her use of marijuana and other hallucinogens. After finishing high school, Miss W. L. left her family in the Midwest and moved to Los Angeles where she began using heroin while living with a group of friends who were also dependent on opiates. She described her life in Los Angeles in the following terms:

> I was the only person there amidst millions of people. Lost all my "rules." Got strung out on junk. Discovered further intensity to despondency and frustration as well as higher highs, but not many. Felt that anything could happen to me. I did think I was dying one night from shooting an impurity. I was nearly busted, my friends actually were . . . enough. Escaped to Florida. Disoriented.

When she moved to Florida she, continued the pattern of heroin dependence previously established in California. "Fell in with Gainesville junkies. They were a lot like the people in L.A." Her feelings of anxiety and depression persisted but were relieved by her use of heroin. The signs of substance abuse quickly became evident and included poor job performance, absenteeism, and multiple crises in interpersonal relationships.

During her initial contact at the Drug Project, Miss W. L. was fully informed of the assessment and treatment procedures employed in the program and, at the conclusion of the meeting, she was instructed to call the Project office immediately prior to her next "fix." When she subsequently called that evening to report that she was preparing to "shoot" heroin, she was kept talking on the telephone while the therapist went to her home. It was expected that such a dramatic and personal intervention would prompt her to make a strong commitment to abstinence from heroin and other drugs. Indeed, she appeared emotionally relieved, cried, and stated that this convinced her to enter the program. The following written commitment was negotiated in her home that evening:

> I have in my possession a hit of heroin. Being weak I'm going to do half of it. The rest, including my works [*paraphernalia*], I'm handing over to Dr. Boudin to do with as he pleases. From this time on, with as much strength as I can muster, I will put my trust in him to handle my case, as he knows more how to stimulate me to help myself towards progress and growth than I do at this stage of my life. I'm trying to say with all good intentions this will be the last time I will do junk.

> Signed: Miss W. L.
> Date: May 2, 1972

At her appointment the next day, Miss W. L. was presented with the other half of her "hit" of heroin. This was done to emphasize to her that her participation in the treatment program was entirely voluntary and that she was not in any way being coerced or manipulated. However it might be accomplished, the development of a trusting relationship and a strong commitment to the goals of therapy, free of duress, are as much essential prerequisites for contingency contracting as they are for any other behavioral intervention. On being presented with the heroin, she promptly flushed it down the toilet.

During the same sessions, a structured interview was administered and Miss W. L. was instructed to continue to record on a daily basis her thoughts, feelings, and significant daily events in her diary. She also was instructed to call the Project office at regular intervals each day to report the frequency of a number of responses that she monitored using wrist counters. By means of these assessment procedures, daily records were obtained on each of the following variables: the use of all drugs including marijuana, hashish, cigarettes, and Quaaludes; her thoughts about using drugs; her urges, including physiological withdrawal symptoms, to use drugs; her thoughts of breaking her initial commitment to abstain from heroin and later of breaking the contingency contract; her frustration in social situations; and what she herself referred to as *karma balance* that essentially was a rating of her feelings of contentment. Finally, the procedures and random scheduling of urine specimen collection were described in detail.

During the eight sessions conducted during the following 2 weeks, the following treatment objectives were identified: (a) to discontinue her use of heroin; (b) to develop appropriate social behaviors that could be used as alternative responses to drug use; (c) to reduce her feelings of anxiety and depression; and (d) to develop self-control through a hierarchical series of contractual obligations and reinforcers. Following is the contract that was completed and signed two weeks after Miss W. L. made her first written commitment to discontinue using heroin:

I. We, _____, _____, and _____, agree to uphold and abide by the following terms and conditions set by this contract, and we acknowledge that this contract is valid and binding.

II. Responsibilities of First Party to Second Party

I, _____, accept the following terms and conditions as necessary for me to change my lifestyle which has been up to this time, determined by my dependence upon and frequent use of dangerous and illicit drugs. The following articles specify the nature of my duties and obligations to Dr. Boudin and the Drug Project. I am wholly accountable for my actions concerning the observance of said responsibilities.

A. I shall no longer use amphetamines, barbiturates, narcotics, tranquilizers, opiates, sedatives, hypnotics, CNS stimulants (except caffeine), analgesics (except over-the-counter preparations such as "aspirin") or any other prescription drug except when specifically dispensed for my use.

B. I shall inform *all persons* about this contract whose presence constitutes a possible or probable threat to my independence from drugs. I shall indicate that I am unable to use drugs at any time, and that I am working in therapy specifically on this problem.

C. I agree to notify a staff member immediately of any intention to use drugs or of any situations involving the use of drugs in my presence. When I am alone and *beginning* to think of acting on an urge to take drugs or to obtain them, I will also contact a staff member.

D. Each day I will contact a staff member by telephone at 12:00 noon, 6:00 P.M., 9:00 P.M., and at bedtime. I will inform him of my activities and use of drugs or thoughts of using or obtaining drugs since my previous phone call. I will also inform the staff member of the activities I am planning for the next interval.

E. I will carry with me at all times wrist counters on which I will record the following: (a) drug thoughts and urges; (b) use of marijuana, hashish, cigarettes, and prescribed Quaaludes; (c) ratings of my discomfort in social situations; (d) opportunities to relax; (e) thoughts of breaking this contract: (f) karma balance (self-rated feelings of contentment); and (g) sexual contact. I also agree to record any additional behaviors which are deemed necessary by the staff.

F. I agree to provide the self-monitored information to a staff member at each telephone call and to enter it on the forms provided for me.

G. I will provide urine specimens for analysis whenever the staff deem it necessary and at randomly scheduled (24 hour) spot checks.

H. I will deposit $10.00 weekly into a joint savings account held by the Project staff and me for the purchase of reinforcers contingent upon my compliance with this contract.

I. I agree to comply with any requests of the staff to provide information, to make appointments, and to change my living conditions.

J. If I am unable to keep an appointment with my therapist or employer, I will provide a legitimate excuse beforehand by telephone.

K. I agree to write daily in my diary.

III. Consequences for Breach of Contract

Failure to meet the above responsibilities will result in the following set of consequences which will be meted out consistently and immediately following any breach of this contract.

A. If I am more than ten minutes late in making the specified phone calls or in keeping any appointment, I will forfeit from my bank account $.50 for the first additional 5-minute interval; $1.00 for the second 5-minute interval; $1.50 for the third 5-minute interval; and my entire weekly allowance of $10.00 if I am more than 25 minutes late.

B. If I am late for two consecutive phone calls or appointments or if I fail to fulfill any of my other responsibilities specified in this contract, I will forfeit $10.00 which will be used for the apprehension and conviction of other local drug abusers.

IV. Privileges and Bonuses Due to the First Party

For compliance with the terms of this contract, I am entitled to the following privileges and bonuses:

A. Mutually agreed upon amendments to this contract may be made.

B. If I abide by all of the terms of this contract for seven consecutive days, I will be given money to buy one record album and $10.00 will be placed into a special account for the purchase of a stereo and clothes.

C. If I abide by this contract for two consecutive weeks, I shall receive a $.50 increase in my daily allowance and $10.00 will be withdrawn from my special account for me to purchase clothes. When I have sufficient earnings, I may also choose and purchase my own stereo.

D. My allowance will be available at the Project office according to the following schedule, provided I continue to observe all the terms of my contract: (a) daily for the first 2 weeks of the contract; (b) alternate days for the second 2 weeks of the contract; (c) at 3-day intervals for the third 2 weeks of the contract; (d) at 4-day intervals for the fourth 2 weeks of the contract; and (e) weekly following two consecutive months of observance. If, however, I break even one term of this contract, I will revert back to my original daily allowance and the schedule for receiving it.

E. I shall be paid $.10 for each page I write in my log.

V. Responsibilities of the Second Party to the First Party

We, _____, and _____, and responsible for the following activities in regard to _____.

A. We agree to monitor her behavior, provide therapy and keep all appointments made with her. We also agree to have a responsible person attend Miss W. L. at her request in a crisis.

B. We assume complete responsibility for the management of joint bank accounts and agree not to use any of her funds except for reasons specified in this contract.

C. We may make mutually agreed upon amendments to this contract at any time.

This contract is valid and binding from this day _____, until such time as both parties mutually consent to dissolve it.

‾‾‾‾‾‾
First Party

‾‾‾‾‾‾
Second Party

‾‾‾‾‾‾
Witness

    After the contract was implemented, treatment sessions were scheduled twice weekly to monitor compliance and to implement additional treatment techniques selected on the basis of a functional analysis of Miss W. L.'s self-reported data. Minor breaches of the contract occurred infrequently, and Miss W. L. stoically accepted imposition of the prespecified fines. A major breach of the contract occurred during Week 8, however, when she failed to notify Project staff that she had found herself in a situation where illicit drugs were available. Later the same

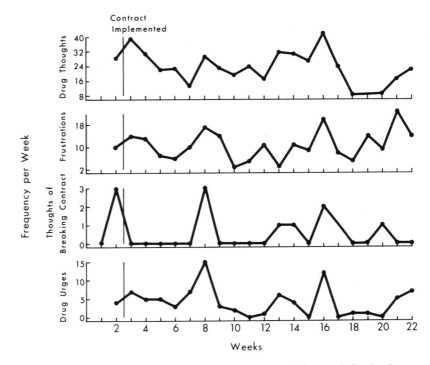

Figure 1. Mean weekly frequency of targeted subjective responses before and after implementation of the contingency contract.

day, she "shot up" with heroin, which was subsequently detected by urinalysis. The consequences specified in the contract were therefore imposed. On two subsequent occasions during the first 6 months of treatment, when drugs were available, Miss W. L. did not self-administer them but instead contacted Project staff by voice pager and requested immediate support. During the last 6 months, Miss W. L. reported two additional "crises," neither of which resulted in heroin use.

Weekly frequency of four of the self-monitored responses are presented in Figure 1. During the first 8 weeks of treatment, drug thoughts, drug urges, and thoughts of breaking the contract appeared to be positively correlated with "frustrations," occasions when Miss W. L. was thwarted in obtaining satisfactory outcomes in interpersonal relationships. As a result of these findings, subsequent treatment sessions focused on the development of social skills, including assertiveness. Although frustrating situations continued to occur and Miss W. L. continued to experience difficulty in them, she also reported during treatment sessions and in her diary that she was gradually becoming more assertive and less likely to consider heroin use as an escape from these situations. Consistent with these reports, it is evident from Figure 1 that subsequent peaks in the frequency of frustrations on Weeks 16 and 21 were not accompanied by increases of the same magnitude in cognitions relating to drug use and contract termination. Moreover, gradual reductions in the frequency of these cognitions are evident during the first 22 weeks of treatment.

After completing 1 year in treatment, Miss W. L. became a regular instructor in the Drug Project's paraprofessional training program, and several months later she became an instructor in a course on drug abuse offered at a local university. She continued to give randomly scheduled weekly urine specimens for 4 years following treatment for which she was paid at the rate of $5.00 per week. No further episodes of heroin self-administration were reported or detected during this period. Eleven years after treatment was initiated, Miss W. L. reported being drug free, fully employed at the managerial level in the entertainment industry, and leading an active social and personal life, devoting much of her time to the Nichiran Shoshu World Peace Organization.

Assessment of Treatment Efficacy

The assessment of treatment efficacy requires the retrieval of valid data on a number of treatment-related dependent variables including work performance, school performance, legal problems, drug use, and emotional stability. The procedures involved in obtaining these data during treatment and at follow-up can be conceptualized as a negotiation process in which the client and the clinician arrive at a mutually acceptable arrangement concerning the validation and continuity of data.

The purpose of this negotiation is to facilitate continuous collection of dependent measures that range on a continuum from "soft" to "hard," depending on the degree of validation inherent in the data-gathering process. For example, "hard" data relating to work performance may consist of daily employer reports regarding the hours of work together with weekly pay stubs collected by the client. "Soft" data in this area would consist of self-reports of the number of hours worked and rate of pay. Obviously, the clinician's objective, within the limits of sound clinical judgment, is to obtain hard data to verify treatment effects. Furthermore, if clients are to be paid for this information, hard data should be regarded as having higher value than soft data. In addition, the length of time a client provides these data continuously can determine the rate of pay as well. Thus, monetary remuneration should be based upon both the quality and continuity of data received.

Table 1 lists in order from hard to soft the parameters used in the negotiation of follow-up contracts between former clients and treatment personnel at the Drug Project in Gainesville, Florida.

An equally important consideration in these negotiations is the schedule that determines the data flow. Data collection schedules can be classified as totally random, partially random, or fixed. A totally random schedule is in effect when the subject is completely unaware of the time the data will be collected. For example, random collection of urine specimens can occur at any time of the day or night on any night of the week. A partially random schedule is in effect when the subject prearranges specific time parameters during which data collection can occur. This type of schedule has elements of randomness and predictability. For example, urine collections may occur between 6:00 P.M. to 12:00 A.M. Monday through Friday but not on weekends. Urine collection and work or school site visits should always be scheduled on a totally or partially random basis. A fixed schedule is one where data collection is in effect at times prespecified by the subject. Weekly fixed

Table 1. Parameters Used in Negotiating Data Collection Procedures

Urine specimen collection	Work performance	School performance	Legal status
Monitored specimen at clinic	Presentation of actual time card	Transcripts and instructor's written report	Court records
Monitored specimen at home	Written employer report	Instructor's verbal report	Probation reports
Personal search and unmonitored sample at clinic	Verbal employer report	Registration cards	Prison records
Personal and bathroom search and unmonitored sample at home	Paycheck stub	School visits	Public records (newspaper)
Unmonitored sample at clinic	Employer receipt	Significant other reports	Significant other reports
Personal search and unmonitored sample at home	Visit to worksite	Unvalidated self-report	Unvalidated self-reports
Bathroom search and unmonitored sample at home	Phone call to worksite		
Sample monitored by collateral	Deposits in bank account		
Unmonitored sample at home	Significant other reports		
	Unvalidated self-report		

schedules are used extensively in gathering information on work, school, and court attendance as well as paper-and-pencil test results.

It is essential to recognize during negotiation about data collection that clients may be justifiably concerned with intrusions into their place of work, school, and social life and that these arrangements must be negotiated with sensitivity. In fact, the clinician must evaluate whether such intrusions themselves will negatively affect treatment outcome.

Summary

Substance abuse and dependence are prevalent, complex disorders that affect not only health, but virtually every other area of functioning. Consequently, clinical assessment must not only include measures of alcohol and drug ingestion but also of interpersonal behavior and cognitive and affective states, all of which may be affected by and/or be functionally related to the use of these substances. Furthermore, because all of the assessment methods described earlier have inherent limitations, it is recommended that a combination of procedures including self-report, observational, and physiological measures be utilized in the assessment of these clients.

Numerous approaches, including aversion therapy, alternative coping skills training, and contingency management have been developed for the treatment of substance abuse and dependence. Given that these disorders have multiple determinants, however, the optimal approach to treatment is one in which a combination of procedures is employed, each selected on the basis of an objective and continuous assessment of the client. Although most of the individual treatment techniques are as yet unsupported by adequately controlled empirical research, the results obtained by multicomponent treatment programs are promising. It is for future clinical research to identify more specifically the effective components used in these programs and to define more precisely the criteria for optimal matching of client and treatment.

ACKNOWLEDGMENTS

We wish to thank Christina McMillan and Barbara Beach who assisted in the preparation of the manuscript.

References

American Psychiatric Association. (1980). *Diagnostic and statistical manual of mental disorders* (3rd ed.). Washington, DC: Author.

Azrin, N. H. (1976). Improvements in the community-reinforcement approach to alcoholism. *Behavior Research and Therapy, 14,* 339–348.

Azrin, N. H., Sisson, R. W., Meyers, R., & Godley, M. (1982). Outpatient alcoholism treatment by disulfiram and community-reinforcement therapy. *Journal of Behavior Therapy and Experimental Psychiatry, 13,* 105–112.

Babor, T. F., Meyer, R. E., Mirin, S. M., McNamee, H. B., & Davies, M. (1976). Behavioral and social effects of heroin self-administration and withdrawal. *Archives of General Psychiatry, 33,* 363–367.

Boudin, H. M. (1980). Contingency contracting with drug abusers in the natural environment: Treatment evaluation. In L. C. Sobell, M. B. Sobell, & E. Ward (Eds.), *Evaluating alcohol and drug abuse treatment effectiveness: recent advances* (pp. 109–128). New York: Plenum Press.

Boudin, H. M., & Valentine, V. E. (1972). *Behavioral techniques as an alternative to methadone maintenance.* Unpublished manuscript, University of Florida.

Boudin, H. M., Valentine, V. E., Ingram, R. D., Brantley, J. M., Ruiz, M. R., Smith, G. G., Catlin, R. P., & Regan, E. J. (1977) Contingency contracting with drug abusers in the natural environment. *The International Journal of Addictions, 12,* 1–16.

Brandsma, J. M., Maultsby, M. C., & Welsh, R. J. (1980). *Outpatient treatment of alcoholism: A review and a comparative study.* Baltimore: University Park Press.

Brown, S. A., Goldman, M. S., Inn, A., & Anderson, L. (1980). Expectations of reinforcement from alcohol: Their domain and relation to drinking patterns. *Journal of Consulting and Clinical Psychology, 48,* 419–426.

Brownell, K. D. (1984). Behavioral medicine. In G. T. Wilson, C. M. Franks, K. D. Brownell, & P. C. Kendall (Eds.), *Annual review of behavior therapy: Theory and practice* (Vol. 9) (pp. 180–210). New York: Guilford Press.

Brownell, K. D., (1982). The addictive disorders. In C. M. Franks, G. T. Wilson, P. C. Kendall, & K. D. Brownell (Eds.), *Annual review of behavior therapy: Theory and practice* (Vol. 8) (pp. 211–258). New York: Guilford Press.

Callahan, E. J., & Rawson, R. S. (1980). Behavioral assessment and treatment evaluation of narcotic addiction. In L. C. Sobell, M. B. Sobell, & E. Ward (Eds.), *Evaluating alcohol and drug abuse treatment effectiveness: Recent advances* (pp. 77–91). New York: Pergamon Press.

Callner, D. A., & Ross, S. M. (1978). The assessment and training of assertive skills with drug addicts: A preliminary study. *International Journal of the Addictions, 13,* 227–239.

Chaney, E. F., O'Leary, M. R., & Marlatt, G. A. (1978). Skill training with alcoholics. *Journal of Consulting and Clinical Psychology, 46,* 1092–1104.

Chaney, E. F., Roszell, D. K., & Cummings, C. (1982). Relapse in opiate addicts: A behavioral analysis. *Addictive Behaviors, 7,* 291–297.

Copemann, C. D. (1976). Drug addiction: II. An aversive counterconditioning technique for treatment. *Psychology Reports, 38,* 1271–1281.

Eisler, R. M., Hersen, M., & Miller, P. M. (1974). Shaping components of assertive behavior with instructions and feedback. *American Journal of Psychiatry, 30,* 643–649.

Foy, D. W., Miller, P. M., Eisler, R. W., & O'Toole, D. H. (1976). Social skills training to teach alcoholics to refuse drinks effectively. *Journal of Studies on Alcohol, 37,* 1340–1345.

Glosser, D. S. (1983). The use of a token economy to reduce illicit drug use among methadone maintenance clients. *Addictive Behaviors, 8,* 93–104.

Götestam, K. G., & Melin, L. (1974). Covert extinction of amphetamine addiction. *Behavior Therapy, 5,* 90–92.

Hay, W. M., & Nathan, P. E. (1982). *Clinical case studies in the behavioral treatment of alcoholism.* New York: Plenum Press.

Hersen, M., & Bellack, A. S. (Eds.). (1981). *Behavioral assessment: A practical handbook* (2nd ed.). New York: Pergamon Press.

Hollonds, G. B., Oei, T. P. S., & Turecek, L. R. (1980). An evaluation of a behavior therapy programme as an intervention treatment for the fear of withdrawal with heroin-dependent persons. *Drug and Alcohol Dependence, 5,* 153–160.

Hunt, G. M., & Azrin, N. H. (1973). A community-reinforcement approach to alcoholism. *Behaviour Research and Therapy, 11,* 91–104.

Knowles, P. L. (1983). Inpatient versus outpatient treatment of substance misuse in hospitals, 1975–1980. *Journal of Studies on Alcohol, 44,* 384–387.

Kwentus, J., & Major, L. F. (1979). Disulfiram in the treatment of alcoholism. *Journal of Studies on Alcohol, 40,* 428–446.

Lawson, D. M., Wilson, G. T., Briddell, D. W., & Ives, C. C. (1976). Assessment and modification of alcoholics' drinking behavior in controlled laboratory settings: A cautionary note. *Addictive Behaviors, 1,* 299–303.

Liebson, I. A., Tommasello, A., & Bigelow, G. E. (1978). A behavioral treatment of alcoholic methadone patients. *Annals of Internal Medicine, 89,* 342–344.

Marlatt, G. A. (1976). The Drinking Profile—A questionnaire for the behavioral assessment of alco-holism. In E. J. Mash & L. G. Terdal (Eds.), *Behavior therapy assessment: Diagnosis, design and eval-uation* (pp. 121–137). New York: Springer.

Marlatt, G. A. (1978). Craving for alcohol, loss of control, and relapse: A cognitive-behavioral analysis. In P. E. Nathan, G. A. Marlatt, & T. Loberg (Eds.), *Alcoholism: New directions in behavioral research and treatment* (pp. 271–314). New York: Plenum Press.

Marlatt, G. A. (1983). The controlled-drinking controversy: A commentary. *American Psychologist, 38,* 1097–1110.

Marlatt, G. A., & Donovan, D. M. (1981). Alcoholism and drug dependence: Cognitive social learning factors in addictive behaviors. In W. E. Craighead, A. E. Kazdin, & M. J. Mahoney (Eds.), *Behavior modification: Principles, issues and applications* (2nd ed.) (pp. 264–285). New York: Houghton Mifflin.

Marlatt, G. A., & Gordon, J. R. (1980). Determinants of relapse: Implications for the maintenance of behavior change. In P. O. Davidson & S. M. Davidson (Eds.), *Behavioral medicine: Changing health lifestyles* (pp. 410–452). New York: Brunner/Mazel.

Miller, P. M. (1975). A behavioral intervention program for chronic public drunkenness offenders. *Archives of General Psychiatry, 32,* 915–918.

Miller, P. M. (1976). *Behavioral treatment of alcoholism.* New York: Pergamon Press.

Miller, W. R. (1982). Treating problem drinkers: What works? *The Behavior Therapist, 5,* 15–18.

Miller, W. R. (1983). Motivational interviewing with problem drinkers. *Behavioral Psychotherapy, 11,* 147–172. (a)

Miller, W. R. (1983). Controlled drinking: A history and a critical review. *Journal of Studies on Alcohol, 44,* 68–83. (b)

Miller, W. R., & Hester, R. K. (1980). Treating the problem drinker: Modern approaches. In W. R. Miller (Ed.), *The addictive behaviors: Treatment of alcoholism, drug abuse, smoking and obesity.* New York: Pergamon Press.

Miller, W. R., & Muñoz, R. F. (1976). *How to control your drinking.* Englewood Cliffs, NJ: Prentice-Hall.

Miller, W. R., Crawford, V. L., & Taylor, C. A. (1979). Significant others as corroborative sources for problem drinkers. *Addictive Behaviors, 4,* 67–70.

Mirin, S. M., Meyer, R. E., & McNamee, B. (1976). Psychopathology and mood during heroin use: Acute vs. chronic effects. *Archives of General Psychiatry, 33,* 1503–1508.

Nathan, P. E., & Briddell, D. W. (1977). Behavioral assessment and treatment of alcoholism. In B. Kissin & H. Begleiter (Eds.), *The biology of alcoholism* (Vol. 5) (pp. 301–349). New York: Plenum Press.

Nathan, P. E., & Lipscomb, T. R. (1979). Behavior therapy and behavior modification in the treatment of alcoholism. In J. H. Mendelson & N. K. Mello (Eds.), *The diagnosis and treatment of alcoholism* (pp. 305–357). New York: McGraw-Hill.

Nathan, P. E., & O'Brien, J. S. (1971). An experimental analysis of the behavior of alcoholics and normal drinkers during prolonged experimental drinking: A necessary precursor to behavioral therapy? *Behavior Therapy, 2,* 455–476.

O'Brien, C. P., Greenstein, R., Ternes, J., McLellan, A. T., & Grabowski, J. (1980). Unreinforced self-injections: Effects on rituals and outcome in heroin addicts. In L. S. Harris (Ed.), *Problems of drug dependence, 1979* (DHEW Publication No. ADM 80–901). Washington, DC: U.S. Government Print-ing Office.

Polich, J. M. (1982). The validity of self-reports in alcoholism research. *Additive Behaviors, 1,* 123–132.

Quayle, D. (1983). American productivity: The devastating effect of alcoholism and alcohol abuse. *Amer-ican Psychologist, 38,* 454–458.

Rankin, H., Hodgson, R., & Stockwell, T. (1983). Cue exposure and response prevention with alcohol-ics: A controlled trial. *Behavior Research and Therapy, 21,* 435–446.

Rosenbluth, J., Nathan, P. E., & Lawson, D. M. (1978). Environmental influences on drinking by college students in a college pub: Behavioral observation in the natural environment. *Addictive Behaviors, 3,* 117–121.

Selzer, M. L. (1971). The Michigan Alcoholism Screening Test: The quest for a new diagnostic instru-ment. *American Journal of Psychiatry, 127,* 1653–1658.

Siegel, J. (1976). Psychological testing and the detection of drug abusers. *The International Journal of the Addictions, 11,* 1031–1043.

Siegel, S. (1979). The role of conditioning in drug tolerance and addiction. In J. D. Keehn (Ed.), *Psy-chopathology in animals: Research and clinical applications* (pp. 143–168). New York: Academic Press.

Skinner, H. A. (1979). A multivariate evaluation of the MAST. *Journal of Studies on Alcohol, 40,* 831–844.

Skinner, H. A. (1982). The drug abuse screening test. *Addictive Behaviors, 7,* 363–371.

Sobell, M. B., & Sobell, L. C. A. (1975). A brief technical report on the MOBAT: An inexpensive portable test for determining blood alcohol concentration. *Journal of Applied Behavior Analysis, 8,* 117–120.

Southwick, L., Stelle, C., Marlatt, G. A., & Lindell, M. (1981). Alcohol-related expectancies: Defined by phase of intoxication and drinking experience. *Journal of Consulting and Clinical Psychology, 49,* 713–721.

Stitzer, M. L., Bigelow, G. E., & McCaul, M. E. (1983). Behavioral approaches to drug abuse. In M. Hersen, R. M. Eisler, & P. M. Miller (Eds.), *Progress in Behavior Modication, 14,* 49–124.

Twentyman, C. T., Greenwald, D. P., Greenwald, M. A., Kloss, J. D., Kovaleski, M. E., & Zibung-Hoffman, P. (1982). An assessment of social skills deficits in alcoholics. *Behavioral Assessment, 4,* 317–326.

Wanberg, K. W., & Horn, J. L. (1983). Assessment of alcohol use with multi-dimensional concepts and measures. *American Psychologist, 38,* 1055–1069.

Wiens, A. N., & Menustik, C. E. (1983). Treatment outcome and patient characteristics in an aversion therapy program for alcoholism. *American Psychologist, 38,* 1096–1098.

Wikler, A. (1965). Conditioning factors in opiate addiction and relapse. In D. Wilner & G. Kassenbaum (Eds.), *Narcotics* (pp. 85–100). New York: McGraw-Hill.

Wilson, G. T. (1978). Alcoholism and aversion therapy: Issues, ethics and evidence. In G. A. Marlatt & P. E. Nathan (Eds.), *Behavioral approaches to alcoholism* (pp. 90–103). New Brunswick, N. J.: Rutgers Center of Alcohol Studies.

Zung, B. J. (1979). Psychometric properties of the MAST and two briefer versions. *Journal of Studies on Alcohol, 40,* 845–859.

12

Insomnia

KENNETH L. LICHSTEIN AND SUZANNE M. FISCHER

Sleep taken at regular intervals has been an indispensable part of human and virtually all mammalian life. Yet its ephemeral and delicate nature remains poised to introduce the pain of insomnia when strained by momentous, but more often, trivial irritants. An extra sip of coffee, an awkward glance by a supervisor, or a barely audible noise in the home at bedtime may steal sleep from us. Left in its place is frustration and the nagging heritage of inadequate sleep that haunts us the next day.

Most simply defined, *insomnia* refers to difficulty in sleeping. Carefully conducted, large-scale surveys disagree on the incidence of chronic insomnia, with estimates ranging from 10% (Kripke, Simons, Garfinkel, & Hammond, 1979) to 30% (Bixler, Kales, Soldatos, Kales, & Healey, 1979) of the adult population. Data on sleep medication consumption gives further insight into the magnitude of the insomnia problem. In 1973, an estimated 3% of the U.S. adult population spent $114 million on 37 million hypnotic prescriptions, and another 6% of adults consumed over-the-counter sleep medications (Balter & Bauer, 1975). By the late 1970s, consumption of hypnotic medications had declined by about one-third but was still alarmingly high in absolute terms (Institute of Medicine, 1979).

Insomnia is not equally distributed throughout the population. It is more frequent among the elderly (Bixler *et al.*, 1979; McGhie & Russell, 1962) and among women (Karacan, Warheit, Thornby, Schwab, & Williams, 1973; Kripke *et al.*, 1979). Childhood insomnia is infrequently encountered by professionals, partly because parents often do not recognize or appreciate the problem and childhood insomnia covaries with other symptomatology, such as hyperactivity, which com-

KENNETH L. LICHSTEIN and SUZANNE M. FISCHER • Department of Psychology, Memphis State University, Memphis, Tennessee 38152.

mand a higher treatment priority (Bergman, 1976; Dixon, Monroe, & Jakim, 1981).

Definition of Insomnia

The reigning sleep classificatory system was published by the Association of Sleep Disorders Centers in 1979. It denotes four broad categories of sleep disturbance: (a) disorders of initiating and maintaining sleep (DIMS); (b) disorders of excessive somnolence (DOES, e.g., narcolepsy and sleep apnea); (c) disorders of the sleep/wake schedule (e.g., shiftwork effects and delayed sleep phase syndrome); and (d) dysfunctions associated with sleep, sleep stages, or partial arousals (heterogeneous disorders of atypical conduct during sleep including sleepwalking, nightmares, and enuresis).

Category A (DIMS) incorporates insomnia, and Categories B, C, and D are tangential to the present discussion. The nine sections of the DIMS category are summarized in Table 1. Section 1, psychophysiological DIMS, corresponds to the customary meaning of the word *insomnia*. Insomnia may take the form of difficulty in falling asleep (sleep-onset insomnia) or in staying asleep (sleep-maintenance insomnia). There are two varieties of the latter type: intermittent awakenings during the night and early morning awakening with the inability to fall back to sleep. Clinicians (e.g., Beutler, Thornby, & Karacan, 1978) rely on the distinction between primary (of psychological origin, see Table 1, Section 1) and secondary (see Table 1, Sections 2 to 8) insomnia. The latter denotes insomnia as the side effect of another disorder (e.g., psychiatric disturbance, pain states) commanding primary attention.

Specific, standardized duration and frequency criteria for insomnia are not available. Most clinicians observe the guideline of latency to sleep exceeding 30 minutes in diagnosing sleep-onset insomnia. Quantitative criteria for sleep maintenance insomnia are less clear. In general, affixing of a diagnosis of insomnia is dependent largely on the urgency of the client's complaint.

Table 1. Subtypes of Insomnia According to the Association of Sleep Disorders Center Nosology[a]

Subtypes	Description
1. Psychophysiological DIMS	Insomnia based on chronic, somatized tension anxiety and negative conditioning. Often diagnosed by exclusion: an objectively verified insomnia that seems unrelated to either medical disease or to serious psychiatric problems. It is postulated that an organic predisposition toward poor sleep and hyperarousal is aggravated, in a vicious cycle, by behavioral factors. Other characteristics of this type of insomnia: patient sleeps better away from the customary sleep environment or falls asleep easily when not trying to sleep.
2. DIMS associated with psychiatric disturbance	Clear psychiatric conditions are present, diagnosable by DSM-III criteria. The insomnia is interpreted as a symptom of the underlying psychopathology, although the precise interactions among psychological processes, biochemical events, and sleep mechanisms are as yet poorly understood.

Table 1. Subtypes of Insomnia According to the Association of Sleep Disorders Center Nosology (cont.)

Subtypes	Description
3. DIMS associated with use of drugs and alcohol use	Chronic ingestion of hypnotic medication, alcohol, or other CNS depressants over weeks and months may lead to tolerance and loss of soporific effects, occasionally even to a paradoxical disruption of natural sleep. Withdrawal symptoms from these CNS depressants include severe sleeplessness. The chronic use of and/or withdrawal from numerous other drugs also may lead to sleep disturbances. Gradual reduction and eventual elimination of the drug is required before diagnosis can be made with confidence.
4. DIMS associated with sleep-induced respiratory impairment	Frequent arousals leading to a complaint of insomnia may be secondary to either a total cessation of breathing or to a severe decrease in ventilation during sleep. In patients complaining of DIMS, this is often a central (brainstem) problem. Less frequently, upper airway obstructions prevent ventilation. In this latter case, intermittent snoring and gasping can be observed. The assessment of severity in respiratory impairment involves the continuous recording of blood gasses (e.g., ear oxymetry). A medical condition, apparently not treatable by behavior therapy.
5. DIMS associated with sleep-related myoclonus and "restless legs"	Nocturnal myoclonus involves periodic episodes of repetitive and highly stereotyped leg muscle jerks that disturb sleep. Patients rarely know of these twitches, but bed partners can describe them. "Restless legs" are defined as extremely disagreeable, deep, creeping sensations inside the calves, thighs, or arms whenever relaxing. These very uncomfortable, but not painful, sensations disappear when exercising the limbs. The condition has to be separated from the agitation and motor restlessness of anxiety. Both nocturnal myoclonus and "restless legs" are medical conditions, apparently not treatable by behavior therapy.
6. DIMS associated with other medical, toxic, and environmental conditions	Many agents in the internal and external environment of the individual can disturb sleep. Elimination of the sleep problem occurs once the source condition has been identified and is removed.
7. Childhood-onset DIMS	A relentless insomnia characterized by a history of unexplained sleep disturbances starting well before puberty. Often associated with other symptoms of arousal difficulties, such as attention-deficit disorders. It is postulated that the basic sleep/wake system is organically (neurologically) disturbed.
8. DIMS associated with other conditions	This category involves a number of sleep disturbances that can only be diagnosed by polygraph, e.g., repeated awakening from REM sleep or the intrusion of waking (alpha) waves into non-REM sleep. This latter condition is often called "nonrestorative" sleep.
9. No DIMS abnormality	Classified here are those patients who present with a convincing and honest complaint of insomnia—made by an individual lacking apparent psychopathology—that is not substantiated by polysomnogram. This involves the relatively large group of poor sleepers discussed in this article as "subjective" insomniacs. Also classified here are short sleepers; i.e., patients who habitually sleep very few hours without apparent effects on wakefulness.

Note. DIMS = disorders of initiating and maintaining sleep (insomnia): DSM-III = third edition of the *Diagnostic and Statistical Manual of Mental Disorders* (American Psychiatric Association, 1980); CNS = central nervous system.

[a]Adapted from "Insomnia" by T. D. Borkovec, 1982, *Journal of Consulting and Clinical Psychology, 50,* 880–895. Copyright 1982 by the American Psychological Association. Reprinted by permission.

Causes of Insomnia

The causes of insomnia are numerous and diverse. At least four independent domains can breed threats to sleep: psychological, psychiatric, chemical, and medical/biological.

Psychological

Monroe (1967) suggested insomniacs were more physiologically aroused before and during sleep than noninsomniacs, and these data have invited relaxation interventions for insomnia. Although some moderately supportive data have since been reported (e.g., Freedman & Sattler, 1982; Haynes, Follingstad, & McGowan, 1974), numerous instances of low correlation between changes in physiological arousal and sleep latency have seriously undermined the applicability of this view for the majority of insomniacs (e.g., Borkovec, Grayson, O'Brien, & Weerts, 1979; Freedman & Papsdorf, 1976; Haynes, Sides, & Lockwood, 1977).

Insomniacs report that intrusive cognitions pose the greatest obstacle to sleep (Lichstein & Rosenthal, 1980; Shealy, 1979). At bedtime, they "think out" family problems, plan budgets, or analyze occupational entanglements (Coursey, Frankel, Gaarder, & Mott, 1980). Often, anticipation of sleep difficulty generates arousal and self-validating insomnia in what has been termed an *exacerbation cycle* (Ascher & Turner, 1980). Effortful thinking beckons coincident increases in sleep-incompatible cognitive and physiological arousal. Data from both clinical (Mitchell, 1979) and laboratory analog (Gross & Borkovec, 1982) studies document the close correspondence between level of intrusive cognitions and sleep-onset difficulty, although some laboratory attempts to verify the disruptive role of noxious thoughts have been unsuccessful (Haynes, Adams, & Franzen, 1981).

The sleep environment itself may challenge the onset of sleep. Uncomfortable variations in physical conditions such as temperature, noise, bed comfort, and the like are often cited as irritants. Engaging in nonsleep activities in the bedroom such as eating, bill paying, and doing homework may establish the bedroom as a conditioned stimulus capable of evoking emotional and cognitive responses unfriendly to sleep. Evidence relating to this theory is presented in the stimulus control treatment section.

Some individuals label themselves as *insomniacs* due to inappropriate sleep goals. Many people do not need 7 or 8 hours of sleep, contrary to common beliefs. Indeed, some people normally function on a few hours of sleep or less with no apparent deleterious effects on wakefulness (Jones & Oswald, 1968; Meddis, Pearson, & Langford, 1973). Misperceived small need for sleep can lead to sleep disturbances as the individual spends many frustrating hours awake in bed (Lichstein, 1980). Perhaps excessive daytime sleepiness should be one of the primary criteria of insomnia, confirming the complaint of insufficient sleep. Recent studies bearing on this question employed the multiple sleep latency test, a series of daytime naps assessing sleepiness. Group comparisons of *insomniacs* and normals did not reveal differences in daytime sleepiness (Stepanski, Lamphere, Badia, Zorick, & Roth,

1984), and some one-third of *chronic insomniacs* may not be insomniac by the day-time sleepiness criterion (Seidel & Dement, 1982). For this subset of the insomniac population, the term *insomnoid state* more accurately characterizes their condition, which presents the appearance of insomnia while still satisfying the individual's biological need for sleep.

Psychiatric

Insomnia is a common symptom of psychiatric dysfunction, particularly among the affective disorders (Crisp & Stonehill, 1976). Emotional disturbance is also elevated among nonpsychiatric insomniacs. Numerous studies (e.g., Coursey, Buchsbaum, & Frankel, 1975; Haynes *et al.*, 1974; Shealy, Lowe, & Ritzler, 1980) reveal insomniacs score higher on such questionnaires as the MMPI (Hathaway & McKinley, 1943) and the Taylor (1953) Manifest Anxiety Scale, compared to non-insomniacs, although a causal role of mild to moderate psychopatholgy in insomnia has yet to be demonstrated.

Chemical

Hypnotic Drugs

For individuals suffering from insomnia, hypnotic medication offers, at first glance, welcomed relief. However, chronic use of nearly all hypnotics usually leads to resumption of the original insomnia problem as tolerance develops for these chemicals (Institute of Medicine, 1979). Thus, drug-dependent insomnia emerges as the patient takes increasingly larger doses of medicine to *maintain* poor sleep and avoid even worse sleep.

Dietary Habits

Chemical stimulants common in foods, most notably caffeine ("Caffeine," 1981), can profoundly affect sleep, dependent on individual tolerance and dose. Coffee is, of course, the primary caffeine culprit, but there are many other sources. A cup of tea and 12 oz of most soft drinks contain about 30% of the caffeine in a cup of coffee. Some over-the-counter pain relievers (e.g., Anacin, Excedrin) approximate the level of caffeine in coffee, and many nonprescription diuretics, stimulants, and weight-control aids have more caffeine than coffee. Contrary to popular belief, chocolate contains very little caffeine but may still disrupt the sleep of sensitive individuals.

Another factor to consider is regularity of chemical intake. Heavy, regular consumers are likely to develop a tolerance and suffer less ill effects on their sleep than sporadic consumers (Bolton & Null, 1981). Similarly, with regard to bedtime snacks, it is not the amount of food consumed but the degree of departure in either direction from one's usual pattern of evening food intake that threatens sleep (Adam, 1980). On the positive side, there are sleep laboratory data confirming the soporific effects of warm milk or comparable preparations, particularly with respect to sleep during the last third of the night (Brezinova & Oswald, 1972).

Medical/Biological

Painful Conditions

There are a number of medical conditions that can impair sleep by leaving the individual uncomfortable (Williams, 1978). Perhaps those conditions taking the greatest toll on sleep, particularly among the elderly, are arthritis and other pain syndromes (Prinz & Raskind, 1978; Wittig, Zorick, Blumer, Heilbronn, & Roth, 1982).

Exercise

Findings in the extant literature on effects of exercise on sleep are inconsistent, although some trends can be discerned. Intense exercise (e.g., jogging, racquetball) can benefit the same night's sleep with respect to increased deep sleep (particularly in the first half of the night) and, to a lesser extent, decreased sleep latency and increased total sleep time. The magnitude of sleep improvement is directly proportional to the regularity with which exercise is taken, the length of the exercise period, and the amount of energy expended during exercise, and is indirectly proportional to the interval between the exercise and bedtime up till about 2 hours prior to bedtime, at which point exercise may adversely affect sleep (Baekeland & Lasky, 1966; Browman & Tepas, 1976; Griffin & Trinder, 1978; Horne & Porter, 1976). However, as Paxton, Trinder, and Montgomery (1983) convincingly pointed out, these relationships may be unreliable and subject to alternative explanations. Clinical prudence demands that the sleep effects of exercise be judged on an individual basis.

Circadian Rhythm Problems

The sleep/wake cycle is subject to the body's circadian rhythm, an internal clock that also regulates, among other things, body temperature and hormonal cycles (Winfree, 1982). Shiftwork schedules, "sleeping in," afternoon naps, and the like can lead to a partial reversal between sleep and wake cycles (e.g., Kamgar-Parsi, Wehr, & Gillin, 1983). Some individuals are naturally inclined to take their sleep at *off* hours, and this may pose serious chronobiological problems when confronted by conventional time schedules. (See *Disorders of the Sleep-Wake Schedule*, Association of Sleep Disorders Centers, 1979.)

Naps

There are few data available on daytime naps and their effects on nighttime sleep. The main study in this area (Karacan, Williams, Finley, & Hursch, 1970) observed disproportionately large amounts of deep sleep (particularly Stage 4) occurring in afternoon naps. In the night following, there was a tendency toward increased latency to sleep and a significant reduction in Stage 4 sleep. We also know that as the time of nap advances into late afternoon and early evening, the Stage 4 sleep content in the nap increases (Webb & Agnew, 1967), although this study did not, unfortunately, evaluate nighttime sleep effects.

Existing data suggest that naps have mild to moderate deleterious effects on nighttime sleep. However, there are clinically important questions as yet unanswered in this domain. The subjects in the aforementioned studies were healthy, young adult, mostly male volunteers. Nap effects on older females, who constitute a large proportion of the insomnia population, are completely unknown. Also unknown are the effects of napping patterns sustained over days, weeks, or longer.

We (Lichstein, Takayama, & Sanders, 1984) have recently collected some of the only epidemiological data available on napping. We surveyed a nonrandom sample of some 1,400 adults and found 20% reported napping frequently (at least three times per week); another 20% nap about once a week. In light of the high frequency of nap behavior and the potential challenge it poses for nighttime sleep, further study in this area is strongly indicated.

Assessment

The interview is the most commonly used method of sleep assessment, particularly by behavioral clinicians. Other assessment methods are polysomnography, observation, self-report, and various sleep assessment devices.

Polysomnography refers to all-night sleep evaluations using multiple physiological measures—electroencephalography (EEG), electromyography (EMG), electrooculography (EOG), and others (Bootzin & Engle-Friedman, 1981). This approach is required in the proper diagnosis of such disorders as nocturnal myoclonus and sleep apnea. However, insomnia is often setting specific, and sleep laboratory evaluations may fail to observe the sleep problem as it occurs in the home (Hauri, 1983; Karacan, 1972). The introduction of telemetry equipment has permitted, at great cost, polysomnographic assessments in the home, thus overcoming the setting specificity problem (Coates, Rosekind, & Thoresen, 1978; Karacan, 1972).

As polysomnography is not conveniently available to most clinicians, alternative, less adequate sources of sleep data have been developed (Bootzin & Engle-Friedman, 1981; Lichstein & Kelley, 1979). Nurses and bedmates have provided observational sleep data of hospital patients and subjects in the home, but this approach is inconvenient and of suspect reliability. Subjects' self-reports of insomnia are what usually initiate professional concern over the problem, and ongoing self-estimates are an important, popular source of clinical and research information, but the inaccuracy of self-report sleep data is well documented. The self-report questionnaire that we have employed, typifying this genre, is duplicated in Figure 1.

In recent years, several devices have been introduced to obtain reliable, empirical sleep data in the natural environment at modest expense. The two most promising approaches monitor wrist activity (Webster, Kripke, Messin, Mullaney, & Wyborney, 1982) and verbal responses to auditory cues (Lichstein, Hoelscher, & Eakin, 1984; Lichstein, Nickel, Hoelscher, & Kelley, 1982).

A detailed sleep interview, including a complete general history, is indispensable in assessing insomnia in that it allows the therapist to obtain the client's per-

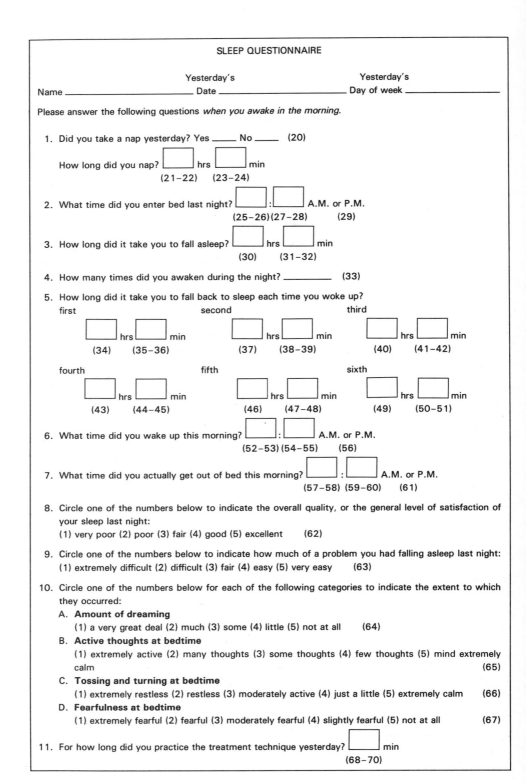

Figure 1. A typical sleep questionnaire completed by clients each morning. This questionnaire yields 14 sleep parameters: naps (Item 1), sleep latency (Item 3), number of awakenings during the night (Item 4), duration of awakenings during the night (Item 5), early morning awakening (Item 7—Item 6), total

Table 2. Outline of Insomnia Assessment Interview

Areas of assessment	Likely interventions

I. Rule out secondary insomnia
  A. Prescribed and nonprescribed drug use
  B. Medical illness
  C. Psychiatric disturbance
	I. A. & B. Medical evaluation and treatment
	  C. Psychological/psychiatric treatment

II. Rule out other primary sleep disorders
  A. Narcolepsy
  B. Sleep apnea
  C. Nocturnal myoclonus
  D. Nightmares
  E. Etc.
	II. A., B., & C. Sleep laboratory evaluation and medical treatment
	  D. & E. Psychological/ psychiatric treatment

III. Specify characteristics of primary insomnia
  A. Incompatible sleep behaviors
  B. Cognitive arousal
    1. Worrying unrelated to sleep
    2. Fears about falling asleep
  C. Somatic arousal
  D. Inappropriate sleep expectations
  E. Disruptive life-style
    1. Napping
    2. Caffeine intake
    3. Excessive physical exercise
	III. A. Stimulus control
	  B. Relaxation/cognitive interventions
	  C. Relaxation/biofeedback
	  D. & E. Life-style management

ceptions about the problem and judge the urgency of the complaint. Table 2 outlines the key points to cover in the interview in order to accomplish three goals: (a) rule out competing explanations for primary insomnia (Table 2, Sections I and II); (b) obtain a detailed description of the insomnia problem (Table 2, Section III); and (c) generate an intervention package (Table 2, second column). Important aspects of the second goal listed include the frequency, severity, and longstanding nature of the insomnia problem and the client's perceptions of its causes.

Medical Treatments

Hypnotic Medication

With the minor exception of electrosleep therapy (discussed later), hypnotic (sleep-inducing) medicines represent the sole medical approach to insomnia treatment, and these have been widely criticized. To varying degrees, chronic use of hypnotics leads to increased dosage due to accumulated tolerance, adverse alteration of sleep stages, daytime grogginess due to residual drug effects, chemical dependence, and, upon drug withdrawal, disrupted sleep (nightmares, insomnia

---

time in bed (Item 7—Item 2), total time slept (total time in bed–(sleep latency, duration of awakenings during the night, and early morning awakening), sleep efficiency percentage (total time slept/total time in bed × 100), and qualitative ratings of six other parameters (Items 8, 9, 10A, 10B, 10C, and 10D). Item 11 monitors homework compliance. The numbers in parentheses in the questionnaire refer to card columns employed for computer analyses.

exacerbation due to REM rebound) and disturbed daytime functioning (nervousness, irritability). In brief, regular use of sleep medications promises serious iatrogenic complications. Medical experts condemn the prescription of hypnotics for chronic insomniacs, recommending their use only in cases of occasional, transitory insomnia (Institute of Medicine, 1979).

Table 3 summarizes the most frequently used prescription sleep medications. As indicated, only a minority of these are primarily hypnotics, as most of the drugs

Table 3. Commonly Employed Hypnotic Drugs

Generic and chemical names	Brand name	Primary use
Barbiturates		
Aprobarbital	Alurate	Sedative, hyponotic
Amobarbital	Amytal	Hypnotic, sedative
Butabarbital Sodium	Butisol Sodium	Sedative, hyponotic
Pentobarbital Sodium	Nembutal Sodium	Hypnotic
Secobarbital	Seconal	Hypnotic, sedative
Amobarbital/secobarbital	Tuinal	Hypnotic
Benzodiazepines		
Lorazepam	Ativan	Tranquilizer
Flurazepam	Dalmane	Hypnotic
Triazolam	Halcion	Hypnotic
Chlordiazepoxide	Librium	Tranquilizer
Temazepam	Restoril	Hypnotic
Oxazepam	Serax	Tranquilizer
Clorazepate	Tranxene	Tranquilizer
Diazepam	Valium	Tranquilizer
Miscellaneous Minor Tranquilizers and Other Chemicals		
Hydroxyzine	Atarax	Tranquilizer
Diphenhydramine	Benadryl	Antihistamine, hypnotic
Glutethimide	Doriden	Hypnotic
Meprobamate	Equanil, Miltown	Tranquilizer
Chloral hydrate	Noctec	Hypnotic, sedative
Methyprylon	Noludar	Hypnotic
Ethchlorvynol	Placidyl	Hypnotic
L-Tryptophan	Tryptacin	Amino acid, hypnotic
Ethinamate	Valmid	Hypnotic
Major Tranquilizers		
Haloperidol	Haldol	Antipsychotic
Thioridazine	Mellaril	Antipsychotic
Thiothixene	Navane	Antipsychotic
Chlorprothixene	Taractan	Antipsychotic
Chlorpromazine	Thorazine	Antipsychotic
Antidepressants		
Amitriptyline	Elavil	Antidepressant
Doxepin	Sinequan	Antidepressant
Amitriptyline/perphenazine	Triavil, Etrafon	Antidepressant, tranquilizer

Note. Drugs are listed alphabetically by brand name within drug families. The *1984 Physician's Desk Reference* was used to compile this table.

target other disorders but are used for insomnia due to their hypnotic "side-effects." Following is a brief overview of the major drug families, within which there is considerable homogeneity of effect.

Barbiturates were some of the earliest drugs employed to induce sleep and are probably the most dangerous. The chronic barbiturate user risks addiction, accidental death by overdose (particularly when mixed with other medications or alcohol), and a severe withdrawal syndrome. The benzodiazepines are milder in their clinical effects and associated risks than barbiturates, but they have a longer half-life in the body, thus increasing the likelihood of a hangover effect. To counteract this problem, short-acting benzodiazepines (e.g., Triazolam) were introduced that minimally disrupt daytime functioning because of their short half-life but worsen sleep during the final hours of the night before arising. The miscellaneous minor tranquilizers listed in Table 3 are a chemically heterogeneous group of hypnotic and antianxiety agents having clinical and risk properties roughly comparable to the benzodiazepines. The remaining groups, major tranquilizers and antidepressants, may be used when the hazards associated with other hypnotics are great with a particular client or when psychosis or depression is present.

Alcohol is a commonly self-prescribed hypnotic, but it, too, is not without hazards. During intoxication, REM is depressed and deep sleep enhanced, and upon withdrawal following chronic use, the reverse occurs within the context of generally disturbed sleep (Pokorny, 1978). There are a small number of drugs among the large number of over-the-counter sleep preparations (summarized in Table 4). Currently, diphenhydramine hydrochloride, an antihistamine with anticholinergic and sedative side-effects, is most popular. In general, the hypnotic effects of over-the-counter drugs are weak, and within a few days, rapidly developing systemic tolerance reduces their potency dramatically.

Electrosleep

Electrosleep involves the induction of sleep by introducing a low-amplitude electrical current through the cranium. Electrosleep therapy was developed in the

Table 4. Over-the-Counter Sleep Aids

Active ingredient	Brand name	Primary use
Diphenhydramine HCL	Compoz	Hypnotic, antihistamine
Diphenhydramine HCL	Cope	Hypnotic, antihistamine
Scopolamine, methapyrilene	Mr. Sleep	Hypnotic, antihistamine
Pyrilamine maleate	Nervine	Hypnotic, antihistamine
Diphenhydramine HCL	Nytol	Hypnotic, antihistamine
Diphenhydramine HCL	Sleep-Eze III	Hypnotic, antihistamine
Diphenhydramine HCL	Sleepinal	Hypnotic, antihistamine
Pyrilamine maleate	Sominex	Hypnotic, antihistamine
Diphenhydramine HCL	Sominex II	Hypnotic, antihistamine
Doxylamine succinate	Unisom	Hypnotic, antihistamine

Note. Products are listed alphabetically by brand name. We surveyed the counters of three major drug stores in compiling this table.

USSR, has received relatively little attention in the United States, and the evidence of its clinical utility is equivocal (Brown, 1975; Von Richthofen & Mellor, 1979).

Psychological Treatments

The literature on psychological interventions for insomnia is large and diverse. Sleep-onset insomnia has received the greatest attention far, and the single-subject and group-design studies in this area are summarized in Tables 5 and 6. Table 5 reviews the individual results of 57 studies, and Table 6 combines outcome data from like treatments across studies in a manner akin to the meta-analysis recommended by Blanchard, Andrasik, Ahles, Teders, and O'Keefe (1980). These tables help crystalize some general conclusions as follows.

First, there is a high frequency of success among distinct treatments for this one disorder (Table 5), suggesting insomnia is a highly reactive condition. This view is supported by the good success of credible placebos (e.g., Lacks, Bertelson, Gans, & Kunkel, 1983; Zwart & Lisman, 1979), and attribution manipulations (e.g., Davison, Tsujimoto, & Glaros, 1973) with insomnia. Second, once treatment gains are attained, they have reasonably good longevity, and there are stronger gains and better longevity associated with the treatments than the placebos (Tables 5 and 6). Third, the sleep-latency benefits are best described as moderate. Often, an insomniac is not converted into a noninsomniac (using the 30-minute criterion), but rather, the insomnia problem is diminished. Averaging (unweighted means) across the 48 studies representing 16 different treatments listed in Table 6, subjects entering psychological treatments for insomnia reported 66 minutes latency to sleep during baseline and 35 minutes at posttreatment. Fourth, chronic insomnia does not abate if not treated, as evidenced by the course of subjects in no-treatment, control conditions (Table 6). Fifth, insomnia research is often criticized for relying too heavily on college student subjects, raising questions about the generalizability of treatment outcomes to insomniacs from the community. The majority of studies in Table 5 (71%) employed insomniacs recruited from the community, thus negating the validity of this criticism. Sixth, we may inquire as to which insomnia treatment is best. In Table 5, there are 34 studies that contained treatment comparisons, and in 23 of these (68%) there were no differences on the primary measure of interest—latency to sleep. In the remaining 11 studies, inconsistent findings prevailed. For example, paradoxical instruction was found to be superior (Ascher & Efran, 1978) and also inferior (Turner & Ascher, 1982) to progressive relaxation. In brief, no particular treatment emerges supreme from Table 5. The average (unweighted means) percentage latency reduction across all treatments (in Table 6) was 45% (excluding placebo and no-treatment data). Only 6 of 16 treatments produced at least a 50% reduction in latency to sleep. Stimulus control produced the largest percentage reduction and was the only treatment for which there are substantial data available (number of studies greater than 5) to still exceed the 50% criterion. Therefore, Table 6 suggests that stimulus control is the most effective insomnia treatment.

The numerous interventions listed in Table 5 can be organized by common procedural or target elements into three classes of approaches: relaxation, cognitive control, and life-style management. The relaxation treatments include autogenic training, three varieties of biofeedback, hypnosis, meditation, passive relaxation, progressive relaxation, and self-control relaxation and are represented in 75% of the studies listed in Table 5, being the most popular insomnia treatment approach. The cognitive control treatments (cognitive restructuring, imagery, ocular relaxation, paradoxical instruction, and systematic desensitization) are represented in 39%, and the life-style management treatments (didactic treatment and stimulus control) in 25%.

Relaxation

This approach has attracted the application of a diverse array of methods. These will now be briefly outlined.

Progressive Relaxation (PR)

As indicated in Table 5, this has been a popular treatment for insomnia. PR involves the tensing and relaxing of about 15 muscle groups covering the body. A typical induction requires about 20 minutes, and details on the clinical procedure are readily available (Bernstein & Borkovec, 1973; Lichstein, in press).

Over the years, Jacobson (e.g., 1920, 1938a, 1970) supplied ample case study data on treating insomnia with the method. A major breakthrough occurred in the treatment of insomnia when Steinmark and Borkovec (1974) introduced two brilliant methodological innovations: (a) counterdemand instructions, whereby subjects are told not to expect improvement for several weeks to control for experimenter demand and placebo influences; and (b) treatment credibility evaluations, whereby subjects rate the expectancy for improvement generated by viable and placebo treatments to verify the placebo control value of the latter.

The success of PR for insomnia is highly consistent. Even those few studies that included pre-post sleep laboratory evaluations (Borkovec & Weerts, 1976; Borkovec *et al.*, 1979; Freedman & Papsdorf, 1976) confirmed the utility of PR, although the magnitude of effects in these studies is somewhat less than that indicated by studies relying on self-report. Nearly all of the PR studies targeted primarily sleep-onset insomnia, although some reported additional benefits for middle-of-the-night awakenings as well (e.g., Carr-Kaffashan & Woolfolk, 1979; Gershman & Clouser, 1974).

Passive Relaxation

This is a variant of progressive relaxation, popularized in a series of studies by Haynes (Haynes, Woodward, Moran, & Alexander, 1974; Haynes *et al.*, 1977), and involves sequentially focusing attention on pleasant feelings in the body musculature without the tensing component. A series of studies by Borkovec (Borkovec & Hennings, 1978; Borkovec, Kaloupek, & Slama, 1975; Borkovec *et al.*, 1979) suggest that progressive relaxation is more effective than passive relaxation, but

Table 5. Controlled Research on Psychological Treatment of Sleep-Onset Insomnia

Study	Ss[c]	AT	CR	Di	EEG-S	EEG-T	EMG	Hy	Im	Med
Alperson & Biglan, 1979	c									+
Ascher & Efran, 1978	c									
Ascher & Turner, 1979	c									
Ascher & Turner, 1980	c									
Bell, 1979	c					+				
Besner, 1978	c					+	+			
Bootzin, 1973	c									
Borkovec & Fowles, 1973	s							+		
Borkovec, Grayson, O'Brien, & Weerts, 1979	s									
Borkovec & Hennings, 1978	s								+	
Borkovec, Kaloupek, & Slama, 1975	s									
Borkovec, Steinmark, & Nau, 1973	c									
Borkovec & Weerts, 1976	s									
Cannici, Malcolm, & Peek, 1983	c									
Carr-Kaffashan & Woolfolk, 1979	c									+
Coursey, Frankel, Gaarder, & Mott, 1980	c	+					+			
Evans & Bond, 1969	c									
Feinstein, Sterman, & Macdonald, 1974	c				+					
Fogle & Dyal, 1983	c									
Freedman, Hauri, Coursey, & Frankel, 1978[d]		+				+	+			
Freedman & Papsdorf, 1976	c						+			
Gershman & Clouser, 1974	s									
Graham, Wright, Toman, & Mark, 1975	s	+						+		
Hauri, 1981	c				+	+	+			
Hauri & Good, 1975	c						+			
Hauri, Percy, Hellekson, Hartmann, & Russ, 1982	c				+	+	+			
Haynes, Price, & Simons, 1975	c									
Haynes, Sides, & Lockwood, 1977	c						+			
Haynes, Woodward, Moran, & Alexander, 1974	s									
Hughes & Hughes, 1978	c						+			
Lacks, Bertelson, Gans, & Kunkel, 1983	c									
Lichstein, 1980	c			+						
Lichstein, 1983	s									
Lichstein & Blew, 1980	c									
Lick & Heffler, 1977	c									
Mitchell, 1979	c			+					+	
Mitchell & White, 1977	s		+						+	
Nicassio & Bootzin, 1974	c	+								
Nicassio, Boylan, & McCabe, 1982	c						+			
Ott, Levine, & Ascher, 1983	c									
Pendleton & Tasto, 1976	s									
Puder, Lacks, Bertelson, & Storandt, 1983	c									
Relinger & Bornstein, 1979	c									
Relinger, Bornstein, & Mungas, 1978	c									
Ribordy, 1976[d]									+	
Shealy, 1979	s									
Steinmark & Borkovec, 1974	s									
Tokarz & Lawrence, 1974	s									
Toler, 1978	c									
Traub, Jencks, & Bliss, 1973	c	+								
Turner & Ascher, 1979a	c									
Turner & Ascher, 1979b	c									
Turner & Ascher, 1982	c									
VanderPlate & Eno, 1983	s						+			
Woolfolk, Carr-Kaffashan, McNulty, & Lehrer, 1976	c									+
Woolfolk & McNulty, 1983	c								+	
Zwart & Lisman, 1979	s									

[a]The treatment group abbreviations signify autogenic training (AT), cognitive restructuring (CR), didactic treatment (Di), Electroencephalographic sensorimotor rhythm biofeedback (EEG-S), electroencephalographic theta rhythm biofeedback (EEG-T), electromyographic biofeedback (EMG), hypnosis (Hy), pleasant imagery (Im), meditation (Med), ocular relaxation (OR), paradoxical instruction (PI), passive relaxation (Pas), progressive relaxation (PR), self-control relaxation (SCR), stimulus control (SC), systematic desensitization (SD), placebo treatment (PL), and no treatment (NT).

Table. 5. Controlled Research on Psychological Treatment of Sleep-Onset Insomnia (cont.)

| | | | | | | | | | Sleep latency improvement[b] | |
OR	PI	Pas	PR	SCR	SC	SD	PL	NT	Posttreatment	Follow-up
					+		+	+	Med/SC=PL>NT	Med/SC=PL
	+		+			+		+	PI>PR/SD=NT	
	+						+	+	PI>PL=NT	
	+						+	+	PI>PL=NT	
			+					+	EEG-T>PR=NT	
							+		EEG-T=EMG=PL	
			+		+		+	+	SC>PR=PL=NT	
			+				+	+	Hy=PR=PL>NT	
		+	+					+	PR>Pas=NT	
			+					+	Im=PR>NT	
		+	+				+	+	Pas=PR=PL>NT	Pas=PR=PL
			+			+			PR=PR/SD=SD	
			+				+	+	PR=PL>NT	PR>PL
			+					+	PR>NT	PR>NT
			+				+		Med/PR>PL	Med/PR>PL
									EMG>AT	
						+		+	SD=NT	
							+		EEG-S>PL	
	+						+		PI=PL	
			+					+	AT=EEG-T=EMG=PR=NT	
			+				+		EMG=PR>PL	EMG=PR=PL
			+			+		+	PR=SD>NT	PR=SD>NT
									AT>Hy	
								+	EEG-S=EEG-T/EMG=EMG=NT	EEG-S=EEG-T/EMG=EMG=NT
								+	EMG=NT	
									EMG/EEG-S=EMG/EEG-T	EMG/EEG-S=EMG/EEG-T
					+			+	SC>NT	
		+					+		EMG=Pas>PL	EMG=Pas>PL
		+					+		Pas>PL	Pas>PL
			+		+		+		EMG=PR=SC=PL	EMG=PR=SC=PL
	+		+		+		+		SC>PI=PR=PL	SC>PI=PR=PL
+					+				Di>OR=SC	
+								+	OR>NT	
+			+				+	+	OR=PR=PL=NT	OR=PR=PL
			+				+	+	PR>PL=NT	
				+				+	Im/SCR>Di=SCR>NT	Im/SCR>Di=SCR>NT
			+					+	Im/PR>CR=Im=PR>NT	
			+				+	+	AT=PR>PL=NT	AT=PR>PL
			+				+	+	EMG=PR=PL>NT	EMG=PR=PL
	+						+	+	PI=PL>NT	
		+	+					+	Pas=PR>NT	PR>Pas
					+			+	SC>NT	
	+							+	PI>NT	
	+							+	PI>NT	
			+			+		+	Im=PR=SD>NT	
		+			+		+	+	Pas=Pas/SC>PL=NT	Pas=Pas/SC>PL=NT
			+			+	+	+	PR=SD=PL>NT	PR=SD>PL
					+		+	+	SC>PL=NT	SC>PL
			+		+			+	PR=SC=NT	PR=SC
								+	AT>NT	
	+		+		+		+	+	PI=PR=SC>PL=NT	
					+		+		SC>PL	
	+		+		+			+	PR=SC>PI=NT	
							+	+	EMG=PL>NT	EMG=PL
			+					+	Med=PR>NT	Med=PR
		+	+					+	Im=Pas=PR>NT	Im>Pas=PR
					+		+	+	SC=PL>NT	SC=PL=NT

[b] The symbol > signifies that the treatment preceding the symbol was more effective than the treatment following it.
[c] Subjects used were either student volunteers (s) or volunteers from the community (c).
[d] Subject type was not indicated.

research from other laboratories (Haynes, Mosely, & McGowan, 1975; Lehrer, Batey, Woolfolk, Remde, & Garlick, 1983; Woolfolk, & McNulty, 1983) suggests the reverse is true. At present, the question is unresolved.

Brady (1973) introduced metronome-conditioned relaxation (MCR), which adds the steady beat of a metronome to enhance the relaxation effects of passive relaxation. Pendleton and Tasto (1976) found two versions of MCR, metronome plus passive relaxation versus metronome only, and progressive relaxation to be comparably effective.

Autogenic Training (AT)

Autogenic training is a method of imaginal relaxation requiring about 20 minutes, in which subjects imagine themselves in peaceful nature scenes while also imagining relaxation-facilitative sensations of the body including warmth and heaviness of the limbs, heart rate slowing, and so forth (see Lichstein, in press, and Schultz & Luthe, 1959, for the particulars of the procedure). The method was developed in Germany some 60 years ago by Schultz, and to this day the bulk of the extensive AT literature is in European journals. A brief summary of research on AT for insomnia found in Luthe and Schultz (1969) is very positive, particularly in regard to sleep-maintenance insomnia, but a recent sleep laboratory study found it successful in only two of six subjects presenting sleep-onset insomnia (Coursey *et al.,* 1980).

Table 6. Mean Sleep-Latency Changes in Controlled Research on Psychological Treatment of Insomnia

	Latency to sleep in minutes			
Insomnia treatment	Baseline (*n*)	Posttreatment (*n*)	Follow-up (*n*)	% Improvement at posttreatment
Autogenic training	56 (3)	28 (3)	50 (1)	50
Cognitive restructuring	24 (1)	16 (1)		33
Didactic treatment	153 (2)	71 (2)	45 (2)	54
EEG-SMR biofeedback	31 (2)	24 (2)	18 (2)	23
EEG-theta biofeedback	39 (2)	21 (2)	17 (2)	46
EMG biofeedback	48 (8)	28 (8)	40 (3)	42
Hypnosis	43 (1)	24 (1)		44
Imagery	84 (4)	40 (4)	34 (2)	52
Meditation	67 (2)	32 (2)	25 (2)	52
Ocular relaxation	63 (2)	32 (2)	30 (2)	49
Paradoxical instruction	63 (9)	34 (9)	22 (3)	46
Passive relaxation	54 (7)	34 (7)	36 (5)	37
Progressive relaxation	68 (24)	39 (24)	39 (12)	43
Self-control relaxation	135 (1)	81 (1)	64 (1)	40
Stimulus control	67 (13)	28 (13)	34 (8)	58
Systematic desensitization	56 (2)	27 (2)	18 (2)	52
Placebo treatment	57 (26)	43 (26)	40 (13)	25
No treatment	64 (28)	62 (27)	73 (5)	3

Note. Under *n* is the number of studies contributing to each mean. *n* is equal to or less than column sums in Table 5 as quantifiable data were unavailable for some studies. Many studies did not include follow-up data. The greater the discrepancy between the follow-up *n* and the baseline and posttreatment *n*'s, the more misleading are the follow-up data for a given treatment.

There are a seemingly endless number of techniques under the meditation rubric. Despite its appearance as a likely candidate for insomnia intervention, there is surprisingly little data available on meditation applications in this area. Indeed, Davidson and Schwartz (1976) recommended meditation for insomnia more than any other method of relaxation because it is well suited to neutralize the intrusive cognitions prevalent in this disorder.

Woolfolk found a form of breath and mantra meditation was effective for insomnia when paired with progressive relaxation (Carr-Kaffashan & Woolfolk, 1979) or presented singly (Woolfolk, Carr-Kaffashan, McNulty, & Lehrer, 1976). There is some data to suggest that both Transcendental Meditation (Miskiman, 1977) and Benson's (1975) method of mantra meditation (Alperson & Biglan, 1979) are helpful for insomnia. The latter study is one of the few that has separately analyzed the treatment response of middle-aged and elderly subjects and found that only the younger subjects benefited from treatment.

Self-Control Relaxation (SCR)

SCR refers to abbreviated, portable forms of relaxation that may be conveniently and unobtrusively employed in the natural environment when confronted with stress (Lichstein, in press). There has been little work with this approach for insomnia, probably due to the narrow limits defining the situational specificity of this disorder. The sole group-design study in this area (Mitchell, 1979) sought to reduce residual anxiety at bedtime, in part by more effective anxiety management during the day, and presented data supporting the efficacy of SCR. Others (Coates & Thoresen, 1979; Thoresen, Coates, Kirmil-Gray, & Rosekind, 1981) have presented data on the successful treatment of sleep-maintenance insomnia, wherein SCR was part of a treatment package.

Hypnosis

There is a paucity of data on hypnosis for insomnia, but anecdotal reports recommend this approach using autohypnosis and posthypnotic suggestion (Fry, 1973; Hanley, 1965). In group design studies, autohypnotic relaxation was equally as effective as progressive relaxation (Borkovec & Fowles, 1973) and less effective than autogenic training (Graham, Wright, Toman, & Mark, 1975).

Biofeedback

Two rationales have been advanced to explain the mechanism of biofeedback treatments for insomnia. One view offered in support of electromyographic (EMG) biofeedback is that a global relaxation effect prepares the individual for sleep. It has also been hypothesized that electroencephalographic biofeedback targeting the sensorimotor rhythm (EEG-S) associated with stage 2 sleep alters specific brain functioning to more closely mimic brain processes during sleep. Theta biofeedback (EEG-T) has been viewed from both perspectives.

EMG biofeedback is the type of biofeedback that has received the most attention in insomnia treatment. Some one dozen group design studies (see Table 5) present ample evidence of its usefulness. Fancy biofeedback equipment may impart strong placebo effects, and the success of placebo biofeedback groups supports this conclusion (Besner, 1978; Hughes & Hughes, 1978; Nicassio, Boylan, & McCabe, 1982; VanderPlate & Eno, 1983). The few sleep laboratory evaluations in this area report supportive (Coursey *et al.*, 1980; Freedman & Papsdorf, 1976) and disconfirming (Freedman, Hauri, Coursey, & Frankel, 1978; Hauri, 1981; Hauri & Good, 1975) data on EMG biofeedback efficacy. Hauri's (1981) data suggest that EMG biofeedback is useful with a subset of insomniacs presenting elevated muscular or experiential tension.

Two studies (Hauri, 1981; Hauri, Percy, Hellekson, Hartmann, & Russ, 1982) trained insomniacs first in EMG and then EEG-T biofeedback. Basic research (Sittenfeld, Budzynski, & Stoyva, 1976) has shown this sequence, compared to theta feedback only, to be more productive of theta waves for subjects with high-EMG but not low-EMG resting levels. The clinical trials cited previously found this strategy to be moderately effective for insomnia. Hauri and his associates (Hauri *et al.*, 1982) obtained particularly interesting results. They found that EMG/EEG-T biofeedback is functionally equivalent to EMG biofeedback only, as is stated in Hauri (1981). Specifically, EMG/EEG-T biofeedback was superior to EMG/EEG-S biofeedback for tense insomniacs, but the reverse held for nontense insomniacs. What remains unclear is if EEG-T adds anything to the clinical potency of EMG biofeedback for tense insomniacs. Trials of EEG-T biofeedback only produced mixed results (see Table 5).

Based upon Sterman's basic research with cats (Sterman, Howe, & Macdonald, 1970), Sterman (Feinstein, Sterman, & Macdonald, 1974) and Hauri (Hauri, 1981; Hauri *et al.*, 1982) cultivated the 12 to 14 Hz EEG activity occurring in Stage 2 sleep (termed *sleep spindles*) through biofeedback training of the same pattern emanating from the sensorimotor cortex during wakefulness. Sleep laboratory evaluations in these clinical trials found EEG-S biofeedback to be clinically effective, but Hauri's data in 1981 and 1982 indicate this to be so only with those insomniacs who do not present experiential or muscular anxiety and tension.

Cognitive Interventions

The methods of this section share both a common assumption about the principal cause of insomnia and a common treatment goal. Unwanted bedtime cognitions, be they fears concerned with sleep or unrelated to sleep, prolong wakefulness when sleep is desired. Treatment is aimed at reducing the impact of these cognitions by neutralizing their valence or diminishing their occurrence.

Cognitive Restructuring (CR)

Under the *cognitive restructuring* rubric fall a variety of techniques designed to alter the frequency and valence of troublesome thoughts. Although this approach holds promise for insomnia, little research has been conducted in this domain. Mitchell (1979; Mitchell & White, 1977) employed several CR techniques including thought stopping, time-out from worry, and training in rational thinking and found CR useful with sleep-onset insomnia. Thoresen *et al.* (1981) employed training in rational thinking as a component in a treatment package successfully targeting sleep-maintenance insomnia.

Imagery

For insomnia (and most other appropriate targets), imagery is employed to promote relaxation and to divert one's attention away from negatively valenced, arousing thoughts (Lichstein, in press). Initially, the therapist may verbally guide the imagery, and its content is usually devoted to a peaceful nature scene (e.g., the sun warms your body at the beach; you listen to the trickle of a mountain brook while strolling through a meadow) familiar to the client's experience. Cotler and Guerra (1976) have produced an excellent imagery tape providing about one-half dozen relaxation scenarioes for clients' self-use.

Mitchell (1979; Mitchell & White, 1977) presented data showing that imagery quiets cognition beyond the effects of progressive or self-control relaxation, and increments in insomnia improvement follow. Coates and Thoresen (1979; Thoresen *et al.,* 1981) successfully employed imagery within a multifaceted treatment package for sleep-maintenance insomnia, although the individual contribution of imagery could not be isolated. Borkovec and Hennings (1978) found pleasant imagery (enhanced by muscle tensing-releasing) to be equally as effective as standard progressive relaxation, and Woolfolk and McNuity (1983) observed imagery to be superior to progressive relaxation on measures of sleep latency and sleep awakenings.

Ocular Relaxation (OR)

Early in his work, Jacobson (1938a) employed eye-movement exercises as part of the progressive relaxation procedure to induce "blank minds" in his subjects. He presented case study data (Jacobson, 1938b) on this method used along with full body progressive relaxation to demonstrate its effectiveness with insomniacs.

Our laboratory has studied OR, adapted from Jacobson, separate from progressive relaxation. OR is considered to be a cognitive technique as it serves primarily to reduce ocular motility (which presumably will suppress cognitive activity), rather than promoting global relaxation (Lichstein & Sallis, 1982).

The technique involves six eye movements—up, down, right, left, around, and around the other way, each held for about 7 seconds and separated by 40 seconds of focusing on relaxing sensations in the eyes. Available data on OR are mixed. OR was ineffective with a single, elderly insomniac, as was stimulus control with the same individual (see Lichstein, 1980, under Didactic Treatment). Five student subjects showed good sleep improvement, and this was maintained in four of them at 10-months follow-up (Lichstein, 1983). In a group design study (Lichstein & Blew, 1980) OR performed equally as well as the veteran progressive relaxation, but neither was superior to placebo or no treatment.

Paradoxical Instruction (PI)

PI (also called paradoxical intention) for insomnia involves instructing subjects to attempt to stay awake for as long as possible at bedtime, ostensibly to become more aware of the thoughts and feelings blocking sleep. Relinger and Bornstein (1979) provide a detailed account of the rationale given subjects.

The purpose of PI is to abate sleep-delaying, anxious thoughts arising from one's concerns about falling asleep. Such thoughts may be viewed as a form of performance anxiety (Ascher & Efran, 1978). Delayed sleep confirms and escalates this anxiety creating a self-energized exacerbation cycle (Relinger, Bornstein, & Mungas, 1978).

Early rigorous case studies, supportive of its efficacy (Ascher & Efran, 1978; Relinger et al., 1978) were soon supplemented by single-subject (Relinger & Bornstein, 1979) and group (Ascher & Turner, 1979; Turner & Ascher, 1979a) design research showing PI to be an effective sleep-induction strategy, although one negative-outcome study of PI has appeared (Turner & Ascher, 1982). Some studies (Ascher & Turner, 1979; Relinger & Bornstein, 1979; Turner & Ascher, 1979a) reported additional benefits accruing to awakenings during the night.

Ascher and Turner (1980) offered an interesting comparison of two methods of administering PI. One method involved explaining the actual therapeutic rationale to the client, that is, anxious thoughts about falling asleep can be dispelled by attempting to stay awake. The second group received the commonly employed fictitious rationale, that is, stay awake to identify problematic thoughts that will then be treated in therapy sessions. Insomniacs receiving the veridical rationale improved significantly more than the nonveridical PI, placebo, and no-treatment groups.

Systematic Desensitization (SD)

Systematic desensitization is the most time-honored behavior therapy technique. It imaginally pairs a graded sequence of anxious events with a response incompatible with anxiety (usually progressive relaxation) to reduce the noxious properties of the target situation (Wolpe, 1982). For insomnia, anxiety hierarchy items are associated typically with going to bed, such as putting on nightclothes, turning the lights out, and so on. Most of the insomnia studies (Borkovec, Steinmark, & Nau, 1973; Evans & Bond, 1969; Ribordy, 1976; Steinmark & Borkovec, 1974) repeated a single image encompassing a series of bedtime events instead of using a hierarchy.

As indicated in Table 5, the bulk of the evidence supports the efficacy of SD. Borkovec et al. (1973) provided suggestive evidence that SD, when combined with home practice of relaxation, is particularly useful for severe insomnia, and SD alone profits sleep-maintenance insomnia. However, other studies (Gershman & Clouser, 1974; Steinmark & Borkovec, 1974) failed to replicate this latter finding.

Life-style Management

The life-style management orientation considers sleep problems within the context of the entire day. Other treatments emphasize internal obstacles to sleep onset arising at bedtime (i.e., cognitive and somatic arousal), whereas life-style management approaches examine environmental factors, attitudes unrelated to sleep, and daily living routines that may be temporally and physically removed from the bedtime setting but still influence its proceedings.

Broad Spectrum Treatment Packages

In their self-help book, Coates and Thoresen (1977) advocate careful scrutiny of daytime and nighttime habits that might adversely affect sleep. Included in their array of recommendations are several methods of relaxation, daytime stress management, arranging the bedtime environment so that it is conducive to sleep, neutralizing bedtime cognitions, stimulus control procedures, and the scheduling of more leisurely and recreational activities during the day. Coates and Thoresen (1979; Thoresen *et al.*, 1981) tested this approach in carefully documented case studies of sleep-maintenance insomniacs. Polysomnographic evaluations verified therapy progress in these studies that are some of the very few published attempts to treat this type of insomnia. Employing a somewhat similar treatment package, Mitchell (1979; Mitchell & White, 1977) obtained positive results with sleep-onset insomniacs.

Didactic Treatment

This approach argues that insomnia may arise from a variety of factors, for example, inappropriate sleep goals, exercise and dietary habits, napping, and the like, maintained by the client due to incorrect or insufficient information. Client education is provided to encourage habits and attitudes more friendly to sleep.

There has been little study of the usefulness of didactic treatment. In the sole group design study of this approach, Mitchell (1979) found that randomly selected insomniacs administered general sleep information showed significant sleep improvement to the same extent as self-control relaxation subjects, but less improvement than self-control relaxation and cognitive control procedures combined. This study may have underestimated the value of didactic treatment for particular insomniacs, as this treatment strategy might be less suited to group design research than other psychological interventions. Clinical assessment should guide decisions as to who could profit from this approach.

Bootzin, Engle-Friedman, and Hazelwood (1983) provided some encouraging anecdotal data with an elderly subject. In a carefully documented case study, Lichstein (1980) began didactic treatment with a 59-year-old individual exhibiting chronic, severe insomnia, after ocular relaxation and stimulus control treatments failed. Didactic treatment was motivated by the observations that (a) over several months, average time slept per night was highly consistent at about 4½ hours, despite extreme sleep variability from one night to the next; and (b) daytime sleepiness was not a problem. We concluded that the subject artificially induced an insomnoid state by seeking 7½ hours of sleep per night. Treatment mainly consisted of gradually advancing bedtime and backing up time of morning arising. Over about 3 months, the subject established a stable sleep routine with latency to sleep now 53 minutes (174 minutes during baseline), few awakenings during the night (82 minutes awake during the night in baseline), and sleep efficiency percentage at 71% (49% during baseline). Total sleep time per night actually decreased from 4½ to 3½ hours, but sleep variability between nights was dramatically decreased, day-time sleepiness still presented no problem, and rated quality of sleep improved. At 5-months follow-up, all treatment gains had maintained or improved, with latency to sleep down to 18 minutes and sleep efficiency reaching 82%.

Stimulus Control (SC)

The stimulus control operant approach, introduced by Bootzin (1972), asserts that the stimulus properties of the bedroom for insomniacs are no longer discri-minitive cues for sleep but have become cues for wakefulness. This results from habitually engaging in sleep-incompatible behaviors (e.g., watching television, eat-ing, school- or employment-related work) in the bedroom. The treatment is designed to reestablish the bedroom as a discriminitive stimulus for sleep by elim-inating all sleep-incompatible behaviors from that setting.

The SC rationale predicts a higher rate of sleep-incompatible behaviors in the bedroom among insomniacs than noninsomiacs, but basic research examining the occurrence of such behavior has obtained weak (Kazarian, Howe, & Csapo, 1979) or no (Haynes, Adams, West, Kamens, & Safranek, 1982; Haynes *et al.,* 1974) sup-port for this thesis. One could argue that the same incompatible behaviors exert a differential influence on individuals and thereby cause insomnia in some persons and not others, but this alternative explanation awaits validation. Another view (Turner & Ascher, 1979b; Zwart & Lisman, 1979) holds that SC procedures dis-rupt noxious cognitions that impede sleep onset.

The thrust of the method is a simple prescription: "Don't go to sleep unless tired, don't stay in bed if you can't fall asleep, and don't engage in nonsleep-related activities in the bedroom" (Bootzin, 1972, 1973). Daytime napping is usually pro-hibited as well. Most SC regimens (e.g., Lacks, Bertelson, Sugerman, & Kunkel, 1983; Zwart & Lisman, 1979) place a 10-minute limit on awake time in bed before the subject should get up, but Bootzin (personal communication, January 9, 1984) cautions against "clock watching" and does not recommend a strict time period. Our own experience with this method suggests that an upper limit of *about* 20 min-utes seems to work best with most insomniacs.

SC has fared well as a sleep-induction strategy in well-controlled single-subject design research (Haynes, Price, & Simons, 1975; Turner & Ascher, 1979b), but the results of group design research have been inconsistent (e.g., Hughes & Hughes, 1978; Turner & Ascher, 1982; Zwart & Lisman, 1979). Lacks and her associates presented interesting data indicating SC aids sleep-onset insomnia in the elderly (Puder, Lacks, Bertelson, & Storandt, 1983) and sleep-maintenance insomnia in a middle-aged sample (Lacks, Bertelson, Sugarman, & Kunkel, 1983), although the placebo group also did well in the latter study. Tokarz and Lawrence (1974) found SC to be effective for both onset and maintenance aspects of insomnia but no more so than separate tests of the sleep-incompatible behavior or temporal regularity of bedtime components.

SC treatment can be readily added to relaxation interventions to form a com-plementary two-pronged approach. The few studies that have tested this combi-nation documented modest additional benefits over relaxation alone (Shealy, 1979; Toler, 1978).

Although psychological interventions for insomnia have obtained generally favorable results, more specific information would be useful to clinicians in guiding their prescriptions for individual clients. To this end, efforts have been made to identify predictors of successful outcome and to determine which treatments are the most powerful. Unfortunately, there are many more questions than answers in both cases.

Client characteristics have received the most attention as predictor variables, but this has not been fruitful. Neither insomnia severity (Carr-Kaffashan & Woolfolk, 1979; Lacks, Bertelson, Gans, & Kunkel, 1983; Lick & Heffler, 1977; Shealy *et al.*, 1980), insomnia chronicity (Shealy *et al.*, 1980), client gender (Shealy *et al.*, 1980), nor client psychopathology (Carr-Kaffashan & Woolfolk, 1979; Lick & Heffler, 1977; Nicassio & Bootzin, 1974) has proved to be influential. In disagreement with the preceding, some studies (Freedman *et al.*, 1978; Nicassio & Bootzin, 1974) observed a better treatment response among females than males.

The most reliable finding in this area concerns the client's age. Three studies (Alperson & Biglan, 1979; Lick & Heffler, 1977; Nicassio & Bootzin, 1974) documented a weaker treatment response among elderly than middle-aged insomniacs.

Borkovec (1979) has drawn attention to the distinction between idiopathic insomnia (insomnia complaint confirmed by sleep laboratory assessment) and pseudoinsomnia (insomnia complaint disconfirmed by sleep laboratory assessment: also called *subjective insomnia,* see Table 1, Section 9). His data suggest that relaxation treatments improve the self-reported sleep of both groups, but actual sleep improves only among the idiopathic insomniacs (Borkovec *et al.*, 1979).

Attempts to determine which treatments are best have generally not been fruitful, probably because of the heterogeneity of insomnia subtypes. Along these lines, Hauri's research matching EMG biofeedback with tense insomniacs and SMR biofeedback with nontense insomniacs appears very promising.

Case Study Illustration

My (Lichstein) initial impression of Jennifer is that I have treated scores of individuals just like her before. Jennifer is a 41-year-old, divorced white woman, employed in a low-level managerial position, and seemingly victimized by two children with more energy and mischievous inclinations than is reasonable. Jennifer's complaint is a familiar one. Despite her efforts, which include extra exercise during the day and boring reading material at bedtime, she cannot get to sleep in less than an hour.

In treating insomnia (or any other focal disorder), the total person bearing the complaint must not be neglected. Thus, the principal goal of the first few therapy sessions is to establish a positive interpersonal relationship between myself and the client, and, having accomplished this, benefits will accrue to numerous and varied aspects of the emerging therapy. Secondarily, I will obtain a comprehensive social history as well as a general outline of the presenting problem. This second-order priority serves the goal of collecting information sufficient to confirm or rule out, at least on a preliminary basis, the diagnosis of secondary insomnia (Table 2, Numbers I and II).

We join the current case early in the third session. At this juncture, the diagnosis of primary insomnia appears appropriate. Prescribed and nonprescribed chemical use is minimal; Jennifer is in good physical health; she enjoys at least adequate psychological adjustment in important spheres; and indicators of other primary sleep disorders such as heavy snoring (sleep apnea) and daytime sleep attacks (narcolepsy) are absent. Jennifer is feeling at ease in the therapy, and a trusting relationship is solidifying.

DR. LICHSTEIN: When, exactly, did your difficulty falling asleep begin?

JENNIFER: It must have been about 8 years ago. My marriage was falling apart and my little one was driving me crazy. It was late in my pregnancy and even though I felt tired, I was having the hardest time getting to sleep. I figured it had to do with being pregnant and I looked forward to sleeping well again after giving birth, but it never changed.

DR. LICHSTEIN: You say it never changed. Does that mean that every night for 8 years you've had trouble getting to sleep? [I'm mixing intervention with assessment as I begin to expose to Jennifer her own exaggerated self-perception which probably fuels an exacerbation cycle.]

JENNIFER: No. Of course not. That's just an expression I use.

DR. LICHSTEIN: But expressions are not always harmless. They can serve to cement unhelpful attitudes and focus undue attention on problems.

JENNIFER: Well, I'm not making up that I have insomnia (stated harshly). The sleep problem is really there. [I may have challenged Jennifer too forcefully. She's on the defense now.]

DR. LICHSTEIN: I know it's there and I definitely did not mean to say that it wasn't. However, I do know that when people use shorthand expressions to give general descriptions to complicated situations, the expressions sometimes capture only the negative aspects of the situation and make the situation heavy on our minds.

JENNIFER: Are you saying that I think my insomnia problem is worse than it is?

DR. LICHSTEIN: Partly. But I also suspect that if you believe you have a bad insomnia problem, this belief can lead to disruption of sleep and make your sleep worse than it has to be. To illustrate what I mean, tell me the typical thoughts you have while lying in bed on bad insomnia nights.

JENNIFER: Well, I'll think about things like an employee who's giving me fits at work, or problems with math that my youngest is having, or how I'm going to meet some upcoming bills.

DR. LICHSTEIN: I don't hear too many pleasant thoughts.

JENNIFER: That's true.

DR. LICHSTEIN: What about on nights when you fall asleep easily.

JENNIFER: That's a tough one. I'm not sure. I might not be so preoccupied with all these worries when I fall asleep quickly.

DR. LICHSTEIN: One more point and this is an important one. Among the worrisome thoughts you listed, you did not mention concerns about falling asleep, which is what I was talking about a few minutes earlier.

JENNIFER: Well, that's a given. Every time I enter bed, that is almost every time, I dread that I won't be able to fall asleep.

DR. LICHSTEIN: And that very concern about falling asleep is at least as disruptive to your sleep as your concerns about daytime events. This is what I meant when I said your conviction that you are an insomniac helps create the insomnia. [I pause and allow the silence to help drive home this point.] One of your main tasks in this therapy is to become less concerned about your sleep problem. The more you can take the attitude "I'll just let my sleep take care of itself," the better you'll sleep.

The remainder of this interview collected additional data on changes in sleep pattern over the years, major life events and daily routines that appear to affect Jennifer's sleep, her bedtime phenomenology, and her bedtime routines. I gave Jennifer a stack of sleep questionnaires (Figure 1), which she will fill out as long as therapy addresses her sleep, and seven questionnaires surveying sleep-incompatible behaviors (Kazarian *et al.*, 1979) to be filled out 1 week only. I also loaned her a sleep assessment device (SAD, Lichstein, Hoelscher, & Eakin, 1984) for 1 week to verify her self-report.

The early part of the fourth session was devoted mainly to carefully reviewing the sleep data Jennifer collected during the week. This is done, in part, to demonstrate to Jennifer that this information is important and to reinforce her compliance to homework assignments. Following are some interesting aspects of the data and their implications that we explored.

1. Jennifer reported difficulty falling asleep on four nights only, which conflicts with her previous global report.
2. The SAD tape record, which Jennifer dropped off at my office the day before our fourth session, confirmed no sleep difficulty on the nights Jennifer reported having no problems, but revealed about a 20-minute latency to sleep over-estimation by Jennifer on the problem nights.
3. Jennifer had evening telephone conversations on three nights last week, all of which were bad sleep nights.

The latter part of the fourth session focused on the critical subject of daytime sleepiness.

DR. LICHSTEIN: Are you sleepy during the day?

JENNIFER: Very.

DR. LICHSTEIN: How do you know you're sleepy?

JENNIFER: I just feel like I didn't get the sleep I needed the night before. I feel worn out, jumpy, irritable.

DR. LICHSTEIN: People can feel worn out, jumpy, and irritable for lots of reasons. How do you know that sleepiness is causing these feelings?

JENNIFER: It just seems like I feel that way more on days following a poor night's sleep than a good one, and it's obviously caused by not getting enough sleep.

DR. LICHSTEIN: I think we may be heading in the same direction as last week when I suggested that your defining yourself as an insomniac helps create the insomnia.

JENNIFER: This time, I think I'll not get annoyed at you until I hear what you have to say.

DR. LICHSTEIN: I appreciate the more open stance you're taking. [*I just dropped another food pellet in the Skinner box.*] Two things happen on nights you sleep poorly. One, you're getting less sleep. Two, you're spending more awake time in bed. Awake time in bed is boring, frustrating, and irritating. The way you describe your daytime sleepiness, it sounds like much of it could be caused by frustrating awake time as opposed to insufficient sleep. Daytime sleepiness is usually accompanied by drowsiness, the eyelids feeling heavy, difficulty maintaining visual focus while reading, and sometimes naps. You identified none of these.

JENNIFER: Now that you mention it, I do have some of those sleepy feelings too, but you're right, I'm more exasperated than sleepy. After not getting the sleep I need, I wake up in the morning dreading the day, convinced that I won't be able to function. I guess that's a pretty sour attitude.

DR. LICHSTEIN: I certainly agree with you there, but I must challenge you on something else you just said. That is, "after not getting the sleep I need." I'm not sure you *need* all the sleep you're wanting to get. One of the problems may be that you are trying to get more sleep than you need.

Toward the end of this session, I formulated a tentative treatment plan in my mind and will share it with Jennifer the following week after evaluation of her second week of sleep data and further exploration of relevant variables.

By midway in the fifth session, I feel confident with a treatment plan (highlighted next) that I describe and explain in detail to Jennifer.

1. In therapy sessions, I will continue to explore and challenge Jennifer's attitudes toward sleep that may be contributing to an exacerbation cycle at bedtime.
2. Jennifer will attempt to standardize the time she enters bed in the evening and leaves bed in the morning. Every 4 days she will advance by 15 minutes (i.e., 11:00 P.M., 11:15 P.M, and so on) the time she enters bed while keeping the morning time constant, as early morning awakenings are not a problem for her. This is done to reduce sleep variability between nights and decrease awake time in bed.
3. Jennifer will institute a stimulus control regimen.
4. I will describe several different relaxation methods, and Jennifer will select the one she prefers. This will be trained in session and practiced at least once a day. One practice must occur in bed while trying to fall asleep. Jennifer will institute Items 2 and 3 immediately. Relaxation will be taught in Session 6. Also in Session 6, I will begin carefully monitoring her implementation of treatment and its effects.

If the treatment package is appropriate, we should observe unambiguous improvement within 3 weeks. Additional gains may occur over 1 or 2 months. Much depends on clients' willingness to reassess their sleep beliefs and their diligence in following through on home assignments. In Jennifer's case, we terminated by mutual consent after the 12th session. Therapy had progressed at a reasonably lively pace with Jennifer. Had she been less intelligent and less psychologically minded, my explanations and analyses would have consumed more time, and the length of treatment would have been extended.

At the time of termination, Jennifer's sleep routines had stabilized and her self-reported latency to sleep was well below 30 minutes on most nights. What is most important, she no longer defined herself as an insomniac, and this change was due as much to revising her attitudes as to revising her sleep behavior.

Routine problems present themselves in treating insomnia. Clients may provide inadequate information, be hostile to the treatment plan, or fail to implement treatment satisfactorily at home. These are the sorts of problems common to most behavioral therapies, and they must be actively addressed in session.

One of the major challenges facing insomnia treatment is gerontologic insomnia. Sleep patterns naturally change across the life span (Williams, Karacan, & Hursch, 1974). During early childhood, sleep is characterized by long periods of continuous sleep largely composed of REM, moderately deep sleep (Stage 2), and delta EEG waves, or Stage 4. By adulthood, sleep duration gradually shrinks to about 7 hours, light sleep (Stages 1 and 2) increases to claim about 60% of sleep time, REM declines somewhat to about 25%, and deep sleep to about 15%. As one's age approaches 60, the relative sleep pattern stability of the past four decades yields to expanding light sleep (particularly Stage 1), slightly decreasing REM, greatly decreasing deep sleep (down to about 2%), and a discontinuous sleep pattern marked by multiple awakenings during the night. In part due to increased Stage 1 sleep, the elderly may be condemned to more daytime sleepiness than middle-aged normal sleepers (Carskadon & Dement, 1982). Furthermore, the elderly are at greater risk for chronic diseases that may disrupt sleep. The reader is referred to Bootzin *et al.* (1983), Miles and Dement (1980), Prinz and Raskind (1978), and Siegel and Lichstein (1980) for extended discussions of sleep in the elderly. Clinically salient, changing trends in sleep across the age span are highlighted in Figure 2.

What was defined as an insomnia pattern in middle age—abbreviated, light, discontinuous sleep—is now the norm. Failure to recognize and adjust to one's changing sleep needs may create a highly distressful, insomnoid state in the elderly. Most psychological treatments for insomnia contrive to increase sleep, which is an inappropriate goal for an unknown number of elderly insomniacs. Not surprisingly, the elderly respond poorly to insomnia treatments designed for middle-aged subjects (Alperson & Biglan, 1979; Nicassio & Bootzin, 1974), suggesting that existing treatments require modification and novel treatments need to be developed.

Sleep efficiency percentage, the ratio of time slept to total time in bed, has received relatively little attention in studies of middle-aged insomniacs, but it may be the key dependent measure in gerontologic insomnia. Treatments that manipulate the sleep efficiency denominator (time in bed) may prove more useful for the elderly than those targeting sleep latency with an emphasis on extending sleep (sleep efficiency numerator).

Life-style management, discussed previously, is deserving of further investigation for this problem. It has already logged several successes with the elderly (Lichstein, 1980; Puder *et al.*, 1983) and is sufficiently flexible to test new avenues of intervention. For example, napping may be deleterious to middle-aged people's sleep by suppressing deep sleep, but it may be a desirable therapeutic strategy for

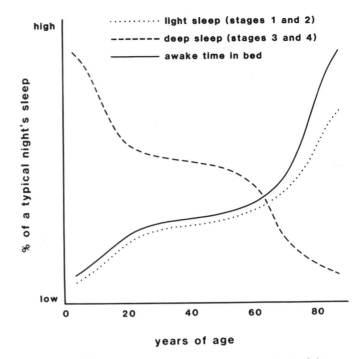

Figure 2. Life span changes in clinically relevant aspects of sleep.

the elderly where deep sleep has all but vanished anyway. Sleeping in two or three short (2 to 3 hours) blocks of time distributed throughout a 24-hour period may neatly conform to the biological sleep needs of the elderly. As a cautionary note, elderly subjects may require considerable sleep education and aid in scheduling sleep routines and shifts in awake time.

General Summary

Insomnia may exert a substantive impact on one's mood and performance and is prone to developing a chronic status. Nevertheless, it is often responsive to treatment. In most cases, a functional analysis of insomnia will dictate an effective treatment regimen. There remain many important, outstanding issues in the behavioral treatment of insomnia that merit the systematic attention of clinicians and researchers alike. Some of these are outlined next.

As revealed by Tables 5 and 6, most psychological treatments for insomnia are helpful, and no one treatment clearly emerges as superior to others, although stimulus control has an edge. Accumulating evidence points toward the heterogeneity of insomnia subtypes, and it is becoming less tenable to apply uniformly any one insomnia treatment to all subjects. Researchers and clinicians need to define more clearly the client's insomnia profile (e.g., age considerations, incompatible behaviors, cognitive arousal, etc.) and select treatments accordingly. Under these conditions, particular insomnia interventions may well emerge as the treatment of choice for specific insomnia subtypes.

Insomnoid states, as described herein, are a distinct clinical entity from pseudo- and idiopathic insomnia, although they share some of the features of each. Insomnoid states require interventions of a life-style management sort and would not be expected to respond to treatments aimed at helping people sleep longer (e.g., relaxation treatments). Although insomnoid states may occur in any age group, they are most likely to occur among the elderly. In general, insufficient attention has been devoted to the sleep problems of the elderly, despite a great need in this age group.

More than 80% of the studies of the psychological treatment of insomnia relied on highly suspect, self-report data to determine treatment efficacy. Scientific progress in this area will be retarded as long as unreliable dependent measures predominate. The recently emerging genre of empirical devices outlined in this chapter offer a desirable compromise between scientific rigor and expense. Future research is obliged to shift toward more reliable dependent measures in the form of devices such as these or polysomnography.

Relaxation therapy constitutes the most popular insomnia treatment approach. In these treatments, one or two treatment sessions are usually scheduled a week, but the bulk of the treatment is self-administered via home practice. Recent studies prescribing home practice of taped relaxation for hypertensive (Taylor, Agras, Schneider, & Allen, 1983) and anxious (Hoelscher, Lichstein, & Rosenthal, 1984) clients, documented low compliance of home practice assignments with the use of unobtrusively rigged tape recorders. Many of these individuals received a subtherapeutic dosage of relaxation despite high levels of *self-reported* relaxation practice. A valid evaluation of the efficacy of relaxation therapy (or any other insomnia treatment) awaits empirical determination of actual level of treatment implementation.

References

Adam, K. (1980). Dietary habits and sleep after bedtime food drinks. *Sleep, 3,* 47–58.

Alperson, J., & Biglan, A. (1979). Self-administered treatment of sleep onset insomnia and the importance of age. *Behavior Therapy, 10,* 347–356.

Ascher, L. M., & Efran, J. S. (1978). Use of paradoxical intention in a behavioral program for sleep onset insomnia. *Journal of Consulting and Clinical Psychology, 46,* 547–550.

Ascher, L. M., & Turner, R. M. (1979). Paradoxical intention and insomnia: An experimental investigation. *Behaviour Research and Therapy, 17,* 408–411.

Ascher, L. M., & Turner, R. M. (1980). A comparison of two methods for the administration of paradoxical intention. *Behaviour Research and Therapy, 18,* 121–126.

Association of Sleep Disorders Centers. (1979). Diagnostic classification of sleep and arousal disorders. *Sleep, 2,* 1–137.

Baekeland, F., & Lasky, R. (1966). Exercise and sleep patterns in college athletes. *Perceptual and Motor Skills, 23,* 1203–1207.

Balter, M. B., & Bauer, M. L. (1975). Patterns of prescribing and use of hypnotic drugs in the United States. In A. D. Clift (Ed.), *Sleep disturbance and hypnotic drug dependence* (pp. 261–293). Amsterdam: Excerpta Medica.

Bell, J. S. (1979). The use of EEG-theta biofeedback in the treatment of a patient with sleep-onset insomnia. *Biofeedback and Self-Regulation, 4,* 229–236.

Benson, H. (1975). *The relaxation response.* New York: Morrow.

Bergman, R. L. (1976). Treatment of childhood insomnia diagnosed as "hyperactivity." *Journal of Behavior Therapy and Experimental Psychiatry, 7,* 199.

Bernstein, D. A., & Borkovec, T. D. (1973). *Progressive relaxation training: A manual for the helping professions.* Champaign, IL: Research Press.

Besner, H. F. (1978). Biofeedback—Possible placebo in treating chronic-onset insomnia. *Biofeedback and Self-Regulation, 3,* 208.

Beutler, L. E., Thornby, J. I., & Karacan, I. (1978). Psychological variables in the diagnosis of insomnia. In R. L. Williams & I. Karacan (Eds.), *Sleep disorders: Diagnosis and treatment* (pp. 61–100). New York: Wiley.

Bixler, E. O., Kales, A., Soldatos, C. R., Kales, J. D., & Healey, S. (1979). Prevalence of sleep disorders in the Los Angeles Metropolitan Area. *American Journal of Psychiatry, 136,* 1257–1262.

Blanchard, E. B., Andrasik, F., Ahles, T. A., Teders, S. J., & O'Keefe, D. (1980). *Behavior Therapy, 11,* 613–631.

Bolton, S., & Null, G. (1981). Caffeine: Psychological effects, use and abuse. *Journal of Orthomolecular Psychiatry, 10,* 202–211.

Bootzin, R. R. (1972). Stimulus control treatment for insomnia. *Proceedings of the 80th Annual Convention of the American Psychological Association, 7,* 395–396.

Bootzin, R. R. (1973, August). *Stimulus control of insomnia.* Paper presented at the meeting of the American Psychological Association, Montreal.

Bootzin, R. R., & Engle-Friedman, M. (1981). The assessment of insomnia. *Behavioral Assessment, 3,* 107–126.

Bootzin, R. R., Engle-Friedman, M., & Hazelwood, L. (1983). Insomnia. In P. M. Lewinsohn & L. Teri (Eds.), *Clinical geropsychology: New directions in assessment and treatment* (pp. 81–115). New York: Pergamon.

Borkovec, T. D. (1979). Pseudo (experiential)-insomnia and idiopathic (objective) insomnia: Theoretical and therapeutic issues. *Advances in Behaviour Research and Therapy, 2,* 27–55.

Borkovec, T. D. (1982). Insomnia. *Journal of Consulting and Clinical Psychology, 50,* 880–895.

Borkovec, T. D., & Fowles, D. C. (1973). Controlled investigation of the effects of progressive and hypnotic relaxation on insomnia. *Journal of Abnormal Psychology, 82,* 153–158.

Borkovec, T. D., & Hennings, B. L. (1978). The role of physiological attention-focusing in the relaxation treatment of sleep disturbance, general tension, and specific stress reaction. *Behaviour Research and Therapy, 16,* 7–19.

Borkovec, T. D., & Weerts, T. C. (1976). Effects of progressive relaxation on sleep disturbance: An electroencephalographic evaluation. *Psychosomatic Medicine, 38,* 173–180.

Borkevec, T. D., Steinmark, S. W., & Nau, S. D. (1973). Relaxation training and single-item desensitization in the group treatment of insomnia. *Journal of Behavior Therapy and Experimental Psychiatry, 4,* 401–403.

Borkovec, T. D., Kaloupek, D. G., & Slama, K. M. (1975). The facilitative effect of muscle tension-release in the relaxation treatment of sleep disturbance. *Behavior Therapy, 6,* 301–309.

Borkovec, T. D., Grayson, J. B., O'Brien, G. T., & Weerts, T. C. (1979). Relaxation treatment of pseudoinsomnia and idiopathic insomnia: An electroencephalographic evaluation. *Journal of Applied Behavior Analysis, 12,* 37–54.

Brady, J. P. (1973). Metronome-conditioned relaxation: A new behavioral procedure. *British Journal of Psychiatry, 122,* 729–730.

Brezinova, V., & Oswald, I. (1972). Sleep after a bedtime beverage. *British Medical Journal, 2,* 431–433.

Browman, C. P., & Tepas, D. I. (1976). The effects of presleep activity on all-night sleep. *Psychophysiology, 13,* 536–540.

Brown, C. C. (1975). Electroanesthesia and electrosleep. *American Psychologist, 30,* 402–410.

Caffeine: What it does. (1981, October). *Consumer Reports,* pp. 595–599.

Cannici, J., Malcolm, R., & Peek, L. A. (1983). Treatment of insomnia in cancer patients using muscle relaxation training. *Journal of Behavior Therapy and Experimental Psychiatry, 14,* 251–256.

Carr-Kaffashan, L., & Woolfolk, R. L. (1979). Active and placebo effects in treatment of moderate and severe insomnia. *Journal of Consulting and Clinical Psychology, 47,* 1072–1080.

Carskadon, M. A., & Dement, W. C. (1982). Nocturnal determinants of daytime sleepiness. *Sleep, 5* (Suppl. 2), 73–81.

Coates, T. J., & Thoresen, C. E. (1977). *How to sleep better: A drug-free program for overcoming insomnia.* Englewood Cliffs, NJ: Prentice-Hall.

Coates, T. J., & Thoresen, C. E. (1979). Treating arousals during sleep using behavioral self-management. *Journal of Consulting and Clinical Psychology, 47,* 603–605.

Coates, T. J., Rosekind, M. R., & Thoresen, C. E. (1978). All night sleep recording in clients' homes by telephone. *Journal of Behavior Therapy and Experimental Psychiatry, 9,* 157–162.

Cotler, S. B., & Guerra, J. J. (1976). *Self-relaxation training* [Audiotape]. Champaign, IL: Research Press.

Coursey, R. D., Buchsbaum, M., & Frankel, B. L. (1975). Personality measures and evoked responses in chronic insomniacs. *Journal of Abnormal Psychology, 84,* 239–249.

Coursey, R. D., Frankel, B. L., Gaarder, K. R., & Mott, D. E. (1980). A comparison of relaxation techniques with electrosleep therapy for chronic, sleep-onset insomnia: A sleep-EEG study. *Biofeedback and Self-Regulation, 5,* 57–73.

Crisp, A. H., & Stonehill, E. (1976). *Sleep, nutrition and mood.* London: Wiley.

Davidson, R. J., & Schwartz, G. E. (1976). The psychobiology of relaxation and related states: A multi-process theory. In D. I. Mostofsky (Ed.), *Behavior control and modification of physiological activity* (pp. 399–442). Englewood Cliffs, NJ: Prentice-Hall.

Davison, G. C., Tsujimoto, R. N., & Glaros, A. G. (1973). Attribution and the maintenance of behavior change in falling asleep. *Journal of Abnormal Psychology, 82,* 124–133.

Dixon, K. N., Monroe, L. J., & Jakim, S. (1981). Insomniac children. *Sleep, 4,* 313–318.

Evans, D. R., & Bond, I. K. (1969). Reciprocal inhibition therapy and classical conditioning in the treatment of insomnia. *Behaviour Research and Therapy, 7,* 323–325.

Feinstein, B., Sterman, M. B., & Macdonald, L. R. (1974). Effects of sensorimotor rhythm biofeedback training on sleep. *Sleep Research, 3,* 134.

Fogle, D. O., & Dyal, J. A. (1983). Paradoxical giving up and the reduction of sleep performance anxiety in chronic insomniacs. *Psychotherapy: Theory, Research and Practice, 20,* 21–30.

Freedman, R. R., & Papsdorf, J. D. (1976). Biofeedback and progressive relaxation treatment of sleep-onset insomnia: A controlled all-night investigation. *Biofeedback and Self-Regulation, 1,* 253–271.

Freedman, R. R., & Sattler, H. L. (1982). Physiological and psychological factors in sleep-onset insomnia. *Journal of Abnormal Psychology, 91,* 380–389.

Freedman, R. R., Hauri, P., Coursey, R., & Frankel, B. (1978). Behavioral treatment of insomnia: A collaborative study. *Biofeedback and Self-Regulation, 3,* 208–209.

Fry, A. (1973). Hypnosis in the treatment of insomnia. *British Journal of Clinical Hypnosis, 4,* 23–28.

Gershman, L., & Clouser, R. A. (1974). Treating insomnia with relaxation and desensitization in a group setting by an automated approach. *Journal of Behavior Therapy and Experimental Psychiatry, 5,* 31–35.

Graham, K. R., Wright, G. W., Toman, W. J., & Mark, C. B. (1975). Relaxation and hypnosis in the treatment of insomnia. *American Journal of Clinical Hypnosis, 18,* 39–42.

Griffin, S. J., & Trinder, J. (1978). Physical fitness, exercise, and human sleep. *Psychophysiology, 15,* 447–450.

Gross, R. T., & Borkovec, T. D. (1982). Effects of a cognitive intrusion manipulation on the sleep-onset latency of good sleepers. *Behavior Therapy, 13,* 112–116.

Hanley, F. W. (1965). Modern hypnotherapy. *Applied Therapeutics, 7,* 625–628.

Hathaway, S. R., & McKinley, J. C. (1943). *Minnesota Multiphasic Personality Inventory: Manual.* New York: Psychological Corporation.

Hauri, P. (1981). Treating psychophysiologic insomnia with biofeedback. *Archives of General Psychiatry, 38,* 752–758.

Hauri, P. J. (1983). A cluster analysis of insomnia. *Sleep, 6,* 326–338.

Hauri, P., & Good, R. (1975). *Frontalis muscle tension and sleep onset.* Paper presented at the meeting of the Association for the Psychophysiological Study of Sleep, Edinburgh, Scotland.

Hauri, P. J., Percy, L., Hellekson, C., Hartmann, E., & Russ, D. (1982). The treatment of psychophysiologic insomnia with biofeedback: A replication study. *Biofeedback and Self-Regulation, 7,* 223–235.

Haynes, S. N., Follingstad, D. R., & McGowan, W. T. (1974). Insomnia: Sleep patterns and anxiety level. *Journal of Psychosomatic Research, 18,* 69–74.

Haynes, S. N., Woodward, S., Moran, R., & Alexander, D. (1974). Relaxation treatment of insomnia. *Behavior Therapy, 5,* 555–558.

Haynes, S. N., Price, M. G., & Simons, J. B. (1975). Stimulus control treatment of insomnia. *Journal of Behavior Therapy and Experimental Psychiatry, 6,* 279–282.

Haynes, S. N., Moseley, D., & McGowan, W. T. (1975). Relaxation training and biofeedback in the reduction of frontalis muscle tension. *Psychophysiology, 12,* 547–552.

Haynes, S. N., Sides, H., & Lockwood, G. (1977). Relaxation instructions and frontalis electromyographic feedback intervention with sleep-onset insomnia. *Behavior Therapy, 8,* 644–652.

Haynes, S. N., Adams, A., & Franzen, M. (1981). The effects of presleep stress on sleep-onset insomnia. *Journal of Abnormal Psychology, 90,* 601–606.

Haynes, S. N., Adams, A. E., West, S., Kamens, L., & Safranek, R. (1982). The stimulus control paradigm in sleep-onset insomnia: A multimethod assessment. *Journal of Psychosomatic Research, 26,* 333–339.

Hoelscher, T. J., Lichstein, K. L., & Rosenthal, T. L. (1984). Objective vs. subjective assessment of relaxation compliance among anxious individuals. *Behaviour Research and Therapy, 22,* 187–193.

Horne, J. A., & Porter, J. M. (1976). Time of day effects with standardized exercise upon subsequent sleep. *Electroencephalography and Clinical Neurophysiology, 40,* 178–184.

Hughes, R. C., & Hughes, H. H. (1978). Insomnia: Effects of EMG biofeedback, relaxation training, and stimulus control. *Behavioral Engineering, 5,* 67–72.

Institute of Medicine. (1979). *Sleeping pills, insomnia, and medical practice.* Washington, DC: National Academy of Sciences.

Jacobson, E. (1920). Use of relaxation in hypertensive states. *New York Medical Journal, 111,* 419–422.

Jacobson, E. (1938a). *Progressive relaxation* (2nd ed.). Chicago: University of Chicago Press.

Jacobson, E. (1938b). *You can sleep well.* New York: Whittlesey House.

Jacobson, E. (1970). *Modern treatment of tense patients.* Springfield, IL: Charles C Thomas.

Jones, H. S., & Oswald, I. (1968). Two cases of healthy insomnia. *Electroencephalography and Clinical Neurophysiology, 24,* 378–380.

Kamgar-Parsi, B., Wehr, T. A., & Gillin, J. C. (1983). Successful treatment of human non-24-hour sleep-wake syndrome. *Sleep, 6,* 257–264.

Karacan, I. (1972). Symposium: The evaluation and treatment of sleep disorders: Pharmacological and psychological studies. In M. H. Chase (Ed.), *The sleeping brain* (pp. 461–467). Los Angeles: Brain Information Service/Brain Research Institute.

Karacan, I., Warheit, G. G., Thornby, J. I. Schwab, J. J., & Williams, R. L. (1973). Prevalence of sleep disturbance in the general population. *Sleep Research, 2,* 158.

Karacan, I., Williams, R. L., Finley, W. W., & Hursch, C. J. (1970). The effects of naps on nocturnal sleep: Influence on the need for Stage-1 REM and Stage-4 sleep. *Biological Psychiatry, 2,* 391–399.

Kazarian, S. S., Howe, M. G., & Csapo, K. G. (1979). Development of the sleep behavior self-rating scale. *Behavior Therapy, 10,* 412–417.

Kripke, D. F., Simons, R. N., Garfinkel, L., & Hammond, E. C. (1979). Short and long sleep and sleeping pills. *Archives of General Psychiatry, 36,* 103–116.

Lacks, P., Bertelson, A. D., Gans, L., & Kunkel, J. (1983). The effectiveness of three behavioral treatments for different degrees of sleep onset insomnia. *Behavior Therapy, 14,* 593–605.

Lacks, P., Bertelson, A. D., Sugerman, J., & Kunkel, J. (1983). The treatment of sleep-maintenance insomnia with stimulus-control techniques. *Behaviour Research and Therapy, 21,* 291–295.

Lehrer, P. M., Batey, D., Woolfolk, R. L., Remde, A., & Garlick, T. (1983, December). *Does tensing muscles help to relax them? Does thinking about muscle tension increase it? A test of some procedural variables in progressive relaxation therapy.* Paper presented at the meeting of the World Congress on Behavior Therapy, Washington, DC.

Lichstein, K. L. (1980, November). *Treatment of severe insomnia by manipulation of sleep schedule.* Paper presented at the meeting of the Association for Advancement of Behavior Therapy, New York.

Lichstein, K. L. (1983). Ocular relaxation as a treatment for insomnia. *Behavioral Counseling and Community Interventions. 3,* 178–185.

Lichstein, K. L. (in press). *Clinical relaxation strategies.* New York: Wiley.

Lichstein, K. L., & Blew, A. (1980, November). *Ocular relaxation and progressive relaxation treatments for insomnia.* Paper presented at the meeting of the Association for Advancement of Behavior Therapy, New York.

Lichstein, K. L., & Kelley, J. E. (1979). Measuring sleep patterns in natural settings. *Behavioral Engineering, 5,* 95–101.

Lichstein, K. L., & Rosenthal, T. L. (1980). Insomniacs' perceptions of cognitive versus somatic determinants of sleep disturbance. *Journal of Abnormal Psychology, 89,* 105–107.

Lichstein, K. L., & Sallis, J. F. (1982). Ocular relaxation to reduce eye movements. *Cognitive Therapy and Research, 6,* 113–118.

Lichstein, K. L., Nickel, R., Hoelscher, T. J., & Kelley, J. E. (1982). Clinical validation of a sleep assessment device. *Behaviour Research and Therapy, 20,* 292–297.

Lichstein, K. L., Hoelscher, T. J., & Eakin, T. L. (1984, May). *Insomniacs' empirical self-assessment of sleep in the home.* Paper presented at the meeting of the Society of Behavioral Medicine, Philadelphia.

Lichstein, K. L., Takayama, M., & Sanders, J. (1984, November). *Napping: Some epidemiological data.* Paper presented at the meeting of the Association for Advancement of Behavior Therapy, Philadelphia.

Lick, J. R., & Heffler, D. (1977). Relaxation training and attention placebo in the treatment of severe insomnia. *Journal of Consulting and Clinical Psychology, 45,* 153–161.

Luthe, W., & Schultz, J. H. (1969). Applications in psychotherapy (Vol. 3). In W. Luthe (Ed.), *Autogenic therapy* (pp. 141–143). New York: Grune & Stratton.

McGhie, A., & Russell, S. M. (1962). The subjective assessment of normal sleep patterns. *Journal of Mental Science, 108,* 642–654.

Meddis, R., Pearson, A. J. D., & Langford, G. (1973). An extreme case of healthy insomnia. *Electroencephalography and Clinical Neurophysiology, 35,* 213–214.

Miles, L. E., & Dement, W. C. (1980). Sleep and aging. *Sleep, 3,* 119–220.

Miskiman, D. E. (1977). The treatment of insomnia by the Transcendental Meditation program. In D. W. Orme-Johnson & J. T. Farrow (Eds.), *Scientific research on the Transcendental Meditation program: Collected papers* (Vol. 1, 2nd ed., pp. 296–298). Livingston Manor, NY: Maharishi European Research University Press.

Mitchell, K. R. (1979). Behavioral treatment of presleep tension and intrusive cognitions in patients with severe predormital insomnia. *Journal of Behavioral Medicine, 2,* 57–69.

Mitchell, K. R., & White, R. G. (1977). Self-management of severe predormital insomnia. *Journal of Behavior Therapy and Experimental Psychiatry, 8,* 57–63.

Monroe, L. J. (1967). Psychological and physiological differences between good and poor sleepers. *Journal of Abnormal Psychology, 72,* 255–264.

Nicassio, P., & Bootzin, R. (1974). A comparison of progressive relaxation and autogenic training as treatments for insomnia. *Journal of Abnormal Psychology, 83,* 253–260.

Nicassio, P. M., Boylan, M. B., & McCabe, T. G. (1982). Progressive relaxation, EMG biofeedback and biofeedback placebo in the treatment of sleep-onset insomnia. *British Journal of Medical Psychology, 55,* 159–166.

Ott, B. D., Levine, B. A., & Ascher, L. M. (1983). Manipulating the explicit demand of paradoxical intention instructions. *Behavioural Psychotherapy, 11,* 25–35.

Paxton, S. J., Trinder, J., & Montgomery, I. (1983). Does aerobic fitness affect sleep? *Psychophysiology, 20,* 320–324.

Pendleton, L. R., & Tasto, D. L. (1976). Effects of metronome-conditioned relaxation, metronome-induced relaxation, and progressive muscle relaxation on insomnia. *Behaviour Research and Therapy, 14,* 165–166.

Pokorny, A. D. (1978). Sleep disturbances, alcohol, and alcoholism: A review. In R. L. Williams & I. Karacan (Eds.), *Sleep disorders: Diagnosis and treatment* (pp. 233–260). New York: Wiley.

Prinz, P. N., & Raskind, M. (1978). Aging and sleep disorders. In R. L. Williams & I. Karacan (Eds.), *Sleep disorders: Diagnosis and treatment* (pp. 303–321). New York: Wiley.

Puder, R., Lacks, P., Bertelson, A. D., & Storandt, M. (1983). Short-term stimulus control treatment of insomnia in older adults. *Behavior Therapy, 14,* 424–429.

Relinger, H., & Bornstein, P. H. (1979). Treatment of sleep onset insomnia by paradoxical instruction: A multiple baseline design. *Behavior Modification, 3,* 203–222.

Relinger, H., Bornstein, P. H., & Mungas, D. M. (1978). Treatment of insomnia by paradoxical intention: A time-series analysis. *Behavior Therapy, 9,* 955–959.

Ribordy, S. C. (1976). The behavioral treatment of insomnia. *Dissertation Abstracts International, 37,* 477B. (University Microfilms No. 76–16, 769).

Schultz, J. H., & Luthe, W. (1959). *Autogenic training: A psychophysiologic approach in psychotherapy.* New York: Grune & Stratton.

Seidel, W. F., & Dement, W. C. (1982). Sleepiness in insomnia: Evaluation and treatment. *Sleep, 5* (Suppl. 2), 182–190.

Shealy, R. C. (1979). The effectiveness of various treatment techniques on different degrees and durations of sleep-onset insomnia. *Behaviour Research and Therapy, 17,* 541–546.

Shealy, R. C., Lowe, J. D., & Ritzler, B. A. (1980). Sleep onset insomnia: Personality characteristics and treatment outcome. *Journal of Consulting and Clinical Psychology, 48,* 659–661.

Siegal, G. S., & Lichstein, K. L. (1980). The treatment of gerontologic insomnia. *Canadian Counsellor, 14*, 121–126.

Sittenfeld, P., Budzynski, T., & Stoyva, J. (1976). Differential shaping of EEG theta rhythms. *Biofeedback and Self-Regulation, 1*, 31–46.

Steinmark, S. W., & Borkovec, T. D. (1974). Active and placebo treatment effects on moderate insomnia under counterdemand and positive demand instructions. *Journal of Abnormal Psychology, 83*, 157–163.

Stepanski, E., Lamphere, J., Badia, P., Zorick, F., & Roth, T. (1984). Sleep fragmentation and daytime sleepiness. *Sleep, 7*, 18–26.

Sterman, M. B., Howe, R. C., & Macdonald, L. R. (1970). Facilitation of spindle-burst sleep by conditioning electroencephalographic activity while awake. *Science, 167*, 1146–1148.

Taylor, C. B., Agras, W. S., Schneider, J. A., & Allen, R. A. (1983). Adherence to instructions to practice relaxation exercises. *Journal of Consulting and Clinical Psychology, 51*, 952–953.

Taylor, J. A. (1953). A personality scale of manifest anxiety. *Journal of Abnormal and Social Psychology, 48*, 285–290.

Thoresen, C. E., Coates, T. J., Kirmil-Gray, K., & Rosekind, M. R. (1981). Behavioral self-management in treating sleep-maintenance insomnia. *Journal of Behavioral Medicine, 4*, 41–52.

Tokarz, T. P., & Lawrence, P. S. (1974, November). *An analysis of temporal and stimulus factors in the treatment of insomnia.* Paper presented at the meeting of the Association for Advancement of Behavior Therapy, Chicago.

Toler, H. C. (1978). The treatment of insomnia with relaxation and stimulus-control instructions among incarcerated males. *Criminal Justice and Behavior, 5*, 117–130.

Traub, A. C., Jencks, B., & Bliss, E. L. (1973). Effects of relaxation training on chronic insomnia. *Sleep Research, 2*, 164.

Turner, R. M., & Ascher, L. M. (1979a). Controlled comparison of progressive relaxation, stimulus control, and paradoxical intention therapies for insomnia. *Journal of Consulting and Clinical Psychology, 47*, 500–508.

Turner, R. M., & Ascher, L. M. (1979b). A within-subject analysis of stimulus control therapy with severe sleep-onset insomnia. *Behaviour Research and Therapy, 17*, 107–112.

Turner, R. M., & Ascher, L. M. (1982). Therapist factor in the treatment of insomnia. *Behaviour Research and Therapy, 20*, 33–40.

VanderPlate, C., & Eno, E. N. (1983). Electromyograph biofeedback and sleep onset insomnia: Comparison of treatment and placebo. *Behavioral Engineering, 8*, 146–153.

Von Richthofen, C. L., & Mellor, C. S. (1979). Cerebral electrotherapy: Methodological problems in assessing its therapeutic effectiveness. *Psychological Bulletin, 86*, 1264–1271.

Webb, W. B., & Agnew, H. W., Jr. (1967). Sleep cycling within twenty-four hour periods. *Journal of Experimental Psychology, 74*, 158–160.

Webster, J. B., Kripke, D. F., Messin, S., Mullaney, D. J., & Wyborney, G. (1982). An activity-based sleep monitor system for ambulatory use. *Sleep, 5*, 389–399.

Williams, R. L. (1978). Sleep disturbances in various medical and surgical conditions. In R. L. Williams & I. Karacan (Eds.), *Sleep disorders: Diagnosis and treatment* (pp. 285–301). New York: Wiley.

Williams, R. L., Karacan, I., & Hursch, C. J. (1974). *Electroencephalography (EEG) of human sleep: Clinical applications.* New York: Wiley.

Winfree, A. T. (1982). Circadian timing of sleepiness in man and woman. *American Journal of Physiology, 243*, R193–R204.

Wittig, R. M., Zorick, F. J., Blumer, D., Heilbronn, M., & Roth, T. (1982). Disturbed sleep in patients complaining of chronic pain. *Journal of Nervous and Mental Disease, 170*, 429–431.

Wolpe, J. (1982). *The practice of behavior therapy* (3rd ed.). New York: Pergamon.

Woolfolk, R. L., Carr-Kaffashan, L., McNulty, T. F., & Lehrer, P. M. (1976). Meditation training as a treatment for insomnia. *Behavior Therapy, 7*, 359–365.

Woolfolk, R. L., & McNulty, T. F. (1983). Relaxation treatment for insomnia: A component analysis. *Journal of Consulting and Clinical Psychology, 51*, 495–503.

Zwart, C. A., & Lisman, S. A. (1979). Analysis of stimulus control treatment of sleep-onset insomnia. *Journal of Consulting and Clinical Psychology, 47*, 113–118.

13

Pain

K. Gunnar Götestam and Steven J. Linton

Introduction

Chronic pain is a multifaceted and complex phenomenon, and although advancements have been made, it remains a difficult problem for the health care system. Pain is one of the most frequent complaints that doctors encounter, but it is by no means a well-defined disorder. Pain ususally occurs as a result of noxious stimulation; however, sometimes it occurs or remains without apparent cause. This has resulted in much speculation about psychological mechanisms. Although psychological theories perhaps originated to account for cases that doctors could not successfully understand or deal with, a behavioral approach is interested in the behaviors associated with pain and how these may be influenced by learning.

A distinction between *acute* pain and *intractible* or *chronic* pain is usually made. Acute pain occurs as a result of some trauma and disappears when the injury has healed. Intractable or chronic pain is quite different. The pain occurs or persists even though healing should have occurred or even if no trauma has been observed. (Chronic pain is defined as that lasting 3 to 6 months or more.) Even if acute pain is believed to serve the function of a warning, signaling body damage, chronic pain may no longer serve any useful function. From a behavioral standpoint, chronic pain is interesting because the time involved in the development of the problem allows for much learning. Most of the literature dealing with behavioral approaches to pain are concerned with chronic pain. However, behavioral programs may also be used to influence acute pain, usually by dealing with the fear, anxiety, and ten-

K. GUNNAR GÖTESTAM • Department of Psychiatry and Behavioural Medicine, University of Trondheim, N-7001, Trondheim, Norway. STEVEN J. LINTON • Department of Occupational Medicine, Örebro Medical Centre Hospital, 701 85 Örebro, Sweden.

sion aspects of it; several examples are provided by Turk and Genest (1979). The fact remains, though, that the most difficult cases and most frequently encountered problems are with chronic pain patients. As a result, we intend to concentrate on chronic pain problems in this chapter, even if the techniques may, in general, be applied to acute pain situations as well.

Chronic pain is indeed a problem for individuals as well as society. In the United States, 700 million working days are lost, and the cost is estimated to be between $50 and $100 billion annually (Bonica, 1981; Brena, Chapman, & Decker, 1981). The individual consequences also are considerable. Patients may become depressed, over use analgesics, become inactive socially and physically, have problems sleeping and enjoying sex, have interpersonal difficulties, and generally develop a "passive" life-style (Linton, Melin, & Götestam, 1984).

Considering the magnitude of the problem, it is not surprising that much attention is being paid to it. Conventional medical treatments have advanced so that, for example, they are of some help for most instances of acute back pain (Nachemson, 1983). The trouble for the medical system is to deal effectively with the development of chronic pain problems. Preventing the development of chronic pain as well as treating fully developed cases has not been negotiated very effectively in the medical system. Behavioral psychologists began analyzing the problem, and the revolutionary idea that resulted was to look at pain as a set of behaviors rather than as a neurological state. Early books on the subject (Fordyce, 1976; Sternbach, 1974) stressed that pain consisted of several behaviors and that these behaviors could be influenced by systematically applying the principles of learning. Today, behavioral programs for the treatment of chronic pain have been incorporated into a large number of rehabilitation projects and pain clinics. The efficacy of these programs is reviewed elsewhere (e.g., Linton, 1982a; Turner & Chapman, 1982), but it may be said here that such behavioral programs seem to be clearly warranted for clinical use. The remainder of this chapter is oriented toward assessment and treatment methods that may be used in clinical work with this pain population. It should be noted that the chapter is organized around an example of back/joint pain and that methods for other types of chronic pain (e.g., headache or cancer) may require adaptation of the procedures.

Assessment

Despite the fact that most attention in the literature is given to treatment, a good assessment is a prerequisite for successful remediation of chronic pain. In fact, inaccurate or poor assessment seems to be a major reason for treatment failures (Follick, Zitter, & Ahern, 1983). The evaluation helps to identify problem behaviors, and it should indicate conditions for relief in a manner that allows for matching of the most efficacious treatment procedures to an individual patient. In this section guidelines for evaluating chronic pain patients will be outlined. The general approach for behavioral assessment described by Keefe, Kopel, and Gordon (1978) is used. Critical reviews of methods for assessment may be found elsewhere (Keefe, 1982; Keefe, Brown, Scott, & Ziesat, 1982; Linton, in press; Sanders 1979).

Behavioral assessment of chronic pain is in its infancy, and it would be unfair to present this information as a finalized, rigid program. Instead, the basic methods are described along with some alternative ones. Methods thought to be most useful are highlighted. A clinician's final decision about which methods and instruments to use will in part be guided by practical needs and in part by the patient's problem. We do not recommend any one given "assessment" or battery of tests but suggest that the assessment be designed for individuals. The rules that need to be stressed are (a) use a broad range of variables tapping several aspects (physiology, behavior, cognitions) of the problem; (b) emphasize the importance of a functional analysis; (c) conduct the behavior analysis in conjunction with medical evaluations. This final point need not be dwelled upon here, but it is obvious that a current, thorough medical examination needs to be conducted. Unlike some authors (e.g., Follick *et al.*, 1983), however, we see no need to automatically exclude patients for whom medical treatments may also be recommended. Indeed, a closer working relationship between medical and behavioral approaches is recommended.

The goal of assessment is to identify problem behaviors, to measure and analyze them functionally, to select and match treatment to the individual client, and to assess how well the therapy works (Kanfer & Saslow, 1976). With this in mind we proceed to the evaluation.

Problem Identification

For pain patients the problem would seem to be obvious: pain. As pointed out earlier, things are not that simple. Pain and suffering have many behavioral aspects, and these may or may not be related to organic processes. Not infrequently the complaint of pain may actually be secondary to other problems. This is seen, for example, in depression, where pain is of secondary importance. The idea, then, is to obtain specific information about problem behavior.

Interview

The initial interview provides the opportunity to define the pain problem operationally in behavioral terms. This includes specifying problem behaviors, desirable behaviors, and activities one is hindered from participating in, and exploring other consequences of the problem that the patient may not have previously considered. A list of general interview topics for use with chronic pain patients is provided in Table 1. Examples of interview questions are provided in Table 2. A history of the problem can be important in helping to determine if learning factors are helping to maintain the current problem. (The specific format and questionnaires are described later.) A look at frequency, intensity, and duration of responses should give an initial indication of whether the response is in deficit or excess. Through self-reports during the interview, one can also obtain preliminary information about the antecedents and consequences of problem behaviors. This is facilitated by asking the patient about a "typical" day (yesterday) and the last one or two occurrences of each problem/target behavior.

Interview Formats

Though reliability, validity, and compliance data are lacking, several interview formats are available (e.g., Cautela, 1977; Heaton, Getto, Lehman, Fordyce, Brauer, & Groban, 1982; Melzack, 1975; Mooney, Cairns, & Robertson, 1976; Relinger, 1980). Most are designed for self-administration, although we suggest that they be used as a structure for the first interview. Which format is used is largely a matter of personal preference and of how much detail is desired. It is important to keep in mind, though, that patients cannot answer too many questions or fill in too many questionnaires. Thus, many questions in the interview formats may not be necessary for some patients.

Assessment Instruments

In this phase of the assessment, attention is focused on refined measurement of problem behaviors and factors controlling them. The patient may be given questionnaires to fill in at the conclusion of the first interview, and observation may begin via self-monitoring or having significant others monitor behavior. Observation *in vivo* usually occurs a little later in the assessment.

Questionnaires

Standardized psychological questionnaires and tests also are available. Occasionally some testing may be indicated after problem identification, but many clinics seem to administer tests routinely as a prelude to the first interview. The most widely used tests are the Minnesota Multiphasic Personality Inventory (MMPI), Ill-

Table 1. List of Points That Should Be Covered during Initial Interview

1. Current problem behaviors and their background
2. Pattern of current problem behaviors
   (a) description of behavior
   (b) intensity, duration, frequency etc.
   (c) antecedents and consequences
3. Avoidance and escape behaviors
4. Body image/handicap conceptions
5. "Denial" of other problems
6. Expectations and goals of treatment
7. Information deficits
8. Communication skills (social, assertion)
9. Screening of possible related problems
   (a) anxiety/fear
   (b) depression
   (c) guilt
   (d) marital
   (e) substance abuse
   (f) others

ness Behavior Questionnaire (IBQ) (Pilowsky & Spence, 1976), Eysenck Personality Inventory (EPI) (cf. Bond, 1971), and Cornell Health Index (Bond, 1971). Despite frequent use of these tests, their utility has not yet been established, particularly for clinical work with individuals (e.g., Sanders, 1979). If such testing is to be done, it is imperative that the reason for their use be clear so that the "cause" of the pain not be confused with the answers on the test. Although physical exams may be able to identify "exaggerators" (Waddell, McCulloch, Kummel, & Wenner, 1980), psychological tests cannot identify malingerers or separate "organic" from "psychogenic" pain with any reliability. Nor can they identify causes of the pain. As an example of this sort of problem, an elevated neurotic triad is often found for pain patients on the MMPI. The pain, then, may be thought to be of psychological nature. However, research shows that such "psychopathology" disappears when the patients are treated for pain behavior (Roberts & Reinhardt, 1980). On the other hand, tests such as Beck's Depression Inventory (Beck, Ward, Mendelson, Mock, & Erbaugh, 1961) might be used for screening purposes and as an outcome measure.

The McGill Pain Questionnaire (Melzack, 1975) was specifically designed to evaluate qualitative aspects of pain on sensory and affective dimensions. The test may give some insights into the problem, and it also has been used as an evaluation of therapy outcome. But its use in assessment aimed at designing treatments is not yet clear.

Finally, laboratory tests may occasionally be undertaken in a behavior analysis. These ordinarily have to do with measuring physiological "stress" indicators (e.g., EMG levels or temperature).

Rating Scales

For the assessment of pain, activity, and other variables, both in the assessment of the problem and of treatment progress, several rating scales have been constructed.

Which questionnaires one chooses depends, of course, on which behaviors are problematic. For many potential "secondary" problems, questionnaires or inventories have been developed; some of these are shown in Table 2.

Physical activity is a vital part of the pain problem, and some scales are available. The Activity Pattern Indicator (Fordyce, Lansky, Calsyn, Shelton, Stolov, & Rock, 1984) has been developed to assess what activity changes have taken place after the onset of pain. Its primary use is with patients whose pain is of recent onset and who risk developing chronic problems.

Sarno, Sarno, and Levita (1973) developed the Function Life Scale to assess rehabilitation patients' abilities to manage daily activities. Although reliability and validity are reportedly satisfactory, its disadvantage is that staff are required to rate 44 items. Thus, its use is limited to patients in the hospital.

Another scale is being developed, and it consists of 10 behaviorally oriented questions concerning daily activities (e.g., being able to sit, shop, and do housework) (Linton & Melin, 1984). Patients rate their abilities to participate in the activ-

Table 2. Common Problems Associated with Pain and Examples of Assessment Techniques

Problem	Interview Questions	Tests/Instruments	Monitoring
Pain experience (quality, intensity)	Describe pain intensity, frequency, duration, quality (general, yesterday). Describe in relation to specific activities (name, e.g., lifting, resting). Pain sites	McGill Pain Questionnaire, Visual Analogue Scales; Verbal (behavioral) rating scales	Self-monitoring of intensity, duration, quality, etc. (Caution: do not reinforce pain behavior!)
Activity (e.g., low levels or difficulties with specific ones)	How does your pain specifically affect your activities? (probe) What things do you do less/more of? Tell me how it affects you in the following areas: (a) work, (b) cook, (c) sit, (d) walk, (e) vacuum, this week? Spouse: same questions as above.	Activities of Daily Living tests; Test of Physical Condition (doctor / physical therapist); Activity Hierarchy; Pedometer; Actometer; Up-time units	Self-monitoring of frequency of general/specific activities; observation of ADL and/or problem situations; spouse monitoring of frequency and quality
Depression	Has the pain affected your mood? How? How do you feel about your future? Do you wake up early? Do you have trouble getting started to do things? Have you ever thought about taking your own life?	Beck Depression Inventory; Other inventories (e.g., Hamilton, MMPI)	If problem warrants it, self-monitoring of mood (Caution: do not reinforce depression!); spouse monitor patient's mood; note also that activity and sleep methods may be helpful
Medicine use	What do you do when you have a lot of pain? Do you ever use pain killers or any other type of medicine? What type? How often this week/yesterday? When did you take them? Did they help? How long? Are you satisfied with them? Do you ever take pain pills in anticipation of pain, e.g., before participating in activities?	With consent of patient if narcotic abuse is suspected, may use urine or blood test; automatic recording pill bottles	Self-monitoring type, frequency, when, effect (e.g., pill counts)

Fear, anxiety, muscle tension	Does the pain ever make you feel uptight? Are you unsure about why you have pain/what activities you may do? Do you worry about getting more pain if you do certain things (list)? Do you feel like you have tight muscles/that you are stressed? Tell me how you feel when _____ (e.g., name activity).	EMG; fear/anxiety scales: S-R Inventory of Anxiety Affect; Adjective Checklist	Self-monitor subjective state; observe patient in test or *in vivo* situations
Sleep	Is the pain affecting your sleep? Difficulty (a) getting to sleep, (b) waking up at night, (c) early morning awakening. Do you feel rested in the morning? What do you think about when go to bed? How long does it take for you to fall asleep?	Sleep onset units; sleep questionnaires, sleep laboratory (EEG)	Self-monitor of sleep onset, duration, awakenings, time up in morning, etc.
Cognitions/ coping style	Why do you think you have the pain? On a personal level, how do you handle the pain when it's at its worst/usual/best? What do you think about when in pain (e.g., when waiting today for appointment/during episode described earlier)?	Thought listing; inventories	Monitor thoughts periodically or in relation to situation/pain
Social skills, assertion	How are you in group situations (e.g. party, meeting, etc.)? Do you ever have problems saying no or telling people what you think (use examples, e.g., waiting in line, someone butts in)?	Wolpe-Lazarus Assertiveness Questionnaire; Rathus Assertiveness Scale; Social Avoidance and Distress Scale; Social Activity Questionnaire	Observe during interview, roleplay or *in vivo*; self-monitoring of problem situations
Marital	Do you feel that the pain is affecting your marriage in any way? How? How often do you do things as a couple/family?	Marital Pre-Counseling Inventory; Marital Adjustment Scale.	Observe couple in office in problem-solving task; Observe *in vivo* affectionate exchanges, S^+/S^- given to spouse. Self monitor number of S^+ given by spouse or touching, complaining, compliments, demands, etc.

ities on a 10-point scale from "cannot participate because of pain" to "can participate without pain being a problem." Research underway suggests that the scale is both reliable and valid. It provides a quick and economical look at the patients' activities in the home environment and may be used to evaluate outcome of therapy.

Inventories and scales can be of help in isolating target behaviors and determining their severity as well as in evaluating the outcome of therapy. However, they are of most help when the information is used as a supplement to other information that is collected.

Observation

Refined measurements of the behavior targeted are monitored *in vivo* to obtain information about its frequency, intensity, and duration.

Self-Monitoring

Pain has a clear, subjective aspect. This experience often is why the patient seeks help, and it therefore is of considerable importance. Patients may be asked to monitor their pain by making ratings to tap the subjective side of the pain experience. But care needs to be taken so that patients do not receive inadvertent reinforcement for pain behavior. On the contrary, this is an opportunity to shape intensity decreases and appropriate "paintalk" (Linton & Götestam, 1985).

A variety of pain rating scales have been used. A 0–5 point scale that has behavioral definitions for each category is preferable (Collins & Martin, 1980; Linton & Götestam, 1983; Sjödén & Bates, 1984). Although ratings are sometimes obtained hourly (e.g., Fordyce, 1976), four times per day provides adequate information (Collins & Martin, 1980) and probably increases compliance considerably. Other data may also be obtained on the same blank (e.g., medication use, sleep patterns, mood, or other target behaviors). An example of the monitoring blank is shown in Figure 1. It is important that the blank be designed so that it can be carried in a pocket or wallet. Further, to assure good compliance, it is essential that the blanks be thoroughly described—including reasons why they are to be used, instructions for how to fill them in, samples actually being filled in, and times and places where the blank will be used (agreed upon before the patient starts the monitoring).

Filling in these blanks should be reinforced. Priority should be given in the beginning of therapy sessions for examining the blanks, and correct monitoring should be verbally reinforced. Another way of reinforcing such behavior is to relate therapy progress (assessment and treatment) to the monitoring. Graphs and the like are often helpful in this respect.

In Vivo Observation

It can be important to observe behavior *in vivo* to obtain a clear picture of the problem and its controlling factors. Activity problems and pain communication behaviors are particularly suitable because other measures of them may be unreliable. It is helpful to develop a system of observing problem behaviors.

Occasionally, a person close to the patient may be asked to monitor certain behaviors. This may be a sensitive issue, and the patient and potential observer should both be consulted and agree to the procedure. The observer may be asked to make ratings or monitor behavior in a manner similar to how the patient is asked to self-rate.

Card page 4 (Reminders):

Reminders:

Practice relaxation 2 × day —
at 7:00 a.m. and 9:00 p.m.

Sit in chair and have your eyes open.

Use positive self-statements!

You can influence your pain!

Card page 1 (Pain Card):

Pain Card

Name: John Jones

Date out: September 13, 1985

Date in: September 21, 1985

Next appointment: September 28, 1985

Please fill this card in according to our agreement, four times everyday. Bring this card with you to your next appointment!

Further instructions:

Card page 2 (Pain Scale):

Pain Scale

to be used in judging your pain level

0 = No pain

1 = Pain present, but can be ignored

2 = Pain present, cannot be ignored, but does not interfere with everyday activities

3 = Pain present, cannot be ignored, interferes with concentration

4 = Pain present, cannot be ignored, interferes with all tasks except taking care of basic needs (eating, toilet visits)

5 = Pain present, cannot be ignored, rest or bedrest required

Card page 3 (Data table):

	Pain (0–5)	Duration (hours)	Medicine type/number		Sleep A time to sleep (min) B quality of sleep (good or poor) C number of awakings D hours slept	
Date Sept 22 Time 8:00 a.m.	4	2	Aspirin	2	A	45
11:30 a.m.	3	2½		0	B	good
5:00 p.m.	4	1	Tylenol	2	C	3
					D	7
Date ——— Time ——— ——— ———					A B C D	
Date ——— Time ——— ——— ———					A B C D	
Date ——— Time ——— ——— ———					A B C D	
Date ——— Time ——— ——— ———					A B C D	
Date ——— Time ——— ——— ———					A B C D	
Date ——— Time ——— ——— ———					A B C D	

Figure 1. Sample of a Pain Card in 3 × 5 format with details of each page.

Laboratory or Clinic Observations

Because it often is not practical to conduct *in vivo* observation, observations in the clinic are frequently carried out. These are made during interviews or in contrived situations (e.g., during activities or a conversation). Pain communication behavior, activity level, assertion, and coping styles are among the many behaviors that lend themselves to assessment with this method. Here again, it is advisable to develop an observational system.

Functional Analysis

To develop a treatment plan, it is necessary to pinpoint factors controlling and maintaining the patient's problem. A functional analysis is designed to isolate learning processes that may be relevant. All of the interview and observational techniques described before may be used, but attention shifts from merely describing the problem behavior to analyzing its function in relation to the discriminative stimuli of environmental situations (S^ds) in which it occurs as well as its consequences of positive and negative reinforcement (S^{r+-}) and punishment (S^-).

Self-Monitoring

Self-monitoring is an "old standby" method for functional analysis in behavior therapy. One or two problem behaviors at a time are selected, and the patient is asked to monitor the problem behavior, its antecedents, and consequences. Cognitive patterns and fear/anxiety are also monitored because they may be relevant for therapy. A sample form is shown in Table 3.

Table 3. Patient Form for Assessment of Pain

Time	Pain situation	Pain description		Pain consequences
		Behavior	Thoughts	

A great strength of observing the patient directly is that functional relations may emerge even if they are subtle or unknown to the patient. Again, target behaviors should be selected before observation takes place. Care should also be taken in arranging the observation situation so that the behavior of interest will occur. Clinic observations, for example, might include exercise in the gym (bike riding, running, etc.), an interview, and the spouse–patient relationship in several situations (conversation, while doing simple tasks: e.g., walking, vacuuming). Some sort of rating scale for observation should be designed to monitor the target behavior and look at antecedants and consequences. An example for pain behavior is shown in Figure 2. Another system has been developed by Keefe and Block (1982).

Observation can be especially fruitful for pain communication behavior, avoidance of activity, and spouse interaction. During or immediately after each observation period, the patient may be questioned about feelings and cognitions experienced during the course of the activity in question.

All recordings need to be charted so that relationships may be easily seen. They are also useful in motivating the patient and in demonstrating the progress of therapy.

Designing a Treatment for the Individual Client

By this time, much information has been collected. Whether learning processes are important in the pain problem should become clear. Usually, some tentative hypotheses concerning problem behaviors and their controlling factors emerge. Treatment is designed to test these hypotheses, and continuous measurement throughout treatment helps us in deciding if therapy is in fact working. Sometimes assessment needs to be continued because the hypotheses are not yet clear enough to generate a treatment plan, but they nonetheless may help guide further evaluation. For some patients, learning factors may not contribute significantly to their problem, and they may be referred for conventional medical care.

Conducting a functional analysis is like solving a puzzle. It takes time and patience, but putting the bits together is quite satisfying. Pain problems are unique to each individual, and a functional analysis is necessary to identify specific learning processes.

Therapy Techniques

Since specific pain centers and clinics have been established, psychological principles have been included both in diagnosis and treatment of chronic pain (Sternbach, 1974). Practical clinical treatment approaches have mainly been based on behavioral theories. Reviews of such procedures have been published by Linton (1982a) and Turner and Chapman (1982). Three approaches seem to have adequate theoretical foundation, empirical evidence to motivate clinical use, and to be widely accepted and followed by clinicians working with chronic pain patients.

Target person ___Fred___   Observer ___SJL___
                                  Length of intervals _30 sec_

Spouse/others present ___Susan___   Data sheet no._1_
                                    Date _July 23, 1985_

Setting: Home or Lab (describe): _Patient and spouse are to read instructions and carry out: get up, walk, lift, carry, etc._

Behavior Codes

I = Inappropriate: would not ordinarily be done by a person not having chronic pain

A = Appropriate: would be likely to be done by nonchronic pain person

Pain Behaviors (specific behaviors may be specified)

F = Facial, e.g., grimace
V = Verbal, pain statement

B = Body, e.g., limp, gating, holding, rubbing

Response of Spouse/Others

− = Disapproval, e.g., facial/verbal expression

+ = Approval, e.g., attention sympathy, help

0 = Nonevaluative comment or expression

Observation

Setting 1 _read/discuss_

	1	2	3	4	5	6	7	8	9	10
Patient	F/I	V/I	V/A	B/I	B/I	V/A	V/A	V/I		
Spouse	−	O	−	−	−		O	−		

Setting 2 _lift/carry_

	1	2	3	4	5	6	7	8	9	10
Patient	V/I	V/I	F/I	B/A	B/A	B/I	F/I	B/I	V/I	V/I
Spouse	+	+	+	O		−		+	+	O

Setting 3 _____

Patient										
Spouse										

Setting 4 _____

Patient										
Spouse										

Comments:

Figure 2. An example of a coding system for observing pain behavior.

These approaches include (a) relaxation procedures; (b) operant procedures; and (c) cognitive procedures.

365

PAIN

Relaxation Procedures

Relaxation procedures are founded on the respondent (or Pavlovian) conditioning model and constitute a counterconditioning of pain experience in different pain situations. Through relaxation (preferably applied relaxation in special situations), the individual becomes less tense and vulnerable to noxious stimuli in general and exhaustion and fatigue in particular (cf. Linton, 1982a; Turner & Chapman, 1982).

The training of applied relaxation should proceed as follows: intensive training in relaxation (cf. Jacobson, 1938) is provided 2 to 3 times per week for 45 minutes. During therapy, patients practice relaxation techniques, and homework assignments are given and discussed. In addition, written information concerning medications and activity performance is provided. This information sheet could explain that there is often no direct link between pain and activity levels nor between pain and medicine use. The sheet suggests that patients try increasing activity levels and decreasing medicine levels.

Because standard relaxation is of questionable help for chronic back pain patients (Linton, 1982a; Turner & Chapman, 1982), applied relaxation, as a coping skills approach, should be employed. The patient is first taught to relax using standard relaxation methods. Then, the amount of time required to relax is systematically shortened by decreasing the length of instructions and through practice. At the same time, conditioned relaxation exercises are implemented by having patients say *relax* while they exhale. When patients are able to relax in a short period of time, they practice in a variety of situations (e.g., while sitting, standing, walking). Finally, patients identify bodily feelings and environmental situations in which they begin to feel pain (or worse pain). They then are taught to apply such relaxation strategies to either prevent the pain from starting or to control it. Further details concerning the procedure may be found elsewhere (Linton 1982b; Linton & Melin, 1983). The main point is that patients are taught an active coping skill to prevent or control their pain.

Operant Procedures

Fordyce *et al.* (1973) have outlined a treatment program from an operant or instrumental (i.e., Skinnerian) conditioning perspective. This has been further developed by others as well as Fordyce (1976) himself. Based on this approach (as described in detail by Fordyce) several operant conditioning procedures are employed in the treatment of chronic pain patients.

One aspect of such a program is an optimization of medicine use. After explaining the program and obtaining consent, patients are informed that they will receive medications in capsules in a pill box and that the amount has been altered to optimize effects. These boxes are marked and patients are instructed to take their medication at the times designated on the box each day. This substitutes medication on a time rather than pain contingency. Subsequently, the content of analgesic medication is systematically reduced, until a zero level is reached or just above where the patient reports a decrease in its effectiveness.

A program for increasing physical activity is another aspect of the operant approach. Patients participate in a physical therapy exercise program patterned after Fordyce (1976), in which activity-level goals are gradually increased and success is reinforced with verbal praise and a chance to rest. In addition to physical therapy, participation in occupational therapy, where the same reinforcement parameters are employed, is advisable. Patients also engage in various other activities on the ward (e.g., coffee parties, games, cooking, dancing, and outings).

In order to minimize "sick" behavior, it is important to give personnel a short course in behavioral pain treatment and instruction to encourage "well" behavior by reinforcing it systematically.

Cognitive Procedures

Theoretically, cognitive procedures have both respondent and operant features. The most important area of application and of empirical results for cognitive procedures is in the treatment of depression (Beck, Rush, Shaw, & Merey, 1979), where it has stood up well in comparison to tricyclic antidepressants (Kovacs, Rush, Beck, & Hollon, 1981). They also have recently been applied in the treatment of chronic pain (Turk, Meichenbaum, & Genest, 1983).

The cognitive strategy applied to pain by Meichenbaum and Turk (1976) and Turk, Meichenbaum, and Genest (1983) is the SIT (Stress Inoculation Technique). It starts with training in imagery practice of pain. Following an information component, patients are told that they will experience much less "pain" and find it easier to tolerate "pain" if they vividly involve themselves in imaginal practice. This involves focusing on a pleasant exerpience that is incompatible with pain. The therapist should also describe to the patient the kind of pleasant events he or she himself or herself might try to imagine (e.g., lying on a beach on a hot summer day). The therapist instructs the patient to relax while a vivid description about being on a beach is narrated. This involves visual, auditory, olfactory, and kinesthetic qualities. Following these examples of the technique it is explained to patients that this coping technique would make them less bothered by the pain because it allows them to defocus their attention from the unpleasant experience and to focus on a pleasant experience that is incompatible with pain experience.

Adjunct Procedures

In addition to the specific procedures addressed to the problem of chronic pain and its concomitants, some adjunct procedures might be of help in improving the functioning of the chronic pain patient.

The behavioral pattern of a chronic pain patient often includes a low level of assertive behavior and a decreased ability to say *no*. When the patient is asked to do something she or he does not want to, she or he refers to or shows pain to avoid the situation. An increased ability to say *no,* and to assert oneself, therefore, means a real increase in choices for the patient. Assertive training procedures, which eventually may lead to reduced pain, are described elsewhere (Alberti & Emmons, 1970; Smith, 1975).

Social Skills Training

The chronic pain patient typically is withdrawn from social interaction. This may be due to his or her lack of social skills. Often the chronic pain patient evidences pain behaviors to manipulate his or her environment. But when reinforced for his or her efforts he or she tends to experience even more pain.

Social skills training aims at increasing adequate social skills behavior and is often directed toward the job situation (job-seeking skills, job performance skills), home situation, and other social situations (development of social competence, hobby interests). The procedures were originally applied mainly to the treatment of alcoholism. Description and review of social skills training or assertiveness training with alcoholics has been published by Miller and Hester (1980).

Other Problem Areas

Anxiety and fear are important problems in pain, especially in acute pain, and depression and guilt are said to be present in at least 20% of patients with chronic pain. Marital problems often result from long-term pain states. Overdependence on medicines, and even drug or substance abuse can develop in conjunction with a chronic pain problem. These and other problems can be effectively treated by a wide range of behavioral therapies (Leitenberg, 1976).

Program Tailoring and Multimodal Programs

In the clinical setting it is important to adapt the treatment to individual needs. One patient may have intensive pain but with restricted social and work invalidity. This type of patient might profit considerably from a relaxation therapy. Another patient may have less pain, but an almost total invalidity and a highly restricted level of activity. A third patient may experience the problem of high medicine consumption. These latter two types of patients might profit most from operant therapies.

Götestam (1983) has described a three-dimensional program for the operant treatment of chronic pain. This program addresses three of the general pain problems and aims to (a) increase activity; (b) decrease medication; and (c) decrease the pain experience. Increased activity and decreased medication seem to be most effectively handled through operant procedures (Linton & Götestam, 1984), whereas the reduction of subjective pain is more effectively attacked with a combination of relaxation training and cognitive procedures (Linton & Melin, 1983; Turk, Meichenbaum, & Genest, 1983).

Problems and Limitations of Treatment

In the practice of behavior therapy for chronic pain, several problems may arise that will limit the effects or lead to a complete treatment failure. Follick *et al.* (1983) have listed six factors related to failure in operant programs, and Linton (1982b) has listed problems associated with the use of relaxation. These two sources are heavily relied upon in this section.

General Problems

Although some problems are specific to the technique employed, the majority are related to doing therapy with chronic pain patients in general.

Misclassification

Not all pain patients can be treated optimally with the behavioral approach. If operant pain behaviors are not present and if the pain does not involve the muscles or an anxiety/fear component, then behavioral treatments may have little to offer the patient. Unfortunately, we know little about prognostic variables, so that one must often rely on two factors: (a) whether a clear medical intervention is available; and (b) on the results of the behavioral analysis. The behavioral analysis also tests the important therapy prerequisite of the patient's ability to carry out assignments.

"Disease Conviction"

As a rule, chronic pain patients are quite convinced that their pain is caused by organic processes or disease (Chapman, Sola, & Bonica, 1979), and this has been termed *disease conviction*. Occasionally, patients feel very strongly about this; if so, it may be very difficult to start tratment. To avoid problems, the existence and extent of the belief should be evaluated during the first interviews. Several tactics may help. Information concerning the "realness" of their pain and the futility of organic-nonorganic distinctions can be provided. Going through previous records concerning medical examinations and treatments (with the presiding doctor present) may also be helpful. A "hands on" method of examining the patient even by the psychologist (muscle tension, etc.) tends to communicate to the patient empathy concerning the realness of the pain and suffering.

Low Motivation/Failure to Practice

Chronic pain patients almost invariably have undergone a long series of treatments for their pain with little success. It is not surprising, then, that they are described as having "given up." The problem, of course, can undermine the entire program, especially if the patient does not carry out the homework assignments. Basically, one needs to reinforce these patients on a rich schedule for their participation. In the beginning of therapy, assignments should be very simple and not very time consuming to help insure success. Clear instructions should be given, including times and places decided upon for the completion of assignments. Contracts may even be used. Reminders (S^d) may be employed, and it is important to give priority during therapy to reviewing and reinforcing completed assignments. Detailed techniques for this appear in Shelton and Levy (1981).

Incomplete Problem List

Chronic pain patients are characterized by multiple problems. Sometimes, these problems do not seem to be directly related to pain. However, if a significant problem is overlooked in the treatment program, it may lead to poor results. For instance, a marital problem may not seem to be related to the pain, but resolution of the marital problem may nevertheless be required before successful pain remediation can be accomplished. This may be a result of indirect variables concerned with motivation, but it also may be the function of a "direct" link between pain and the marital problem. Initial evaluation should therefore concern itself with obtaining information about all problems experienced. Direct questioning (e.g., "Are you currently experiencing any type of marital problem" or "How do you get along with your spouse?") is usually helpful. If therapy is not proceeding very well, one should consider the possibility of having missed the essence of the problem.

Covert Pain Behaviors

Because the traditional behavior analysis of pain specifically concentrated on observable pain behaviors, cognitive behaviors were not always evaluated. Although almost exclusive concern with observables is desirable in the first formulations of the theoretical analysis, such exclusive concern is a mistake in the clinic. Covert behavior, including the experience of pain, is probably the single reason why the patient is seeking help. It seems unwise to ignore this because it may decrease motivation and cause conflicts in goal setting. Furthermore, covert behaviors may reflect tendencies for overt behaviors. Consequently, patients may sometimes harbor "attitudes" or self-statements that are in conflict with the goals of the treatment program. Evaluation should include questions about pain experience and about interpretations, beliefs, and the like that are associated with pain or with specific pain-related behaviors (e.g., carrying out an activity). One may target this problem by making the experience of pain the focus of evaluation and by allowing it to become the main goal of treatment if the patient so desires.

Attributional Problems

Most patients possess a disease model orientation to their problem. This was earlier described in the section on problems with "disease conviction." Another aspect of the problem reflects responsibility for treatment and the nature of treatment. The patient's beliefs and goals may not be in line with a behavioral approach. If this is so, it will be difficult to motivate the patient to actively participate, unless, of course, the "attitude" can be altered. Providing a conceptual basis for a behavioral program can help a lot as can the recommendations in the disease conviction section. Furthermore, treatment should allow for reinforcement of verbal statements and overt behaviors that demonstrate that the *patient can alter his or her situation*. However, firm beliefs that a pill or surgery is needed or goals that are not consistent with behavioral intervention may not be easily changed. It is questionable whether such patients will benefit fully from the treatment. Follick *et al.* (1983) argue that these patients will report little or no improvement, even if the objective data are clearly and significantly positive because the treatment has not provided the client with what he or she wanted. Fortunately, this group seems to be fairly small. The presence of such problems, however, does indicate that treatment effects will probably be of limited value (i.e., some behaviors unaffected, poor maintenance).

Leveling of Treatment Gains

With a severe pain problem and a high degree of invalidism, treatment gains are easily recognized. However, once some improvement is achieved, a ceiling effect might reduce the contrast possibilities, and the treatment process therefore often slows down or ceases.

Maintenance and Generalization

Because patients usually have a long history of the problem and because interventions are typically of short duration, there may be a tendency for high recidivism. Generalization may be improved by focusing treatment on everyday situations. Maintenance techniques generally used in behavior therapy are also applicable. The important point is that maintenance does not automatically occur; it has to be built into the treatment regime.

Package Problems

Research in the area of chronic pain has shown a tendency to use package programs in the hope of obtaining a broad-based treatment. Although using multicomponent treatments is almost always necessary for this patient category, the blind administration of "package" treatments can lead to limited effectiveness or even failure. Basically, components must be relevant to the patient, and they should be carefully selected on the basis of the behavior analysis. Otherwise, one runs the risk of using components that are not effective, or even worse, those that decrease the utility of the other components. Furthermore, compliance seems to be related to the number of components one employs and to how relevant the patient experiences them (Hall, 1980). Consequently, packages that include components not indicated may actually decrease overall effectiveness and compliance.

Economy

Sternbach (1974) speaks about the "professional" patient (i.e., the patient who has his or her income or pension secured as long as he or she has the chronic pain problem). The only possibility here is to sever the contingencies between the chronic pain and the pension, so that the pension no longer is dependent on the pain, or the patient is no longer dependent on the pension.

Problems Related to Relaxation Training

One problem with progressive relaxation is that patients may feel additional pain from tensing their muscles. Also, there is some risk that tension may cause organic damage. Other relaxation procedures involving breathing exercises and imagery may be used.

Difficulty in Relaxing Affected Muscles

If the patient has had chronically tensed muscles over a long period, and particularly if the pain is in the back or shoulders, she or he may have great difficulty in relaxing the muscles in the affected body site. This may be true even if the patient reports deep levels of general relaxation. Therefore, relaxation levels need to be physically checked periodically (see Marquis, Ferguson, & Taylor, 1980) by observing the patient and by feeling the various muscles in question. If muscles are tense, special efforts focusing on the particular muscle groups in question may be started. If additional focusing does not work, tensing drills might be tried; and for difficult cases the therapist can massage the affected muscles. This is done by placing the thumb on the muscle and stroking with the grain of the muscles. At first it is done lightly, and gradually more pressure is applied. It may require several minutes to obtain satisfactory results. Care should be taken to use this procedure primarily to teach the patient how to experience the tension relaxation sequence, not to achieve it for him or her. In extremes cases, the muscles may actually have become shortened, and physical therapy may be required to help stretch out the muscles again.

Difficulties in Discriminating Relaxation/Tension States

Some patients may have great trouble in discriminating when their muscles are relaxed or tensed. This prevents optimal use of relaxation and may cause difficulties in identifying body signals' "warning" that pain is coming. The patient should rate his or her bodily state for tension as well as the probability of having pain periodically, before and after relaxation. Training with EMG biofeedback also may be indicated.

Patient Has Constant Pain

A number of patients frequently state that they have "constant pain," making preventive measures impossible. If these patients rate their pain four times per day, for example, it will be discovered that the majority actually do have considerable variations in their pain intensity. A small number will rate their pain as always being of the same intensity. Although the accuracy of their pain-intensity ratings may be questioned, we have not found any especially helpful method for dealing with this problem. On the contrary, constant pain seems to be related to a poor prognosis.

However, one may change tactics and concentrate on obtaining some pain reduction during relaxation exercises. If that works, one can then begin with generalization to other situations.

Difficulties in Relaxating during "Pain" Situations

Patients are taught to relax as soon as they feel the pain starting or as soon as they come into a situation where they usually have additional pain. Occasionally patients have difficulties in relaxing in these "pain situations." This is an indication that therapy has proceeded too rapidly and/or that one has selected incorrect situations for them to practice. Extra practice with the therapist using easy situations and with extensive guidance should be of help.

Problems Related to Operant Programs

Administration

An operant program for outpatients or hospitalized patients requires much administration and cooperation. Absence of such compliance may sabotage the goals of the program. Such a program requires economic resources, an educational program to teach staff members the behavioral principles, and much cooperation among staff members. It is not always easy to accomplish this, but, in general, it demands careful long-term planning with all of the involved parties.

Gaining Control of Reinforcers

A successful operant program is based on identifying and altering the prevailing contingencies of reinforcement. Sometimes it is difficult to identify potent reinforcers; at other times it may be troublesome to gain enough control over a reinforcer so that it may be effectively altered. For instance, a spouse that responds to pain behavior may be receiving much reinforcement for doing so. Consequently, it may be complicated to alter the spouse's behavior (i.e., reinforcing patient's pain behavior). The best advice here is to do a thorough behavior analysis so that such factors may be taken into consideration before any treatment is offered to the client.

Problems Related to Cognitive Programs

Difficulties in Imagining Situations

Some patients have difficulties in imagining pain situations and pain experience when in the therapy setting. Intensified training may increase such imagery skill by using different sense modalities (e.g., visual, auditory, tactile, and olfactory).

An Illustrative Case Study

In this section, we will present a case study illustrating the different stages in diagnosis and treatment. We include a dialogue between therapist (T) and patient (P) as well as a commentary on the dialogue.

The patient, who has undergone several surgical procedures for his severe back pain, is now referred from the general practitioner (GP) as pain (for some time relieved by surgery 5 months ago) has returned, greatly incapacitating him. His GP is now thinking of supporting his obtaining a pension, as he seems unable to work any longer.

The patient is a 56-year-old man, married, with three grown children who have moved from the parents' home (the last one 3 years ago). The patient is a worker in a factory for metal equipment. He has had several different positions in this factory throughout his entire working life. His wife previously was employed as a nursing assistant in the local hospital but has been at home since the children were born. She now is thinking about going back to work but has not yet done so.

The pain began in connection with a back trauma while carrying a heavy instrument some 15 years ago. At first the patient's back pain was not too severe. However, subsequent to a second traumatic incident carrying heavy equipment some 4 years ago, the lower back pain intensified. Since then, the patient has had three surgical procedures for disc prolapse. He also has had trials of several analgesic drugs, mostly of the weaker type. While hospitalized he was given opiate analgesics. In addition, he has tried acupuncture, with some short-lived relief.

First Interview

T: Could you tell me what are your most severe problems just now?
P: The pain during daytime is not so disturbing as it was, but I am really disturbed when I cannot go to work without having severe pain.
T: What kind of activities and movements are giving you pain?
P: Especially when I am carrying things, even rather light things, I feel the pain in the back.
T: What are your thoughts when you feel that pain?
P: I am worried about the future, and I am afraid that the back is broken or so, and I fear that I will have to undergo another surgery, which so far has not helped me. At least not helped me enough.
T: Are there any ways you could avoid pain in the working situation?
P: At work, that is is really difficult. When it is necessary to carry things, it is very difficult just to say I cannot. I always give a hand, and there it comes.
T: What other possibilities do you have to avoid pain? What about in your home situation?
P: At home it is rather easy to avoid pain, and I quite seldom experience severe pain at home.
T: What is the most effective way to avoid pain at home?
P: If I don't carry things, it is rather easy. Of course, it is sometimes difficult not to give a hand, but I feel I get more understanding now at home, from my wife, when I am not helping.
T: When you feel pain at home, could you do anything about it, to reduce it, I mean?
P: Well, I could lie down and rest for a while. That is mostly quite effective to relieve the pain.
T: How does your pain problem affect your working ability?
P: Just now, it prevents me totally from going to my job!
T: Do you think it is possible to be at work, restrict some of the activities which induce pain, and still function satisfactorily?

P: Well, it might be possible, although I think it should be quite difficult, in a practical way, I mean.

T: Do you feel your pain problem has affected your social life?

P: No, I don't think so.

T: What about your interactions with your wife. Are your discussions centered around the pain problem, or are you totally avoiding that subject in your discussions?

P: No, of course we speak of my pain problem.

T: Do you think your wife sometimes gets bored with these discussions?

P: No, she is a very understanding woman, and a real support to me.

T: What about your sex life. Do you have intercourse as often as you did before your pain problem?

P: No, not really. But that's also a question of age, isn't it?

T: What are your expectations with regard to treatment?

P: I don't really know. I suppose I want to be able to go back to my job, and perform a pretty good job.

T: What about your pain in the future? Do you think you will be totally free of pain?

P: Of course I would like to! But I don't really know if that is realistic, after such a long time with pain. I would be quite satisfied if I could function in my job, even if I have some pain.

T: What about other problems? Do you have much anxiety or feel depressed at times?

P: In the beginning I had quite a lot of anxiety. Then after some time I felt very depressed for a while. I suppose I still feel depressed now and then, but not as much as before.

T: I want you to fill in this form for me by the next time we meet [*Seven daily forms of Table 3 handed out*]. This will allow us to trace situational factors, and what happens when you get pain. You are to indicate when you have pain, in what situation, and how you behave and think in that situation. I also want you to estimate your pain intensity, and for that you should use this 0–5 point scale [*Figure 1, page 2*].

P: OK, I will try my best.

Comments

It appears that the patient has a severe pain problem that incapacitates him at work as well as affects his social situation. However, he seems to have some difficulties accepting the latter. Much of the pain is related to the work situation, where it is easily elicited. On the other hand, at home there are some possibilities to avoid it, and also to cope with it, by resting.

The general scheme of the interview follows the list of points outlined in Table 1. Most of the questions are covered during the first interview; those remaining are dealt with in Interview 2 after the patient has filled in the forms.

• *Medical Diagnosis*

A physical examination revealed severe pain when the patient leaned forward, and also when he lifted his left leg upward (positive Lasègue). He also had some reduced mobility in his left leg and in the hip. Otherwise, the examination was within normal limits. A neurological examination was also conducted to further try to identify the possible damage or disturbance in the spinal chord. The patient evidenced reduced sensibility in his leg and foot, corresponding to the two discs (L5 and S1) and also reduced force in the left foot. X-rays showed a small disc prolapse between the L5 and S1 discs, but no visible organic change in the next disc (S1–S2).

The condition was diagnosed as low back pain (LBP), or an L5–S1 syndrome of ischias.

Assessment

When the patient was asked about his pain, he had difficulties indicating when, how much, how severe, and so on it was. Therefore, he was asked to rate his pain at predetermined times during the day (see Figure 1, page 2). He also was asked to describe the situations in which pain occurred, the antecedents, and the consequences that followed (see Table 3).

A behavioral analysis was also performed. It revealed excesses in pain behavior and rather extensive use of medication, above what was medically advisable. The patient also showed severe withdrawal with regard to normal social activity, and advanced inactivity; most of the time he lay on his bed or a sofa. Analysis of the interaction in the family (determined through home visits) revealed that generally there was a minimum of contact between the patient and his spouse. However, such interaction tended to increase when the patient showed or spoke about his pain. Some of this attention was of a positive nature, but for an external observer, some of it seemed to be aversive (e.g., hostility from the wife). However, our impression was that all this attention served as a positive reinforcer for pain behaviors (which increased in these situations).

Treatment

Several types of treatment approaches were considered. However, because the functional analysis showed a strong reinforcement component, the treatment package eventually chosen for this patient consisted of a combination of respondent and operant strategies in a three-dimensional treatment program (see Götestam, 1983). Treatment involved (a) reduction of pill taking; (b) increase of activity; and (c) reduction of pain behavior and experience.

The results are shown in a multiple-baseline analysis across behaviors in Figure 3.

Treatment Outcome

Empirical Support for Treatment Effect

Although several reports on the use of behavioral procedures for chronic pain have been published, relatively few studies have been conducted as controlled experiments with adequate design (Linton, 1982a; Turner & Chapman, 1982). Even when adequately designed as single-case experimental designs, the small samples only allow for tentative conclusions.

Relaxation Procedures

In a controlled study conducted by Linton and Melin (1983) with 17 patients, use of an applied relaxation procedure (AR) proved superior to a waiting list control on the following measures: subjective pain, medicine intake, activity, and over-all evaluation of treatment. In another controlled study by Linton and Götestam (1984), AR was superior both to a waiting list control group and a group receiving a combination of applied relaxation and operant treatment on measures of subjective pain, activity of daily living, and depression.

Operant Procedures

In the previously mentioned study by Linton and Götestam (1984), the applied relaxation plus operant treatment was superior to the waiting list or applied relaxation only in activity and in medicine intake reduction. Furthermore, it was superior to the waiting list control on an exercise test, activities of daily living, and depression.

Cognitive Procedures

Cognitive procedures have been shown to be superior to tricyclic antidepressants in the treatment of depression (Kovacs *et al.*, 1981). They also have been touted as effective in the treatment of chronic pain (Meichenbaum & Turk, 1976; Turk, Meichenbaum, & Genest, 1983), but so far no controlled experimental study has been published.

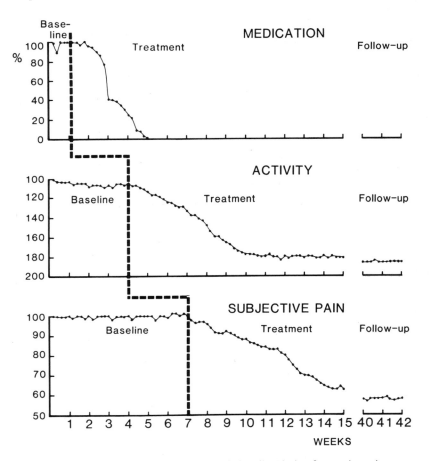

Figure 3. Treatment results from a multiple baseline design for a pain patient.

Adjunct Procedures and Multimodal Programs

The adjunct procedures previously mentioned have been empirically evaluated for single symptoms or problems (Leitenberg, 1976), but not in relation to chronic pain. Although simple components in multimodal programs have been evaluated separately, the evaluation of a multimodal program package raises several methodological problems, thus far not tackled.

Assessment of Therapy Process

In the clinical setting, assessment to determine the efficacy of the treatment under controlled conditions may not be totally realistic. However, some kind of repeated assessment might be useful, such as that of subjective pain (i.e., the 0–5 point scale previously described). Also, a gross measure of activity level or work adaption might be taken as well as measure of social functioning.

Immediate and Long-Term Outcome

In addition to targeted measures, immediate and long-term outcome follow-ups should involve an evaluation of medicine use and satisfaction with treatment. Also, in order to ensure maintenance of treatment gains on a long-term basis, preplanned booster treatment should prove to be useful.

Summary

This chapter has focused on the assessment and behavioral treatment of chronic pain. Following our analysis of problem identification and interview formats, we have examined the use of a variety of assessment instruments and observation methods. Also, the importance of functional analysis has been highlighted.

The main therapy techniques reviewed were (a) relaxation procedures; (b) operant procedures; and (c) cognitive procedures. In addition, we considered a variety of adjunct procedures to be applied for specific problems in individual cases. In a section on problems and limitations, general problems were presented, followed by specific problems related to the three main therapy procedures.

A case study was presented, including the referral assessment and diagnosis, and treatment and follow-up. Most of the first interview was presented for illustrative purposes. Empirical support for the different treatment procedures was presented, in addition to recommendations to ensure the long-term benefits of treatment.

References

Alberti, R. E., & Emmons, M. L. (1970). *Your perfect right.* San Luis Obispo, CA: Impact.

Beck, A. T., Ward, C. H., Mendelson, M., Mock, J., & Erbaugh, J. (1961). An inventory for measuring depression. *Archives of General Psychiatry, 4,* 561–571.

Beck, A. T., Rush, A. J., Shaw, B. F., & Merey, G. (1979). *Cognitive therapy of depression*. New York: Guilford Press.

Bond, M. R. (1971). The relation of pain to the Eysenck Personality Inventory, Cornell Medical Index, and Whiteley Index of Hypochondriasis. *British Journal of Psychiatry, 119,* 671–678.

Bonica, J. J. (1981). Preface. In K. Y. Lorenz (Ed.), *New approaches to treatment of chronic pain: A review of multidisciplinary pain clinics and pain centers.* (Research Monograph 36, pp. 7–10). Washington, DC: National Institute on Drug Abuse.

Brena, S. F., Chapman, S. L., & Decker, R. (1981). Chronic pain as a learned experience: Emory University Pain Control Center. In K. Y. Lorenz (Ed.), *New approaches to treatment of chronic pain: A review of multidisciplinary pain clinics and pain centers* (Research Monograph 36). Washington DC: National Institute on Drug Abuse.

Cautela, J. R. (1977). The use of covert conditioning in modifying pain behavior. *Journal of Behavior Therapy and Experimental Psychiatry, 8,* 45–52.

Chapman, R. C., Sola, A., & Bonica, J. J. (1979). Illness behaviour and depression compared in pain center and private practice patients. *Pain, 6,* 1–7.

Collins, F. L., & Martin, J. E. (1980). Assessing self-report of pain: A comparison of two recording procedures. *Journal of Behavioral Assessment, 2,* 55–63.

Follick, M. J., Zitter, R. E., & Ahern, D. K. (1983). Failures in the operant treatment of chronic pain. In E. B. Foa & P. M. G. Emmelkamp (Eds.). *Failures in behavior therapy.* New York: Wiley.

Fordyce, W. E. (1976). *Behavioral methods for chronic pain and illness.* St. Louis: C. V. Mosby.

Fordyce, W. E., Fowler, R. S., Lehmann, J. F., DeLateur, B. J., Sand, P. L., & Trieschmann, R. B. (1973). Operant conditioning in the treatment of chronic pain. *Archives of General Psychiatry, 54,* 399–408.

Fordyce, W. E., Lansky, D., Calsyn, D. A., Shelton, J. L., Stolov, W. C., & Rock, D. L. (1984). Pain measurement and pain behavior. *Pain, 18,* 53–69.

Götestam, K. G. (1983). A three-dimensional psychological programme for chronic pain. *Acta Psychiatrica Scandinavica, 67,* 209–217.

Hall, S. M. (1980). Self-management and therapeutic maintenance: Theory and research. In P. Karoly & J. J. Steffan (Eds.), *Improving the long-term effects of psychotherapy* (pp. 263–300). New York: Gardner Press.

Heaton, R. K., Getto, C. J., Lehman, R. A., Fordyce, W. E., Brauer, E., & Groban, S. E. (1982). A standardized evaluation of psychosocial factors in chronic pain. *Pain, 12,* 165–174.

Jacobson, E. (1938). *Progressive relaxation.* Chicago: University of Chicago Press.

Kanfer, F. H., & Saslow, G. (1976). An outline for behavioral diagnosis. In E. S. Mash & L. G. Terdal (Eds.), *Behavior therapy assessment, diagnosis, design, and evaluation.* New York: Springer.

Keefe, F. J. (1982). Behavioral assessment and treatment of chronic pain: Current status and future directions. *Journal of Consulting and Clinical Psychology, 50,* 896–911.

Keefe, F. J., & Block, A. R. (1982). Development of an observation method for assessing pain behavior in chronic low back pain patients. *Behavior Therapy, 13,* 363–375.

Keefe, F. J., Kopel, S. A., & Gordon, S. B. (1978). *A practical guide to behavioral assessment.* New York: Springer.

Keefe, F. J., Brown, C., Scott, D. S., & Ziesat, H. (1982). Behavioral assessment of chronic pain. In F. J. Keefe & J. A. Blumenthal (Eds.), *Assessment strategies in behavior medicine.* New York: Grune & Stratton.

Kovacs, M., Rush, A. J., Beck, A. T., & Hollon, S. D. (1981). Depressive outpatients treated with cognitive therapy or pharmacotherphy. *Archives of General Psychiatry, 38,* 33–39.

Leitenberg, H. (Ed.). (1976). *Handbook of behavior modification and behavior therapy.* Englewood Cliffs, NJ: Prentice-Hall.

Linton, S. J. (1982,a) A critical review of behavioural treatments for chronic benign pain other than headache. *British Journal of Clinical Psychology, 21,* 321–337.

Linton, S. J. (1982,b) Applied relaxation as a method of coping with chronic pain: A therapist's guide. *Scandinavian Journal of Behaviour Therapy, 11,* 161–174.

Linton, S. J. (in press). A critical look at techniques for a behavioral assessment of chronic pain patients. *Behavioral Engineering.*

Linton, S. J., & Götestam, K. G. (1983). A clinical comparison of two pain scales: Correlation, remembering chronic pain, and a measure of compliance. *Pain, 17,* 57–65.

Linton, S. J. & Götestam, K. G. (1984). A controlled study of the effects of applied relaxation and applied relaxation plus operant procedures in the regulation of chronic pain. *British Journal of Clinical Psychology, 23,* 291–299.

Linton, S. J., & Götestam, K. G. (1985). Controlling pain reports through operant conditioning: A laboratory demonstration. *Perceptual and Motor Skills, 60,* 427–437.

Linton, S. J., & Melin, L. (1983). Applied relaxation in the management of chronic pain. *Behavioural Psychotherapy, 11,* 337–350.

Linton, S. J., & Melin, L. (1984). An Activities of Daily Living Scale for chronic pain patients. Unpublished manuscript.

Linton, S. J., Melin, L., & Götestam, K. G. (1984). Behavioral analysis of chronic pain and its management. In M. Hersen, R. Eisler, & P. M. Miller (Eds.), *Progress in behavior modification* (Vol. 18, pp. 1–42). New York: Academic Press.

Marquis, J., Ferguson, J., & Taylor, C. (1980). Generalization of relaxation skills. *Journal of Behavior Therapy and Experimental Psychiatry, 11,* 95–99.

Meichenbaum, D., & Turk, D. (1976). The cognitive-behavioral management of anxiety, anger and pain. In J. Davison (Ed.), *The behavioral management of anxiety, depression and pain.* New York: Brunner/Mazel.

Melzack, R. (1975). The McGill Pain Questionnaire: Major properties and scoring methods. *Pain, 1,* 277–299.

Miller, W. R., & Hester, R. K. (1980). Treatment the problem drinker: Modern approaches. In W. R. Miller (Ed.), *The addictive behaviors. Treatment of alcoholism, drug abuse, smoking, and obesity.* Oxford: Pergamon Press.

Mooney, V., Cairns, D., & Robertson, J. A. (1976). A system for evaluating and treating chronic back disability. *Western Journal of Medicine, 124,* 370–376.

Nachemson, A. (1983). Work for all: For those with low back pain as well. *Clinical orthopaedics and related research* (Lippincott series), No. 179, 77–85.

Pilowsky, I., & Spence, N. D. (1976). Illness behavior syndromes associated with intractable pain. *Pain, 2,* 61–71.

Relinger, H. (1980). Pain evaluation form. *Catalogue of Selected Documents in Psychology. 10,* 15.

Roberts, A., & Reinhardt, L. (1980). The behavioral management of chronic pain: Long-term follow-up with comparison groups. *Pain, 8,* 151–162.

Sanders, S. H. (1979). Behavioral assessment and treatment of clinical pain: Appraisal of current status. In M. Hersen, R. Eisler, & P. M. Miller (Eds.), *Progress in behavior modification* (Vol. 8). New York: Academic Press.

Sarno, J. E., Sarno, M. T., & Levita, E. (1973). The Functional Life Scale. *Archives of Physical Medicine and Rehabilitation, 54,* 214–220.

Shelton, J. L., & Levy, R. L. (1981). *Behavioral assignments and treatment compliance: A handbook of clinical strategies.* Champaign, IL: Research Press.

Sjödén, P. O., Bates, S., & Nyrén, O. (1984). Continuous self-recording of epigastric pain on two rating scales: Compliance, authenticity, reliability, and sensitivity. *Journal of Behavioral Assessment.*

Smith, M. J. (1975). *When I say no, I feel guilty.* New York: Dial Press.

Sternbach, R. (1974). *Pain patients: Traits and treatment.* London: Academic Press.

Turner, J. A., & Chapman, C. R. (1982). Psychological interventions for chronic pain: A critical review. I, II. *Pain, 12,* 1–46.

Turk, D. C., & Genest, M. (1979). Regulation of pain: The application of cognitive and behavioral techniques for prevention and remediation. In P. Kendall & S. Hollon (Eds.), *Cognitive behavioral interventions: Theory, research, and prevention.* New York: Academic Press.

Turk, D. C., Meichenbaum, D., & Genest, M. (1983). *Pain and behavioral medicine.* New York: Guilford Press.

Waddell, G., McCulloch, J. A., Kummel, E., & Wenner, R. M. (1980). Nonorganic physical signs in low back pain. *Spine, 5,* 117–125.

Cardiovascular Disorders

MARGRET A. APPEL, PATRICE G. SAAB, AND
KENNETH A. HOLROYD

Introduction

Diseases of the heart and blood vessels account for a large proportion of illness and are a major cause of death in the United States. Cardiovascular diseases cover a broad assortment of disorders including hypertension, coronary heart disease (CHD), cerebrovascular disease, arteriosclerosis, arrhythmias, heart failure, rheumatic heart disease, Raynaud's phenomena, and migraine headache. The behavioral treatment of each disorder may involve the application of a number of different interventions to distinct targets. Rather than briefly mentioning all possible cardiovascular disorders and behavioral treatments, we have chosen to focus on the methods used to reduce two cardiovascular risk factors—essential hypertension and the coronary-prone behavior pattern. Judging from the volume of literature, these two disorders have elicited considerable interest among behavioral researchers. In addition, we present a brief discussion of a new direction in behavioral intervention for one sequela of cardiovascular disease, namely neuromuscular complications following a cerebrovascular accident.

Essential Hypertension

Hypertension, or high blood pressure, is a chronic disorder affecting approximately 15% of the population. It is a major risk factor for cardiovascular and renal

MARGRET A. APPEL • Department of Psychology, Porter Hall, Ohio University, Athens, Ohio 45701.   PATRICE G. SAAB • Department of Psychiatry, University of Pittsburgh, Pittsburgh, Pennsylvania 15261.   KENNETH A. HOLROYD • Department of Psychology, Porter Hall, Ohio University, Athens, Ohio 45701.

diseases such as myocardial infarction, congestive heart failure, cerebrovascular disease, and renal failure. About 10% of cases of hypertension occur secondary to an identifiable cause, such as renal disease, endocrine disorder, coarctation of the aorta, or pregnancy. The remaining 90% are of unknown cause and are designated *idiopathic* or essential hypertension.

A wide range of factors has been implicated in the etiology and maintenance of essential hypertension. These include genetic predisposition, sedentary life-style, high sodium intake, low potassium and calcium intake, heavy alcohol consumption, personality traits, and stress (Kaplan, 1982; Shapiro & Goldstein, 1982).

Treatment articles generally define *hypertension* in terms of *diastolic* blood pressure (DBP) levels using the following categories and cutoffs: mild, either 90 or 95 to 104 mm Hg; moderate 105 to either 114 or 119 mm Hg; and severe, 115 or 120 and higher. *Hypertension* is also defined as *systolic* blood pressure (SBP) of 160 mm Hg or greater, with 140 to 159 labeled *borderline hypertension*. Although the criteria of the World Health Organization are based on diastolic levels, the Framingham data suggest that systolic pressure may be a better predictor of overall risk (Kaplan, 1982). In addition, the cutoffs are artifactual because a continuous gradient links blood pressure to risk: the higher the pressure, the higher the risk.

Blood pressure is a function of systemic blood flow (cardiac output) and resistance to blood flow in the peripheral vasculature (peripheral resistance). In hypertension, arterial pressure is raised due to increases in cardiac output, peripheral resistance, or both. The roles of these hemodynamic factors vary across individuals and, possibly, at different stages of the disorder in any one individual. For example, a common pattern is elevated cardiac output and normal peripheral resistance in the early development of hypertension, followed by high resistance and normal cardiac output when hypertension becomes established.

Essential hypertension appears to be a heterogeneous disorder. In the medical literature, hypertensive individuals have been divided into subgroups on the basis of variables such as renin system activity (Cody, Laragh, Case, & Atlas, 1983) and sodium sensitivity (Kawasaki, Delea, Bartter, & Smith, 1978). Such subgroups may have significant implications for treatment. For example, renin–sodium profiling predicted the effectiveness of five major types of antihypertensive medication (Cody *et al.*, 1983). Similar subgrouping has not been applied yet to research on behavioral treatment.

The major treatment for hypertension is pharmacological. The benefits of drug therapy for moderate and severe hypertension have been recognized for some time. Aggressive pharmacological treatment of mild hypertension has been recommended recently as a result of major clinical trials (e.g., Hypertension Detection and Follow-up Program Cooperative Group, 1979). However, caution should be used in the long-term pharmacological treatment of mild hypertension because almost all antihypertensive drugs have some potential for worsening cardiovascular risk. Some groups of individuals whose blood pressures were reduced while on drug treatment fared worse than individuals whose blood pressures were reduced without active drug treatment or with less aggressive regimens (Kaplan, 1982, 1983). These findings lend support to the search for effective nonpharmacological interventions for hypertension.

Blood pressure is used both as a diagnostic measure to determine whom we should treat and as an outcome measure to assess the effectiveness of intervention. Blood pressure is most accurately measured by direct intraarterial readings. However, this invasive method is impractical for regular use. Therefore, blood pressure is usually assessed indirectly with a mercury or aneroid sphygmomanometer.

When blood pressure is measured with a sphygmomanometer, it is important to use a cuff of the proper size for the individual's arm. A cuff that is too short or too narrow will give erroneously high readings, whereas an oversized cuff will give erroneously low readings. The cuff is inflated to about 30 mm Hg above SBP and then deflated at the rate of about 2 to 3 mm Hg per second. SBP is read at the pressure where Korotkoff sounds (which occur with each heartbeat) are first heard with a stethoscope placed over the brachial artery. DBP can be read either as the pressure where muffling of the sounds occurs (Phase IV), or where sound disappears (Phase V). The World Health Organization (Guidelines, 1983) recommends using Phase V because the epidemiological and medical treatment literatures are based mainly on these readings.

For the diagnosis of hypertension, repeated measurements are recommended (e.g., more than three occasions over a period of several weeks with at least three readings per occasion). When assessing treatment effectiveness in diagnosed hypertensives, at least three readings should be taken at each assessment. The first reading is discarded, and the average of the second and third readings is reported. Some research studies use mean arterial pressure (MAP), which is DBP plus one-third of the difference between SBP and DBP. Useful information about blood pressure measurement may be found in Guidelines (1983), Kaplan (1982), and Kirkendall, Feinleib, Freis, and Mark (1980).

In addition to the usual mercury and aneroid sphygmomanometers, a number of semiautomated devices are available. Many of these tend to underestimate SBP and to overestimate DBP, but they are fairly accurate when the concern is with changes in blood pressure from one occasion to another (Kaplan, 1982). Automated ambulatory systems, such as the Del Mar Avionics Pressurometer, are sometimes used in research to obtain 24-hour blood pressures while individuals engage in routine activities (e.g., Pickering, Harshfield, Kleinert, Blank, & Laragh, 1982).

The prediction of cardiovascular risk is based on casual blood pressure readings. However, casual readings obtained in the physician's office may not be representative of the individual's usual blood pressure. In a large proportion of patients, both SBP and DBP decrease over repeated office measurements, and some patients may never habituate to the office setting. Pickering and his colleagues (Harshfield, Pickering, Kleinert, Blank, & Laragh, 1982; Kleinert *et al.*, 1984; Pickering *et al.*, 1982) found that blood pressures obtained in the home correlated with office blood pressures for both normotensives and established hypertensives but not for borderline and mild hypertensives: about one-third of mild hypertensives had average 24-hr DBPs of less than 85 mm Hg, which are in the normotensive range. In addition, basal (measured upon awakening), automated 24-hr, and patient-measured home and work blood pressure readings are all more predictive of target organ damage than are office readings (Devereux *et al.*, 1983; Kleinert *et al.*, 1984; Laughlin, 1981). Therefore, it is desirable to measure blood pressure in the person's usual environment (home and work).

The inherent variability of blood pressure, together with the possible non-representativeness of office readings, indicates that thorough assessment should be carried out before treatment is initiated, especially for mild hypertensives. Pickering *et al.* (1982) suggest that 24-hr blood pressure may be used to identify those individuals who are most at risk and, hence, in need of treatment. Patients' home recordings provide an adequate approximation to automated 24-hr pressures (Kleinert *et al.*, 1984). Kaplan (1982, 1983) has suggested that those mild hypertensives who are at increased risk and need aggressive treatment might be identified by the use of an overall cardiovascular risk profile derived from the Framingham data. This profile considers the factors of age, sex, SBP, serum cholesterol, cigarette smoking, glucose tolerance, and left ventricular hypertrophy. Tables to determine relative risk for coronary disease and stroke are available from the American Heart Association. Problems related to the assessment of treatment outcome are discussed in a later section.

Nonpharmacological Treatment

The goal of treatment of hypertensive individuals is to reduce cardiovascular risk by lowering DBP below 90 mm Hg with pharmacological or nonpharmacological methods, or both. Behavioral techniques may be used (a) as a first step before pharmacological treatment in newly diagnosed mild or moderate hypertensive individuals; (b) to provide further control in patients who respond inadequately to drugs or in whom dosage is limited because of adverse side effects; (c) in conjunction with drug treatment even in well-controlled patients to reduce drug requirements and, thereby, the iatrogenic consequences of medication; and (d) as preventive measures for at-risk individuals. The following sections describe techniques used mainly with diagnosed hypertensives. These techniques attempt to reduce blood pressure either indirectly by modifying contributing factors such as diet, exercise, medication compliance, and response to stress, or directly through physiological self-control procedures such as biofeedback and relaxation training.

Life-Style Modification

The recommendation that one alter one's life-style has become routine in the treatment of hypertension. The hypertensive individual is encouraged to change a variety of behaviors in the hope that the changes will reduce blood pressure and with the assumption that, even if the changes do not help, they will not hurt. Unfortunately, the list of changes is often difficult to implement and even more difficult to maintain, with some physicians advocating fairly Spartan life-styles. This section describes some of the more common recommendations and discusses their effectiveness.

Diet. The need to restrict salt as a way to decrease blood pressure has gained wide acceptance among both medical practitioners and the lay public. Initial support for the value of sodium reduction was provided by the effectiveness of the Kempner rice and fruit diet that restricted sodium to 10 mEq per day (less than 1 g sodium chloride). However, the diet was so unpalatable that patients had difficulty adhering to it for long. The data obtained with the Kempner diet are also difficult to evaluate because the diet altered many other nutrients that may have been as important as sodium in blood pressure regulation (McCarron, Henry, & Morris, 1982).

The current recommendation is to reduce sodium intake by 50% (e.g., to approximately 5 or 6 g sodium chloride per day). Reduction may be achieved by having patients avoid salty foods, such as pickles, and add little or no salt in preparation of food and none at the table. A 50% reduction in salt intake will be associated with a modest blood pressure decrease (about 6%) in mild and moderate hypertension but will be less likely to affect severe hypertension (MacGregor, 1983). However, blood pressure reductions obtained with moderate salt restriction may not be different from those obtained with a general health package (Silman, Locke, Mitchell, & Humpherson, 1983) or other credible placebos (Andrews, MacMahon, Austin, & Byrne, 1982). In addition, a number of studies have failed to find a dose-response relation between the degree of sodium intake and the fall of blood pressure (e.g., Silman *et al.,* 1983).

It is likely that some hypertensive individuals are salt sensitive, whereas others are not. For example, Kawasaki *et al.,* (1978) categorized about half of a group of mild and moderate hypertensives as salt sensitive on the basis of their blood pressure responses to successive 1-week periods of sodium restriction and loading on a dietary sodium challenge. Salt restriction may be effective only for those patients who are demonstrated to be salt sensitive. In addition, blood pressure reactivity to dietary challenge, if feasible, may provide feedback that will increase compliance in salt-sensitive individuals whose adherence to sodium restriction is poor.

When sodium restriction is indicated, the dietitian should provide more than a list of foods and recipes. Specific information is helpful on where to procure particular low-sodium foods such as bread. An attempt should be made to tailor the recommendations to the patient's life-style (e.g., low-sodium sandwich fillings for work lunches, how to cope with eating out, etc.). In addition to methods for reducing sodium, recommendations should be made to increase potassium because potassium appears to provide a protective effect against high sodium intake (McCarron *et al.,* 1982). Effects of sodium restriction on blood pressure tend to be fairly rapid. In addition, sensory adaptation occurs quickly to the lower sodium intake and, when taste sensitivity to salt has increased, patients often find heavily salted foods to be unpleasant. Unfortunately, adaptation to higher sodium intake occurs as quickly.

In contrast to the debate over sodium, there is considerable agreement about the role of excess weight in hypertension. McCarron *et al.* (1982) suggest that "caloric intake may be the single most important nutritional consideration in the pathogenesis of hypertension" (p. III-4). The relationship between hypertension and overweight appears to be bidirectional: in addition to overweight being a risk factor for hypertension, hypertensives may have an increased tendency to become overweight (Majais, Tarazi, Dustan, Fouad, & Bravo, 1982).

Typical procedures for the treatment of overweight include caloric restriction, alteration in eating style, changing stimulus control of eating, and exercise (see Chapter 9, this volume). For overweight hypertensive patients, a weight loss program is a desirable first step in intervention and may prove beneficial even for individuals who have as little as 10% excess weight. The positive correlation between reduction in blood pressure and reduction in body weight is independent of the amount of salt in the diet (Pickering, 1982). Therefore, weight loss should be attempted initially in overweight patients without adding salt restriction. Patients will probably find it less bothersome to adhere to a diet permitting normal salt intake. Salt restriction can be added if required at a later time.

Sizable decreases in blood pressure occur in overweight hypertensives with moderate weight loss of about 5% of total body weight, and normal pressure may be achieved with loss of only half of the excess weight. The blood pressure reduction persists as long as body weight is maintained at the lower level. However, because cardiovascular risk in the overweight is dependent on factors other than hypertension, treatment may be required until normal weight is reached in order to normalize other important obesity-related cardiovascular risk factors such as glucose intolerance (Berchtold, Jörgens, Kemmer, & Berger, 1982).

Alcohol and Smoking. Heavy alcohol use, defined as five or more drinks a day, is associated with increases both in hypertension and in the complications of hypertension, especially cerebrovascular disease (Larbi, Cooper, & Stamler, 1983). The determinant of the relationship is current consumption: when drinking is discontinued, blood pressure decreases. Procedures for the treatment of substance abuse are discussed in Chapter 11 in this volume. There is some disagreement whether moderate alcohol users should be encouraged to continue intake (Kaplan, 1982) or to curtail it (Larbi *et al.,* 1983). Data on the relationship of moderate alcohol use to blood pressure are conflicting, but moderate consumption appears to be related to decreased coronary risk.

Smoking is a significant risk factor for many cardiovascular diseases, especially CHD. However, smoking does not appear to be correlated with essential hypertension, and data are conflicting on the effect of quitting smoking on blood pressure in hypertensive patients (Nicholson *et al.,* 1983). Nonetheless, a smoking cessation program should be recommended for a hypertensive patient who has a high overall cardiovascular risk profile. In this case, the clinician should be aware that blood pressure may actually increase due, in part, to the weight gain that often accompanies smoking cessation (Kaplan, 1982). A number of intervention strategies are available including progressive reduction (fading) of nicotine; nicotine chewing gum; and self-management training, which combines procedures such as self-monitoring, stimulus control, relaxation training, and contingency contracting (Glasgow, in press; Lichtenstein, 1982).

Exercise. Physical training is often recommended due to the relationship between hypertension and sedentary life-style and the observation that people who are physically fit tend to have lower resting blood pressure and less blood pressure reactivity to stress than those who are not fit. Exercise programs for hypertensives are based on isotonic rather than isometric training. Although guidelines for exercise prescriptions are available (e.g., American College of Sports Medicine, 1981), hypertensive individuals should be referred to a cardiologist or an exercise physiologist for exercise testing and development of a physical training program. The exercise prescription should specify the frequency, intensity, duration, and type of activity. Attempts should be made to tailor the program to the individual's skills, preferred activities, and life-style. Many patients need a program that shapes the exercise habit by starting with small goals and increasing these goals in gradual steps (Dubbert, Martin, & Epstein, in press).

Data on the effect of physical training on hypertension are inconclusive (Pickering, 1982). When changes in blood pressure are found, they tend to be small (Reeves & Victor, 1982) and to be no different from those produced by plausible placebo treatment (Andrews *et al.*, 1982). Blood pressure reductions that occur as a result of physical training are associated with decreases in heart rate and cardiac output. Peripheral resistance does not change (Björntorp, 1982). Therefore, exercise may be more effective for borderline hypertensive individuals who have hyperkinetic circulation at rest (high cardiac output and tachycardia) than it will be for patients with increased peripheral resistance and normal cardiac output (Björntorp, 1982; Pickering, 1982). However, decreased levels of blood viscosity that appear to accompany training may benefit peripheral resistance. Patients with volume-dependent hypertension would not be expected to benefit because physical training tends to increase plasma volume (Pickering, 1982). The small changes in blood pressure usually found after physical training suggest that the effectiveness of exercise in reducing cardiovascular risk is probably more attributable to its effects on risk factors other than high blood pressure (e.g., increases in high-density lipoproteins). In addition, some of the effects of exercise are psychological rather than physiological. Exercise permits distraction from daily routine and refocusing of attention. Some individuals may experience an enhancement of self-efficacy due to success at achieving new or increased abilities (Dubbert *et al.*, in press).

Medication Compliance

Data on long-term medication compliance suggest that approximately 50% of hypertensive patients do not comply with drug regimens (Sackett & Snow, 1979). In general, the probability of noncompliance with medical regimens increases with the complexity, duration, and cost of therapy (Haynes, 1979a) and decreases with the amount of regimen-specific information provided to the patient (Hulka, 1979). An additional detriment to compliance in hypertensive patients is the essentially asymptomatic nature of the disorder. A small number of individuals experience hypertension-related symptoms such as headache. However, for most patients, there are no readily perceptible symptoms of high blood pressure and, therefore, no immediate symptom-related consequences of compliance and noncompliance. Cardiovascular and cerebrovascular complications may not be apparent until many years later. On the other hand, some hypertensive medications result in immediate, unpleasant side effects including fatigue, dizziness, nausea, palpitations, dry mouth, skin rash, and impotence (Kaplan, 1982).

Noncompliance can be prevented to some degree at the time that the medication is prescribed. It is helpful to provide detailed oral instructions that are backed up by written instructions. The dosage regimen should be simplified as much as possible, and an attempt should be made to tailor the regimen to the individual's daily routine (Dunbar, Marshall, & Hovell, 1979; Haynes, 1979b). Some patients comply more if given regular pill containers rather than safety containers (Hulka, 1979). Finally, obtaining a verbal commitment by simply asking the patient "Will you do this?" increases compliance (Levy, Yamashita, & Pow, 1979).

If noncompliance appears to be a problem, several interventions are often beneficial. The first step is to insure that patients understand the instructions for taking the medication. Cards or calendars listing times and dosages, with a space for the individual to mark when the medication is taken, provide useful reminders for some patients. Additional tailoring and reminders can be provided. For example, twice-daily medications may be prescribed in the morning and evening at mealtimes and the medication kept at the table (Dunbar et al., 1979). Ingenious pill containers have been devised with timed alarms to remind patients to take medication (Azrin & Powell, 1969). A family member can be enlisted to help monitor the patient's behavior. This person also may dispense reinforcement when behavioral goals are met (Ziesat, 1982). In addition to monitoring medication adherence, patients can be encouraged to monitor blood pressure to provide feedback about symptom control.

Some therapists use a formal, written contract to enhance compliance (Dunbar et al., 1979; Ziesat, 1982). The contract specifies behavioral goals within the client's capabilities and reasonable medical requirements. For example, Sackett and Snow (1979) found that the hypertensives in their samples had to take at least 80% of the prescribed medication to demonstrate systematic blood pressure response to therapy, and this rate was used as the minimum required to define compliance (Haynes et al., 1980). A good contract delineates both the patient's responsibilities in meeting the goals and the responsibilities of others in helping the patient. For example, if the therapist is the contract partner, he or she may make available a blood pressure monitor for the patient's use. A family member may be the contract partner and assist in monitoring or provide reminders and reinforcement for the patient. The contract specifies reinforcement contingencies for meeting behavioral goals. A response-cost procedure may be incorporated, such as forfeiting part of a monetary deposit if goals are not met.

Educational programs alone have been notoriously unsuccessful across a range of compliance problems (Epstein & Cluss, 1982). Haynes and his colleagues (Haynes, 1979b) found that compliance was significantly improved in hypertensive patients with a program combining a medication regimen tailored to the patient's daily routine and habits, self-monitoring of pill consumption and blood pressure, positive reinforcement, and increased supervision. Unfortunately, individual components of this program may not be successful when used in isolation. For example, neither self-monitoring of blood pressure nor frequent monitoring by home visitors increased compliance.

A major problem in the clinical evaluation of compliance is adequate measurement of compliance. Research programs often rely on measures such as pill counts, serum and urine tests, and chemical markers. However, these are not readily available in many clinical settings and are costly in time, personnel, and money (Haynes *et al.*, 1980). Therefore, they are recommended only with recalcitrant cases (Ziesat, 1982). Blood pressure control is often used as an outcome measure. However, blood pressure is an imperfect correlate of compliance. Some compliant patients do not show the expected blood pressure decrease, and some noncompliant patients show improvement. For example, Haynes *et al.* (1980) found that 43% of their subjects did not achieve good blood pressure control despite high compliance. Interestingly, Haynes *et al.* found that self-reports on a structured interview correlated more highly with compliance than did blood pressure and several serum and urine assessments. The structured interview was introduced with the statement "people often have difficulty taking their pills for one reason or another, and we are interested in finding out any problems that occur so that we can understand them better" (p. 758). The patients were then asked to provide specific information about their compliance. Patients overestimated their compliance by an average of 17%. Only half of the patients who said they were compliant were found to be compliant (taking at least 80% of their medications); however, 90% of those who admitted to being noncompliant were found to be reporting accurately. Our experience suggests that a combination of daily self-recording of medication usage and regular blood pressure monitoring by the patient and therapist provide adequate measures of compliance in clinical practice for most patients.

Physiological Regulation

A major thrust of behavioral intervention is to lower blood pressure by helping individuals to gain direct control of physiological activity. The two procedures commonly used for this purpose are *relaxation training* and *biofeedback*.

Relaxation Training. Relaxation training attempts to lower physiological arousal and, thereby, to reduce the somatic consequences of stress. The two relaxation procedures that have been used most frequently with hypertensive individuals are progressive muscle relaxation and meditation. In progressive muscle relaxation, the individual is taught to alternately relax and tense the major muscle groups and to focus attention on the somatic cues involved in each state. As the individual develops the muscle relaxation skills, the tension component is gradually decreased and finally eliminated. Progressive relaxation training may be modeled after protocols developed by Bernstein and Borkovec (1973) and Marquis (1974). Meditation subsumes a variety of techniques in which the individual focuses on a constant and repetitive stimulus while in a comfortable position. Two therapy procedures based on transcendental meditation are the respiratory-one method, which involves silent repetition of the word *one* during the exhalation portion of each respiratory cycle (Benson, 1975), and clinically standardized meditation, in which a sound is repeated silently at its own pace without being linked to respiration (Carrington, 1977). Patel (1977) includes yoga-based training in passive mental concentration as part of her treatment package. Relaxation may also be induced with autogenic training (Schultz & Luthe, 1969), in which the individual is required to concentrate on psychophysiological functions such as feelings of heaviness and warmth in the extremities. In research, autogenic training has been used in conjunction with thermal biofeedback, but its independent effect on blood pressure lowering has not been assessed with hypertensive individuals.

Relaxation training is usually presented to clients in one of two ways. One approach is to have clients set aside time from daily activities to practice relaxation, on the assumption that one or two relaxation breaks of 15- to 30-minutes' duration each day will restore autonomic balance and provide protection against the effects of sympathetic arousal (e.g., Benson, 1975). The other approach is to present relaxation as a coping skill that clients can use to relieve tension in stressful situations. Clients are encouraged to use relaxation throughout the day and to use physiological arousal or environmental stimuli as cues for relaxation (e.g., Patel, 1977). These two approaches are not mutually exclusive, and many therapists instruct patients to practice regularly at home and to attempt to relax during daily activities by using either differential muscle relaxation or control of respiration.

The potential effects of relaxation extend beyond simply reducing physiological arousal (Appel, 1984). Relaxation has cognitive and emotional effects, such as decreased worry and feelings of increased calmness. It provides the opportunity for distraction from daily activities and refocusing of attention as well as giving structure and purpose to these breaks from daily activity when practiced regularly. The availability of relaxation as a coping skill may enhance self-efficacy and encourage individuals to attempt other changes in their habitual coping styles or life-style.

To date, the most consistent results for relaxation treatment of hypertension have been reported by Agras's group. They have found that blood pressure reductions produced by progressive muscle relaxation not only persisted throughout the day but were particularly evident in nighttime readings (Agras, Taylor, Kraemer, Allen, & Schneider, 1980). Blood pressure reductions obtained in the clinic also generalized to the work setting (Southam, Agras, Taylor, & Kraemer, 1982) and persisted in both the clinic and the work setting at a 15-month follow-up (Agras, Southam, & Taylor, 1983).

When conducting relaxation training, it is important to train subjects intensively. At least six to eight sessions are usually required (Agras, 1981). Therapist-conducted relaxation training, supplemented with relaxation tapes for home practice, appears to be more effective than relaxation therapy conducted mainly by home use of tapes (Brauer, Horlick, Nelson, Farquhar, & Agras, 1979). Part of the advantage of live training is that the trainer can individually tailor the procedures, pace the instruction to the progress of the client, and provide feedback on performance (Lehrer, 1982).

Although a dose-response relationship has not been demonstrated for relaxation and blood pressure reduction (Peters, Benson, & Peters, 1977), blood pressure appears to be lower only during those phases of treatment when subjects practice relaxation, and it returns to baseline when subjects stop practicing the techniques (Brady, Luborsky, & Kron, 1974). Relaxation training is contraindicated for some individuals because they find the procedure to be anxiety arousing (Agras, 1981). Such relaxation-induced anxiety appears to be more likely to occur with meditation than with progressive relaxation training (Heide & Borkovec, 1983). Other individuals who do not respond to therapist-administered relaxation instructions may be able to learn to relax when therapist instructions are supplemented with muscle tension biofeedback (Lehrer, 1982).

Biofeedback. In biofeedback training, information about a physiological function is presented to enable the individual to gain increased control of that function. Biofeedback is used to achieve two major purposes: either to gain control of a specific physiological function or to induce a generalized state of relaxation. Due to the nature of the response and its measurement, it is difficult to provide continuous, analog feedback of blood pressure. The standard methods of blood pressure measurement can provide measures only a few times a minute. A system that is frequently used in research is the constant-cuff method (Kristt & Engel, 1975). With this method, a blood pressure cuff is placed around the upper arm and inflated to a fixed pressure (either average SBP or average DBP), where it is maintained for about 30 seconds at a time. The subject receives binary information indicating whether blood pressure is above or below the fixed pressure on each heartbeat. On successive trials, the pressure in the cuff is changed to shape the desired blood pressure response. Recently, a tracking-cuff system has been developed (Shapiro, Greenstadt, Lane, & Rubinstein, 1981) in which pressure in the cuff is automatically readjusted during each interval between heartbeats to provide better tracking of blood pressure. It should be noted that both frequently repeated cuff inflation and the presence of a partially inflated cuff left on the arm for several recording periods are uncomfortable for many individuals.

In general, the changes in blood pressure that result from biofeedback have been modest (Pickering, 1982). In addition, blood pressure reductions obtained in the laboratory often do not generalize to the home situation (Goldstein, Shapiro, Thananopavarn, & Sambhi, 1982). Finally, biofeedback is frequently found to be no more effective than relaxation training (White & Tursky, 1982). Therefore, relaxation training is preferable to the more costly and cumbersome blood pressure biofeedback procedures.

Hypertensive individuals have also been treated with biofeedback for skin resistance (Patel, 1977) and fingertip temperature (Green, Green, & Norris, 1979). Because both responses appear to be under sympathetic nervous system control, it has been hypothesized that these training procedures may enable patients to control excessive sympathetic activity that contributes to the hypertensive disease process. Although neither of these biofeedback procedures has yet been adequately evaluated, recent findings suggest that thermal training may prove more effective than blood pressure biofeedback for the treatment of hypertension (Blanchard *et al.*, 1983).

Stress Management

Stress management focuses on improving the patients' abilities to cope with stressful events in their lives, thereby reducing stress-related fluctuations in sympathetic activity (Holroyd, Appel, & Andrasik, 1983). Stress management has two potential advantages that biofeedback and relaxation training do not have. First, attempts to control physiological responses to stress may fail because the individual continues to cope with stressful events in ways that generate the very responses he or she is attempting to control (Holroyd, 1979). To the extent that stress management training can alter the way that the individual copes with stressful events, it may enable him or her to control stress responses in situations where biofeedback or relaxation training is ineffective. Second, biofeedback and relaxation training provide clients with only a single coping response (e.g., relaxation). The complex stresses encountered in everyday life generally require more flexible coping strategies. Therefore, coping skills training that is more broadly based may enhance effectiveness for some individuals.

Stress management training teaches patients to monitor overt and covert events that precede, accompany, and follow stressful interactions and to employ various coping skills to manage stress responses and to eliminate environmental sources of stress. Because blood pressure and other indexes of cardiovascular reactivity are only weakly related to self-reports of emotion and stress, self-assessments of stress may not be good indicators of stress-related cardiovascular responses. Therefore, we recommend that patients both record their responses to events that are experienced as stressful and monitor pulse rate and/or blood pressure. Information obtained through self-monitoring can then be used to assist the client in identifying relationships between situational variables (e.g., criticism from the boss), thoughts (e.g., I'm going to lose my job), and emotional, behavioral, and cardiovascular responses (e.g., anxiety, cardiovascular reactivity).

As the patient becomes adept at self-monitoring, treatment focuses on altering his or her cognitive and behavioral responses to stressful events. Because stress responses are often mediated by the individual's appraisal of events, cognitive restructuring may help to control stress responses. If appraisal processes play an important role, this is frequently evident in the self-monitoring data. The recognition that particular beliefs and expectations (e.g., unrealistically high expectations for job performance) affect stress responses helps to motivate clients to examine and alter stress-inducing patterns of thought and behavior.

Coping strategies are tailored to the specific stressful situations that confront the client and to the particular problems that the client experiences with these situations. Clients may be taught to use relaxation as a coping skill to control arousal and rumination. Self-instructional training can be used to guide coping efforts, to maintain a coping orientation, and to combat anxiety-arousing rumination. Some patients may benefit from the application of rational problem-solving skills to practical problems (e.g., time management). Skills for self-assertion and for negotiating interpersonal conflicts also can be useful in managing particular stressful interactions. Where chronic conflict in a marital relationship or in the larger family appears to be a major source of stress for the client or where family members undermine the autonomous coping efforts of the patient, it may be helpful to include his or her partner or other family members in treatment (Coyne & Holroyd, 1982).

Unfortunately, the use of stress management interventions with essential hypertension has received little systematic research attention. The few small-scale studies that have compared stress management with other nonpharmacological interventions have failed to provide convincing evidence that stress management is more likely than relaxation training to benefit the average patient (Crowther, 1983; Drazen, Nevid, Pace, & O'Brien, 1982). The adequacy of these studies as tests of cognitive-behavioral interventions may be questioned. For example, Crowther's (1983) stress management group differed from the relaxation group mainly in receiving specific instruction on the use of relaxation as a coping response and on the application of positive self-statements. Additional data on the effectiveness of stress management will undoubtedly be forthcoming as investigators attempt to enhance effects that have been reliably produced with relaxation training. Until such data are available or until we are better able to identify those patients most likely to benefit from stress management, we suggest that stress management interventions be used in cases where patients appear to be unable to generalize the effects achieved with relaxation training beyond the laboratory or clinic setting. This may occur when patients report that chronic stresses at home or at work limit the effectiveness of relaxation training in those environments, when stress responses are repeatedly generated by the cognitive activity or behavior of the patient, or when the patient fails to practice relaxation training.

Case Illustration

The following case describes the treatment of a patient with mild hypertension using a multidisciplinary approach. The program combined relaxation training, diet, and exercise. In addition to describing the contribution of the various disciplines to the intervention, the case illustrates compliance problems that may be encountered in treatment.

W was a 23-year-old, white male with mild essential hypertension who was referred to determine if behavioral methods of controlling blood pressure could prevent or postpone the initiation of drug therapy. Biweekly blood pressure readings obtained for 6 months by the referring physician revealed labile borderline hypertension ($M = 148/98$, Range $= 132/92$ to $160/113$ mm Hg). On weekly laboratory assessments, pressures were in essentially the same range. Background information suggested several possible contributors to W's hypertension. W reported a family history of hypertension (father, grandfather, two aunts). He was about 20 lb overweight (245 lb, 39% fat, compared to a desirable weight of 225 lb). Estimated caloric intake was slightly high (2,780 calories, 50% carbohydrate, 44% fat, 14% protein), and estimated energy expenditure was somewhat low (2,300 calories). Cardiovascular fitness was low average for a young adult (maximum oxygen consumption $= 27.8$ ml/kg/min). Cholesterol was normal (170 mg/100 ml), but high-density lipoproteins were lower (35 mg/100 ml) and triglycerides were higher (130 mg/100 ml) than might be desired. W reported that social anxiety, insomnia, and chronic tension had been longstanding problems for him. He impressed both the referring physician and the evaluating psychologist as highly motivated to control his blood pressure through nonpharmacological methods and thus as an excellent candidate for behavioral intervention.

Initial interventions involved alterations in W's diet, a progressive aerobic exercise regimen, and relaxation training. In consultation with a dietitian, a flexible diet (1,000 calories, 225 g carbohydrate, 90 g protein, 60 g fat) was developed, incorporating as many of W's preferred foods as possible. Salt restriction was not included beyond what would normally accompany the decrease in food intake. An exercise physiologist prescribed a graduated exercise program with the goal of 30 minutes of aerobic exercise at 70% of maximum oxygen consumption (target heart rate of 138 bpm) 5 days per week. Because W chose to exercise by jogging, the first step of this exercise program alternated 30 seconds of jogging with 2 minutes of brisk walking for 30 minutes.

Progressive muscle relaxation training, modeled after Bernstein and Borkovec (1973), was also begun. Instructions to tense and relax 16 muscle groups were abbreviated over the course of six sessions until relaxation could be achieved by focusing on four muscle groups. Relaxation tapes were recorded during each session, and W was instructed to practice relaxation twice a day, once with and once without a tape (to facilitate independence from the tape recording). Cue-controlled and self-control relaxation procedures were introduced in the subsequent four sessions. In cue-controlled relaxation, the cue word *relax* was repeatedly paired with the taking of a deep breath and the recall of the sensations of relaxation. Once W appeared to have mastered this skill, he was instructed to use a variety of stimuli occurring throughout the day as signals to engage in cue-controlled relaxation. Self-control relaxation training involved guided imagination of himself in progressively more tension-arousing situations until tension and worry were evoked, followed by the active use of relaxation to control this tension and worry. During Sessions 8 through 11, self-control relaxation training was practiced with six progressively more tension-arousing situations. Consultation on problems encountered in the implementation of the dietary and exercise programs was also provided at weekly relaxation training sessions.

Two months after the start of treatment, it was evident that W was not complying adequately with the dietary and exercise components of the program and was practicing relaxation only irregularly. However, W continued to express enthusiasm for the prescribed program and was highly critical of himself for failing to comply. To provide support for the desired changes in behavior, W was enrolled in a structured exercise program that provided the daily supervision of an exercise physiologist and group support. The psychologist spoke to W's roommates to elicit their cooperation with the dietary changes and with providing reminders to W to practice relaxation regularly. These interventions increased W's compliance with exercise somewhat (70% class attendance) but increased only minimally his cooperation with the other components of the program. The partial failure of these interventions did not dampen W's enthusiasm for the recommended program, but it further increased his self-depreciation.

Given W's expressed enthusiasm for the program and the presence of reasonable environmental support for the proposed activities, explanation of W's noncompliance required further exploration of his thoughts and feelings about the program. This revealed that W possessed a very negative body image and little ability to imagine himself in a physically more healthy state. This problem was evident in the following dialogue that immediately followed an exercise in which W was instructed to imagine himself and his daily routine following the proposed behavior changes.

T: You didn't have much trouble imagining other people engaging in these activities, but it was a problem to imagine yourself doing them.

W: I got upset. . . . I couldn't stay relaxed when I tried to imagine myself.

T: What prevented you? What were the thoughts and images that came into your mind instead?

W: I couldn't imagine myself not tense and sort of agitated. . . . I guess I just really feel ugly, and to see myself run like I could do it right. . . . I just couldn't do it.

T: Even just in your imagination?

W: That's obviously not part of how I see myself, even though I can imagine myself doing other things that are even more impossible.

T: Maybe if we can change that first in your head, in your imagination, so you can imagine and begin to accept yourself doing these things, then they will be a little easier to do regularly.

Three interventions were employed in an attempt to alter W's self-depreciation and negative view of the possibility of behavior change. Meetings were arranged with two individuals who had made difficult but successful changes in health behaviors and who could serve as models. These potential coping models were asked to describe both the setbacks and the successes they had experienced on the road to behavior change. W was assisted in working through a hierarchy of images that progressively depicted him engaging in closer approximations to the desired behavior changes. Finally, W was taught to interrupt and dispute negative thoughts about his body and his ability to engage in healthy behavior. These interventions appeared to reduce W's self-depreciation. Within 1 month (five treatment sessions), W's compliance with the prescribed regimen also increased dramatically (approximately 90% compliance in all three areas). This produced objective feedback of successful performance that further enhanced his self-confidence. At the end of 1 year, compliance was still high, although there had been some slippage with the dietary program. W remained somewhat above optimal weight (235 lb), but his blood pressure was in the normotensive range (138/84 mm Hg); cardiovascular fitness had improved (maximum oxygen consumption = 40 ml/kg/min), and triglycerides and high-density lipoproteins were optimum (92 and 40 mg/100 ml, respectively).

Problems and Limitations of Treatment

Relative Effectiveness

The major limitation of nonpharmacological treatments of hypertension is the modest blood pressure reductions that are achieved. Medication typically produces a 10% to 30% reduction in blood pressure (Kaplan, 1983), whereas nonpharmacological interventions typically yield less than 10% reduction. Some nonpharmacological interventions appear to be more effective than others. Results of a meta-analytic comparison of drug and nondrug treatments (Andrews *et al.*, 1982) are presented in Table 1. (Meta-analysis is a statistical procedure that facilitates comparison across studies by expressing the size of the treatment effect for each study in standard deviation units.) On the basis of the meta-analysis, Andrews *et al.* concluded that none of the nonpharmacological interventions were as effective as drug treatment. Only weight reduction, muscle relaxation, and yoga produced greater blood pressure reductions than credible placebo treatments, whereas meditation, biofeedback, exercise, and salt restriction were no better than placebo. Our survey of the literature is consistent with the conclusions of this metaanalysis, with one caveat: the effect size for yoga was based largely on Patel's research that used a treatment package combining meditation, muscle relaxation, biofeedback, and generalization training; hence, characterizing the intervention as yoga is misleading.

Compliance

Compliance may be as much (if not more) of a problem for nonpharmacological interventions as for pharmacological treatment. In addition to the problems attendant on treating an asymptomatic disorder, adherence may be decreased due to the greater effort required and the greater disruption of the patient's life-style with nonpharmacological interventions than with drug therapy. Patients are often more willing to take a pill than to change long-standing dietary and exercise habits (Kaplan, 1983). Nonpharmacological interventions also may require more time and effort from the medical practitioner, with no guarantee of effectiveness even in highly compliant patients. Therefore, the physician may be less than enthusiastic in recommending such measures to the patient, providing a further deterrent to compliance.

Table 1. Mean Effect Sizes and Standard Errors of Measurement (SEM) for Pharmacological and Nonpharmacological Treatments of Hypertension

Treatment	n^a	Effect size Mean	SEM
Drugs	14/6	2.9	0.35
Weight loss	8/5	1.6	0.16
Yoga	23/8	1.4	0.12
Muscle relaxation	9/5	1.3	0.29
Meditation	21/7	0.7	0.11
Biofeedback	13/8	0.7	0.14
Exercise	6/3	0.7	0.22
Salt restriction	10/6	0.6	0.11
Placebo	5/3	0.6	0.32
Mean of all treatments	109/51	1.2	0.20
Mean of nondrug treatments	90/42	1.0	0.16

Note. From "Hypertension: Comparison of Drug and Non-Drug Treatments" by G. Andrews, S. W. MacMahon, A. Austin, and D. G. Byrne, 1982, *British Medical Journal, 284*, pp. 1523–1526. Copyright 1982 by the British Medical Journal. Adapted by permission.
^{a}Number of effect sizes calculated/number of groups.

Few indexes of compliance to nonpharmacological interventions are available other than self-reported compliance and blood pressure reduction. Self-report is subject to distortion, although, as in medication compliance, individuals who report themselves to be noncompliant are likely to be reporting accurately. Because of the limited effectiveness of nonpharmacological interventions and the inherent variability of blood pressure, reduction or lack of reduction in blood pressure is an imprecise reflection of compliance. Alternate compliance measures have been developed for a few nonpharmacological interventions. Use of tapes for home practice of relaxation can be monitored by tape recorders designed to measure when a tape with a superimposed signal is turned on and off (Taylor, Agras, Schneider, & Allen, 1983), but this requires special equipment. Subjects can be asked more readily to monitor tone cues dubbed onto relaxation tapes (Martin, Collins, Hillenberg, Zabin, & Katell, 1981). A rapid, reasonable estimate of adherence to dietary sodium restriction is provided by testing overnight urine specimens with easily obtainable chloride titrator strips (Kaplan *et al.*, 1982).

Methods to enhance medication compliance can be applied to nonpharmacological interventions. A minimum requirement is an introductory educational program that includes discussions of the rationale for nonpharmacological treatment and of the cost and side effects of medication. Later in treatment, the potential problem of noncompliance and techniques to avoid, or at least not to escalate, lapses, such as overeating or failure to practice relaxation, are discussed, possibly modeled after Marlatt and Gordon's (1980) relapse prevention methods. Self-monitoring of blood pressure is highly recommended. Self-monitoring of target behaviors is useful to enhance compliance and, when combined with notations of mood and circumstance, provides information that can be quite helpful in addressing compliance problems. These interventions are best presented in the context of a self-management program where the patient assumes responsibility for, and becomes an active participant in, treatment (Appel, in press).

Both externally and self-administered reinforcement can be provided contingent on meeting adherence or adherence-related goals such as daily practice of relaxation or weight loss. Making reinforcement contingent only on blood pressure reduction should be avoided due to the problems in using blood pressure as a reflection of compliance. Compliance may also be facilitated by involving family members or others in the person's daily environment in the treatment process or by arranging social support among individuals who are following similar regimens.

Generalization

Although blood pressure reductions resulting from interventions such as weight loss will be apparent across situations, reductions achieved by methods such as relaxation and biofeedback often do not generalize outside of the treatment setting (e.g., Goldstein *et al.*, 1982). For these interventions, specific generalization training must be included. Patel (1977) encourages patients to incorporate relaxation into their daily activities by using stimuli such as red dots attached to their watches, red traffic lights, and ringing telephones as signals to check for tension and to relax. Patients are told also to relax during personally stressful situations such as before an interview or while waiting in a dentist's office. Motivation to use relaxation techniques during daily activities can be enhanced by demonstrating to patients the blood pressure changes that accompany a stress test, such as mental arithmetic under time pressure or a stressful roleplay. Time-sampling of blood pressure at least three times daily over about a 1-week period, combined with self-reports of subjective state and circumstances, can serve a similar purpose (Kallinke, Kulick, & Heim, 1982).

Treatment Packages

Nonpharmacological interventions often are combined into multicomponent treatment packages in the hope of improving effectiveness. The danger of such multicomponent packages is that programs may become unnecessarily complex, so that clients find it difficult to understand or to carry out the recommended activities. In planning treatment, it is important to consider whether some interventions are more likely than others to be indicated as a first step for intervention (e.g., weight loss for overweight patients or alcohol management for excessive users). When beginning a multicomponent program, care should be taken to assess what tasks clients can reasonably be expected to carry out, especially in the early stages of therapy. More demanding and costly procedures should be introduced only as needed (e.g., salt restriction after weight loss for overweight patients or biofeedback after a trial of relaxation training).

Efficacy: Assessment and Problems

Short-Term and Long-Term Goals

The short-term goal of therapy for hypertensive patients is blood pressure control, preferably by a reduction into the normotensive range (i.e., DBP less than 90 mm Hg and SBP less than 140 mm Hg). The long-term goal is the prevention of cardiovascular and cerebrovascular complications, with medical data indicating that blood pressure control may have more effect on stroke and congestive heart failure than on CHD (Paul, 1983; Pickering, 1982). Whereas the short-term goal of blood pressure control is fairly easy to assess, the outcome criteria for the long-term goal may take years to manifest themselves and, hence, are not readily available as measures of treatment efficacy.

Inability to verify long-term goals may be of less concern to the practicing therapist, who is usually presented with the more immediate problem of reducing blood pressure. However, it is an important problem for research: large-scale clinical trials are needed to demonstrate the cost-effectiveness of the more promising nonpharmacological interventions in achieving the long-term goals of antihypertensive treatment. Judging from pharmacological trials, outcome with no treatment is good for mild hypertensives—the group most likely to be referred for nonpharmacological interventions. In a large-scale trial in Australia, about 50% of patients with initial DBPs between 95 and 109 mm Hg (the cutoffs used for mild hypertension in this study) dropped below 95, and about 80% remained below 100 without active treatment over a 4-year period (Management Committee, 1982).

The results were not related to factors such as weight loss and dietary changes. In addition, over 90% of mild hypertensives will not die of hypertension-related causes within a 20-year follow-up period (Kaplan, 1983).

These data have more relevance for pharmacological treatment due to possible side effects and iatrogenic consequences of drugs. However, some behavior therapists and a number of clients may find little solace in the suggestion than even if treatment is not necessary for most mild hypertensives, it will do no harm. The decision to treat mild hypertension, especially when DBP is less than 100 mm Hg, should likely take into consideration concomitant risk factors that identify individuals at high risk for cardiovascular and cerebrovascular disorders.

Blood Pressure Assessment

Returning to the short-term goal of treatment, the assessment of blood pressure reduction requires adequate blood pressure samples to evaluate therapy effects. Care should be taken to establish a stable baseline prior to treatment; otherwise, blood pressure decreases may reflect only an adaptation effect or regression to the mean. Achievement of a suitable baseline may require measurement for several weeks for some patients. Blood pressure should be recorded regularly (e.g., weekly) throughout treatment and at 3- to 6-month intervals for follow-up. It is useful to evaluate treatment effects with clinic and home readings as well as work-site readings, if feasible, to assess the generalization of blood pressure reduction. When patients are on medication, drug usage is recorded concurrently with blood pressure. If the patient's blood pressure was controlled by medication prior to treatment, the maintenance of this control in the context of decreased medication requirements is the major variable of interest for outcome.

Nonspecific Effects of Intervention

When treatment is effective, it cannot necessarily be assumed that this is due to the (presumably) active components of the treatment. For example, in a review of medical compliance research, Epstein and Cluss (1982) noted that adherence *per se* had an effect on outcome that was independent of whether patients adhered to a placebo or to an active pharmacological agent. When placebo-treated patients were divided into adherers and nonadherers, those who adhered had better outcome than those who did not adhere, despite receiving an inactive drug. This result could reflect some preexisting characteristic of the patients that has outcome implications: adherers may be less ill, lead more ordered lives, or engage in better health behaviors than do nonadherers. On the other hand, adherence may also lead to changes that directly or indirectly influence outcome. As a consequence of successfully meeting the goal of adherence, feelings of well-being may be enhanced and psychological side effects of illness reduced, or patients may make changes in illness-related behaviors such as smoking or diet. Anecdotal evidence suggests that hypertensive patients undergoing relaxation training may make symptom-relevant changes in their life-styles and coping activities other than those occasioned by the relaxation procedure (Godaert, 1982), even when such changes have not been discussed in therapy.

The coronary-prone behavior pattern, Type A, refers to a behavioral style that contributes to CHD risk. Research (e.g., Friedman *et al.*, 1982; Rosenman *et al.*, 1975) demonstrated that Type A men were twice as likely as their Type B counterparts to develop CHD and were at considerably greater risk for recurrent myocardial infarction once CHD developed. The relationship between Type A and CHD still obtained when the contribution of other cardiovascular risk factors was statistically controlled. The relative risk associated with Type A is similar in magnitude to that associated with the traditional risk factors of high blood pressure, smoking, and cholesterol (Review Panel, 1981).

The Type A pattern is generally defined in terms of three core characteristics: (a) sense of time urgency and impatience; (b) arousable hostility; and (c) competitiveness and achievement strivings (Rosenman, 1978). The pattern is conceptualized not as a personality trait, but as a behavioral style with which particular individuals react to appropriately challenging situations. Some components of the pattern may be more strongly associated with cardiovascular disease than are other components. Matthews, Glass, Rosenman, and Bortner (1977) identified five factors on a factor analysis of the Type A interview. The factors were competitive drive, past achievements, impatience, nonjob achievement, and speed. Only two of these factors—competitive drive and impatience—were associated with the subsequent occurrence of CHD. Analysis of the individual items that constituted the factors revealed that CHD cases showed higher scores on explosive voice modulation, potential for hostility, vigorous answers, and irritation at waiting in lines. High levels of hostility have also been found to be significant for coronary disease by Williams and his colleagues (Barefoot, Dahlstrom, & Williams, 1983; Williams *et al.*, 1980). Considerable work is still needed to identify the components of Type A that are pathogenic and, hence, are appropriate targets for intervention.

The pathogenic mechanisms by which Type A leads to CHD are unclear, but behaviorally induced neuroendocrine and sympathetic nervous system influences are generally implicated. Although the two groups show similar levels at rest and during nonchallenging activities, Type A individuals display greater physiological responsivity than Type B to behavioral challenges in the laboratory and in the field. This reactivity includes elevations in heart rate, blood pressure, catecholamines, and cortisol (see Matthews, 1982, for a review). Although physiological reactivity to stress is assumed to play a role in the development of CHD, the relationship remains to be established.

Assessment of Type A

Type A is typically assessed by interview and self-report paper-and-pencil measures. The classification into Type A is made on the basis of a preponderance of Type A characteristics on the measure. Alternatively, Type B, which is posited to lie at the opposite end of the continuum, is defined by the absence of Type A characteristics. Of the various Type A measures, the Structured Interview (SI), the

Jenkins Activity Survey (JAS), and the Framingham Type A Scale have been pro-
spectively related to the incidence of CHD. Other measures are available (e.g.,
Bortner, 1969), but they have not demonstrated their predictive ability in the
United States population in any consistent fashion (Matthews, 1983). In clinical
research, the SI and the JAS are favored, particularly the SI.

401

CARDIOVASCULAR
DISORDERS

Structured Interview

The SI constitutes the "standard" for the assessment of Type A. The SI comprises 25 questions that explore content areas relevant to the coronary-prone
behavior pattern including anger/hostility, time urgency, the trait of being hard
driving, and competitiveness (Rosenman, 1978). Although the content of the individual's answers is considered, the interviewer is more interested in eliciting a characteristic behavior sample that can be classified along the Type A–Type B continuum. This is accomplished by conducting the interview in a challenging manner.
To achieve this end, responses are queried, and the pace and tone of the interview
are varied. Compared to Type B's, Type A individuals are more likely to speak
rapidly and explosively in a loud and vigorous voice. Their answers are often terse
and emphatic, and they frequently interrupt or try to hurry the interviewer. They
display vehement reactions to questions about impedance of progress in utilizing
time (e.g., waiting in lines). They may show annoyance or hostility (including the
use of profanity) toward the interviewer or toward the topics of the interview
(Rosenman, 1978). On the basis of ratings of the interview, the individual is given
one of four classifications: A_1 (fully developed Type A); A_2 (incompletely developed
Type A); X (equivalent degrees of Type A and Type B characteristics); and Type B
(the relative absence of Type A). A recent modification of the traditional structured
interview is the Video Structured Interview (Friedman, Thoresen, & Gill, 1981),
which places more emphasis on the hostility and time urgency components of Type
A and takes greater account of overt nonverbal behavior in the expression of the
behavior pattern.

Jenkins Activity Survey (JAS)

The JAS is a self-report scale that has been used extensively to assess Type A
in a variety of populations (e.g., employed, unemployed, and student). In its standard form (for employed adults), the JAS comprises 50 multiple-choice items that
evaluate the content areas associated with Type A. Scores can be obtained for (a)
overall Type A; (b) speed and impatience; (c) being hard driving and competitive;
and (d) job involvement. Agreement of the JAS with the SI for A–B classification
was 73% in samples of middle-aged males (Jenkins, 1978). The advantage of the
JAS over the SI is that it does not require a trained interviewer and, therefore, can
be administered easily.

Difficulties in the Assessment of Type A

Although the measures purport to assess a common dimension, there is some
lack of agreement in the classification of individuals into Types A and B using different methods of assessment (Matthews, 1982, 1983). The lack of concordance

results, in part, from the fact that the measures evaluate Type A from different vantage points (e.g., observable impatience on an interview vs. the endorsement of content suggesting impatience on a self-report scale). Because somewhat different facets of coronary-prone behavior are reflected in the various measures, Matthews (1983) has proposed that Type A be assessed by a multimethod approach in which different measures of Type A are administered to the same individuals. Tasto, Chesney, and Chadwick (1978) recommended the assessment of physiological responses to standardized laboratory stressors and of psychological characteristics such as cognitive style in addition to the typical Type A measures. Such approaches may help to clarify some of the inconsistencies in research relating Type A to CHD.

In actual clinical practice, it is unclear whether a formal Type A assessment is consistently completed prior to intervention with Type A individuals. Instead, clinicians may identify components of the Type A behavior pattern that are problematic (e.g., anger or impatience) and base their interventions on methods to alter these components. Further discussion of assessment issues is beyond the scope of this chapter. Matthews (1983) provides a thoughtful and critical review of Type A assessment.

Treatment Techniques

Behavioral interventions with Type A individuals have attempted either to help the individual to control the harmful consequences of the Type A pattern or to alter the behavior pattern itself. Relaxation training has been used most frequently to control stress-induced arousal in Type A individuals. Alteration of various components of the behavior pattern has been the focus of cognitive-behavior therapy.

Relaxation

Type A individuals are characterized as chronically tense and driven, with a pervasive inability to relax. Relaxation training provides a method to regulate tension. Of the various relaxation techniques, progressive muscle relaxation is used most frequently in Type A interventions. One advantage of muscle relaxation is that it can be practiced unobtrusively throughout the day (Roskies, 1983). Relaxation is more likely to be beneficial if it is combined with self-monitoring and presented as a coping skill. For example, Roskies (1983; Roskies, Spevack, Surkis, Cohen, & Gilman, 1978) taught clients to monitor their tension hourly on a 1–10 scale for a period of 1 week at the beginning of therapy. The clients recorded the level of tension together with the activity currently in progress. Such self-observation increases awareness of tension as well as of the situations that are likely to be associated with increased arousal. Once they mastered the relaxation skill, the participants in Roskies's program were encouraged to use regularly occurring events in their daily routine (e.g., shaving, driving the car, and looking at an appointment book) as signals to check tension level and relax if necessary. It may also be helpful to have clients rehearse the use of relaxation as a coping skill to reduce imagery-induced arousal, as is done in Anxiety Management Training (Suinn & Bloom, 1978). Situations for imagery may be chosen from problematic areas identified through self-monitoring.

In order to make the relaxation procedures more attractive to Type A individuals, the rationales for the procedure should be presented in a way to appeal to Type A characteristics. For example, Roskies capitalized on the Type A's motivational pattern by stressing the inefficiency and the harmful physiological effects of the chronically driven Type A pattern. The program promised to help the participants learn to pace themselves so that they could accomplish more with less strain (Roskies *et al.*, 1978). Such a rationale uses to advantage the Type A's need for control by offering a means to control oneself as well as challenging the individual to learn to maximize productivity while minimizing strain.

Relaxation-based interventions for Type A have been demonstrated to be more effective than no treatment (Jenni & Wollersheim, 1979; Suinn & Bloom, 1978). They offered little advantage over a credible psychotherapy group in the short run (Roskies *et al.*, 1978), although the effects of relaxation were more likely to be maintained at 6-month follow-up (Roskies *et al.*, 1979). Relaxation was somewhat less effective than cognitive restructuring therapy (Jenni & Wollersheim, 1979).

As indicated previously, relaxation offers a valuable, albeit limited, coping skill. Many situations confront the Type A individual in which effective coping requires more than a reduction of immediate arousal (Roskies, 1983). Therefore, more complex programs have been introduced to help Type A clients develop a repertoire of coping strategies.

Cognitive-Behavior Therapy

In addition to helping Type A individuals develop more flexible coping strategies, cognitive-behavior therapy attempts to alter the unreasonable, stereotyped, and nonproductive cognitions that contribute to the Type A's characteristic appraisals of and reactions to environmental events (Friedman *et al.*, 1981; Levenkron, Cohen, Mueller, & Fisher, 1983; Roskies, 1983). A comprehensive cognitive-behavioral intervention incorporates a number of procedures such as self-monitoring, cognitive restructuring, and coping skills training, which are geared toward the problematic components of the Type A pattern (e.g., time pressure and hostility).

Self-monitoring of Type A behavior is important to promote change in the behavioral style. Many Type A individuals have poor awareness of, and insight into, their behavior. In order for Type A individuals to appreciate the pervasiveness of the pattern, it is necessary for them to become aware of the frequency of Type A behavior as well as the situations that elicit it. Self-monitoring of mood and circumstance several times daily, or even hourly, is recommended early in therapy. It is useful during self-monitoring to rate emotion on an arithmetic scale. Although self-monitoring is a relatively easy task to accomplish, it is not uncommon for it to be met with resistance from the Type A individual, who often complains that it requires too much time.

Because Type A behavior is often mediated by the individual's appraisals of the stresses he or she encounters in daily life, cognitive restructuring plays an important role in helping the client to control the behavior pattern. One approach is to identify particular expectations or beliefs that appear to explain the client's

Type A responses across a variety of situations. To illustrate, Type A individuals often believe that whatever occupational success they have obtained is due to the Type A pattern and that unless they continue the behavior (e.g., accomplishing all life activities with the least delay and with an absolute minimum of error), their careers may collapse (Friedman *et al.*, 1981). Another problem is the tendency of some Type A's to perceive a wide range of situations as threatening and to perceive objectively different situations (e.g., an inattentive waiter and an antagonistic co-worker) at the same level of severe threat (Roskies, 1983). Clients are pushed to examine the role that these beliefs play in their typical behaviors. In addition, the reasonableness and productiveness of the beliefs and expectations are challenged. Clients are then taught to rehearse more adaptive cognitions (appraisals and self-statements) for the upsetting situations that confront them.

Coping strategies are tailored to the characteristics of the Type A individual and to the situations that elicit Type A behaviors, as indicated by the daily diaries. Because Type A individuals may perceive prescriptive behavior change instructions as undermining their sense of control, it is advisable to use a problem-solving approach in which the individual participates in generating alternative ways of handling situations that typically elicit Type A behavior (Levenkron *et al.*, 1983). Specific coping skills that prove to be beneficial include self-control relaxation to reduce tension, anger management and communication skills training to reduce interpersonal conflict, and time and environmental management to minimize exposure to situations that elicit Type A behavior. These procedures can be combined with self-administered reinforcement for non-A behavior, such as responding without hostility in a frustrating situation that historically elicited anger and hostility. Response cost can also be implemented for use when the client engages in Type A behaviors. For example, when the individual displays time urgency by increasing speed to get through an intersection as the light turns red, the response cost would require him or her to turn and go around the block again (Rosenman & Friedman, 1977).

Intervention with Type A individuals can be accomplished individually or in groups. The group procedures tend to be particularly attractive and engaging to Type A individuals. The group format facilitates problem solving and the acquisition of new skills as well as providing support for the behavioral changes and for shared problems (e.g., the impact of myocardial infarction [MI] on functioning).

Few data are available on the effectiveness of cognitive-behavioral interventions for Type A behavior. In a group of men who were free of clinical CHD, Levenkron *et al.* (1983) found that comprehensive behavior therapy was more effective than minimal treatment (a brief information control that simulated usual care). However, behavior therapy yielded comparable effects to a condition comprising group support and discussion of stress and coping with no specific training in coping strategies. In the only available study with post-MI patients (Friedman *et al.*, 1982), the behavioral group had a lower rate of recurrent nonfatal infarction than did a group that received cardiologic counseling aimed at enhancing compliance with dietary, exercise, and drug regimens. In addition, the behavioral group had lower rates of nonfatal infarction and cardiovascular death than a no-treatment control group.

The following excerpt is from a therapy session with a post-MI Type A patient. During an interview several days following emergency coronary bypass surgery, it was clear to the rehabilitation team that the patient displayed several characteristics associated with the coronary-prone behavior pattern. He was hostile, achievement oriented and competitive, and extremely frustrated with his job situation. Initially, he refused to participate in behavior therapy, contending that he could make appropriate changes on his own. He entered treatment only after the team confronted him with the potential negative consequences of his behavior.

Upon discharge from the hospital, C was taught to monitor his tension levels and feelings of anger several times daily. Monitoring was achieved with a 0–10 rating scale and continued throughout treatment. Treatment combined relaxation training and cognitive-behavior therapy with special focus on C's easily arousable hostility, especially at work and with family members. After several sessions, little progress had been made. Although he was apparently continuing to monitor his behavior, C was not practicing relaxation regularly. As illustrated in the excerpt, impatience and hostility rendered him unable to make use of relaxation training. The excerpt also illustrates C's tendency to personalize everyday interactions as intrusions and affronts.

T: How has this week been? I see from your diary that you've been somewhat tense through a lot of the week.

C: Yesterday the car went out and cost me. I've also been thinking about my job situation. That's why I put a [*stress rating of*] 7 there. It's not cliff hanging, but there's constant nagging. What will I do?

T: Have the relaxation exercises been any help?

C: The relaxation tapes are fine. I understand the principle behind it. I try to practice twice a day, but sometimes only do it once a day.

T: That's a good start and it may be enough to be helpful.

C: I've begun to know what's coming so I don't have to listen to the tape.

T: If you find yourself mentally skipping ahead, that may get in your way. It's the time urgency issue we spoke about before and it can interfere with your ability to relax. Unfortunately, getting relaxed is not like getting to work—you can't rush and get there a little quicker. If you rush, you may not arrive. Do you feel the difference after the relaxation exercises?

C: Sometimes. Right now, though, I'm a 5 and I think it would be hard for me to get below that.

T: Has feeling angry interfered with your ability to relax at all? Did you record a lot of times in your diary where you were pretty angry?

C: Well, there were some.

T: How about here where you have a rating of 8 in the morning at work.

T: Yeah, but it's so stupid. I haven't seen the sonofabitch [a previous boss] for a year, but every once in a while I imagine him and I know it's stupid.

T: What do you imagine when he comes to mind?

C: I want to give him a knee job [*embarrassed, inappropriate laughter*]. Hire someone to shoot him in the knee. But he's over in Europe enjoying his retirement and I'm a lousy desk clerk making $7,000 a year. And I know it's not productive, but it gets me at weak points and I can't shake it; maybe it's self-pity. I don't know what it is.

T: I'm sure it feels good to get some revenge, even if only in your imagination. I can also see that it would be hard to control your tension when you're imagining a scene like that. What about here later in the afternoon where you have another 8?

C: That's difficult to put into words. I was carrying out my job. He had no business being there. That's what I get paid to do.

T: In your position, you must have to deal with many people walking through the building. What made this man's presence in the building so upsetting to you?

C: I asked him politely to leave and he said no. I started out fairly nicely: I asked if I could help him and found out he was just roaming around. There have been thefts. He could be a thief. Other things too—his flippant way of talking to me. So I started to get defensive and more aggressive.

T: Did the situation escalate?

C: Yeah. I didn't feel in control. Well, I know that if you get aggressive toward another person, his adrenalin starts to flow and he gets mad too and so you build up the frustration level.

T: What went through your mind when you first saw him?

C: Here he was making my job more difficult for me. And he was going to ruin my whole afternoon. I didn't need the hassle so soon after my surgery.

T: You viewed him as doing something that was personally directed at you, rather than being in the building for some unknown reason.

C: OK, uh, that's true. I don't know why I do that. I get very personal about it. I internalize these things. I don't know why.

T: There's a lot of traffic through your building. If you see very many of these people as personally attacking you by being there—and particularly if your way of approaching them elicits defensiveness or hostility—this would make it difficult to control your tension at work. You seem to interpret a fair number of situations in terms of an injury or affront. Sometimes this may be accurate, but other times I think there may be other ways of viewing the same situation that are as accurate, or more accurate. More importantly, this way of viewing events, this slot you put so many situations in, ends up repeatedly generating anger, making it difficult to control your tension and possibly jeopardizing your health. I think we are going to have to deal with this before you will be able to use the relaxation exercises the way I would like you to.

Problems and Limitations of Treatment

Effectiveness

In contrast to the large number of studies delineating Type A characteristics, there has been little evaluative research on methods to alter the Type A behavior pattern. The few studies that are available have often reported unimpressive changes in outcome variables (e.g., Jenni & Wollersheim, 1979; Suinn & Bloom, 1978). In addition, the data have been based mainly on healthy Type A subjects. It is likely that Type A individuals referred for psychological intervention will be those who show evidence of CHD. The one large-scale, controlled investigation with post-MI patients yielded promising results, but, thus far, outcome data have been reported for only the first year of the 5-year project (Friedman *et al.*, 1982). There is also a lack of data on the generalization of behavior change, even though the pervasiveness of the Type A pattern's influence on the individual's functioning requires generalizability across a multitude of situations.

Treatment Targets

In order to develop effective intervention for Type A, treatment targets need to be specified more precisely than has been done to date. Despite suggestive evidence (e.g., Matthews *et al.*, 1977), it has not been demonstrated which of the components that comprise Type A are pathogenic for CHD and which are irrelevant. In addition, there is a lack of information on pathogenic mechanisms through which Type A contributes to CHD, or even whether the relationship between Type A and CHD is causative rather than just associative (Friedman *et al.*, 1981). To some extent, past interventions tended to apply

> more or less haphazardly, a variety of currently fashionable therapies (anxiety management, relaxation, psychotherapy, cognitive therapy, exercise training) to type A individuals in the hope that these treatments would change something in the person's physiological, emotional, or behavioral functioning that would somehow reduce his or her coronary risk. (Roskies, 1983, pp. 265–266)

Motivation for Treatment

A further problem for intervention is the weak to nonexistent motivation of some Type A individuals to change their behavior. The rushed, competitive life-style is viewed as normal and even praiseworthy by the individual and is reinforced by society (Roskies, 1983). Type A individuals resist changing a life-style that they perceive is responsible for their success and fear that modification of Type A characteristics will have adverse occupational and personal consequences. It is difficult for the Type A individual to understand the relationship between his or her behavioral style and increased cardiovascular risk, particularly because many Type A's have strongly entrenched beliefs in their own invulnerability. These beliefs may persist even after an MI in the form of difficulty both admitting that an infarction has taken place and believing that there can be a recurrence (Friedman *et al.*, 1981).

These problems make it unlikely that primary prevention will be implemented on a wide scale. Individuals who have already experienced an MI are more likely to be amenable to treatment than are healthy Type A individuals. To maximize motivation, it is advisable to initiate contact while the MI patient is still hospitalized and in the acute stage. Providing a rationale for psychological intervention close in time to the event cuts through defensive denial and facilitates the patient's evaluation of the impact of his or her life-style in the context of his or her current health situation (Friedman *et al.*, 1981).

Once the individual is involved in treatment, the therapist must be prepared to deal with the impatient Type A, for whom changes are perceived as not occurring quickly enough. The Type A individual who is always in a hurry to get things done may be equally anxious to see immediate therapy results. In this case, it is helpful for the clinician to explain that the Type A behavior pattern is familiar, stable, and well learned and that changing it will require time and practice. In addition, the order of therapy techniques can be geared to both immediacy of benefit and acceptability to the Type A client. Roskies (1983) recommends that relaxation training be the first technique because of its ease of use and quick benefits. Cognitive restructuring is a good second choice because, although clients show some resistance to it, its effective use brings immediate increases in the sense of well-being. Communication and problem-solving skills take longer to learn and to apply and should be presented later in therapy. The client's involvement in, and compliance with, treatment can be enhanced by making him or her an active partner in treatment planning and in the development of coping strategies (Levenkron *et al.,* 1983).

Efficacy: Assessment and Problems

Because the goal of treatment with Type A individuals is the reduction of CHD, the obvious outcome variable to evaluate the effectiveness of intervention is the occurrence of relevant cardiovascular events such as fatal and nonfatal MI. However, assessment of cardiovascular disease outcome requires long-term follow-up that many clinicians are not prepared to provide.

More immediately available outcome measures are changes in Type A behavior components (e.g., time urgency and hostility) and in physiological variables thought to mediate the Type A–CHD relationship (e.g., cardiovascular reactivity and catecholamines). However, the lack of definitive information about what Type A components are pathogenic for CHD and of a model of pathophysiology makes it difficult to know which of these variables are relevant to increased CHD incidence.

In addition to the problem of relevance for CHD, there are problems with the actual assessment of the behavioral and physiological outcome variables. A number of treatment studies assessed resting levels of physiological activity. It is more appropriate to assess physiological reactivity to a stressor because research indicates that physiological differences between Type A and Type B subjects appear only when Type A subjects are challenged, and not at rest or during nonchallenging activities. The design of an appropriately challenging stress test that is also easy to administer in the office remains a challenge in itself. Furthermore, the assessment of neuroendocrine levels is expensive and beyond the ability of most practitioners.

Documenting change on traditional measures of Type A may also be difficult. For example, the SI, because it relies on a five-category classification system rather than a quantified numerical scale, is not very sensitive to change (Razin, 1982). Self-report measures such as the JAS are frequently used as outcome measures, but they are subject to distortion. Anxiety measures are sometimes used to evaluate outcome, but their validity is questionable because anxiety is not one of the components of Type A, as is indicated by the lack of relationship between anxiety and the SI (Chesney, Black, Chadwick, & Rosenman, 1981).

In most clinical settings, the measurement of change in Type A behavior will likely rely on self-report measures. Despite problems with the scale, the JAS is preferable to other self-report measures. Due to demand characteristics for change, the clinician is advised to employ reports by a spouse or others in the person's daily environment to compare with the Type A individual's evaluation. For example, Friedman *et al.* (1982) obtained assessments of participants' behavior from questionnaires completed by the spouse and a business associate or friend of the participant.

Cost Effectiveness

Recently, there has been an increasing trend toward interventions aimed at primary prevention. In light of our current lack of knowledge about the mechanisms leading to CHD, concern has been expressed about the cost-effectiveness of Type A treatment for primary prevention (Appel, 1984; Roskies, 1982). The prevalence of Type A in research studies has ranged between about 50 and 76%. Although Type A is an established risk factor for CHD, only a small proportion of Type A's will develop the disorder. For example, in their sample of middle-aged men, Rosenman *et al.* (1975) found that the annual rate of new cases of CHD was about 1%. Thus, if Type A alone is used as a criterion for inclusion in therapy, over half of the population would be targeted. Most of these individuals would be treated unnecessarily if the goal is to prevent CHD. Adding the traditional CHD risk factors (elevated serum cholesterol, hypertension, smoking, family history of the disorder, and obesity) increases specificity. However, because the traditional risk factors are poor predictors of CHD (Marmot & Winkelstein, 1975), a large number of individuals who will not develop CHD will still be targeted, and many of those who will eventually develop the disorder will not be identified.

Furthermore, indiscriminate modification of the pattern may have undesirable personal and social effects.

> At this point, we can only hope that certain types of individual and/or environmental changes will reduce the coronary risk associated with type A behavior, but we have far more certain knowledge of the personal, familial, and social disruption that can follow any radical change in lifestyle. Under these circumstances there are obvious ethical restrictions on the type of change that the clinician can responsibly advocate. (Roskies, 1983, p. 268)

There is greater justification for intervention once Type A individuals manifest their risk by developing CHD. For example, the recurrence rate for the Type A, post-MI subjects in Friedman *et al.*'s (1982) no-treatment control group was 8.9% in the first year. On the other hand, the first-year recurrence for the behaviorally treated subjects was 2.9%. These data may be somewhat nonrepresentative for the general population because smokers and diabetics were excluded. Despite this problem, the data suggest that intervention is more cost-effective for individuals with established coronary risk. However, prevention of recurrence may appear to some to be a fairly conservative prevention goal.

Cerebrovascular Disease

Although significant numbers of Americans die yearly from cerebrovascular accidents (CVA), many survive. In the United States, it is estimated that there are over two million stroke survivors. A variety of difficulties compromise the functioning of the stroke patient. Neuromuscular complications, however, are the focus of this discussion. After CVA, patients are likely to evidence hemiplegia or evidence of motor weakness or paralysis in the face and the upper and lower extremities on the side contralateral to the lesion. Eventually, spasticity develops in these areas.

Cerebrovascular disease presents a significant challenge for rehabilitation. Unfortunately, many CVA patients have been unresponsive to traditional rehabilitative techniques. In some cases, amelioration has been obtained when behavioral interventions have been implemented.

Assessment

Extent of impairment is assessed with measures of neuromuscular functioning, such as the electromyograph (EMG), range of motion, balance and movement patterns, and manual muscle tests, which are usually administered by medical personnel. In addition, it is advisable to include a behavioral analysis of the patient's functional capacity by observing the individual's behavior in various situations (Cleeland, 1981). The importance of observing the stroke patient's behavior in various situations is illustrated by the case of a woman who, despite being able to meet behavioral demands in her occupational and physical therapy sessions, complained that she was unable to function acceptably at home. These complaints puzzled the rehabilitation team who had observed her behavior only in the hospital. Observation by the therapist in the home revealed that, as expected, the woman could execute the tasks that had been relearned in the rehabilitation program. However, she was unable to adequately meet the demands of taking care of her infant son. This observation prompted the modification of the rehabilitation program to permit her to acquire the skills to feed and nurture her child.

Location of the lesion and the amount of time that has elapsed since the CVA may be important variables to assess. Individuals with less severe lesions or multiple small lesions appear to derive more benefit from treatment than those with single, devastating lesions (Shahani, Connors, & Mohr, 1977). Likewise, spontaneous recovery of some functions within 6 to 12 months following the stroke will occur as the brain stabilizes, whereas spontaneous recovery is less likely after 12 months.

Unfortunately, little systematic work has been done in neurological or psychological assessment to identify those patients who would be most likely to benefit from behavioral neuromuscular intervention (Inglis, Campbell, & Donald, 1976). Though often overlooked, cognitive functioning should be evaluated. Deficits in this realm could severely compromise the patient's ability to comply with treatment. For example, patients who have poor receptive language and memory abilities will have difficulty understanding and following treatment directions.

Biofeedback Treatment

EMG biofeedback is the primary behavioral technique that has been employed to facilitate changes in neuromuscular responses in stroke patients. The goal of EMG training is self-control of motor responses involving appropriate inhibition and excitation of muscle function. Auditory and/or visual feedback from muscle tension provides information to modify EMG responses as well as reinforcement for learning (Brucker, 1980).

Although EMG biofeedback has a relatively brief history of use in stroke rehabilitation, reported gains in functioning have been greater than those often observed with traditional therapy (Basmajian, 1980; Wolf, 1983). These techniques have been applied to upper and lower extremities for a variety of problems including impaired hand function, shoulder subluxation, and foot drop (Baker, 1979; Basmajian, 1982; Brudny, 1982).

Typically, surface electrodes are applied to the involved muscle group. For example, in dealing with shoulder subluxation, the areas of focus include the upper trapezius for elevation, mid-deltoid for abduction, and anterior deltoid for flexion. It is difficult for the CVA patient to minimize synergy, essentially isolating activity in one muscle group and inhibiting activity in others. In the event that the patient is unable to accomplish this task, the therapist may need to shape and eventually fade the inappropriate response (Baker, 1979). Specifically, if the desired goal is to facilitate contraction in one muscle group in the arm while inhibiting contraction in other muscles in order to eventually execute a movement, the therapist might first deal with this by reinforcing the synergistic activity. Once this has occurred, it will be critical to shape the undesired neuromuscular behavior by a series of successive approximations that involve extinguishing the inappropriate contractions and reinforcing the individual's display of control by inhibition of contractions in the appropriate muscles.

As the patient acquires the muscular skills, feedback is eventually faded, and increased demands for self-control are made. Self-observation of muscle activity is facilitated by the use of mirrors or by orienting the patient toward achieving a goal such as placing his or her hand on a table or his or her foot on a stool (Baker, 1979). The latter procedures provide structure and give the stroke patient immediate feedback about his or her performance of the task.

Problems and Limitations

In contrast to the disenchantment that has set in about the effectiveness of biofeedback to alter responses under autonomic nervous system control (e.g., blood pressure), there is considerable optimism about the use of biofeedback to help individuals regain voluntary control of the skeletal musculature (White & Tursky, 1982). Impressive results have been reported even in chronic patients who were unresponsive to traditional physical rehabilitation (e.g., Basmajian, 1982; Brudny, 1982).

However, there is a lack of systematic, well-controlled data on rehabilitation via EMG biofeedback. The data that are available suggest some problems. Training is a slow, painstaking process that requires considerable motivation on the part of the patients. To some extent, discouragement can be mitigated when opportunities for mastery are maximized by procedures such as initially setting goals for small changes in behavior. The development of some skills (e.g., regaining the ability to use a fork) may have obvious reinforcement value for patients that will be sufficient to maintain gains. On the other hand, some patients do not maintain their gains at follow-up (Brudny *et al.,* 1976). Chronicity may be a determinant of cost-effectiveness. A substantial amount of the available data is on long-term patients. It is not clear whether EMG training accelerates recovery of function in acute stroke patients who are likely to experience spontaneous recovery within the 12 months subsequent to stroke (Wolf, 1983).

At present, EMG biofeedback shows promise for neuromuscular rehabilitation of some stroke patients. It appears to be more useful within a comprehensive program of neuromuscular reeducation than when implemented to the exclusion of traditional treatments. For example, the combination of EMG biofeedback and exercise (a major component of traditional physical rehabilitation programs) may be more effective than either procedure used alone (Basmajian, Kukulka, Narayan, & Takebe, 1975; Wolf, 1983).

Summary

This chapter has discussed behavioral treatment techniques for hypertension, the Type A behavior pattern, and neuromuscular complications of stroke. Interventions for hypertension include life-style modification, enhancement of medication compliance, relaxation training, biofeedback, and stress management. Of the various procedures, weight reduction and some forms of relaxation training are more effective for lowering blood pressure than are other interventions. The two major behavioral treatments for Type A are relaxation training and cognitive-behavior therapy. Few data are available on the effectiveness of Type A intervention in reducing coronary heart disease. Biofeedback offers promise for the neuromuscular rehabilitation of stroke victims.

References

Agras, W. S. (1981). Behavioral approaches to the treatment of essential hypertension. *International Journal of Obesity, 5*(Suppl. 1), 173–181.

Agras, W. S., Southam, M. A., & Taylor, C. B. (1983). Long-term persistence of relaxation-induced blood pressure lowering during the working day. *Journal of Consulting and Clinical Psychology, 51,* 792–794.

Agras, W. S., Taylor, C. B., Kraemer, H. C., Allen, R. A., & Schneider, J. A. (1980). Relaxation training: Twenty-four-hour blood pressure reductions. *Archives of General Psychiatry, 37,* 859–863.

American College of Sports Medicine. (1981). *Guidelines for graded exercise testing and exercise prescription* (2nd ed.). Philadelphia: Lea & Febiger.

Andrews, G., MacMahon, S. W., Austin, A., & Byrne, D. G. (1982). Hypertension: Comparison of drug and non-drug treatments. *British Medical Journal, 284,* 1523–1526.

Appel, M. A. (1984). The usefulness of stress reduction methods in psychological practice. In J. R. McNamara (Ed.), *Critical issues, developments, and trends in professional psychology* (Vol. 2, pp. 108–154). New York: Praeger.

Appel, M. A. (in press). Hypertension. In K. A. Holroyd & T. L. Creer (Eds.), *Self-management of chronic disease: Handbook of clinical interventions and research.* New York: Academic Press.

Azrin, N. H., & Powell, J. (1969). Behavioral engineering: The use of response priming to improve prescribed self-medication. *Journal of Applied Behavior Analysis, 2,* 39–42.

Baker, M. P. (1979). Biofeedback in specific muscle retraining. In J. V. Basmajian (Ed.), *Biofeedback: Principles and practice for clinicians* (pp. 81–91). Baltimore: Williams & Wilkins.

Barefoot, J. C., Dahlstrom, W. G., & Williams, R. B. (1983). Hostility, CHD incidence, and total mortality: A 25-year follow-up study of 255 physicians. *Psychosomatic Medicine, 45,* 59–63.

Basmajian, J. V. (1980). Stroke and rehabilitation. In J. M. Ferguson & C. B. Taylor (Eds.), *The comprehensive handbook of behavioral medicine: Vol. 1. Systems intervention* (pp. 139–148). New York: Spectrum.

Basmajian, J. V. (1982). EMG feedback in neuromuscular control. In R. S. Surwit, R. B. Williams, A. Steptoe, & R. Biersner (Eds.), *Behavioral treatment of disease* (pp. 201–213). New York: Plenum Press.

Basmajian, J. V., Kukulka, C. G., Narayan, M. G., & Takebe, K. (1975). Biofeedback treatment of foot-drop after stroke compared with standard rehabilitation technique: Effects on voluntary control and strength. *Archives of Physical Medicine and Rehabilitation, 56,* 231–236.

Benson, H. (1975). *The relaxation response.* New York: Morrow.

Berchtold, P., Jörgens, V., Kemmer, F. W., & Berger, M. (1982). Obesity and hypertension: Cardiovascular response to weight reduction. *Hypertension, 4*(Suppl. III), III-50–III-55.

Bernstein, D. A., & Borkovec, T. D. (1973). *Progressive relaxation training: A manual for the helping professions.* Champaign, IL: Research Press.

Björntorp, P. (1982). Hypertension and exercise. *Hypertension,4*(Suppl. III), III-56–III-59.

Blanchard, E. B., McCoy, G. C., Andrasik, F., Pallmeyer, T. P., Gerardi, R., Acerra, M. R., Halpern, M., & Saunders, N. L. (1983, December). *Thermal biofeedback and progressive relaxation in the treatment of moderate hypertension.* Paper presented at the meeting of the Association for the Advancement of Behavior Therapy, Washington, DC.

Bortner, R. W. (1969). A short rating scale as a potential measure of pattern A behavior. *Journal of Chronic Diseases, 22,* 87–91.

Brady, J. P., Luborsky, L., & Kron, R. E. (1974). Blood pressure reduction in patients with essential hypertension through metronome-conditioned relaxation: A preliminary report. *Behavior Therapy, 5,* 203–209.

Brauer, A. P., Horlick, L., Nelson, E., Farquhar, J. W., & Agras, W. S. (1979). Relaxation therapy for essential hypertension: A Veterans Administration outpatient study. *Journal of Behavioral Medicine, 2,* 21–29.

Brucker, B. S. (1980). Biofeedback and rehabilitation. In L. P. Ince (Ed.), *Behavioral psychology in rehabilitation medicine: Clinical applications* (pp. 188–217). Baltimore: Williams & Wilkins.

Brudny, J. (1982). Biofeedback in chronic neurological cases: Therapeutic electromyography. In L. White & B. Tursky (Eds.), *Clinical biofeedback: Efficacy and mechanisms* (pp. 249–276). New York: Guilford Press.

Brudny, J., Korein, J., Grynbaum, B. B., Friedmann, L. W., Weinstein, S., Sachs-Frankel, G., & Belandres, P. V. (1976). EMG feedback therapy: Review of treatment of 114 patients. *Archives of Physical Medicine and Rehabilitation, 57,* 55–61.

Carrington, P. (1977). *Freedom in meditation.* New York: Anchor Press/Doubleday.

Chesney, M. A., Black, G. W., Chadwick, J. H., & Rosenman, R. H. (1981). Psychological correlates of the coronary-prone behavior pattern. *Journal of Behavioral Medicine, 4,* 217–230.

Cleeland, C. S. (1981). Biofeedback as a clinical tool: Its use with the neurologically impaired patient. In S. B. Filskov & T. J. Boll (Eds.), *Handbook of clinical neuropsychology* (pp. 734–753). New York: Wiley.

Cody, R. J., Laragh, J. H., Case, D. B., & Atlas, S. A. (1983). Renin system activity as a determinant of response to treatment in hypertension and heart failure. *Hypertension, 5*(Suppl. III), III-36–III-42.

Coyne, J., & Holroyd, K. (1982). Stress, coping, and illness: A transactional perspective. In T. Millon, C. Green, & R. Meagher (Eds.), *Handbook of clinical health psychology* (pp. 103–127). New York: Plenum Press.

Crowther, J. H. (1983). Stress management training and relaxation imagery in the treatment of essential hypertension. *Journal of Behavioral Medicine, 6,* 169–187.

Devereux, R. B., Pickering, T. G., Harshfield, G. A., Kleinert, H. D., Denby, L., Clark, L., Pregibon, D., Jason, M., Sachs, I., Borer, J. S., & Laragh, J. H. (1983). Left ventricular hypertrophy in patients with hypertension: Importance of blood pressure response to regularly recurring stress. *Circulation, 68,* 470–476.

Drazen, M., Nevid, J. S., Pace, N., & O'Brien, R. M. (1982). Worksite-based behavioral treatment of mild hypertension. *Journal of Occupational Medicine, 24,* 511–514.

Dubbert, P. M., Martin, J. E., & Epstein, L. H. (in press). Exercise. In K. A. Holroyd & T. L. Creer (Eds.), *Self-management of chronic disease: Handbook of clinical interventions and research.* New York: Academic Press.

Dunbar, J. M., Marshall, G. D., & Hovell, M. F. (1979). Behavioral strategies for improving compliance. In R. B. Haynes, D. W. Taylor, & D. L. Sackett (Eds.), *Compliance in health care* (pp. 174–190). Baltimore: Johns Hopkins University Press.

Epstein, L. H., & Cluss, P. A. (1982). A behavioral medicine perspective on adherence to long-term medical regimens. *Journal of Consulting and Clinical Psychology, 50,* 950–971.

Friedman, M., Thoresen, C. E., & Gill, J. J. (1981). Type A behavior: Its possible role, detection, and alteration in patients with ischemic heart disease. In J. W. Hurst (Ed.), *Update V: The heart* (pp. 81–100). New York: McGraw-Hill.

Friedman, M., Thoresen, C. E., Gill, J. J., Ulmer, D., Thompson, L., Powell, L. Price, V., Elek, S. R., Rabin, D. D., Breall, W. S., Piaget, G., Dixon, T., Bourg, E., Levy, R. A., & Tasto, D. L. (1982). Feasibility of altering type A behavior pattern after myocardial infarction: Recurrent Coronary Prevention Project Study: Methods, baseline results, and preliminary findings. *Circulation, 66,* 83–92.

Glasgow, R. E. (in press). Smoking. In K. A. Holroyd & T. L. Creer (Eds.), *Self management of chronic disease: Handbook of clinical interventions and research.* New York: Academic Press.

Godaert, G. L. R. (1982). Relaxation treatment for hypertension. In R. S. Surwit, R. B. Williams, A. Steptoe, & R. Biersner (Eds.), *Behavioral treatment of disease* (pp. 173–183). New York: Plenum Press.

Goldstein, I. B., Shapiro, D., Thananopavarn, C., & Sambhi, M. P. (1982). Comparison of drug and behavioral treatments of essential hypertension. *Health Psychology, 1,* 7–26.

Green, E. E., Green, A. M., & Norris, P. A. (1979). Preliminary observations on a new non-drug method for control of hypertension. *Journal of the South Carolina Medical Association, 75,* 575–582.

Guidelines for the treatment of mild hypertension: Memorandum from a WHO/ISH meeting. (1983). *Hypertension, 5,* 394–397.

Harshfield, G. A., Pickering, T. G., Kleinert, H. D., Blank, S., & Laragh, J. H. (1982). Situational variations of blood pressure in ambulatory hypertensive patients. *Psychosomatic Medicine, 44,* 237–245.

Haynes, R. B. (1979a). Determinants of compliance: The disease and the mechanics of treatment. In R. B. Haynes, D. W., Taylor, & D. L. Sackett (Eds.), *Compliance in health care* (pp. 49–62). Baltimore: Johns Hopkins University Press.

Haynes, R. B. (1979b). Strategies to improve compliance with referrals, appointments, and prescribed medical regimens. In R. B. Haynes, D. W. Taylor, & D. L. Sackett (Eds.), *Compliance in health care* (pp. 121–143). Baltimore: Johns Hopkins University Press.

Haynes, R. B., Taylor, D. W., Sackett, D. L., Gibson, E. S., Bernholz, C. D., & Mukherjee, J., (1980). Can simple clinical measurements detect patient noncompliance? *Hypertension, 2,* 757–764.

Heide, F. J., & Borkovec, T. D. (1983). Relaxation-induced anxiety: Paradoxical anxiety enhancement due to relaxation training. *Journal of Consulting and Clinical Psychology, 1983, 51,* 171–182.

Holroyd, K. A., (1979). Stress, coping, and the treatment of stress-related illness. In J. R. McNamara (Ed.), *Behavioral approaches in medicine: Application and analysis* (pp. 191–226). New York: Plenum Press.

Holroyd, K. A., Appel, M. A., & Andrasik, F. (1983). A cognitive-behavioral approach to psychophysiological disorders. In D. Meichenbaum & M. E. Jaremko (Eds.), *Stress reduction and prevention* (pp. 219–259). New York: Plenum Press.

Hulka, B. S. (1979). Patient-clinician interactions and compliance. In R. B. Haynes, D. W. Taylor, & D. L. Sackett (Eds.), *Compliance in health care* (pp. 63–77). Baltimore: Johns Hopkins University Press.

Hypertension Detection and Follow-up Program Cooperative Group. (1979). Five-year findings of the Hypertension Detection and Follow-up Program: I. Reduction in mortality of persons with high blood pressure, including hypertension. *Journal of the American Medical Association, 242,* 2562–2571.

Inglis, J., Campbell, D., & Donald, M. W. (1976). Electromyographic biofeedback and neuromuscular rehabilitation. *Canadian Journal of Behavioral Science, 8,* 299–323.

Jenkins, C. D. (1978). A comparative review of the interview and questionnaire methods in the assessment of the coronary-prone behavior pattern. In T. M. Dembroski, S. M. Weiss, J. L. Shields, S. G. Haynes, & M. Feinleib (Eds.), *Coronary-prone behavior* (pp. 71–88). New York: Springer.

Jenni, M. A., & Wollersheim, J. P. (1979). Cognitive therapy, stress management training, and the type A behavior pattern. *Cognitive Therapy and Research, 3,* 61–73.

Kallinke, D., Kulick, B., & Heim, P. (1982). Behaviour analysis and the treatment of essential hypertensives. *Journal of Psychosomatic Research, 26,* 541–549.

Kaplan, N. M. (1982). *Clinical hypertension* (3rd ed.). Baltimore: Williams & Wilkins.

Kaplan, N. M. (1983). Mild hypertension: When and how to treat. *Archives of Internal Medicine, 143,* 255–259.

Kaplan, N. M., Simmons, M., McPhee, C., Carnegie, A., Stefanu, C., & Cade, S. (1982). Two techniques to improve adherence to dietary sodium restriction in the treatment of hypertension. *Archives of Internal Medicine, 142,* 1638–1641.

Kawasaki, T., Delea, C. S., Bartter, F. C., & Smith, H. (1978). The effect of high-sodium and low-sodium intakes on blood pressure and other related variables in human subjects with idiopathic hypertension. *American Journal of Medicine, 64,* 193–198.

Kirkendall, W. M., Feinleib, M., Freis, E. D., & Mark, A. L. (1980). Recommendations for human blood pressure determination by sphygmomanometers: AHA committee report. *Circulation, 62,* 1145A–1155A.

Kleinert, H. D., Harshfield, G. A., Pickering, T. G., Devereux, R. B., Sullivan, P. A., Marion, R. M., Mallory, W. K., & Laragh, J. H. (1984). What is the value of home blood pressure measurement in patients with mild hypertension? *Hypertension, 6,* 574–578.

Kristt, G. A., & Engel, B. T. (1975). Learned control of blood pressure in patients with high blood pressure. *Circulation, 51,* 370–378.

Larbi, E. B., Cooper, R. S., & Stamler, J. (1983). Alcohol and hypertension. *Archives of Internal Medicine, 143,* 28–29.

Laughlin, K. D. (1981). Enhancing the effectiveness of behavioral treatments of essential hypertension. *Physiology and Behavior, 26,* 907–913.

Lehrer, P. M. (1982). How to relax and how not to relax: A re-evaluation of the work of Edmund Jacobson—I. *Behaviour Research and Therapy, 20,* 417–428.

Levenkron, J. C., Cohen, J. D., Mueller, H. S., & Fisher, E. B. (1983). Modifying the Type A coronary-prone behavior pattern. *Journal of Consulting and Clinical Psychology, 51,* 192–204.

Levy, R. L., Yamashita, D., & Pow, G. (1979). The relationship of an overt commitment to the frequency and speed of compliance with symptom reporting. *Medical Care, 17,* 281–284.

Lichtenstein, E. (1982). The smoking problem: A behavioral perspective. *Journal of Consulting and Clinical Psychology, 50,* 804–819.

MacGregor, G. A. (1983). Sodium and potassium intake and blood pressure. *Hypertension, 5*(Suppl. III), III-79–III-84.

Management Committee of the Australian Therapeutic Trial in Mild Hypertension. (1982). Untreated mild hypertension. *Lancet, 1,* 185–191.

Marlatt, G. A., & Gordon, J. R. (1980). Determinants of relapse: Implications for the maintenance of behavior change. In P. O. Davidson & S. M. Davidson (Eds.), *Behavioral medicine: Changing health lifestyles* (pp. 410–452). New York: Brunner/Mazel.

Marmot, M., & Winkelstein, W. (1975). Epidemiologic observations on intervention trials for prevention of coronary heart disease. *American Journal of Epidemiology, 101,* 177–181.

Marquis, J. (1974). Relaxation tape and instruction manual. (Available from [Self-Management School, Los Altos, CA])

Martin, J. E., Collins, F. L., Hillenberg, J. B., Zabin, M. A., & Katell, A. D. (1981). Assessing compliance to home relaxation: A simple technology for a critical problem. *Journal of Behavioral Assessment, 3,* 193–198.

Matthews, K. A. (1982). Psychological perspectives on the type A behavior pattern. *Psychological Bulletin, 91,* 293–323.

Matthews, K. A. (1983). Assessment issues in coronary-prone behavior. In T. M. Dembroski, T. H. Schmidt, & G. Blümchen (Eds.), *Biobehavioral bases of coronary heart disease* (pp. 62–78). Basel: Karger.

Matthews, K. A., Glass, D. C., Rosenman, R. H., & Bortner, R. W. (1977). Competitive drive, pattern A, and coronary heart disease: A further analysis of some data from the Western Collaborative Group Study. *Journal of Chronic Diseases, 30,* 489–498.

McCarron, D. A., Henry, H. J., & Morris, C. D. (1982). Human nutrition and blood pressure regulation: An integrated approach. *Hypertension, 4*(Suppl. III), III-2–III-13.

Mujais, S. K., Tarazi, R. C., Dustan, H. P., Fouad, F. M., & Bravo, E. L. (1982). Hypertension in obese patients: Hemodynamic and volume studies. *Hypertension, 4,* 84–92.

Nicholson, J. P., Teichman, S. L., Alderman, M. H., Sos, T. A., Pickering, T. G., & Laragh, J. H. (1983). Cigarette smoking and renovascular hypertension. *Lancet, 2,* 765–766.

Patel, C. (1977). Biofeedback-aided relaxation and meditation in the management of hypertension. *Biofeedback and Self-Regulation, 2,* 1–41.

Paul, O. (1983). Hypertension and its treatment. *Journal of the American Medical Association, 250,* 939–940.

Peters, R. K., Benson, H., & Peters, J. M. (1977). Daily relaxation response breaks in a working population: II. Effects on blood pressure. *American Journal of Public Health, 67,* 954–959.

Pickering, T. G. (1982). Nonpharmacologic methods of treatment of hypertension: Promising but unproved. *Cardiovascular Reviews and Reports, 3,* 82–88.

Pickering, T. G., Harshfield, G. A., Kleinert, H. D., Blank, S., & Laragh, J. H. (1982). Blood pressure during normal daily activities, sleep, and exercise: Comparison of values in normal and hypertensive subjects. *Journal of the American Medical Association, 247,* 992–996.

Razin, A. M. (1982). Psychosocial intervention in coronary artery disease: A review. *Psychosomatic Medicine, 44,* 363–387.

Reeves, J. L., & Victor, R. G. (1982). Behavioral strategies for treating hypertension. In P. A. Boudewyns & F. J. Keefe (Eds.), *Behavioral medicine in general medical practice* (pp. 166–188). Menlo Park, CA: Addison-Wesley.

Review Panel on Coronary-prone Behavior and Coronary Heart Disease. (1981). Coronary-prone behavior and coronary heart disease: A critical review. *Circulation, 63,* 1199–1215.

Rosenman, R. H. (1978). The interview method of assessment of the coronary-prone behavior pattern. In T. M. Dembroski, S. M. Weiss, J. L. Shields, S. G. Haynes, & M. Feinleib (Eds.), *Coronary-prone behavior* (pp. 55–69). New York: Springer.

Rosenman, R. H., & Friedman, M. (1977). Modifying type A behaviour pattern. *Journal of Psychosomatic Research, 21,* 323–331.

Rosenman, R. H., Brand, R. J., Jenkins, C. D., Friedman, M., Straus, R., & Wurm, M. (1975). Coronary heart disease in the Western Collaborative Group Study: Final follow-up experience of 8½ years. *Journal of the American Medical Association, 233,* 872–877.

Roskies, E. (1982). Type A intervention: Finding the disease to fit the cures. In R. S. Surwit, R. B. Williams, A. Steptoe, & R. Biersner (Eds.), *Behavioral treatment of disease* (pp. 71–85). New York: Plenum Press.

Roskies, E. (1983). Stress management for type A individuals. In D. Meichenbaum & M. E. Jaremko (Eds.), *Stress reduction and prevention* (pp. 261–288). New York: Plenum Press.

Roskies, E., Spevack, M., Surkis, A., Cohen, C., & Gilman, S. (1978). Changing the coronary-prone (type A) behavior pattern in a non-clinical population. *Journal of Behavioral Medicine, 1,* 201–215.

Roskies, E., Kearney, H., Spevack, M., Surkis, A., Cohen, C., & Gilman, S. (1979). Generalizability and durability of treatment effects in an intervention program for coronary-prone (type A) managers. *Journal of Behavioral Medicine, 2,* 195–207.

Sackett, D. L., & Snow, J. C. (1979). The magnitude of compliance and noncompliance. In R. B. Haynes, D. W. Taylor, & D. L. Sackett (Eds.), *Compliance in health care* (pp. 11–22). Baltimore: Johns Hopkins University Press.

Schultz, J. H., & Luthe, W. (1969). *Autogenic therapy* (Vol. 1): *Autogenic methods.* New York: Grune & Stratton.

Shahani, B. T., Connors, L., & Mohr, J. P. (1977). Electromyographic audio-visual feedback training effect on the motor performance in patients with lesions of the central nervous system (Abstract). *Archives of Physical Medicine and Rehabilitation, 58,* 519.

Shapiro, D., & Goldstein, I. B. (1982). Biobehavioral perspectives on hypertension. *Journal of Consulting and Clinical Psychology, 50,* 841–858.

Shapiro, D., Greenstadt, L., Lane, J. D., & Rubinstein, E. (1981). Tracking-cuff system for beat-to-beat recording of blood pressure. *Psychophysiology, 18,* 129–136.

Silman, A. J., Locke, C., Mitchell, P., & Humpherson, P. (1983). Evaluation of the effectiveness of a low sodium diet in the treatment of mild to moderate hypertension. *Lancet, 1,* 1179–1182.

Southam, M. A., Agras, W. S., Taylor, C. B., & Kraemer. H. C. (1982). Relaxation training: Blood pressure lowering during the working day. *Archives of General Psychiatry, 39,* 715–717.

Suinn, R. M., & Bloom. L. J. (1978). Anxiety management training for pattern A behavior. *Journal of Behavioral Medicine, 1,* 25–35.

Tasto, D. L., Chesney, M. A., & Chadwick, J. H. (1978). Multi-dimensional analysis of coronary-prone behavior. In T. M. Dembroski, S. M. Weiss, J. L. Shields, S. G. Haynes, & M. Feinleib (Eds.), *Coronary-prone behavior* (pp. 107–118). New York: Springer.

Taylor, C. B., Agras, W. S., Schneider, J. A., & Allen, R. A. (1983). Adherence to instructions to practice relaxation exercises. *Journal of Consulting and Clinical Psychology, 51,* 952–953.

White, L., & Tursky, B. (Eds.). (1982). *Clinical biofeedback: Efficacy and mechanisms.* New York: Guilford Press.

Williams, R. B., Haney, T. L., Lee, K. L., Kong, Y., Blumenthal. J. A., & Whalen, R. E. (1980). Type A behavior, hostility, and coronary atherosclerosis. *Psychosomatic Medicine, 42,* 539–549.

Wolf, S. L. (1983). EMG biofeedback applications to stroke patients: A critical review. *Physical Therapy, 63,* 1448–1459.

Ziesat, H. A. (1982). Adhering to medical regimen. In P. A. Boudewyns & F. J. Keefe (Eds.), *Behavioral medicine in general medical practice* (pp. 269–294). Menlo Park, CA: Addison-Wesley.

15

Headache

DONALD A. WILLIAMSON, LAURIE RUGGIERO, AND
C. J. DAVIS

Introduction

Surveys of outpatient medical facilities have indicated that headache is one of the most common medical complaints of adults (*National Ambulatory Medical Care Survey*, 1981). Epidemiological studies have reported that the incidence rate of migraine in adults is about 20% (Waters & O'Connor, 1975). The incidence rate for muscle-contraction or tension headache has been found to be approximately 80% (Ostfeld, 1963). However, because infrequent muscle-contraction headache can usually be treated using over-the-counter medications, physicians and other health-care providers usually treat only the more severe cases of chronic (almost daily) tension headache.

Traditional medical treatment of migraine headache has involved the use of vasoconstrictors (ergotamine tartrate), beta blockers (propranolol), or psychotropic medications (usually minor tranquilizers or antidepressants). Although pharmacological treatment of migraine is often successful, side effects of the medications are frequently reported to be more problematic than headaches. Also, a study by Mathew (1981) has reported that behavioral treatment methods in combination with these types of medications are superior to either treatment alone. Therefore, there is a great demand for effective nonpharmacological treatment methods that can be used in isolation or in combination with medical treatment.

Chronic tension headache is usually treated using analgesics, combinations of analgesics and sedatives (e.g., Fiorinal), or psychotropic medications (usually minor

DONALD A. WILLIAMSON, LAURIE RUGGIERO, and C. J. DAVIS • Department of Psychology, Louisiana State University, Baton Rouge, Louisiana 70803-5501.

tranquilizers or antidepressants). Although these types of medications are frequently useful in the treatment of tension headache, most medical authorities have long recommended psychological or psychiatric treatment for this type of headache (Friedman, von Storch, & Merritt, 1954). In response to the need for the development of effective nonpharmacological treatment methods for migraine and tension headache, behavioral researchers have developed several well-validated treatment approaches. Biofeedback, relaxation, and cognitive/behavioral programs are among some of the more extensively researched treatment approaches. The purpose of this chapter is to describe the clinical procedures involved in assessing and treating headache from a behavioral perspective. This chapter will emphasize the clinical aspects of this process. The reader may refer to other sources for more technical reviews of the headache literature (cf., Blanchard, Ahles, & Shaw, 1979; Blanchard, Andrasik, Ahles, Teders, & O'Keefe, 1980; Blanchard & Andrasik, 1982; Williamson, 1981).

Clinical Description

Migraine Headache

For diagnostic purposes, migraine or vascular headache has been separated into five categories: Classic migraine, common migraine, cluster headache, hemiplegic migraine, and lower-half headache (Ad Hoc Committee on Classification of Headache, 1962). Of these five types of migraine, classic and common migraines account for the overwhelming majority of cases. Therefore, only these two types of migraines have been extensively studied by behavioral researchers. For these reasons, cluster headache, hemiplegic migraine, and lower-half headache will not be discussed in this chapter. For further information on these types of headaches, the reader may wish to refer to Diamond and Dalessio (1978).

Classic migraine is usually described as a severe, throbbing pain that has a unilateral (one-sided) location on the head. This type of headache is episodic, usually lasting about 4 to 8 hours. Frequency of headache is quite variable, but it is not uncommon for classic migraineurs to report two to three headaches per week. Nausea and/or vomiting usually accompany classic migraine. The important diagnostic feature for diagnosing classic migraine is the report of consistent neurological prodromes prior to the beginning of pain. These prodromal symptoms usually precede the headache by about 30 minutes. Common prodromes are (a) visual disturbances (e.g., flashing lights, stars, blind spots, or tunnel vision); (b) somatosensory disturbances, (e.g., numbness in a particular part of the body); (c) motor disturbances (e.g., difficulty speaking and muscular weakness); and (d) vertigo. Classic migraine accounts for approximately 10% of all migraine cases.

Common migraine is very similar to classic migraine except that there are no clearly defined prodromal symptoms. Instead, sufferers from common migraine report that pain begins without warning. Common migraine also differs from classic migraine in that the location of pain is often described as bilateral, sometimes affecting the entire head. Common migraine is also more likely to be directly precipitated by hormonal changes and environmental events (e.g., stress, work pressure, family problems, etc.). About 85% of all migraine cases are diagnosed as common migraine.

The pathophysiology of common and classic migraines are thought to be identical. According to the most widely accepted theory of migraine (Diamond & Dalessio, 1978; Williamson, 1981), migraineurs are genetically predisposed to respond with an abnormal cerebral vascular reaction to stress, hormonal changes, and a host of other environmental events. Prior to the advent of head pain, there is a period of localized intracranial vasoconstriction that leads to reduced blood flow to certain brain areas, anoxia, and acidosis. This localized vasoconstriction and associated metabolic changes are thought to produce the prodromes of classic migraine (O'Brien, 1971; Skinhoj, 1973; Skinhoj & Paulson, 1969). This vasoconstriction leads to a rebound response of extracranial vasodilation and the release of histamine and peptide kinins. These vascular and humoral changes are thought to produce a sterile inflammation at the locus of pain. The throbbing pain is then due to the pulsation of blood through an inflamed and distended vessel.

Muscle-Contraction (Tension) Headache

Muscle contraction headache is usually described as a dull, constant (not throbbing) pain that is bilateral across the forehead, occipital, or shoulder/neck regions of the head. In severe cases, the entire head may be affected. Common descriptions of the pain are aggravating, nagging pain that feels like a tightness around the head or "a stiffness or soreness in the neck." The most popular theory of tension headache was first proposed by Wolff (1963). This theory postulates that there are two physiological bases of this type of headache: sustained muscle contraction of the facial or neck muscles and vasocontriction of the nutrient arteries of these muscles. According to Wolff's theory, these physiological responses are usually the result of stress. Thus, Wolff proposed a vascular and a muscle-contraction basis for tension headache.

Combined (Mixed) Headache

Combined headache refers to a description of headaches that includes symptoms of both migraine and muscle-contraction headaches. Some patients report discrete headaches of two types. Others report symptoms of migraine and muscle-contraction headaches that occur concurrently within an attack. The pathophysiology of this type of headache is thought to be a combination of the physiological changes associated with migraine and tension headache.

Assessment

Diagnosis

It is rare that a patient presents a textbook description of migraine, tension, or combined headache. More typically the patient will describe a complex set of symptoms that is meaningful to him or her but does not fit the usual descriptors that are used for headache diagnosis. The reasons for this "confused" description of headache symptoms are probably twofold: (a) headache symptoms do vary considerably; and (b) most people have great difficulty in describing painful sensations and symptoms that are somewhat inconsistent (e.g., location of head pain, presence of neurological signs, and temporal patterns of headaches). Therefore, interviewing the patient for diagnostic purposes is often a difficult and challenging task. In order to minimize the problems associated with the diagnostic interview, we have developed a Headache Questionnaire that is used as a structured interview. This questionnaire represents an extension of the work reported by Blanchard, Theobald, Williamson, Silver, and Brown (1978), Cinciripini, Williamson, and Epstein (1981), and Granberry, Williamson, Pratt, Hutchinson, and Monguillot, 1981. This questionnaire is presented in Table 1.

This questionnaire is comprised of a variety of common symptom reports by patients diagnosed as having migraine headache, tension headache, or temporomandibular joint (TMJ) dysfunction. As noted earlier, many headache symptoms overlap these three diagnoses. The symptoms that are *most* applicable to each of the three sources of head pain are indicated by the provision of blank spaces to the left of each question. Migraine symptoms are indicated by blank spaces under *M* and tension headache symptoms under *T*. Ratings of the duration of headaches are indicated by spaces under *D*. To use this interview format, the diagnostician should ask each question and ask for a rating concerning the frequency of this symptom. The rating should be written in the space(s) to the left of the question. These ratings can be summed and divided by the number of questions pertaining to each diagnosis (43 for migraine, 21 for tension, and 7 for TMJ). The resulting average will then suggest which diagnosis is most appropriate for the patient.

This structured interview is very useful for differentially diagnosing headache. However, it is not foolproof. Therefore, careful attention to the general description of headache symptoms is very important for accurate diagnosis. The following case examples are given to provide further information related to diagnosis.

Case 1

M. J. was a 42-year-old female who described episodic head pain that was localized to the right side of her head. These headaches occurred approximately one to three times per week and generally lasted from 4 to 12 hours. She described the pain as severe and throbbing, "as though someone was jabbing a knife into my right temple." She frequently saw bright spots of light about 20 minutes prior to the onset of a headache. At the onset of the headache she usually felt nauseous and sometimes vomited. Bright lights and loud noises made her headache seem more painful. After her headache ended, M. J. reported that the right side of her head was tender to touch. Medical records indicated that she had been diagnosed as having migraine headaches. This case is a textbook description of classic migraine headache.

Case 2

T. M. was a 33-year-old male who described headaches that usually began in the left or right temple but frequently spread to either side or in rare instances to both sides of his head. He described the pain as severe and throbbing at its peak, but dull, and aggravating at onset. Sometimes the headaches never reached their peak intensity. He often felt nauseous but never experienced warning signs or vomiting. The headaches were very frequent, one to four per week and often lasted for 24 hours. Medical records indicated that T. M. had been diagnosed as having migraine headaches by one physician and tension headaches by another physician.

Our diagnosis of this case was common migraine headache. The rationale for this diagnosis was that T. M. indicated that his headaches always began on one side of his head and then radiated, sometimes becoming bilateral. Also, the pain was not always severe and throbbing, but T. M. reported that most of his headaches began with a dull ache, and *some* headaches progressed to a severe, throbbing quality. This description suggests a continuum of pain descriptors as a function of pain severity. Finally, T. M. experienced nausea, but no prodromal symptoms, which suggests a vascular headache but not classic migraine.

Case 3

D. G. was a 45-year-old personnel manager in a large business firm. He described his headaches as feeling like a dull, constant ache across his forehead or around the top of his head. He never experienced nausea, vomiting, or prodromal symptoms. He indicated that his headaches seemed to be a response to job-related stress because they usually began at work and became more intense as the day went on. He reported that aspirin helped his headaches to some degree and that if he could relax his muscles, for example, via massage, whirlpool bath, and the like, his headaches improved.

This description of headache is a textbook case of muscle-contraction headache that is stress-related.

Case 4

J. L. was a 60-year-old female with a very long history of headache. She remembered having "sick" headaches as a child. These headaches were very severe and were usually associated with severe nausea and vomiting. These headaches occurred infrequently, averaging about four per year. As an adult, the headaches gradually increased in frequency. Furthermore, she recalls that the symptoms of her headaches changed over time. During her 20s, she reported the frequent (almost daily) occurrence of dull, aching pain in her neck and shoulders that occasionally developed into severe throbbing headaches that typically localized in either temple. During her late 30s and early 40s, she began to have very severe sharp pain in her right ear and surrounding areas. Also, she reported tension and soreness in the muscles of her jaw and neck. Currently, she reports almost daily head pain that is present upon awakening and is localized on the right side of her face and neck. Lateral pressure to her jaw produced pain in the TMJ region. If this pain persists, she frequently develops a severe pulsating headache that often involves her entire head.

This case represents a very complex case of headache with features of TMJ dysfunction, migraine, and tension headache. Formulation of the case suggests that the patient had experienced migraine and tension headaches for many years and

Table 1. Headache Questionnaire

NAME ———— DATE ————

DIRECTIONS: Read each question carefully and ask the patient which rating is most descriptive of his/her headaches. The five possible answers are defined as follows: always; occurs without exception; usually; occurs on most occasions with infrequent exceptions; sometimes; occurs approximately half the time; infrequently; occurs only once in a great while; never; absolutely does not occur and has not ever occured. Write the rating in the space(s) to the left of each question.

D	M	T	TMJ			NEVER	RARELY	SOME-TIMES	USUALLY	ALWAYS
—				1.	My headache ends within 1 hour.	1	2	3	4	5
—				2.	My headache ends within 4 hours.	1	2	3	4	5
—				3.	My headache ends within 8 hours.	1	2	3	4	5
—				4.	My headache ends within 12 hours.	1	2	3	4	5
—				5.	My headache ends within 24 hours.	1	2	3	4	5
	—	—	—	6.	I wake up with a headache.	1	2	3	4	5
	—	—	—	7.	My headache is worst at the end of the working day.	1	2	3	4	5
	—			8.	My headache is throbbing or pulsating.	1		3	4	5
	—			9.	My headache feels like a tightness or an external pressure (bandlike or caplike).	1	2	3	4	5
	—			10.	My headache feels like a tightness or an internal pressure (bandlike or caplike).	1	2	3	4	5
	—		—	11.	My headache begins on the left-hand side of my head.	1	2	3	4	5
	—		—	12.	My headache begins on the right-hand side of my head.	1	2	3	4	5
	—			13.	My headache begins behind my eye(s).	1	2	3	4	5
	—			14.	My headache begins behind my temple and/or forehead.	1	2	3	4	5
	—	—		15.	My headache begins in the back of my head.	1	2	3	4	5
	—	—		16.	When I have a headache I hurt over my entire head.	1	2	3	4	5
	—			17.	When I get a headache I have visual changes like seeing stars, blind spots, wavy lines, or double vision.	1	2	3	4	5
	—			18.	Some part of my body becomes numb before my headache begins.	1	2	3	4	5
	—	—	—	19.	My headache gets worse if I cough, strain, or lift objects.	1	2	3	4	5
		—		20.	My headache begins in my neck or shoulders.	1	2	3	4	5
		—		21.	My headache is better if I can loosen up my neck muscles.	1	2	3	4	5
		—		22.	Aspirin, Anacin, Bufferin, Excedrin, BC, Alka Seltzer, or other nonprescription pain medications relieve my headache.	1	2	3	4	5
	—		—	23.	My head hurts all the time.	1	2	3	4	5
	—			24.	I take a prescribed medication to prevent a full-blown attack of a headache.	1	2	3	4	5
	—		—	25.	My headache starts during periods of relaxation or rest.	1	2	3	4	5
	—			26.	My headache begins after exercise.	1	2	3	4	5
	—			27.	I have nausea with my headache.	1	2	3	4	5

Table 1. Headache Questionnaire (cont.)

D	M	T	TMJ		NEVER	RARELY	SOME-TIMES	USUALLY	ALWAYS
—				28. I have nausea and vomiting with my headache.	1	2	3	4	5
—	—	—		29. A headache wakes me up from sleep.	1	2	3	4	5
—				30. Headache delays me from going to sleep.	1	2	3	4	5
—	—	—		31. Strong sunlight triggers my headache.	1	2	3	4	5
—				32. During a headache, I am sensitive to sounds, sunlight, or artificial light.	1	2	3	4	5
—				33. I have warning signs that a headache is coming.	1	2	3	4	5
	—	—		34. My headache occurs when I am under pressure.	1	2	3	4	5
—				35. I have dizziness or difficulty concentrating *before* my headaches.	1	2	3	4	5
—				36. During a headache, I have blind spots in my visual field (what you are looking at).	1	2	3	4	5
—				37. After a headache there are areas of my head that are sensitive to touch.	1	2	3	4	5
—	—	—		38. My headache begins early in the morning and increases in severity as the day continues.	1	2	3	4	5
—				39. My headache starts after smoking.	1	2	3	4	5
—				40. My headache starts after drinking alcoholic drinks.	1	2	3	4	5
—				41. My headache starts after drinking coffee.	1	2	3	4	5
—				42. My headache starts after eating certain kinds of food such as nuts, sour cream, cheese, or Chinese food.	1	2	3	4	5
			—	43. My headache is located near the area where my jaw connects to the skull (near the ear or temple).	1	2	3	4	5
			—	44. I notice (or have been told) that I grind my teeth or clinch my jaws together.	1	2	3	4	5
			—	45. When I get a headache I experience pain in area(s):					
—			—	only 1	1	2	3	4	5
—			—	only 2	1	2	3	4	5
—				only 3	1	2	3	4	5
—				only 4	1	2	3	4	5
—				only 5	1	2	3	4	5
—				only 6	1	2	3	4	5
	—	—		only 1 and 2	1	2	3	4	5
—				only 1 and 4	1	2	3	4	5
—				only 1 and 6	1	2	3	4	5
—				only 1, 4, and 6	1	2	3	4	5
—				only 2 and 3	1	2	3	4	5
—				only 2 and 5	1	2	3	4	5
—				only 2, 3, and 5	1	2	3	4	5
	—			only 5 and 6	1	2	3	4	5
—	—			only 3 and 4	1	2	3	4	5
			—	only 3, 4, 5, and 6	1	2	3	4	5
			—	only 1, 2, 3, and 4	1	2	3	4	5
			—	only 1, 2, 3, 4, 5, and 6	1	2	3	4	5

then developed TMJ dysfunction that now serves as a "trigger" for migraine and tension headaches. Such cases present challenging diagnostic problems and require both medical, dental, and behavioral assessment for proper treatment planning.

Behavioral Assessment

For all headache cases, careful assessment of the antecedents and consequences of pain reports is essential for developing an effective treatment plan. For many cases, stress plays a major role in determining headache occurrence. Evaluation of stress and coping skills is very important for tension headache and TMJ dysfunction. Cases of migraine and combined headaches often appear to be less frequently associated with stress or emotional responses. However, we have seen numerous cases in which stress is a clear antecedent to vascular headache. Migraine is also precipitated by many other factors including alcohol, menstrual cycle, fatigue, and overheating. Therefore, careful evaluation of antecedent conditions is very important for treatment recommendations.

Reporting pain has certain predictable consequences—attention and sympathy from others, medication consumption, and relief from responsibilities. Although the overwhelming majority of headache cases do not involve operant factors (e.g., positive or negative reinforcement for pain behavior) one must be careful to assess for this possibility. To assess these influences, one must evaluate the relative degree of negative (punishment and response cost) versus positive (positive and negative reinforcement) consequences for reporting pain. If pain reports produce considerably greater benefits than costs, then the possibility of conversion headache must be seriously entertained. Further psychological evaluation, as described later, is generally required in such cases.

Self-Monitoring

Self-monitoring is one of the most useful methods of assessing the degree of headache activity prior to treatment and the extent to which headache improves after treatment. The self-monitoring procedure that we use is illustrated in Figure 1. This procedure has been used in a number of treatment outcome studies and has been socially validated using independent judgments of headache activity by significant others (Blanchard, Andrasik, Neff, Jurish, & O'Keefe, 1981). Figure 1 presents the first three pages of a headache booklet (dimensions of 3 $\times$ 4 in.). It is comprised of nine pages, the cover sheet, the rating scale sheet, and seven pages of self-monitoring records (one for each day of the week). Patients are instructed to rate their head pain at breakfast, lunch, dinner, and bedtime. Also, they are instructed to record their medication intake during the day. From these records, measures of headache activity can be derived. These measures are the following:

1. Headache index—Average headache rating (sum of ratings/number of ratings, usually 28).
2. Headache frequency—Number of discrete headaches during a week (rat-

ings greater than zero that occur in a sequence are defined as one headache).

3. Headache duration—Average number of rating intervals per headache (sum of rating intervals/frequency of headache). This number may be multiplied by 4 hours in order to estimate the duration of headaches in units of hours.
4. Peak intensity—Highest headache rating during the week.
5. Average peak intensity—Highest headache rating for each discrete headache divided by headache frequency.
6. Medication index—Measure of medication consumption that takes into account the type of medication and quantity of medication ingested.

This index is computed by multiplying the number of pills taken by the potency rating for the medication. These figures are then summed in order to compute the medication index. Potency ratings for the majority of medications taken by headache patients are listed in Table 2.

Psychological Assessment

Assessment of other psychological problems and evaluation of the determinants of headaches is best accomplished using a behavior analytic interview, as described earlier, and several standardized tests. We prefer to use the Minnesota Multiphasic Personality Inventory (MMPI), Symptom Checklist 90 (SCL-90), and Beck Depression Inventory for screening purposes. In cases where stress or life problems are potential determinants of headaches, the therapist should investigate

---

Headache Record
   Record #
   Week of:
      Beginning _____
      Ending _____
NAME _____

Rating Scale
   0 = No HA
   1 = Very mild HA, aware of it only when attending to it
   2 = Mild HA, could be ignored at times
   3 = Moderate HA, pain is noticeably present
   4 = Severe HA, difficult to concentrate, can do undemanding tasks
   5 = Extremely intense HA, incapacitated
Using the scale above, please rate your head pain at the following times:
   Breakfast _____
   Lunch _____
   Dinner _____
   Bedtime _____
   Medications _____

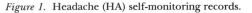

Figure 1. Headache (HA) self-monitoring records.

the nature of these circumstances for consideration of treating them directly. For example, in some cases marital conflict or poor child management skills may contribute much stress to the person's life and may be a direct antecedent of headaches.

Psychological testing is most useful for screening out other forms of psychopathology. In particular, assessing the degree of depression and anxiety of the patient is very important for treatment planning. Also, an accurate diagnosis of the conversion headache, as suggested by a "conversion V" on the MMPI and observations during the interview, is essential for successful treatment. Headache patients usually show elevations of MMPI Scales 1 (Hs), 2 (D), and 3 (Hy). However, the average t scores for these scales are usually between 60 and 65. Therefore, very high (above 70) elevations of these scales should not be dismissed as a typical headache profile. The SCL-90 is especially useful for assessing a wide variety of psychological problems. Headache patients typically show elevations of the Somatic Complaints, Depression, and Anxiety scales. The Beck Depression Inventory is useful for assessment of severe depression. If patients score above 20 on the Beck and

Table 2. *Potency Rating of Drugs Commonly Used by Headache Patients*

Over-the-counter drugs	1. APC	Parafon
	Alka Seltzer	Persistin
	Anacin	Phenaphen
	Aspirin	Robaxisal
	Bufferin	Sinutab
	Cope	Tylenol 1 & 2
	Empirin	Vanquish
	Excedrin	Datril
	Midrin	Percogesics
	Nervine	Comtrex
	Norgesic	Synalgos
Beta blockers	2. Inderal	
	Inderide	
Sedatives & minor tranquilizers	3. Darvon	Mepergan (fortis)
	Fiorinal	Seconal
	Vistaril	Ativan
	Tranxene	Librium
	Triavil	Xanax
	Dalmane	Phenergan
		Valium
Vasoconstrictors	4. Cafergot	
	Gynergen	
	Ergotrate	
	Ergostat	
Prescription analgesics	5. Codeine	Percogesics
	Empirin compound with codeine	Phenergan
	Leritine	Mepergan
	Ponstel	Tylenol #3
	Talwin	Tylenol #4
	6. Demerol	
	7. Dilaudid	
	8. Morphine	

above 70 on the D scale of the MMPI and the Depression scale of the SCL-90, one must strongly consider a primary diagnosis of depression and development of treatment plan for directly treating depression. In general, recent research has shown that high levels of psychopathology and depression are negatively correlated with treatment outcome (Blanchard *et al.*, 1982; Jacob, Turner, Szekely, & Eidelman, 1983). Therefore, use of these instruments is very important for the development of a sound treatment plan.

Treatment Methods

In behavioral treatment of headache, four general methods account for the bulk of the research regarding headache management: biofeedback, relaxation training, cognitive/behavior therapy, and a multimodal approach, including a combination of behavioral techniques. The following discussion will provide a brief summarization of the literature regarding each treatment approach as well as the successes and problems of each.

General Considerations

For many cases of headache, treatment using biofeedback or relaxation may be very straightforward. By following a treatment protocol of about 10 treatment sessions over a 2- to 3-month period, one can often successfully treat 50 to 70% of headache patients. The basic procedure for this type of treatment is (a) training in relaxation or biofeedback; (b) home practice of this relaxation skill; and (c) training in the use of this skill for reducing stress or aborting headaches during onset of head pain or during the prodromal period of the classic migraine. For other cases, significant life problems may be contributing to life stress. In such cases, direct intervention to modify these other problem areas may be required.

Biofeedback

Biofeedback has been defined as

> a special case of feedback where the system is a biologic system and where the feedback is artificially mediated by man-made detection, amplification and display instrumentation rather than being present as an inborn feedback loop within the biologic system. (Diamond, 1976, p. 136)

Simply put, biofeedback is a system that allows for the self-modification of biological responses within the patient's body. In the treatment of headache, biofeedback typically has taken one of three forms: (a) peripheral skin temperature biofeedback; (b) vasomotor response (VMR) biofeedback; or (c) electromyographic (EMG) biofeedback. The following sections will discuss the most pertinent findings regarding the clinical utility of these three approaches.

Skin Temperature Biofeedback

In one of the first biofeedback studies applied to the treatment of headache, Sargent and his collegues at the Menninger Clinic found that thermal biofeedback, when combined with autogenic training, led to a reduction of migraine headache activity (Sargent, Green, & Walters, 1972). This combination of procedures has been termed *autogenic feedback training.*

Since this initial investigation, several controlled group outcome studies evaluating the efficacy of autogenic feedback training have been conducted (Blanchard *et al.,* 1978; Jessup, Neufeld, & Merskey, 1979; Jurish *et al.,* 1983). The first of these studies (Blanchard *et al.,* 1978) found that autogenic feedback training was superior to a waiting-list control group but was comparable to relaxation in the treatment of migraine. A 2-year follow-up study (Silver, Blanchard, Williamson, Theobald, & Brown, 1979) indicated that improvement of headache was maintained, especially for patients who continued to practice autogenic training.

Recent research has shown that skin temperature biofeedback may contribute more to treatment success than simple relaxation in some cases (Blanchard *et al.,* 1982).

Cephalic VMR Biofeedback

Since the demonstration by Snyder and Noble (1968) that biofeedback training could be utilized in modifying VMR, there have been attempts to treat headaches (especially migraines) with VMR biofeedback training. This procedure is designed to train the patient to control the vasodilation of extracranial arteries. Because migraine headache has been postulated to be caused, in part, by vasodilation, training to constrict these arteries is a logical choice.

The procedure is designed to be implemented in the first phases of migraine. A photoplethysmograph is usually placed over the supraorbital branch of the temporal artery, and a binary (yes/no) feedback signal is provided to the patient. A signal (light or tone) is provided, dependent on the degree of vasoconstriction of the temporal artery and the threshold set by the clinician.

Several studies have investigated the effects of cephalic VMR biofeedback in the treatment of headache (Bild & Adams, 1980; Cohen, McArthur, Feurstein, Adams, & Beiman, & Rickles; 1976; Elmore & Tursky, 1976; Feuerstein & Adams, 1977; Friar & Beatty, 1976; Quintanar, Cacioppo, & Monyak, 1980; Sturgis, Tollison, & Adams, 1978). The existing literature suggests that this type of biofeedback may be especially useful in treatment of migraine. Cephalic VMR biofeedback has been found to be superior to placebo (Friar & Beatty, 1976), frontalis EMG biofeedback (Bild & Adams, 1980), skin temperature biofeedback (Elmore & Tursky, 1981), paced breathing (Quintanar *et al.,* 1980), and relaxation training (Zamani, 1974). A study by Cohen *et al.* (1980), however, indicated that cephalic VMR feedback was effective in reducing headache activity, but was equal to skin temperature, EMG, and alpha wave feedback.

The research to date has been very encouraging regarding the efficacy of cephalic VMR feedback in treating adult migraines. In general, the effectiveness of cephalic VMR biofeedback appears to be roughly comparable to other established treatment approaches for migraine (Blanchard *et al.,* 1980).

EMG Biofeedback

A third type of biofeedback involves modifying facial muscle tension or EMG. EMG biofeedback has been used most effectively for tension headache and pain associated with TMJ dysfunction. For those with muscle-contraction headache, surface electrodes are placed over the frontal muscles (Williamson, Epstein, & Lombardo, 1981), or the trapezius muscles (Gray, Lyle, & McGuire, 1980). The most common electrode placement for treatment of TMJ pain is over the masseter muscles (Gale, 1979).

Numerous studies have investigated the utility of EMG biofeedback as a treatment of tension headache. The first controlled group outcome study in this area was reported by Budzynski, Stoyva, Adler, and Mullaney (1973). This study reported a significant advantage for EMG biofeedback over no treatment for tension headache.

Since this initial study, there have been many studies investigating the utility of EMG biofeedback (e.g., Cox, Freundlich, & Meyer, 1975; Haynes, Griffin, Mooney, & Parise, 1975; Philips, 1977). These studies generally showed that EMG biofeedback was superior to placebo and no-treatment conditions, but was equivalent to relaxation training.

A significant study questioning the mechanisms facilitating change with EMG feedback was published in 1980 by Andrasik and Holroyd. Subjects were assigned to one of four conditions: (a) traditional EMG feedback; (b) feedback actually training subjects to maintain EMG levels, although being deceived into thinking that they were lowering EMG; (c) feedback training subjects to increase EMG levels, again being deceived; and (d) a no-treatment control. All three treatment conditions, surprisingly, led to significant reductions in headache activity. Andrasik and Holroyd suggested that the feedback process may have taught the subjects awareness of techniques for decreasing headache activity. Subjects, regardless of group assignment, reported various methods of minimizing headaches, including controlled breathing, praying, fantasy, and refocusing of attention. The authors (1980) concluded that

> it may be less crucial that headache sufferers learn to modify EMG activity than
> it is that they learn to monitor the insidious onset of headache symptoms and
> engage in some sort of coping response incompatible with the further exacer-
> bation of symptoms. (p. 584)

This important study indicates that further research is needed to understand mechanisms underlying treatment efficacy.

Relaxation Training

Progressive muscle relaxation training (PRT) was first described by Jacobson in 1938. The exercise consists of instructions to tense, then relax, different muscle groups of the body. Since the development of PRT, 26 other methods of inducing relaxation have been described (Hillenberg & Collins, 1982). However, PRT continues to be the most widely used relaxation treatment method for treating migraine and tension headaches (Blanchard *et al.,* 1978; Fitcher & Zimmerman; 1973; Hay & Madders, 1971; Lutker, 1971; Tasto & Hinkle, 1973; Warner & Lance, 1975; Williamson *et al.,* 1984). This research has demonstrated that PRT is an effective treatment for both migraine and muscle-contraction headaches. In most studies, relaxation training has been found to produce reduction of headache activity that is comparable to that of the biofeedback procedures.

Cognitive-Behavior Therapy

In the treatment of headache, cognitive procedures are used to train or educate the patient in behaviors facilitating coping skills. As noted by Lake (1983, p. 234), cognitive procedures emphasize

> more adaptive thinking patterns . . . including the recognition of connections between thought, emotion, behavior, and headache, and the identification of thoughts and assumptions that may trigger or sustain headache activity.

Development of new behaviors (e.g., communication skills, stress management training, changes in Type A life-style) are also emphasized in cognitive-behavioral approaches for managing headaches.

As pointed out by Lake (1983) and Bakal (1982), assessment must be multimodal, including behavior, physiology, and cognitions. Cognitive-behavioral treatment may be required in one, two, or all of the response areas.

The most structured cognitive-behavioral treatment program for headache has been described by Bakal (1982). The objectives of this program are twofold: (a) education of patients in the psychobiology of headaches; and (b) development of strategies to regulate headaches. The process of treatment is conducted in three phases, consisting of observation, education, and acquisition of skills. The observation phase is for data collection of headache activity. During the education phase, a rationale of the problem and the treatment process is presented. This phase is very important for compliance with treatment. During the last phase, the patient learns to change his or her behaviors or thoughts that facilitate headache. Bakal utilizes relaxation training, attention-diversion training, imagery, and thought management in the third phase of treatment.

Most of the research on cognitive-behavioral treatment of headache has focused upon tension headache (Holroyd & Andrasik, 1978; Holroyd, Andrasik, & Westbrook, 1977). These studies have found cognitive approaches to be superior to no treatment and to EMG biofeedback alone. Bakal, Demjen, and Kaganov (1981) utilized a cognitive-behavioral treatment approach with 45 subjects diagnosed as having either muscle-contraction, migraine, or mixed headaches. The study found that headache activity was significantly decreased across headache groups at 6-month follow-up. Those with migraine responded as well as those with muscle-contraction headache, supporting the psychobiological model of headache presented by Bakal. In general, the degree of improvement reported for cognitive-behavioral treatments appears to be roughly comparable to other treatment methods.

431

HEADACHE

Multimodal Approach

The major contributor to the investigation of a comprehensive behavioral package in the treatment of headache has been Kenneth Mitchell and his colleagues. The primary focus of Mitchell's work has been with migraineurs, although he has reported some preliminary research with muscle-contraction headache as well.

In 1971, Mitchell published a report of three subjects treated over 15 sessions (2 per week). The treatment consisted of assertion training, reeducation training, systematic desensitization, and progressive muscle relaxation training. These three subjects were significantly improved at the end of treatment and at 2-month follow-up, over three control subjects. A second report by Mitchell and Mitchell in 1971 validated the findings of the first study. Also, the second report indicated that the comprehensive behavioral package was more effective than relaxation training alone or systematic desensitization alone.

A systematic investigation of the contributions of the different components of the behavioral treatment package was reported by Mitchell and White in 1977. The components were self-monitoring of headache, self-monitoring of stressful events, systematic desensitization, progressive muscle relaxation training by audiotape, and self-management skills such as assertion training and stress management. Self-monitoring had no significant effect; relaxation and desensitization resulted in approximately 70% of the subjects' experiencing a 50% reduction in headache activity. Addition of the self-management component resulted in 100% of the subjects' experiencing reduction in headache activity.

A single-case study with a patient's experiencing muscle-contraction headache was reported by Mitchell and White (1976). A program identical to that used by Mitchell and associates with migraineurs was used. At 1-year follow-up, headache activity was negligible.

At this time, little research exists, other than that of Mitchell, investigating the application of a comprehensive treatment package to headache. Research related to the clinical efficacy of the total package, as well as the individual components, is needed. Perhaps the biggest drawback of this approach is the relative lack of controlled, systematic research. To date, the total of subjects who receive this comprehensive treatment package is approximately 20, although 100% of these have shown significant reductions in headache activity. Replication with more controlled group outcome studies to confirm this level of treatment success is needed.

Limitations of Behavioral Treatment Methods

Although there is a plethora of studies investigating the utility of various treatment procedures for headache, many problems exist regarding the clinical utility of the previously mentioned procedures. The initial behavioral procedures (biofeedback, relaxation training) were found to be promising treatments of headache. However, it soon became evident that these treatments were not effective for everyone. For example, a meta-analytic study by Blanchard *et al.* (1980), found that biofeedback and relaxation training averaged about 50% improvement. There was no significant difference between the two treatments. The finding suggests that other methodologies should be investigated for the treatment of those who do not benefit from the aforementioned treatment procedures.

In the treatment of both muscle-contraction and migraine headaches, biofeedback plus pharmacotherapy has been shown to be more effective than biofeedback treatment or pharmacological treatment alone (Diamond, Diamond-Falk, & Largen, 1981; Lake, 1983, Mathew, 1981). However, research investigating the efficacy of drug therapy in combination with other therapies needs much more investigation.

Treatment approaches utilizing a combination of cognitive-behavioral techniques and relaxation/biofeedback training may be more effective than the success rates of singular treatment approaches (Bakal *et al.,* 1981; Mitchell & White, 1976, 1977; Reeves, 1976). The cognitive/behavioral approach is based on the premise that treatment must be individually tailored for each patient in order to be most effective (Bakal, 1982). Significant reductions in headache activity have been reported in the work by Mitchell as well as Bakal. However, additional theoretical and clinical research is needed.

At this time, the major limitation of the existing treatment approaches for headache is that there are still very many individuals who improve very little, if at all, with the application of these procedures. The current trend of investigating the utility of combination of treatments is proving successful, but more work is needed to confirm the treatment combinations on a sound empirical basis.

Case Example

Identifying Information

Mrs. Hill was a 42-year-old white female who was referred from a local physician for biofeedback treatment of headaches after long-term treatment with medication had produced only slight improvement. Mrs. Hill had been a housewife all her life, and her husband was an engineer at a local oil company. Their three children included a married 22-year-old son, a married 18-year-old daughter, and a 12-year-old daughter who resided in their home. Mrs. Hill was very active in various community activities.

Assessment

An intake interview was conducted to collect information on Mrs. Hill's presenting problem, treatment history, and other current problems in her life. Because she was being followed by a physician for her headaches, her medical reports were obtained, including her neurological exam in order to rule out organic causes of her headaches. Three self-report questionnaires, the MMPI, the SCL-90, and the Beck Depression Inventory (BDI), were administered to supplement the interview information in screening for psychopathology. In order to collect daily information concerning headache activity, Mrs. Hill was instructed to complete the headache self-monitoring forms described earlier. These monitoring forms were to be completed daily throughout the assessment period and treatment program to evaluate Mrs. Hill's headache activity pattern and to evaluate the effects of treatment.

Intake Interview

After greeting the client and obtaining general identifying information, the therapist assessed headache symptoms and patterns. This interview was followed by completion of the Headache Questionnaire in order to quantify her headache symptoms. Portions of the interview follow.

T: Mrs. Hill, Doctor Green asked me to talk with you to evaluate your headaches and to recommend an appropriate behavioral treatment program since you do not seem to be responding to medical treatment. In order to recommend the best approach to treating your headaches, I will need to gather a lot of information about your headaches. First of all, can you tell me when your headaches first began?

C: I began having occasional headaches about 12 years ago. After about a year I began having them more often and sometimes spent the whole day in bed because of them. I finally asked my doctor about them and he presecribed a number of pain killers and headache medicines through the years. Some of these medicines helped a little but none really helped much and I don't really like to take drugs anyway. I hope that you can help me with biofeedback or something.

T: What medications are you taking now?

C: I'm taking Inderal a couple times a day for migraines. I take Valium about once a month, and I take Cafergot when they're real bad. I also take a lot of Tylenol.

T: Do these medicines help your headaches at all?

C: Sometimes they help but usually they just make them a little more tolerable. I've never been able to get rid of them.

T: Are you taking medication for anything else?

C: No, I really don't like to take medicine unless I really need it.

T: How often do you get headaches?

C: I've been getting them about 2 to 3 times per week for several years now.

T: How long do these headaches usually last?

C: They always last at least a few hours but sometimes they last all day.

T: Can you describe the headaches? Point to where you usually feel the pain.

C: Usually they begin around my temple and then they move around to the back of my head.

T: Are they always on one side?

C: No, but they almost always start on one side or the other and then move around.

T: What is the pain like, is it pulsating or is it a dull aching pain?

C: It's usually a throbbing pain but I also get tension headaches sometimes. When I get these headaches, it's more like a tightness right here [*pointing to her forehead*].

The client seemed knowledgeable about her headaches and was reporting the symptoms of both migraine and muscle-contraction headaches, in confirmation of her physician's diagnosis of combined headache. Therefore, the interview questioning was directed toward focusing on each type of headache separately.

T: It sounds as though you may get both migraine and tension headaches. Let's talk more about the migraines first. Can you tell ahead of time when you are going to get a migraine? For instance, do you have any warning signs?

C: Yes, I can usually tell when a migraine is coming on but I'm not sure how I can tell. I do act differently; my husband can tell when I'm going to get a headache because I get irritable, he says.

The presence of mood changes can be prodromal symptoms indicative of classic migraine. These types of vague prodromes are rare.

T: When do your migraines usually start? Do you wake up with them or do they start later in the day?

C: I often wake up with the migraines; sometimes I get headaches starting in the early evening, but these usually feel like tension headaches.

T: I'd like to focus for a little while longer on your migraines; then we can find out more about your tension headaches. When you have a migraine, do you ever have accompanying symptoms like nausea, vomiting, increased sensitivity to light or sound, or loss of appetite?

C: Yes, when I have real bad migraines, I can't eat. Sometimes I feel nauseous and I have even vomited a few times. When they're this bad any sound seems real loud and light bothers me too. When I feel like this, I usually can't do anything but lay down, which usually doesn't help. I can never seem to find a position that makes my head feel any better.

T: How often are your headaches that bad that you just go to bed all day?

C: That usually happens about once or twice per month. However, sometimes it may not happen for several months.

T: What do you usually do when you get a migraine?

C: I take medicine but that usually doesn't help very much or for very long if it does help.

T: How long do your migraines last?

C: They usually last most of the day and sometimes straight through to the next day.

T: When the pain goes away do you usually notice any soreness or tenderness in the areas where you felt the pain?

C: Yes.

T: Have you noticed any kind of pattern to your headaches or any times when you have more headaches?

C: Not really, but I do seem to have more during periods when things don't seem to be going right for me.

T: Do they seem to increase during stressful periods?

C: Yes, when the kids I sit for are acting up they seem to be worse.

T: Are there any other situations that seem to lead to more or worse headaches?

C: Yes, thinking about it, they do seem to be worse when I worry about my kids or when I have a lot of work to get done for the women's club.

T: Mrs. Hill, what do your children and your husband do when you have a headache?

C: They usually don't know when I have a headache unless its a real bad one; then they can tell. But my husband says he can tell when I have a migraine, and he usually tells me to relax. He thinks that I get headaches because I worry too much.

T: Do you agree with him?

C: I guess that worrying may help bring them on sometimes but they also happen other times.

T: Mrs. Hill, have you ever noticed any changes in your headaches associated with menstruation?

C: I haven't had a period for several years but I never noticed any changes in my headaches during that time.

T: Did you notice any changes in your headaches when you stopped menstruating?

C: No.

T: Have you ever noticed that you get headaches after eating certain foods like chocolate, cheese, or alcohol?

C: No, not really.

T: Now that we covered a lot of information concerning your migraines, let's talk a little more about your tension headaches. Can you describe these for me?

C: They usually begin in the late afternoon or early evening. I usually feel tension in my forehead and sometimes in my neck and shoulders.

T: What is the pain like?

C: Like a tightness or pressure in these areas [*pointing to forehead and neck*].

T: What do you do when you get them?

C: I take Tylenol and that usually helps somewhat.

T: How long do these headaches last and is there anything else that has helped with them?

C: Sometimes relaxing or taking a hot bath helps a little. They last for several hours usually.

T: Do they usually last less than 4 hours?

C: Yes, they don't last as long as my migraines and sometimes I can even forget about them when I have them.

T: Have you ever noticed that these headaches occur more often or are worse during stressful periods?

C: Yes, they do seem to happen more when I'm upset or under pressure.

T: Do any other members of your family or any of your parents have migraines or frequent tension headaches?

C: No, I'm the only one that gets bad headaches. They get headaches once in a while like most people, but not migraines.

T: Has there been any change in your headaches lately? For instance, are you getting them any more or less often, are they lasting longer lately?

C: Well, since I began my term as president of the women's club I seem to get them more often than usual.

T: Have you ever had any headache-free periods? When have they occurred?

C: I sometimes have long periods without tension headaches like sometimes on vacations but I can't remember any long periods without migraines.

T: Have you ever had any other types of treatment for your headaches besides medication?

C: No, but I hope that you can suggest something that will help.

Following this assessment of the headache symptoms, the therapist continued to assess for other significant problems in the client's life. Although no major problems were identified that could qualify for a separate clinical diagnosis, further assessment revealed a number of other problems that have important implications for treatment planning. The problems identified included mild depression (BDI = 14); increased worrying during the past few months, especially concerning her children's problems (e.g., marital problems of her older daughter), and increased anxiety during the past 6 months, especially associated with her performance as president of her women's club. In addition, although Mrs. Hill's MMPI did not indicate any clinically elevated scales, her profile pattern revealed moderate elevations (t scores of 65, 70, and 67) on the Hs(1), D(2), and Hy(3) scales (Neurotic Triad), common in individuals with somatic disorders. Although none of the SCL-90 scales clinically elevated, three of the scales were moderately elevated, including the Obsessive-Compulsive, Interpersonal Sensitivity, and Depression scales (t scores of 68, 65, 69, respectively). This profile characterizes an individual who is perfectionistic, very sensitive to criticism by others, and presently experiencing moderate depression. This profile provided converging information on Mrs. Hill's reports of increased anxiety and mild depression. Examination of Mrs. Hill's recent medical reports and phone contacts with her physician ruled out medical explanations for her headaches. Additionally, the daily headache self-monitoring revealed that Mrs. Hill had an average of three headaches per week that lasted an average of 8 hours. The pain intensity of the headaches was usually moderate to severe and reached a peak intensity after approximately 4 hours. Examination of the antecedents of Mrs. Hill's headaches revealed that they often began following times when she had experienced problems with the children for whom she baby-sat or when she had rushed to complete work for the women's club, suggesting that stressors were antecedents of headaches. Examination of the consequences of Mrs. Hill's headaches did not indicate any identifiable pattern except the use of medication.

Formulation and Treatment Plan

Completion of the assessment led to a diagnosis of combined headache, as indicated by the frequent occurrence of vascular (migraine) headaches and tension headaches. Mrs. Hill was provided with a formulation of her headache pattern indicating an association between increased stressors in her life and increased headache activity. For example, the recent increases in anxiety, depression, and worry had been accompanied by increases in both migraine and tension headaches. A two-component treatment program was recommended for Mrs. Hill, including skin temperature biofeedback to specifically target her migraines and a stress management program, including relaxation training, to assist her in effectively coping with the significant stressors in her life. Although depression was not chosen as a treatment target, it was regularly monitored for changes that would indicate the need for direct treatment. The observed association between the depressive symptoms and increased headache activity and stress suggested that these symptoms would diminish with successful implementation of the treatment plan. The specific treatment plan included two weekly sessions for the first 2 months followed by a third month of only one meeting each week and two biweekly sessions for the fourth month. Following completion of the program, 3-, 6-, and 12-month follow-up contacts were planned to assess maintenance of treatment effects.

Self-monitoring data were reviewed at the beginning of each treatment session, and changes from the previous week were discussed. During the first 2 months, one weekly biofeedback session was devoted to training Mrs. Hill to increase the temperature in her hands as a method of aborting or decreasing the severity of her migraines. After she achieved success in this procedure in the clinic, she was instructed to practice at home and implement this procedure at the first sign of a headache. The second weekly session for the first 2 months focused on teaching the skills necessary to effectively cope with anxiety and stress. Specifically,

Mrs. Hill was taught relaxation techniques to help her to relax; assertion training was conducted to help her deal more effectively with the members of her women's club; cognitive restructuring was implemented to modify her maladaptive cognitions; and behavioral management techniques were taught to help her to better control the children for whom she baby-sat. The relaxation technique employed included progressive muscle relaxation followed by pleasant imagery. The assertion component focused on teaching her to interact more effectively with her group by delegating more of the work and not giving in to unreasonable demands. Cognitive restructing was conducted to alter her irrational cognitions and self-denigrating thoughts, especially concerning others' feelings about her performance in the women's club. Lastly, the behavioral management component included instructing the children in the rules that they were to follow and in attending only to positive behaviors while ignoring undesirable behaviors. Each of these components included weekly homework assignments to practice applying these skills and to enhance their effectiveness and generalization. The third month included two sessions devoted to the continued application of the hand-warming procedure to insure maintenance and two sessions devoted to continued implementation of the stress management techniques and discussion and problem solving about problems encountered in applying these procedures. The two final sessions were scheduled to fade out treatment and focused primarily on maintenance of the achieved treatment effects and anticipating future problems. To insure continued maintenance of treatment effects, booster sessions would be conducted following treatment if needed.

Problems Encountered

A number of difficulties were encountered over the course of the treatment program. Initially, Mrs. Hill was very lax in completing her daily headache monitoring forms, but following a review of the importance of daily monitoring to assess changes in her headache activity and to evaluate the effectiveness of treatment she complied with this procedure. Furthermore, a number of problems were encountered during the practice and application of the treatment components. At first, Mrs. Hill reported little success in achieving relaxation during her home practice sessions. An analysis of her practice sessions indicated that she was often bothered by a number of distractions during her designated practice time. This problem was overcome by planning a different practice time during which she would be less likely to be distracted, and in addition, asking her family not to disturb her during her scheduled practice time. During the third and fourth weeks of treatment, Mrs. Hill had to entertain a number of houseguests and experienced a dramatic increase in stress that necessitated flexible implementation of the treatment plan to include dealing with her current stressors. An evaluation of Mrs. Hill's success in applying the hand-warming procedure revealed that, instead of employing this procedure at the first sign of a headache, she was waiting until she had a full-blown migraine. She was reminded of the importance of applying this technique as early as possible in order to abort her headaches, and subsequently she reported better success with this procedure. A further problem in implementing a treatment component was experienced during the sixth week of treatment. When Mrs. Hill attempted to apply her newly learned assertion skills in actual interactions with the members of her women's club, she experienced a marked increase in anxiety that was accompanied by increased headache activity. This problem was alleviated by planning further assertion homework assignments to start at a level that was not anxiety producing for her, and then gradually increasing to the level of assertion with her club members. Last, Mrs. Hill became discouraged with her progress in treatment. During these times it was helpful to inform her of the improvements that she actually accomplished and to remind her that she was experiencing improvement at a rate equal to or better than that expected at that particular point in the treatment program. These claims were supported by illustrating the reduction of her headache activity using graphic presentation of her headache data.

Outcome and Follow-Up

The outcome of treatment is illustrated in Figure 2. After initial fluctuations in her headache activity, Mrs. Hill experienced a marked decrease in headache occurrence, especially following the eighth week of treatment. Compared to the average of three headaches per week during the pretreatment assessment, she experienced an average of 2.75 headaches each week during the first month, 2 per week the second month, 1.7 the third month, and 1 during the fourth month of treatment. In addition, Mrs. Hill experienced a significant decrease in the pain intensity of the headaches she did experience as demonstrated by the changes in her headache index following baseline. However, no significant changes were observed in the duration of the headaches Mrs. Hill experienced. Follow-up data indicated that Mrs. Hill had an average of one weekly headache or less at 3-, 6-, and 12-month follow-up periods. Along with decreases in headache frequency and severity, treatment also led to significant decreases in medication use for headaches. The continued assessment of her depressive symptoms indicated a decrease during treatment to minimal level at the end of treatment (BDI = 5). Evaluation of her satisfaction with the treatment program indicated that she was very pleased with the outcome of treatment. She further reported that she felt much more capable of coping with the stressors in her life and also felt that she could now better control her headaches with much less use of medication.

Summary

Behavioral treatment of migraine and tension headaches has been extensively researched. At this time, a number of effective treatment methods have been developed and validated using controlled group outcome studies. These treatment methods generally produce significant improvement for 50 to 70% of the cases treated. Therefore, the place of behavioral methods in the treatment of headache is now well established. The major remaining task of behavioral researchers and

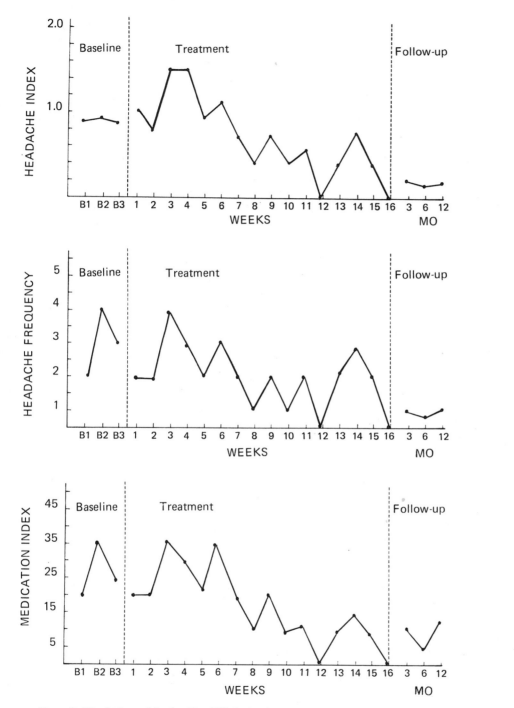

Figure 2. Headache activity for Mrs. Hill during baseline, treatment, and follow-up.

clinicians is to devise treatment methods that are effective with the more difficult, complicated cases that to date have shown poor response to behavioral or pharmacological treatments.

References

Ad Hoc Committee of Classification of Headache. (1982). *Journal of the American Medical Association, 179,* 717–718.

Andrasik, F., & Holroyd, K. A. (1980). A test of specific and nonspecific effects in the biofeedback treatment of tension headache. *Journal of Counsulting and Clinical Psychology, 48,* 575–586.

Bakal, D. A. (1982). *The psychobiology of chronic headache.* New York: Springer.

Bakal, D. A., Demjen, S., & Kaganov, J. A. (1981). Cognitive behavioral treatment of chronic headache. *Headache, 21,* 81–86.

Bild, R., & Adams, H. E. (1980). Modification of migraine headaches by cephalic blood volume pulse and EMG biofeedback. *Journal of Consulting and Clinical Psychology, 48,* 51–57.

Blanchard, E. B. & Andrasik, F. (1982). Psychological assessment and treatment of headache: Recent developments and emerging issues. *Journal of Consulting and Clinical Psychology, 50,* 859–879.

Blanchard, E. B., Theobald, D. E., Williamson, D. A., Silver, B. V., & Brown, D. A. (1978). Temperature biofeedback in the treatment of migraine headaches. *Archives of General Psychiatry, 35,* 581–588.

Blanchard, E. B., Ahles, T. A. & Shaw, E. R. (1979). Behavioral treatment of headaches. In M. Hersen, R. M. Eisler, & P. M. Miller (Eds.), *Progress in behavior modification* (Vol. 8). New York: Academic Press.

Blanchard, E. B., Andrasik, F., Ahles, T. A., Teders, S. J., & O'Keefe, D. (1980). Migraine and tension headache: A meta-analytic review. *Behavior Therapy, 11,* 613–631.

Blanchard, E. B., Andrasik, F., Neff, D. F., Jurish, S. E., & O'Keefe, D. M. (1981). Social validation of the headache diary. *Behavior Therapy, 12,* 711–715.

Blanchard, E. B., Andrasik, F., Neff, D. F., Arena, J. G., Ahles, T. A., Jurish, S. E., Pallmeyer, T. P., Saunders, N. L., Teders, S. J., Barron, T. P., & Rodichock, L. D. (1982). Biofeedback and relaxation training with three kinds of headache: Treatment effects and their prediction. *Journal of Consulting and Clinical Psychology, 30,* 562–575.

Blanchard, E. B., Andrasik, F., Neff, D. F., Teders, S. J., Pallmeyer, T. P., Arena, J. G., Jurish, S. E., Saunders, N. L., & Rodichok, L. D. (1982). Sequential comparison of relaxation training and biofeedback in the treatment of three kinds of chronic headache or the machines may be necessary some of the time. *Behaviour Research and Therapy, 20,* 469–481.

Budzynski, T. H., Stoyva, J. M., Adler, C. S., & Mullaney, D. J. (1973), EMG biofeedback and tension headache: A controlled outcome study. *Psychosomatic Medicine, 6,* 509–514.

Cinciripini, P. M., Williamson, D. A., & Epstein, L. H. (1981). Behavioral treatment of migraine headache. In J. M. Ferguson, & C. B. Taylor (Eds.), *The comprehensive handbook of behavioral medicine* (Vol. 2) (pp. 207–227). New York: Spectrum.

Cohen, M. J., McArthur, D. L., & Rickles, D. L. (1980). Comparison of four biofeedback treatments for migraine headache: Physiological variables. *Psychosomatic Medicine, 42,* 463–480.

Cox, D. J., Freundlich, A., & Meyer, R. G. (1975). Differential effectiveness of electromyographic feedback, verbal relaxation instructions and medication placebo. *Journal of Consulting and Clinical Psychology, 43,* 892–898.

Diamond, S. (1976). Psychogenic headache: Treatment, including biofeedback techniques. In O. Appenzeller (Ed.), *Pathogenesis and treatment of headache* (pp. 135–154). New York: Spectrum.

Diamond, S., & Dalessio, D. J. (1978). *The practicing physician's approach to headache.* Baltimore: Williams & Wilkins.

Diamond, S., & Franklin, M. (1975). Autogenic training with biofeedback in children with migraine. In W. Luthe & F. Antonelli (Eds.), *Therapy in psychosomatic medicine* (pp. 190–192). Proceeding of the Third Congress of the International College of Psychosomatic Medicine, Rome.

Diamond, S., Diamond-Falk, J., & Largen, J. W. (1981). Update: Biofeedback in the treatment of vascular headache. In R. J. Mathew (Ed.), *Treatment of migraine* (pp. 37–66). New York: SP Medical and Scientific Books.

Elmore, A. M., & Tursky, B. (1981). A comparison of two psychophysiological approaches to the treatment of migraine. *Headache, 21,* 93–101.

Feuerstein, M., & Adams, H. E. (1977). Cephalic vasomotor feedback in the modification of migraine headache. *Biofeedback and Self-Regulation, 2,* 241–254.

Fitcher, H., & Zimmerman, R. R. (1973). Change in reported pain from tension headaches. *Perceptual and Motor Skills, 36,* 712.

Friar, C. R., & Beatty, J. (1976). Migraine: Management by a trained control of vasoconstriction. *Journal of Consulting and Clinical Psychology, 44,* 46–53.

Friedman, A. P., von Storch, J. C., & Merritt, H. H. (1954). Migraine and tension headache: A clinical study of two thousand cases. *Neurology, 4,* 773–779.

Gale, E. M. (1979), The effectiveness of biofeedback treatment for temporomandibular joint pain. *Journal of Research in Dentistry* (Special Issue A), *58,* 217.

Granberry, S. W., Williamson, D. A., Pratt, J. M., Hutchinson, F., & Monguillot, J. (1981). *An investigation of empirically derived catagories of headache.* Paper presented at the annual Meeting of the Association for Advancement of Behavior Therapy, Toronto, Canada.

Gray, C. L., Lyle, R. C., & McGuire, R. J. (1980). Electrode placement, EMG feedback, and relaxation for tension headaches. *Behaviour Research and Therapy, 18,* 19–23.

Hay, K. M., & Madders, J. (1971). Migraine treated by relaxation therapy. *Journal of the Royal College of General Practioners, 21,* 664–669.

Haynes, S. N., Griffin, P., Mooney, D., & Parise, M. (1975). Electromyographic biofeedback and relaxation instructions in the treatment of muscle contraction headaches. *Behavior Therapy, 6,* 672–678.

Holroyd, K. A., & Andrasik, F. (1978). Coping and the self-control of chronic tension headache. *Journal of Consulting and Clinical Psychology, 46,* 1036–1045.

Holroyd, K. A., Andrasik, F., & Westbrook, T. (1977). Cognitive control of tension headache. *Cognitive Therapy and Research, 1,* 121–133.

Jacob, R. G., Turner, S. M., Szekely, B. C., & Eidelman, B. H. (1983). Predicting outcome of relaxation therapy in headaches: The role of depression. *Behavior Therapy, 14,* 457–465.

Jacobson, E. (1938). *Progressive relaxation.* Chicago: University of Chicago Press.

Jessup, B. A., Newfeld, R. W. J., & Merskey, H. (1979). Biofeedback therapy for headache and other pain: An evaluative review, *Pain, 7,* 225–270.

Jurish, S. E., Blanchard, E. B., Andrasik, F., Teders, S. J., Neff, D. F., & Arena, J. G. (1983). Home-versus clinic-based treatment of vascular headache. *Journal of Consulting and Clinical Psychology, 51,* 743–751.

Lake, A. E., (1983). Cognitive-behavior therapy for headache: Assessment and treatment considerations. In J. R. Saper (Ed.), *Headache disorders* (pp. 233–251). Boston: John Wright.

Lutker, E. R. (1971). Treatment of migraine headache by conditional relaxation: A case study. *Behavior Therapy, 2,* 592–593.

Mathew, N. T. (1981). Prophylaxis of migraine and mixed headache: A randomized controlled study. *Headache, 21,* 105–109.

Mitchell, K. R. (1971). Note on treatment of migraine using behavior therapy techniques. *Psychological Reports, 28,* 171–172.

Mitchell, K. R., & Mitchell, D. M. (1971). Migraine: An exploratory treatment application of programmed behavior therapy techniques. *Journal of Psychosomatic Research, 15,* 137–157.

Mitchell, K. R., & White, R. G. (1976). Control of migraine headache by behavioral self-management. A controlled case study. *Headache, 16,* 178–184.

Mitchell, K. R., & White, R. G. (1977). Behavioral self-management: An application to the problem of migraine headaches. *Behavior Therapy, 8,* 213–221.

Mitchell, K. R., & White, R. G. (1977). Behavioral self-management: An application to the problem of migraine headaches. *Behavior Therapy, 8,* 213–221.

National Ambulatory Medical Care Survey: 1981 Summary United States. (1981). Rockville, MD: U.S. Department of Health, Education, and Welfare, Public Health Service, Health Resources Administration, National Center for Health Statistics.

O'Brien, M. D. (1971). Cerebral blood flow changes in the migraine headache. *Headache,* 1971, *10,* 139–143.

Ostfeld, A. M. (1963). The natural history and epidemiology of migraine and muscle-contraction headache. *Neurology, 13,* 11–15.

Philips, C. (1977). The modification of tension headache pain using EMG biofeedback. *Behaviour Research and Therapy, 15,* 119–129.

Quintanar, L. R., Cacioppo, J. T., & Monyak, N. (1980). The effects of cranial vasoconstriction and paced respiration of migraine. *Psychophysiology, 17,* 284.

Reeves, J. L. (1976). EMG-biofeedback reduction of tension headache: A cognitive skills-training approach. *Biofeedback and Self-Regulation, 1,* 217–225.

Sargent, J. D., Green, E. E., & Walters, E. D. (1972). The use of autogenic feedback training in a pilot study of migraine and tension headaches. *Headache, 12,* 120–125.

Silver, B. V., Blanchard, E. B., Williamson, D. A., Theobald, D. E., & Brown, D. A. (1979). Temperature biofeedback and relaxation training in the treatment of migraine headache. *Biofeedback and Self-Regulation, 4,* 359–366.

Skinhoj, E. (1973). Hemodynamic studies within the brain during migraine. *Archives of Neurology, 29,* 95–98.

Skinhoj, E., & Paulson, O. B. (1969). Regional blood flow in internal carotid distribution during migraine attack. *British Medical Journal, 3,* 569–570.

Snyder, C., & Noble, M. (1968). Operant conditioning of vasoconstriction. *Journal of Experimental Psychology, 77,* 263–268.

Sturgis, E. T., Tollison, C. D., & Adams, H. E. (1978). Modification of combined migraine-muscle contraction headache using BVP and EMG biofeedback. *Journal of Applied Behavior Analysis, 11,* 215–223.

Tasto, D. L., & Hinkle, J. E. (1973). Muscle relaxation treatment for tension headaches. *Behaviour Research and Therapy, 11,* 347–349.

Warner, G., & Lance, J. W. (1975). Relaxation therapy in migraine and chronic tension headache. *Medical Journal of Australia, 1,* 298–301.

Waters, W. E., & O'Conner, P. J. (1975). Prevalence of migraine. *Journal of Neurology, Neurosurgery, and Psychiatry, 38,* 613–616.

Wolff, J. G. (1963). *Headache and other head pain.* New York: Oxford University Press.

Williamson, D. A. (1981). Behavioral treatment of migraine and muscle-contraction headaches: Outcome and theoretical explanations. In M. Hersen, R. M. Eisler, P. M. Miller (Eds.), *Progress in behavior modification* (Vol. 11) (pp. 163–201. New York: Academic Press.

Williamson, D. A., Epstein, L. H., & Lombardo, T. W. (1981). EMG measurement as a function of electrode placement and level of EMG. *Psychophysiology, 17,* 279–282.

Williamson, D. A., Monguillot, J. E., Jarrell, M. P., Cohen, R. A., Pratt, J. M., & Blouin, D. C. (1984). Relaxation for the treatment of headache: Controlled evaluation of two group programs. *Behavior Modification, 8,* 407–424.

Zamani, R. (1974). *Treatment of migraine through operant conditioning of vasoconstriction.* Ann Arbor, MI: University Microfilms.

V

Schizophrenia

Inpatient Approaches

JAMES P. CURRAN, ROBERT G. SUTTON,
STEPHEN V. FARAONE, AND SIMONE GUENETTE

Introduction

In concordance with the editors' intention of providing a handbook detailing the "nitty-gritty" of daily practice, we will describe our own clinical work on our inpatient unit at the Providence Veterans Administration Medical Center. Obviously, the type of treatment implemented in any clinical setting will be partially a function of the treatment unit. Our treatment environment is a moderate-size (bed capacity 35), acute (average length of stay less than 30 days) psychiatric treatment unit for veterans experiencing a wide variety of behavioral disorders. Hence, our discussion is not a comprehensive review of all behavioral procedures that may be used with schizophrenic populations in different types of treatment settings. However, we feel that our description is representative of many of the major behavioral treatment modalities used with schizophrenics. Before discussing our treatment procedures *per se* we would like to begin with a description of schizophrenia, present a conceptual model for schizophrenia, and discuss strategies used to assess the disorder.

Descriptive Features of Schizophrenia

The descriptive features that have been thought to demarcate schizophrenia have varied throughout its history, often reflecting major cultural differences

JAMES P. CURRAN • Veterans Administration Medical Center, Brown University Medical School, Providence, Rhode Island 02908. ROBERT G. SUTTON • Veterans Administration Medical Center, Davis Park, Providence, Rhode Island 02908. STEPHEN V. FARAONE • Veterans Administration Medical Center, Brown University Medical School, Providence, Rhode Island 02908. SIMONE GUENETTE • Veterans Administration Medical Center, Davis Park, Providence, Rhode Island 02908.

(Neale & Oltmanns, 1980). Although obscuring more subtle issues, these various definitions can generally be classified as belonging to either a narrow or broad view of schizophrenia. Europeans following the tradition of Kraepelin have generally emphasized a descriptive, atheoretical, narrow view of schizophrenia, mainly limiting this diagnostic category to patients with a poor prognosis. Americans, on the other hand, have generally followed Bleuler's psychoanalytic-theoretical notions of schizophrenia and have favored a broader conceptualization of the diagnostic category. In the United States more emphasis was placed on the presence of loosely defined cognitive and emotional disturbances, whereas in Europe the emphasis was on specific symptoms such as hallucinations and delusions.

The prevailing attitude today is for a narrower definition of schizophrenia. This narrower view of schizophrenia is reflected in the tighter diagnostic criteria for schizophrenia in the *Diagnostic and Statistical Manual of Mental Disorders* (DSM-III) (American Psychiatric Association, 1980) as opposed to the looser criteria found in DSM-II (American Psychiatric Association, 1968). DSM-III criteria for schizophrenia require each of the following:

1. A symptom reflecting a major marker for schizophrenia, including a delusion, hallucination, or a formal thought disorder
2. Deterioration from previous level of functioning in such areas as work, social relations, and self-care
3. Continuous signs of the illness for at least 6 months at some time during the person's life with some signs of the illness at present
4. The full depressive or manic syndrome if present, developed after any psychotic symptoms or was brief in duration relative to the duration of psychotic symptoms
5. Onset of prodromal or active phase of the illness before age 45
6. Not due to any organic mental disorder or mental retardation

Course and Outcome

Kraepelin's term *dementia praecox* conveys what he regarded as two major features of this disorder, that is, early onset (praecox) and a progressive intellectual deterioration (dementia). Bleuler, using a broader definition of schizophrenia, had a more optimistic viewpoint regarding the course of schizophrenia and perceived it as considerably more variable. Bleuler felt that although some schizophrenics definitely follow a progressively deteriorating course, others may have only one or two episodes and achieve a good recovery.

One conclusion that could be drawn would be that the prognostic variability observed may be due to differences in the definition of schizophrenia. However, attempts to relate the breadth of the schizophrenia concept to prognosis have not yielded consistent data (Hawk, Carpenter, & Strauss, 1975; Strauss & Carpenter, 1974). Symptoms do not appear to be especially useful prognostically, although periods of prior hospitalization and premorbid history do yield somewhat better results.

The process-reactive dimension has been used to describe the variability in the course of schizophrenia. Process schizophrenics evidence a poor premorbid history (i.e., socially and sexually inadequate) and demonstrate a slow developmental deterioration. Reactive schizophrenics evidence a good premorbid history and show a rapid onset usually precipitated by some environmental stress. There does not appear to be a single course for schizophrenia. Some individuals with good premorbid adjustment experience an acute onset of symptoms precipitated by major stressors in their environment. They have complete remissions and never experience any other psychotic episodes or have long periods of remission followed by brief episodes of schizophrenia. Other individuals with a poor premorbid history experience a slow onset of symptoms with no clear precipitants and continue to experience severe symptoms for the remainder of their lives. Between these two extremes exists a variablility such that one cannot describe a typical course. Thus, some individuals are "more schizophrenic" than others, which raises the debate over whether schizophrenia is one illness, a group of illnesses, or a syndrome with multiple etiologies.

Another useful distinction to make with respect to schizophrenic symptomatology is the distinction between positive and negative symptoms. Positive symptoms are those most usually associated with schizophrenia, that is the principal markers for schizophrenia, including delusions, hallucinations, and formal thought disorders. Negative symptoms include social isolation, withdrawal, impairment of role functioning, deterioration of personal hygiene, grooming, and the like. The phenothiazines are often useful in ameliorating positive symptoms of schizophrenia and in maintaining a remission of these disabling schizophrenic symptoms. However, the phenothiazines are not, in and of themselves, the answer to the treatment of schizophrenia. Some schizophrenics just do not respond well to phenothiazines (Goldstein, Judd, Rodnick, & LaPolla, 1969). Patients often do not comply with their phenothiazine regime because of their negative side effects. Even when patients take their medication regularly, about 50% of them relapse within 2 years (Hogarty, Goldberg, Schooler, *et al.*, 1974). Although the phenothiazines are useful in treating the positive symptoms of schizophrenia, they are not as effective with the negative symptoms. In fact, there is some evidence (Van Putten & May, 1978) that they may contribute to some negative symptomatology. Neuroleptics neither completely prevent relapse nor maintain schizophrenics' adaptation to community living. Drugs by themselves do not teach the coping skills that are often necessary for a schizophrenic's survival and maintenance in the community. Paul (1969), in his view of the treatment of chronic schizophrenics, noted that the greatest treatment need was the teaching of instrumental skills. We shall return to this point later in the chapter. Now we would like to present a conceptual model of schizophrenia that we find useful in treating our patients.

Conceptual Model for Schizophrenia

We regard schizophrenia, as do others (Kendall, 1975; Meehl, 1972; Neale & Oltmanns, 1980), as being an *open-ended hypothetical construct*. A hypothetical construct is an explanatory device, an abstract internal event whose existence is inferred on the basis of observed behaviors and the context in which they occur. Hypothetical constructs do not exist; they are simply more or less useful. Constructs are more or less useful to the extent to which they enter into relationships with other constructs and related observable events. In the case of schizophrenia, there are a number of statements that can be made in support of its utility. Neale and Oltmanns (1980, p. 20) list some of these relationships supporting the utility of the construct of *schizophrenia:* (a) although the exact etiology remains unspecified, it is clear that genetic factors play an important role in determining a predisposition for development of schizophrenia; (b) there appear to be a number of reliable biochemical, physiological, and behavioral correlates of the overt symptoms by which schizophrenia is orginally identified; and (c) there are specific drugs that have a beneficial effect in the alleviation of schizophrenic symptomatology.

We regard schizophrenia as multiply determined and multiply maintained. Our model is basically the diathesis–stress model proposed by Meehl (1972), Zubin and Steinhauer (1981), and others. The diathesis–stress model assumes that individuals inherit a predetermined degree of vulnerability that will make them more likely to demonstrate schizophrenic symptomatology. Whether the phenotype of schizophrenic symptomatology is displayed is dependent upon environmental stress. Schizophrenia is seen as a product of interaction between a constitutional predisposition toward the disorder and environmental experiences.

Zubin and Steinhauer (1981) present evidence supporting a number of constructual factors that may be important to both the etiology and maintenance of schizophrenia. These constructual factors are genetic, biochemical, neurological, developmental, learning, and ecological. There is evidence supporting each of these, although much of the evidence is rather tentative. The firmest evidence lies in the area of genetics. We do know that the incidence of schizophrenia in the population is approximately 1 in 100 (Zerbin-Rudin, 1972). However, for first-degree relatives, if one has schizophrenia, chances increase to 1 in 10 (Hanson, Gottesman, & Meehl, 1977; Zerbin-Rudin, 1972). Genetic twin studies (Fisher, Harvald, & Hauge, 1969; Gottesman & Shields, 1972; Kringlen, 1967b, 1968) point conclusively toward a much higher rate of concurrence in monozygotic twins than in dyzygotic twins. Studies of biological and adoptive families of schizophrenics have also provided strong evidence for the importance of genetic factors (Heston, 1966; Kety, Rosenthal, Wender, Schulsinger, & Jacobsen, 1975; Rosenthal, Wender, Kety, Schulsinger, Welner, & Ostergaard, 1968; Rosenthal, Wender, Kety, Welner, & Schulsinger, 1971). However, the specific nature of these genetic factors has eluded definition. We cannot yet identify any individuals who are predisposed to this disorder before they develop overt psychotic symptoms. Valid indicators of the schizogenetic type have not been found. Without this information, it is difficult to answer several important questions. For example, are there forms of schizophrenia in which a genetic predisposition is or is not necessary? Is or is not sufficient? Likewise, the stress component of the diathesis–stress model is not well specified. Various stressors that have been suggested in the literature vary from certain child-rearing practices, diet, high levels of criticism, and overinvolvement in the family (Neale & Oltmanns, 1980). *Stress* is a construct just as schizophrenia is a construct, and there is no generally agreed upon definition of it. For example, are we talking about presumptive stress, that is, major noxious events that can be regarded as stressful on a normative basis? Or should stress be more idiosyncratically defined on the basis of personal reactions to events? Obviously, there are multiple ways of constructing the possible effects of the environment, and any of them may be important in unraveling the etiology of schizophrenia.

In any case, although the specific components of the diathesis–stress model have not yet been identified, it appears to us to be a useful model with which to conceptualize the data regarding the etiology and the maintenance of schizophrenia. The various data fit into this model and, more importantly, treatment strategies that flow from this model demonstrate some utility in the treatment of schizophrenia. Let us now turn our attention to assessment issues.

Assessment

Our assessment program outlined in this section delineates four major areas of measurement: (a) differential diagnosis and symptom measurement of schizophrenia; (b) vulnerability or predisposition to schizophrenia; (c) life stress; and (d) moderating variables.

Differential Diagnosis

In recent years, with the development of structured interviews, the art of the diagnostic interview has become increasingly rigorous and standardized. An excellent comparative review of structured interviews is provided by Hedlund and Vieweg (1981). Our assessment program utilizes the National Institute of Mental Health's Diagnostic Interview Schedule (DIS). The DIS is a highly structured interview that provides reliable and valid diagnoses of a variety of psychiatric disorders according to DSM-III (Robins, Helzer, Croughan, & Ratcliff, 1981). Because the complete wording of all questions is given along with a competely structured system of probes, minimal clinical experience is needed for its administration. One advantage of this structure is that nonprofessional interviewers can be trained to interview patients in a reliable and valid fashion.

In addition to its diagnostic function, the 263 items of the DIS provide information about a variety of prognostic factors. Most importantly, the comprehensiveness of the DIS ensures that the interviewer inquire about symptoms unrelated to schizophrenia that may exacerbate the course of the disorder. Knowledge of these prognostic symptoms provided by the DIS can aid the clinician's preparation of long-term case management and rehabilitation plans.

The DIS is less useful for monitoring the course of the disorder. This is so because the DIS records only if a psychiatric symptom exists; it does not assess the severity of symptoms. In addition, the approximately 1 to 2 hours required to administer the DIS is not practical for multiple longitudinal assessments of course.

A convenient alternative that provides ratings of severity is a psychiatric rating scale. One scale that has been used extensively in the psychiatric literature is the Brief Psychiatric Rating Scale (BPRS). A comprehensive review of the BPRS is provided by Hedlund and Vieweg (1980). The version used in our assessment program was developed by several individuals at the Mental Health Clinical Research Center (Lukoff, personal communication, 1983). It uses questions from the Present State Examination (Wing, Cooper, & Sartorious, 1974) to collect the information needed to rate each of 21 dimensions of psychopathology on 7-point anchored scales. The interview usually lasts for about 20 minutes. Dimensions of psychopathology that are broader than individual scales yet narrower than the total score can also be derived from the BPRS. Goldstein, Rodnick, Evans, May, and Steinberg (1975) give rules for summing scales into four factors: (a) Anxiety and Depression; (b) Schizophrenic symptoms; (c) Hostility and Suspiciousness; and (d) Withdrawal. The rating scale format of the BPRS allows a clinician to monitor fluctuations in the course of a schizophrenic disorder. Periodic BPRS ratings will document patient responsiveness to therapeutic interventions. They can also be used to validate clinical hypotheses. For example, if a clinician suspects that certain aspects of the patient's psychopathyology are functionally related to specified antecedent and consequent conditions, the BPRS can be used as a dependent measure in an attempt to verify the suspicion.

In addition to the standard BPRS, our assessment program includes the Target Symptom Rating suggested by Falloon, Doane, and Pederson (1982). For each patient, we specify three schizophrenic symptoms that are characteristic of his or her disorder. During the BPRS interview, questions are asked to enable the interviewer to rate these "target symptoms." Because these three scales are individualized, the ratings can be based solely on the unique phenomenology of each patient's symptoms. Although the incremental validity of using target symptoms in addition to the BPRS has yet to be established, their sensitivity to treatment-induced changes has been demonstrated (Falloon *et al.*, 1984).

Assessment of Vulnerability

Theoretically, the assessment of vulnerability should provide valuable prognostic information. Highly vulnerable individuals should be more reactive to the vicissitudes of life stress. This should result in poorer long-term outcome and the need for more intensive rehabilitation programs. An accurate vulnerability measure would also provide a means of selecting individuals to receive prophylactic interventions. Unfortunately, such a measure does not exist. Therefore, our assessment program is attempting to "bootstrap" the assessment of vulnerability by measuring a variety of factors that are linked, empirically or theoretically, to vulnerability. A relatively direct indicator of vulnerability is the existence of a family history positive for schizophrenia. Because it is rarely practical and sometimes impossible to interview all of a patient's relatives, the family history method is the method of choice. For this purpose, we use a semistructured interview known as the Family History-Research Diagnostic Criteria (FH-RDC) (Andreasen, Endicott, Spitzer, &

Winokur, 1974). The FH-RDC can be administered to patients or other informants to collect information enabling diagnoses of family members to be made using modified RDC criteria. It has proven to be a reliable and cost-effective alternative to interviewing relatives directly.

Evidence from studies indicates that genetic factors are more prominent among severely than less severely ill schizophrenics (Gottesman & Shields, 1972). This has been interpreted to mean that severity increases with genetic vulnerability. The implication is that the measurement of vulnerability can be bootstrapped with the use of known prognostic indicators. A review of such indicators concluded that

> ratings of social-interpersonal and work-related skills and activities rather than diagnostic labels and symptomatology are the best predictors of rehabilitation outcome. (Anthony, Cohen, & Vitalo, 1978, p. 372)

Foremost among these predictors is the patient's premorbid level of social adjustment. Numerous studies indicate that, among schizophrenics, a history of poor social functioning during adolescence is predictive of poor outcome (Gittelman-Klein, 1969; Stoffelmayr, Dillavou, & Hunter, 1983; Strauss & Carpenter, 1972). Several instruments have been developed to assess premorbid social competence (Kokes, Strauss and Klorman, 1977). Our assessment program uses the UCLA Social Attainment Survey (Goldstein *et al.*, 1975) and the abbreviated form of Phillip's Premorbid Adjustment Scale (Harris, 1975). The Social Attainment Survey provides seven well-anchored rating scales that cover peer relations, sexual experience, and participation in social activities during adolescence. The abbreviated Phillip's scale has only two items but provides for a rating of marital status—an item that is not covered by the UCLA survey. The second item covers peer relations and participation in social activities.

In addition to premorbid adjustment, two other sources of prognostic information are the patient's history of psychiatric treatment and history of employment. A greater number of previous hospitalizations predicts future hospitalizations; poor work performance predicts future hospitalizations; and both variables predict poor overall outcome (Anthony *et al.*, 1978; Strauss & Carpenter, 1974). Items measuring these predictors have been compiled with items measuring social adjustment to form prognostic scales (Kokes *et al.*, 1977). The 19-item prognostic scale of Strauss and Carpenter (1974) should be suitable for most purposes. It covers current occupational and social functioning, history of psychiatric treatment, family history of psychiatric hospitalization, presence of affective symptoms, and the patient's reported satisfaction with life in the past year. The items have well-defined anchor points that facilitate the expeditious and reliable use of the scale in a clinical setting.

Assessment of Stress

Life stress is defined as a fluctuating characteristic of the environment that, in the presence of inadequate coping resources, will trigger a schizophrenic episode in a vulnerable individual. For the purpose of our assessments, two areas of life stress have been delineated: life change events and the family environment. Life change events are those that modify the environment and require the patient to mobilize coping resources in order to adapt to the modifications. Life events may be desirable (e.g., marriage, birth of a child, promotion at work) or undesirable (e.g., death of a close friend, financial loss, failure in school). Although the data do not support the hypothesis that life events are either necessary or sufficient causes of schizophrenic relapse, they do indicate that life events increase the likelihood of relapse (Day, 1981).

Our assessment program uses the psychiatric Epidemiology Research Institute's (PERI) Life Events Scale (Dohrenwend, Kransoff, Askenasy, & Dohrenwend, 1978). The PERI-Life Events Scale consists of 102 "events" that cover the following areas of psychosocial functioning: school, work, love and marriage, family, children, residence, legal matters, finances, social activities, and health. We have found that a 20-minute interview allows enough time for the patient to recall if these factors were important in the previous 3 months. Although there are no strict guidelines for choosing the length of the recall period, it should be noted that the reliability of life event's reporting decreases as the length of the recall period increases (Neugebauer, 1983). Life events interviews are clinically useful for two reasons. First, they provide a comprehensive, structured means of determining areas of psychosocial functioning where the patient has found it difficult to make needed adaptations. This will help the clinician identify a patient's specific coping skill deficits and may suggest areas where the mobilization of social resources will be useful. For example, the occurrence of life events related to financial hardship would motivate a clinician to examine the patient's money management skills and the need for financial support from social services. Another clinical use of life events inventories involves the assessment of prognosis. The vulnerability model hypothesizes that patients who develop schizophrenic episodes in the absence of life stress should be more vulnerable than those who relapse in the presence of life stress. Because the former are more vulnerable, their outcome should be worse and their illness more severe. This hypothesis was supported by Hardner, Gift, Strauss, Ritzler, and Kokes (1981), who found that higher levels of life events antecedent to first-time hospitalization predicted better outcome.

The second major area of stress assessment examines the family environment. Three measures are currently used in our assessment program, expressed emotion (EE), affective style, and problem-solving style. EE is a measure of the degree of critical comments and/or emotional overinvolvement expressed about the patient by a relative during a 1- to 2-hour interview known as the Camberwell Family Interview (CFI) (Brown & Rutter, 1966). Patients who live with high-EE relatives are at a significantly greater risk for relapse than those without high-EE relatives (Vaughn & Leff, 1976; Vaughn, Snyder, Freeman, Jones, Falloon, & Liberman, 1982). The degree of risk associated with high-EE relatives increases among patients who have more than 35 hours of contact per week with their relatives and among patients who do not take their antipsychotic medication regularly. On the other hand, medication regularity and amount of family contact do not strongly influence relapse risks among patients from low-EE families.

The clinical implications of these findings are evident; patients living with high-EE families would appear to require a family therapy intervention to either decrease the level of EE in the family or decrease the amount of patient–family contact. An assessment procedure that could be used to select families in need of family treatment would, of course, be clinically useful. The CFI is a semistructured interview that encourages relatives to discuss the impact that the patient's disorder has had on them and the emotional atmosphere of the home while the interviewer probes for details about the onset and course of the disorder. Complete descriptions of bothersome episodes along with the relatives' reactions are elicited with the goal of allowing relatives to ventilate negative feelings about the patient without explicitly urging them to do so. Interviews are audiotaped for later coding by a trained rater.

An alternative to the CFI is the Direct Family Interaction (DFI) procedure used by the UCLA family project (Doane, West, Goldstein, Rodnick, & Jones, 1981; Valone, Norton, Goldstein, & Doane, in press). The major difference between the DFI and the CFI is that whereas the CFI rates attitudes that the relative expresses about the patient to an interviewer, the DFI rates the actual behavior of the relative in the presence of the patient. Ratings made from the DFI have been shown to be significantly related to ratings of EE (Valone *et al.*, 1984). They are also predicitive of subsequent schizophrenia spectrum disorders in vulnerable adolescents (Doane *et al.*, 1981). The DFI procedure has been standardized for both the parents and the spouses of schizophrenics. A detailed exposition of the procedure is provided by Valone (1983). Briefly, the DFI is composed for four steps. First, each family member is individually asked to identify two family problems. The patient identifies problems created by other family members, and they identify problems created by the patient. The respondent is asked to roleplay a statement that describes the issue to the offending party. These statements are audiotaped. The second step requires family members to respond to audiotaped problem statements about their behavior. Their responses are audiotaped contiguously to the original problem statement. The audiotapes corresponding to the two most emotionally laden problem areas are played for the entire family as a stimulus for two separate 10-minute family discussions that are videotaped. Finally, these two discussions are coded for affective style (AS) and problem-solving style (PSS). The AS codes are described by Doane *et al.* (1981). They include supportive, critical, guilt-inducing, and intrusive statements. PSS includes codes such as statement of problem, solution proposals, plan for implementation, paraphrase of feelings, and seeking clarification. It has been hypothesized (Falloon *et al.*, in press) that "expressed emotion" is a result of the family's being overwhelmed by the stress of supporting a schizophrenic. As such, it may be derivative of ineffective problem-solving and coping styles.

The DFI shares with the CFI a complexity of adminstration and coding that limits their clinical utility. Ongoing research is attempting to develop assessment tools that are more practical for regular clinical usage. Until these tools are developed, we suggest that the clincian do the following: (a) become familiar with the structure and style of the CFI so as to be able to interview relatives in a manner that allows for expression of criticism and emotional overinvolvement without directly eliciting such expression; (b) become familiar with the definitions of criticism and overinvolvement used in the EE studies and use these dimensions to structure one's evaluation of the patient's relatives; (c) observe the entire family's attempting to resolve one or more problems; (d) become familiar with the AS and PSS codes and use them to structure your evaluation of the family interaction.

Assessment of Moderating Variables

Moderating variables are factors that serve to mitigate or potentiate the effects of stress on a vulnerable individual. In this section we discuss two moderating variables that have important treatment and case management implications: social support and social skills. There is no consensus as to how social support should be measured. Our assessment program uses a semistructured interview to collect the following information about patients: (a) the size of their social network; (b) the degree of interconnectedness of their network members; (c) the average duration that others have been in their network; (d) the average amount of contact they have with the network; (e) the degree to which they enjoy the company of network members; (f) the degree of frankness with which they can discuss problems with network members; and (g) the degree to which their network members are helpful.

The comprehensive assessment of social support is a useful clinical tool. At the molar level it enables one to classify patients into one of three groups: those who need to develop a support network, those who need to repair an existing network, and those who need to maintain an existing network. This means of classification has specific treatment implications, inasmuch as the development, repair, and maintenance of networks require different behavioral skills. At a more molecular level the social support assessment provides information about the details of a support network's functioning. This provides further information about skills deficits. For example, patients who receive little enjoyment from their network may need to learn leisure skills, whereas patients who cannot discuss their problems frankly may need to learn the skills underlying self-disclosure. Another benefit of a comprehensive social support assessment is that it identifies individuals who may help the patient's treatment by entering into family therapy, helping with case management decisions, and providing needed resources (e.g., housing, money, transportation).

As the preceding discussion implies, development and maintenance of a social support network is, in part, a function of one's level of social competence. Social skills can also mitigate life stress in other ways. For example, an effective repertoire of assertiveness skills will help patients cope with potentially stressful business transactions; learning how to give and receive criticism will help patients to avoid escalations of hostile interactions. Our assessment program incorporates two modes of evaluating social competence: self-report inventory and videotaped roleplay interaction. For self-report of social skills, Lowe and Cautela (1978) have developed the Social Performance Survey Scheduel (SPSS). The SPSS can also be administered in a form that asks relatives of patients to report on the social competence of the patient. The SPSS contains "positive" and "negative" subscales. The positive subscale reflects the degree to which a patient performs socially appropriate behaviors. The negative subscale reports the degree to which a patient does not perform socially appropriate behaviors. Knowledge of a patient's standing on these subscales can aid the clinician in the development of individual treatment programs. It also provides a means for forming treatment groups of patients with common skill deficits. However, there are currently no consensually accepted rules that determine how these clinical decisions should be made.

Our roleplay measure of social skills is the Simulated Social Interaction Test (SSIT) (Curran, 1982). The SSIT procedures are straightforward. The patient is videotaped while responding to a series of eight standardized situations. Each videotaped situation is then rated for social skill and anxiety by trained judges. The sums of these ratings produce global measures of skill and anxiety. The SSIT can be used by a clinician to determine which situations are most difficult for a given patient. Social skills programs can be designed in accordance with this assessment by using knowledge of patient–situation interactions to chose roleplays during therapy sessions and to assign between-session practice tasks. The major disadvantage of the SSIT is that most clinicians will not have the resources needed to administer it. For the practicing clinician, a less rigorous but practical approach may be taken. First, the clinician should become familiar with the range of situations covered by the SSIT (cf. Curran, 1982). The clinician can then use these situations to engage in roleplays with the patient. The informal observations of these roleplays can provide the clincian with a guide for assessing the situation specific skill needs of the patient.

For practical reasons, informal behavioral observations of social skills play a substantial role in the selection and treatment of patients. For example, on an inpatient unit, patients are often referred to the social skills group based on informal observations made by hospital staff that led them to suspect that the patient has a deficient skills repertoire. Similarly, social skills therapists will make treatment decisions based upon their informal observations during and between treatment sessions. The usefulness of these observations can be increased if the observers learn a conceptual structure within which observations can be organized. A useful organizational scheme is provided by Curran's (1979) minimodel of social skills performance. The minimodel requires the observer to answer two questions: (a) Are social skills present? and (b) Are interference mechanisms present? An *interference mechanism* is a response "which inhibits and/or disrupts the effective application of social response capabilities" (Curran, 1979, p. 60). Examples include anxiety, cognitive distortion, and depression. Based on answers to the minimodel questions, patients can be classified into four groups: (a) adequate skills/interference absent; (b) adequate skills/interference present; (c) inadequate skills/interference absent; and (d) inadequate skills/interference present. Ideally, such a classification should be made specific to each of the range of situations covered by the SSIT. The implications of the classificatory system are obvious. Patients from group (a) do not require a skills treatment. Neither do group (b) members, but they probably need some other treatment (e.g., exposure therapy, cognitive therapy). Group (c) patients are candidates for social skills therapy, and group (d) patients require skills training in conjunction with some other therapy.

Case Illustration: Assessment of Henry K.

Diagnosis and Psychopathology

Scoring of the DIS indicated that this 25-year-old man was positive for two DSM-III diagnoses: Schizophrenic Disorder and Simple Phobia. He reported a moderate level of affective symptomatology and had no paranoid symptoms.

Vulnerability and Prognosis

Family history assessment with the FH-RDC found Henry K. to have one schizophrenic sibling, and there were no other psychiatric disorders among first-degree relatives. His responses to the UCLA Social Attainment Survey revealed an adolescence marked by social isolation, lack of heterosexual contact, and a passive involvement in friendships and group activities. His relatively poor premorbid social adjustment combined with a low SES, a long history of psychiatric treatment, and a poor employment history resulted in a poor score on the Strauss-Carpenter Prognostic Scale.

Stress

The PERI-Life Events Inventory indicates that no stressful life events occurred during the 3 months prior to hospitalization. However, a comprehensive assessment of the family revealed some substantial stressors in the home environment. Mr. K. currently lives with his mother and father. The Camberwell Family Interview (CFI) revealed his mother to be highly critical and moderately overinvolved. Her scores on these two factors define her as a High-EE parent; she has approximately 45 hours of contact per week with her son. Her husband was equally high on criticism but low on emotional overinvolvement; he, too, can be classified as a High-EE parent; and he has approximately 25 hours of contact per week with his son. The results of the Direct Family Interaction Test are consistent with the information provided by the CFI. Both parents were highly critical during the DFI. The father tended to be guilt inducing, whereas the mother made intrusive statements. Neither parent was supportive of the patient. Furthermore, the problem-solving codes indicate the family have poor problem-solving skills.

Moderating Variables

Mr. K. is of low socioeconomic status. His employment history suggests that he has only a small potential for future gainful employment. Because his family cannot continue to support him, he is in need of community financial support. His poor money management skills aggravate his financial situation. This lack of skill also encourages his mother to involve herself in his affairs.

In addition to his parents, Mr. K.'s social support network includes an older brother and a younger sister. Mr. K. sees his brother at least once a week and describes the relationship as enjoyable and helpful. The younger sister lives with the family; Mr. K. sees here on a daily basis but finds their interaction to be aversive. Like his parents, his sister rarely helps Mr. K. solve his daily problems.

Measures of social skill indicate that Mr. K.'s social competence is poor. The positive subscale Social Performance Survey Schedule indicates that his lack of competence reflects a deficit in adequately performing socially appropriate behaviors. The negative subscale indicates that he does not perform overtly inappropriate behaviors such as aggressiveness. The Simulated Social Interaction Test found the patient's lack of skill to be extreme in all of the situations sampled. He was rated as only moderately anxious during his SSIT performance. In terms of the minimodel of social skills performance, this patient is classified as having inadequate skills and interference mechanisms are present.

Treatment Implications

The following treatment package is suggested by this assessment:

1. Neuroleptic medication to deal with acute florid symptoms
2. Exposure therapy for his simple phobia
3. Family therapy to reduce critical, overinvolved style of parents and increase family problem-solving ability
4. Social skills training to increase social competence and provide the skills needed to increase the size and quality of the patient's social support network
5. Social service case management to secure community financial support

Interventions

Treatment Philosophy and Structure of Inpatient Unit

Before describing the two behavioral interventions that we emphasize in our treatment of schizophrenics on our inpatient unit, it is necessary to describe both the philosophy and structure of our clinical unit. Our inpatient unit has 35 beds and provides acute psychiatric treatment and intermediate rehabilitative services to voluntary patients. It is a very general psychiatric unit in that a variety of psychiatric disorders are treated, varying from alcoholism and drug abuse, depression secondary to medical illnesses, major depressions, manic-depressive illness, people in crisis, and of course the schizophrenias. The unit is not a custodial care facility. As a facility it provides a setting not only for treating veterans but for studying and learning about psychiatric patients, their disorders, and their social settings. It is also a training facility for psychiatric residents, psychology interns, nurses, social workers, and occupational therapy students.

Philosophy

Several unifying principles guide the operation of our clinical unit. The first and most important of these is a biopsychosocial model of illness. The biopsychosocial model recognizes that most psychiatric disorders are complex, and often are long standing, thus requiring attention to biological, psychological, and social factors. It takes into account the patient's need for lifelong adaptation to the community, and as such it dictates assessment of the patients' assets as well as problems. The biopsychosocial model asserts that any model that ignores the complexity of biological, psychological, and social factors in attempting to understand human interactions would be inadequate for understanding psychiatric disorders. It emphasizes a comprehensive evaluation of all factors, with the need to choose specific models for each individual patient.

The second principle dominating our inpatient care is the philosophy of the patient as a co-participant in his or her treatment. Patients are encouraged not to think of themselves as passive recipients of treatment but as co-participants in their care. Patients participate in their treatment planning during team and community meetings and during care-planning rounds.

A third principle is an emphasis on interactional patterns. We regard our clinical unit as a 24-hour living environment. It is assumed that hospital social behavior reflects behavior outside the hospital. Interpersonal problems and conflicts are inherent in any interactional patterns whether they be staff/patient, patient/patient or staff/staff. As such, they provide both a source of tension and a source of opportunity. We acknowledge the presence of these tensions openly and discuss them so that these very conflicts and problems become therapeutic tools for learning experiences and opprotunities for problem solving.

A fourth principle is that although quality patient care is seen as the primary task that takes precedence over other areas, it is not always appropriate to meet all of our patients' expressed needs. All patients are regarded as "good" patients; it is not for the staff to make value judgments. Decisions about allocation of resources are not based on "goodness" or "badness" but on the severity of the illness, treatability, available resources, and institutional demands.

The fifth principle is the value that teaching and research both enhance patient care and promote staff growth. Research and teaching are not regarded as competing with clinical care but complementing it.

Structures of Inpatient Unit: Step Levels and Clinical Teams

Two basic and most fundamental structures on our inpatient unit are our step levels and clinical teams. Our step levels are basically a gross contingency system, whereas our clinical teams are on outgrowth of milieu principles. Our contingency and milieu principles are interwoven, and it is difficult to speak of one without involving the other. The idea behind the step levels is that patients should progress through them as a means for preparation for discharge. At each step more is required from the patient, and more privilieges are available. The earlier steps are more restrictive, whereas the higher step levels are more consistent with community functioning. All patients, when they enter the community, are restricted to step Level I. As a patient stabilizes with initial care he gradually assumes more responsibility. Activities of daily living are addressed, such as eating, sleeping, personal hygiene, and basic socialization. It is at the discretion of the patient's clinical team and community to decide when he or she has met basic criteria in these activities of daily living so that he or she may be advanced to Level II.

Advancement to Level III, the highest level, requires not only appropriate behavior in activities of daily living but also active involvement with the devised treatment plan. Again, the patient's team and the community make the decision regarding entry into Level III. With advancement to Levels II and III comes greater access to both hospital grounds and the outside community. Contingencies are arranged so that advancement through the step levels encourage patient interaction and return to the community. For example, in order to be maintained on Level III, the patient is required to take both day and overnight passes, hence fostering a return to the community.

Each patient is assigned to a clinical team consisting of both patients and staff members. Each team is captained by a patient who records patient-level status and changes. Walking rounds three times weekly provides the treatment team the opportunity to make the necessary observations and assessments and to negotiate level changes. Patient government meets twice a week. All decisions for advancement to the step levels are discussed with the patient government. All advancement must be approved by the patient government and staff. Care planning also takes place on individual teams, and patients are encouraged and are frequently involved with their care planning.

Professional members of the clinical team consist of psychiatrists, psychologists, social workers, occupational therapists, and nurses. Although patients are assigned one primary therapist, all treatment decisions are made in the context of the team. Schizophrenic patients in our treatment programs are assigned to the psychologist on the team. The psychiatrist on the team manages the patient's medication. Nearly all of our schizophrenic patients are managed on neuroleptic medications, and medication compliance is a integral part of our two behavioral programs. The nurses on the unit often serve as co-therapists with our psychologist in our intervention programs and deserve special mention.

In the description of inpatient treatment protocols, nursing service is often neglected. This is rather surprising given that nursing service has a 24-hour-a-day, 7-days-a-week responsibility for patient care. The sheer volume of contact necessitates one to view nursing as having a significant impact on an inpatient experience. Nurses come to mean many things to psychiatric patients. In the past, where the treatment of schizophrenia was generally long term, nurses came to take on the role of "caretaker" that fostered a dependency in patients. Now with the norm of brief hospitalization for the treatment of schizophrenia, nurses are moving away from the role of caretaker to the more active participant role of care provider. Nursing staff as well as all mental health staffs have had to make considerable adjustments in their view of the management of schizophrenia. For example, it has not been that long ago that nursing students were taught that the relatives of schizophrenic patients were responsible for the etiology of schizophrenia. Continuing educational programs are needed in order to help nursing staff become updated regarding their views of schizophrenia and its treatment. We have found that the nurses on our inpatient unit readily appreciate the vulnerability–stress model of schizophrenia. In fact, this vulnerability–stress model is a very familiar model to them, with perhaps the best example being in the area of diabetes. Just as in diabetes, it would follow naturally that nurses are involved in the teaching of the families and patients about the illness and plan an active role in its treatment. We have found our nursing staff extremely useful in teaching families and patients about schizophrenia; nurses are involved in all aspects of our treatment program including our social skills program, our family intervention program, and our relatives support group.

Contexts of Treatment

As already mentioned, we feel that both the philosophy and structure of our clinical unit are not only compatible with, but facilitate our two primary treatments for schizophrenic patients. With less complementary backdrops we would not anticipate as much success with our behavioral program. Our two behavioral programs consist of social and task-functional skills training and a family intervention program. The goal of social and task-functional skills training is to teach patients coping strategies in order that they may better handle environmental stress. The goal of the family intervention program is to teach the family coping and problem-solving strategies to decrease the amount of stress experienced by the patient.

Social and Task-Functional Skills Training

Definition and Assumptions

Skills training is a response acquisition approach to the treatment of disordered behavior (Goldsmith & McFall, 1975). That is, in skills training, a direct and systematic attempt is made to teach behaviors that, when learned, will help the disordered conditions. The skills to be taught are generally used in a descriptive sense to define the treatment (e.g., social skills training if the skills to be taught are interpersonal in nature; academic skills training if the skills to be taught are related to academic achievement, etc.). In our own work (Monti, Corriveau, & Curran, 1982) with schizophrenic patients, we teach both social skills (which we feel have a wide degree of applicability in social situations) and more task-functional skills (e.g., job-interviewing skills) that have a narrower band of application. The assumptive basis (Curran, 1982) behind our skills training program is that some minimal level of competency in social and task-functional situations is required from our patients in order for them to function and remain in the community. Failures in these situations lead to interpersonal disharmony and psychological distress. It is felt that certain behavioral styles and strategies are more adaptive than other styles and strategies in these various situations. It is also believed that these skills can be specified and taught. It is felt that once these skills are learned they will lead to competence, which will consequently lead to improvement in psychological functioning.

Presentation of Rationale to Patients

Before beginning treatment, we make a sincere effort to convince the patient that skills treatment is a viable treatment strategy for his particular set of problems. Some time is spent explaining the diathesis–stress model of schizophrenia. In fact, most of the information reported in our education model for family treatment is discussed with individual patients. We explain to the patients that his medication is prescribed in order to correct a biochemical imbalance that has left him vulnerable to schizophrenia. The stress side of the equation is then emphasized, and the patient is told that it is important for him to learn strategies for decreasing the stress level in his life. Because a large part of our environment consists of interpersonal interactions, it is important for patients to learn skills that will promote gratifying social encounters. It is also emphasized that it is critical for the patients to obtain minimal levels of competency in several task-functional situations if they are to have a successful community stay after their release from the hospital. We have patients specify goals for themselves to be obtained after the release from the hospital. We try to demonstrate to them that successful attainment of the goals could be facilitated by the acquistion of skills taught in the program.

We explain the purpose of the skills program to the patient as an attempt to teach alternate strategies for handling problematic situations. We tell patients that like learning any other type of skill it may be awkward at first, but with practice proficiency is increased. We state that the program is a practical problem-solving approach focusing on the here and now. The goal is not to teach patients how to behave but to increase options. We tell them we do not have all the answers. In fact, what we are trying to do is to discuss their probability of success in these situations. We explain to them that even a "perfect" performance does not guarantee success.

Skills Trainers

Our groups are led by two experienced therapists. We found it exceedingly difficult to run a group with just one therapist. Just completing the lesson plans and running the videotape equipment practically require two therapists. But more important, it is wise to have two therapists to monitor very closely the changes in the patients' condition. At times, other members of our inpatient staff join the group and help with the roleplays. Often, these individuals are in training to become social skills therapists.

One important point that needs to be mentioned again is that our social skills trainers are also the primary therapists for the patients. The therapists meet with the patients on a daily basis outside of the group and consequently know them quite well. Having the skills therapist also serve as the primary clinician obviously makes for better continuity of care. However, we have conducted other social skills groups when this was not the case, and it is possible to conduct skills treatment in such a fashion. However, it is our feeling that it is preferable to have the social skills trainer function as the primary therapist, especially in dealing with the severely disturbed schizophrenic patients. Frequently, in the case of very disturbed or regressed patients, a therapist may spend time with the patient outside of the group and provide individual training.

Program Format

Our social skills training program for schizophrenic inpatients requires a period of 6 weeks. It is a group-based program, with the group meeting twice a day, Monday through Friday. On Monday through Thursday the group meets for

1 hour in the morning and 1 hour in the afternoon. On Friday there is an hour review in the morning, with the afternoon session consisting of a "community trip" that may last 2 hours or longer. The community trip is organized in such a way as to provide patients an opportunity to practice the skills they have learned earlier in the week. These trips are often to restaurants, shopping plazas, bowling alleys, and the like. It is our subjective feeling that these trips are good for the morale of both the patients and staff.

Our skills program is a group-based program. Our groups generally consist of four patients, primarily because this is about the number of schizophrenics that can be found on our unit at any particular point in time. In the past, when we were conducting social skills group for a heterogeneous group of psychiatric patients, we were able to accommodate six to eight patients and found that range to be a good group size. However, our experience with severely disturbed schizophrenic patients tends to make us think that the smaller number of four might be more ideal for this population.

Patients begin the group only after they have been stabilized on medication and their florid symptomatology is under control. We feel that for a skills program to have impact on schizophrenia it should be fairly intense. However, ours is an acute, short-stay clinical unit, and retaining patients for much longer than our 6-week program would be particularly problematic. It can be argued that severely disturbed schizophrenic patients might actually need more time than the 60 hours contained in our program. However, our format was dictated by clinical practicalities. As mentioned, our inpatients unit is an acute unit with an average length of stay of less than 30 days. The patients in our program are essentially in the hospital for twice the average length of stay, and we feel that this is probably the maximum that we could achieve. In fact, some patients are discharged before the program is completed but continue in the program as outpatients.

Two hours a day does not appear to be particularly taxing for most of our patients. Having lunch between intervening sessions offers a nice break. Even though schizophrenics appear to be particularly sensitive to overstimulation, social skills training does not generally produce an exacerbation of schizophrenic symptoms. We think this is because our therapists are well trained and are very sensitive to the overstimulation issue. Consequently, the trainers "back off" at times if they think that "pushing" will lead to an exacerbation of symptoms. The goals of training are broken down into small steps so the performance demands at any one time are manageable. The training format itself is quite predictable, repetitive, and explained well in advance. Patients, with therapist assistance, select their own role-plays, and if a roleplay appears to be too highly emotional, another roleplay situation will be substituted. Group cohesiveness and support are developed, and consequently patients are likely to take risks in this environment. We foster a large degree of positive feedback and positive reinforcement in the group; hence patients feel safe there.

Training Procedures

Our training routine for each session (except for the Friday community trip) generally consists of the following components: (a) a review of the previous session and the homework assignment issued at that session; (b) a didactic presentation of the day's lesson with its accompanying rationale; (c) modeling either via videotape or live modeling of the major points of the lesson; (d) a discussion and some quizzing of the patients on the major points; (e) behavioral rehearsal and roleplaying; (f) both videotape and group members' feedback; (g) mastery of the lesson via repeated trials; and (h) finally, practice assignments to promote transfer of learning.

In order to provide an illustration of how we present our lessons we will review "giving criticism." First, the trainers present the rules of the lesson to the group members. This is usually accomplished by distributing to the members a handout with the rules printed on it and with the leaders going over each rule on a blackboard. Rules for giving criticism are as follows:

1. State the criticism in terms of your own feelings, not in terms of absolute statements.
2. Try not to criticize the entire person but rather try to direct your criticism at the specific aspects of his or her behavior.
3. Try to request specific behavior change. If there is something specific the other person can do to ameliorate the situation, try to request that specifically. Do not assume that he or she will know how to please you.
4. Within the conversation, try both to start and finish on a positive note. In other words, try to diminish the overall negativeness of your conversation by sandwiching statements with either compliments or some type of positive regard.
5. Do not let your tone of voice become angry. If your goal is to actually change the other person's behavior, a heated argument probably will not result in obtaining both your short- and long-term goals.

Therapists review these rules several times, explaining the rationale for them and asking for comments from group members. Modeling demonstrations are then provided. These demonstrations are sometimes videotaped depictions; at other times, they are demonstrated by the therapists themselves. When providing an appropriate model, the therapist should try to demonstrate each of the rules. Sometimes, for a change of pace, therapists will demonstrate inappropriate behavior and ask the group members for feedback. We have found the live models to be more personal, dramatic, and attention holding. However, videotaped models have the advantage of allowing careful preparation and can be more easily replayed in whole or in part. To illustrate any particular skills, several demonstrations may be undertaken.

Next, we ask one or several members of the group to rehearse the lesson. At times, we merely have them imitate the same situation where it would be appropriate to display such behaviors. Often the situation chosen is one that occurred in the not so distant past and one in which they felt they failed to perform adequately. The situation is constructed, and perhaps several members take part by playing different roles. These role rehearsals are obviously critical. They give the therapist an idea as to how the patient has handled these situations in the past and the difficulties he or she may have in carrying out the lesson in these situations in the future. Because these situations are relevant to the patient's life, we feel that they probably foster better generalization than if we used standard roleplays.

At times during these role rehearsals, therapists may request that the patient switch roles. That is, the therapist will request a role reversal where the patient will play a protagonist in the situation, and either another patient or the therapist will play the subject. This is usually done when the patient is having a difficult time in the situation or in order to give him or her an idea of how he or she may be perceived by the other individual if he or she behaved in a more appropriate fashion. This is a particularly good strategy if patients balk at trying out a new skill because they do not feel it will work in the situation. By employing the role reversal, therapists are basically challenging the pessimism of the patients and demonstrating to them how it may work. If patients cannot generate situations themselves, we can draw from a standard stock of situations. But, in most cases, it is not necessary to pull a situation from the standard stock because most patients have no difficulty in generating those that are particularly relevant to them.

Two types of feedback are generally provided: videotaped and verbal. Most of the roleplays are videotaped and played back to the patients in order for them to observe their performance. Video feedback has the advantage of providing immediate, descriptive, and objective feedback, and it can be repeated quite frequently. A series of videotaped rehearsals might be used to show improvement from the patient's first attempt to the last. It has been our experience that patients initially appear to be somewhat anxious about observing themselves on videotape but soon adapt. Of course, there is always the danger that individuals may become distraught at their lack of competency, especially if there has been a markedly noticeable decline from their premorbid competency level. Obviously, such reactions should be monitored quite carefully. However, we have rarely experienced this type of reaction, and in fact, most people really seem to enjoy the videotape playback.

At the beginning of the program, the therapists are usually the ones who provide feedback. We found it best for the therapist to model how to provide this feedback in the beginning stages before letting other members of the group do so. It is always important to provide some positive feedback no matter what the level of competency demonstrated in the performance. We always try to give at least two to three times more positive feedback than negative feedback. The feedback should be specific, detailed, and highly focused. It should be given in nontechnical language and should concentrate on those behaviors over which the subject has some control. Of course, one of the by-products of this feedback is that patients in the group learn how to give both positive feedback in high dosages and also how to give critical feedback in an appropriate and constructive fashion.

At the end of the lesson we provide practice assignments. The purpose of these assignments is to promote transfer of learning from the group situation to the community environment. Patients practice these new skills on the inpatient unit and in other areas of the hospital, such as the cafeteria. As mentioned previously, on Fridays we arrange a community trip in order for patients to practice their skills in community settings. In addition, we encourage our patients who are eligible for weekend passes to take them and practice their new skills in their community environment.

The homework for a particular lesson is reviewed in detail to promote understanding of the assignment. Patients are given homework sheets that are placed in their notebooks. These sheets outline the major points of the lesson. The assignment sheets contain some space for patients to write in the results of their practice. The therapist tries to insure that before the patients leave the group they have formulated a plan to practice their homework. As might be expected, we sometimes encounter motivational problems on the part of some of our patients with respect to their completion of homework assignments. If patients refuse to do their assignments we treat that as a problem and try to do some problem solving in the group. Objections such as "I feel awkward carrying my notebook around" or "I can't write very well" usually can be problem solved fairly easy. The first 15 minutes or so of the next session are devoted to a discussion of the practice assignment. Here all patients are required to discuss their attempts. All attempts are reinforced, even unsuccessful attempts. What we frequently find is that patients tend to be too critical of their performance. Here it is important for the therapist to intervene and try to change these negative evaluations to more positive ones.

Training Content

We divide the content of our skills program into three relatively arbitrary areas: (a) generic communication skills (skills that we feel have a wide range of applicability across situations) (b) general task-functional skills (skills required in particular discrete situations that we feel are important for all our patients); and (c) individual task-functional skills (again here we are talking about skills required for a particular type of situations, but here the skills may be pertinent to only some patients in the group). Examples of generic communication skills would be giving and receiving compliments, active listening skills, giving and receiving criticism, and so on. General task-functional skills would include such skills as money management, use of leisure time, building of social support networks, and so forth. Some patients may also be taught individualized task-functional skills. For example, job-seeking and job-interviewing skills are not universally taught because many of our patients have a service-connected disability and will probably never return to work. Other individualized skills, such as self-help and food preparation, are not universally taught because most patients do not have deficits in these areas. Most of these individualized skills are not taught directly by members of the skills program; rather, other units in the hospital are utilized. For example, job-interviewing skills are taught by occupational therapy, food preparation by the dietary services, and so on. We have worked in the past with these units in order to develop skills programs, and now we are able to refer certain patients to these units if there appears to be a need.

Generative Processes

What may or may not be apparent from our description of our training process is that much more than just discrete behavioral skills are taught. What follows is a partial list of skills (many of which are cognitive) that we teach in our skills training program in addition to discrete component behaviors:

1. The process of generating response options
2. The importance of sequencing behavior
3. General rules and strategy of conduct
4. Social norms and social discourse rules
5. Cue reading and social perception
6. External and internal monitoring
7. "Reality testing"
8. Goal setting both short and long term
9. Problem-solving strategies
10. Estimation of outcome probability and expectancy
11. Examination of self-statements and modification toward more positive statements
12. Process of logical disputing and empirically disproving invalid inferences and illogical assumptions

Trower (1982) has criticized social skills training programs that just teach discrete component behaviors. He feels that skills programs need to teach the process of generating social skills performance rather than just the components. We agree with him and think it is important that trainers pay attention to these generative processes and systematically include them in their skills package. We have mentioned that in our own program we systematically include in our lesson plan some of these generative processes, such as goal setting. However, others such as disputing illogical assumptions, while not formally included, often appear in the course of group discussion.

Integration and Focal Treatment

One point that we should stress is the need to integrate the skills program into the larger clinical unit. It is our contention that if the skills program is not integrated into the larger clinical unit it will be a less effective program. As mentioned previously, our skills therapists are members of a clinical treatment team. They are regarded by the team as the primary clinicians for the patients involved in the group. They attend rounds and care-planning meetings. Other staff on the inpatient unit are encouraged to participate in the group, and information regarding a patient's progress in the group is shared with other members of the unit.

Our skills training program is perceived by members of the clinical unit as a focal point of therapy for the group members. The skills training program is viewed by our staff as a means to teach patients strategies to prevent psychotic relapse. The skills program is frequently applied in conjunction with other treatment modalities. For example, almost all our schizophrenic patients are treated by the team's psychiatrist with neuroleptic mediciaton. The neuroleptic medication is used to control for some of the positive symptoms of schizophrenia, whereas the skills program is used as an opportunity for the patients to improve on the negative symptomatology.

An Overview

The importance of the family in the treatment of schizophrenia cannot be overestimated. With deinstitutionalization of patients with psychological disorders came the realization that families are major caregivers in the mental health system. This realization has led to a revolution in treatment philosophy with a shift in focus, from isolating family members to their full participation in treatment planning. Indeed, McFarlane (1983) has recently labeled a variety of these divergent family treatment methods as the *psychoeducational approaches to schizophrenia.* Our family treatment program is modeled after such psychoeducational approaches (Anderson, 1983; Falloon & Liberman, 1983). It involves a 12-session intensive phase (weekly or twice weekly meetings) consisting of three modules (education, communication, and problem solving).

Schizophrenic patients are enrolled in our family program if family members are willing to participate in treatment. Family membership is very broadly defined to include siblings, spouses, girlfriends, parents, and even surrogate families such as boarding home operators. Most of our experience to date has been with parents and siblings. Family members choose to meet once or twice a week until the 12-session intensive phase is completed. After completion of the intensive treatment, families are followed for 1 year and receive at first bimonthly and then monthly booster sessions. Each session lasts 1½ hours. The program also allows for additional "crisis" sessions as needed.

The 12-session intensive phase is divided into three modules. The education module is covered in two sessions and has as its goal educating family members about the nature and treatment of schizophrenia. The next five sessions are devoted to Module 2: social/communication skills training. This is similar to our social skills training discussed previously. The last module contains five sessions devoted to helping families develop problem-solving skills. Although it has been helpful for us to organize our program into three modules, it should be noted that material from earlier modules may be incorporated into later modules. For example, we frequently find ourselves discussing educational material from the first phase during our problem-solving module.

Before the program actually begins, a separate session is held with the family to describe the program and explain its rationale. We feel that our presentation of the family program to the relatives is critical to its success. Henceforth, careful attention and planning should be given to the initial encounter with the family.

Our rationale to family members is based on the vulnerability/stress model of schizophrenia as outlined in the beginning of this chapter. Two key ideas of this model provide a way for the treatment team to approach family members in a non-accusatory and nonthreatening way that facilitates forming the necessary treatment alliance with the family. Schizophrenia is presented as a mental illness with a biological etiology. Family members are informed that they did not cause the illness. Psychotic symptoms are explained as part of a serious mental illness that would have occurred regardless of what child-rearing practices were used. In addition, the "sick" family member is described as highly vulnerable to stress; family members are told that although they did not cause the illness, they can protect their ill member by providing a home environment more accommodating to his or her individual needs.

Furthermore, statements are made about the effectiveness of family treatment. Essentially, families are told that the treatment program has been found to be effective in keeping schizophrenic patients out of the hospital and helpful to families coping with the exhausting responsibility of having to care for the patient. In attempting to instill an attitude of hopefulness, specific examples of problems we have tackled successfully are discussed. The family is told that they will be given information about the patient's treatment plans, including medication. Moreover, they will be consulted when passes are issued and discharge planning takes place. They are informed that we recognize them as major caregivers and as partners in the patient's ongoing care. The final point to be made is a delicate one; families are told that although they are not responsible for causing the patient's mental illness, they must often change their behavior toward him or her in order to decrease the probability of relapse. We tell families that the patient will have the best chance to avoid rehospitalization if they can lower the stress level in the home. It is the treatment team's responsibility to instruct families as to how to lower the stress level and provide the necessary support while these changes are taking place.

Education Module

Most of the material we cover in the first two sessions is taken directly from other programs (Anderson, 1983; Falloon & Liberman, 1983) and modified to meet the particular needs of our patient population. Our goal in these two sessions is to begin to create "cognitive mastery" over the set of puzzling behaviors associated with schizophrenia by providing family members with information about the illness. The selection of our current educational material has been shaped by the reception that family members have given us and by what we believe is the critical information needed to cope effectively with schizophrenia.

The style of presentation also is important. Perceived expertise has long been known to affect attitude change, and we are careful to underscore the credentials and experience of each of our therapists. Presentations are made in a professional manner, using graphs, statistics, tables, and so forth to increase the family's perception of expertise. The following description of our education module is organized around what we consider to be some of its major goals.

Resolution of Family Guilt

Two areas of information seem particularly helpful in resolving the guilt of family members. These areas involve a discussion of the genetic basis of schizophrenia and the neurochemical problems associated with schizophrenia. The genetic basis of schizophrenia is supported with a description of the twin and adoption studies, including the experimental design and results (Rainer, 1980). In addition, the dopamine hypothesis of schizophrenia is explained, complete with a diagram of the synapse as an audiovisual aid (Kaplan & Sadock, 1980). The sophistication of the presentation varies according to the particular family. Generally, questions and comments from family members demonstrate a paucity of previous knowledge about these topics. Emotional reactions to the material are usually strong. One father said: "I never knew that before [referring to the dopamine hypothesis]; I always thought it was the mother that made him sick." Another mother described lying awake at night trying to determine what she might have done differently to have prevented her son from becoming schizophrenic. Several mothers have said: "The doctor always made me feel like I was to blame." The treatment team's response to comments like these is to strengthen the new knowledge by stating flatly that there is no proof that family members' have caused schizophrenia.

Realization of Handicap

Frequently, family members believe that the ill member's symptoms are volitional and can be brought under control with some effort. A discussion of phenomenology, information-processing deficits, etiology, and prognosis challenges the belief that the patient is "putting on the rest of the world." It is critical for family members to believe that there is a true handicap in order for them to decrease expectations and make a commitment to support the patient at times of increased symptomatology. We realize that this emphasis on handicap risks exposing the family to manipulation by the patient. We believe, however, that this is a necessary risk, and obvious attempts at manipulation can be brought under control during the other modules of the therapy program.

Importance of Neuroleptic Medications

Clearly, the most potent treatment for the positive symptoms of schizophrenia is antipsychotic medication (May & Simpson, 1980). Therefore, compliance with medications should be a major goal in any treatment program for schizophrenia. Roughly 30 to 40% of the time in the educational presentation is spent providing information about medication. It is time well spent. Family members are often effective allies in reinforcing or directing medication compliance. In order to effect an alliance with family members around medication compliance, they must know, at a minimum, the drug's purpose, effectiveness, dose requirements, and side effects. We feel strongly that some plan equally satisfying to patient and family regarding medication compliance should be worked out before the patient is discharged. This helps to prevent the issue of medication compliance from becoming a battleground between patient and family.

Identification of Stressors

The work on "expressed emotion" (Brown & Rutter, 1968) has demonstrated that the family may play an important role in the prevention of a relapse of schizophrenia. Starting with the premise that the patient is vulnerable to stress because of an illness that the family did not cause, family members are taught that there are ways they can behave toward the handicapped member that will decrease the probability of relapse. In particular, family members are told that high levels of criticism and too much emotional involvement are toxic to the patient. In order to make this point very clear, a number of examples of what is meant by criticism and emotional overinvolvement are described. Obviously, lectures and discussions are often not enough to create significant changes in fixed behavioral patterns. But didactic instruction is an important beginning and lays the groundwork for further work in the communication skills and problem-solving modules.

Discussion of criticism and overinvolvement can elicit guilt in family members. To decrease these feelings we have developed methods for teaching the effects of stress without making families defensive. Family members often will be puzzled as to how their behavior can affect the patient now but not have caused the illness. We answer this through the use of metaphor: for example, floods are caused by something beyond human control, but we can have an effect on how much damage floods cause by building effective dams. We also let families know that overinvolvement and criticism are natural responses to a sick person. When a child is physically ill we shower him or her with attention (e.g., with chicken soup, alcohol rubs, reading stories, taking his or her temperature, etc.). We also may admonish the child to stay in bed, rest, take medication, dress warmly, drink fluids, and the like. These explanations seem to help family members accept their own past behaviors and get on with building the needed skills to decrease stress.

Management of Disruptive Behavior

If caretakers feel intimidated by the patient, the utility of family therapy will markedly decrease. It is difficult for family members to persuade a patient to take his or her medication if they feel frightened of him or her or if they feel they have been unable to effect any control of his or her behavior in other areas. In order to help family members regain control of the patient's behavior, we teach them to respond effectively to undesirable and threatening behaviors. We provide and model effective responding to such problems as paranoid delusional thinking and violent behavior. For example, family members are told that violence cannot be tolerated and are urged to call the police if such behavior is exhibited. Similarly, families are told not to argue with or confront paranoid thinking but rather to take a benign, indifferent attitude toward it and accept it as part of the illness.

Communications Skills Module

It is not uncommon for family members to enter this part of the treatment program unable to make the simplest statements to one another without creating an all-out confrontation. This should be of little surprise because communication skills deficits have long been identified in distressed families (Jacobsen & Martin, 1976). In particular, communication deviance has been found in families of patients with schizophrenia (Singer & Wynne, 1966). Borrowing from the findings of this basic communication research, other treatment programs (Falloon & Liberman, 1983), and our clinical experience, we have developed a communication module geared toward making communication among family members of schizophrenics more effective. This module is not independent of the education module. Gains made in communication skills training is dependent on the family's having an accurate understanding of schizophrenia. It is difficult if not impossible for family members to communicate effectively if the patient is believed to be a malingerer or the husband still believes that his wife made his son or daughter schizophrenic. The communication skills module also prepares the family for the problem-solving module because effective communication is a prerequisite for effective negotiation.

A careful assessment of each family's communication problems should be made and the treatment intervention developed on the basis of this assessment. There are several areas, however, that frequently are found to be deficient in these families. Included are listening skills, giving and receiving positive feedback (compliments), giving and receiving criticism, feeling talk, making requests, assertive behavior, and reciprocity of conversation. Communication lessons on these topics are similiar to those given to patients in the individual skills training. However, because of the better information-processing capacity of family members, we are able to cover the material in a shorter time period than we do with the patients (five sessions, 1½ hours long).

Problem Solving

Falloon *et al.* (1984) have found that relapse among schizophrenic patients is strongly associated with their families' abilities to solve problems effectively. Borrowing from Falloon and Liberman (1983), our program uses a six-step approach to teach problem-solving skills:

1. We pinpoint and specify problems.
2. We develop several options or alternative responses.
3. We evaluate each option in terms of its possible consequences.
4. We choose the option that maximizes positive consequence and minimizes negative consequences.
5. We plan how to implement that option as a family.
6. We review the problem after the selected option has been implemented.

These steps appear to be deceptively simple. However, effective family use of the model requires organization, commitment, and the ability to compromise with one another. These skills are usually lacking in the families we have seen. In order to help the family use the model effectively, a fair amount of experience and therapy skill is needed. However, in contrast to the more traditional insight-oriented approach to the family treatment of schizophrenia, there is a clear direction during treatment for therapist and patient alike. Each session has a specific agenda. Concrete problems are defined (e.g., a family telephone bill is too high; the mother is overburdened with housework; a decision needs to be made about where a sibling will live, etc.). As a result of using the problem-solving model, families gain enthusiasm and hopefullness as each problem is solved. Our problem-solving training covers the last five sessions of the intensive treatment phase and continues through the follow-up period. Each session should begin with an update on the implementation of the solutions to the previous session's problems. The family usually designate a member to keep a record of problems and plans for their solution. It is imperative that the therapists insure that each problem is resolved before going on to a different one. The temptation is always there to begin work on new problems before solving old ones. However, frequent sidetracking leads to disorganization and defeats the purpose of the problem-solving treatment program. The goal during the problem-solving module is not to deal with all of the family members' problems but to teach them the process and skills involved to the point where they can be used independently.

Problems with the Treatment Program

We have experienced some problems with family reactions to the model of schizophrenia taught in the first phase of our program. As explained before, we rely heavily on the construct of *illness* as an explanation for the etiology of schizophrenia and as a means to understand the recurrent behavioral problems of the patient. There are a number of troubling consequences of this model. Family members have complained about feeling like they are "walking on eggshells" in their attempts to avoid stressing the ill family member. One sibling complained that she was afraid to talk to the patient for fear of confusing him and causing his rehospitalization. Another patient was accused of "tyrannizing" his family by making extraordinary demands on their time and energy and justifying the demands because he is "sick." These problems are substantial but can be addressed effectively in the ongoing family therapy.

Teaching family members that the patient is "ill" sometimes fosters withdrawal and isolation for some patients. We teach families that schizophrenic patients need a convalescence period (6 months to a year) after a psychotic episode (Anderson, 1983). Family members will usually cooperate with a "hands-off" or "benign indifferent" attitude toward the patient. However, at times it is upsetting for family and treatment team members alike to observe this withdrawal process. This is a problem area that the authors have not resolved and continue to work on with our families. One strategy that we have found helpful involves making the issue an open one for the family, while enlisting the patient in the resolution of the problem.

Aftercare

The skills trainer or family therapist who served as the patient's primary therapist during the intensive phase of the program remains as therapist during the aftercare phase of the program. Aftercare visits are twice monthly the first 2 months after discharge and monthly visits thereafter. Unscheduled visits may be warranted and will be arranged as needed. If a patient in our program presents in our outpatient clinic for whatever reason, his or her primary therapist is contacted. The primary therapist will meet with the patient the same day if at all possible.

Aftercare therapy sessions are consistent with treatment received on the inpatient unit. That is, aftercare visits for people in the skills program will often involve goal setting, behavioral rehearsal, roleplays, and so on. Likewise, patients in the family program will have sessions dealing with communication training and problem solving.

Whenever possible, we attempt to have our therapist visit with patients in their home or residence at least once or twice during our 1-year aftercare phase. Falloon *et al.* (1982) make the point that home visits promote better compliance and give the therapist a first-hand look at the problems confronting patients and their families. Home visits often help the therapist to understand the family's perspective. That is, a family may not be all that concerned about a patient's socializing when their roof is literally falling in on them. Our resources do not permit all of our aftercare visits to take place in the patient's home, but we attempt at least one or two, particularly at the beginning of aftercare. Once a policy of home visits is established, they can provide a unique opportunity to prevent relapses and resulting hospitalizations.

We have also established twice-monthly relatives' support groups that many of the relatives of our schizophrenic patients attend (Atwood, 1983; Hatfield, 1983). Here relatives talk with each other, share their difficulties, and develop strategies to solve their problems. For our patients, we have a day treatment program that they may attend on a daily basis. In many ways, the day treatment program serves as a social club wherein trips to ballgames, fishing expeditions, and the like are planned. A work program can also be found in the day treatment program, and some patients earn money by fulfilling job contracts.

When family placement is not possible we have available to us several community residential programs. We have attempted to form liaisons between our treatment staff and the caregivers in these treatment programs. We have run seminars for the staff of these programs, teaching them our model of schizophrenia and the techniques from the skills and family programs. The vast majority of our patients either return to their families or are in these residential programs. If independent living is a reasonable alternative for a particular patient, we prepare him or her for it. If more than one patient appears appropriate for independent living, we prepare them as a cohort with the intention of having them support each other in the community. Another alternative is the halfway house. For example, in a skills program directed by M. Brown (1982), patients discharged from the hospital are placed in these halfway houses for a contracted 2-month period. Patients participate with the staff in setting goals and are responsible for the housekeeping, meals, and so forth. Two mental health workers are involved at the halfway house and are on call 24 hours a day. Patients are urged to spend time with nonpatients and get out into the community.

As a means to illustrate how our treatment principles translate into everyday clinical care, we will describe the treatment of two of our patients. Both received the social skills and family programs. In one of the cases we have met with much success, whereas our success has been more limited in the other case. Both are good examples of how we adapt our general program to fit the individual needs of each case.

Case Illustrations

Case 1: Ken B.

Ken B. is a 31-year-old unemployed white male with a diagnosis of schizophrenia. He went through both the social skills training and the behavioral family therapy during his third hospitalization. His predominant symptoms at the time of admission were inappropriate, angry affect and the belief that the Virgin Mary took on the identity of people around him. He was hospitalized at the request of his mother when she became frightened of his threatening behavior and preoccupation with homosexuality.

Ken is the youngest male in an French Catholic family that includes five children. He dropped out of a state university after 1 year and entered the Marines, where he had his first psychotic breakdown. The family lives in an affluent suburb, and they spend much time and effort "keeping up with the Jones." Both parents work for large governmental agencies in middle management positions. Ken's youngest sister, who also lives at home with him and her parents, is employed as a clerk at the same government agency as her father. The family describes two of Ken's older brothers as "not settled down" because they change jobs frequently and have many girlfriends. The oldest brother lives close by the parents and visits home frequently, whereas a second brother has lived in Asia for 6 years.

Ken can be described as a thin, attractive man who is meticulous about his dress and grooming, works hard at staying in good physical shape, and has good verbal skills. Despite these strengths he had a lot of difficulty, while hospitalized, getting along with other patients because he was stongly opinionated. He would frequently criticize other patients in an abrasive way at inappropriate times. He also would frequently attempt to convince others of his delusions. Surprisingly, Ken was able to avoid physical confrontations with other patients, but he did not enjoy his unpopularity. He would express guilt and helplessness about his behavior and often dealt with this by withdrawing from interpersonal situations.

Before being hospitalized, Ken was taking Navane, 5 mg b.i.d., and Artane, 2 mg a day. Ken was also taking 125 mg of Antabuse a day for his alcohol problem. Upon entering the hospital his Navane was increased to 10 mg b.i.d., and he was switched from Artane to Cogentin, 2 mg a day. Antabuse was prescribed as before. Our patient continues to be maintained with the same medications and levels as prescribed in the hospital.

At the beginning of the social skills training program, the following goals were mutually set with Ken:

1. To learn what personal information to share with others and where and when to share it
2. To decrease his nonverbal angry behavior, particularly his tone of voice and facial scowling, and increase the amount of positive socializing with others
3. To maintain longer eye contact with others
4. To listen longer to others without changing the topic of conversation to something more personally interesting to him

From the therapist's viewpoint, the nonverbal expression of anger was the most difficult change to achieve. The patient frequently reached levels of anger where his face flushed, at times he became tremulous, and his voice became loud. Roleplays, videotape feedback, and persistence eventually paid off, and expressions of Ken's anger decreased sharply. We found it helpful to avoid insisting on rapid change and to keep focusing on specific behavior (e.g., scowling, as opposed to motives for the anger). Challenging his reasons for the anger only prolonged it and made it more intense. Our instructions and modeling were consistently clear and simple:

> You want people to like you. Scowling and raising your voice scares people or makes them want to fight back. If you want people to like you better you must lower your voice and stop scowling.

Ken also became a much better listener. It seemed helpful to him to learn through group discussion and modeling that other people enjoyed being listened to attentively. As he became able to frame his listening as helpful or charitable to others and practiced these skills with other group members, his listening skills increased. Prior to discharge from the psychiatric unit, Ken himself, along with unit staff members, reported much progress toward reaching the goals he had set. In fact, his increase in skills was rewarded by being elected a team captain in patient-government meetings.

Family treatment with the B. family was equally effective and rewarding. The initial assessment of the family disclosed many serious problems. There was a serious marital schism with a reported history of the father's infidelity. This had led to a virtual "cold war" between the parents, with each of them sleeping in separate rooms and generally avoiding one another. The tension would also erupt into frequent verbal arguments between the parents during which both of them would threaten divorce. In fact, both Ken and his sister Kathy stated flatly that they were continuing to live at home to prevent the parents from divorcing.

The household seemed organized around Ken's mother, who demanded and received control over most of the important and routine family activities. She budgeted the family money, cooked the evening meals, made herself responsible for cleaning and laundry, planned family parties and holidays, and made the decisions to seek hospitalization for Ken. Not surprisingly, when given the Camberwell Family Interview, she was found to be emotionally overinvolved with the patient. For example, at the beginning of the family treatment program she frequently spoke for Ken, often telling the therapists and other family members how he felt. In addition, she clung to high achievement goals for Ken. She wanted him to date, socialize at family get-togethers, go to law school, and change his paranoid beliefs. The father shared the mother's expectation of high functioning for Ken. These high expectations put Ken in an impossible bind because he was forced to pretend that he was well when he was in fact quite psychotic. On one occasion his mother accused him of being lazy because he had refused to go to a nightclub with his sister. With the therapist's help, Ken was able to verbalize how paranoid he became at such places (e.g., thinking frequently that he should murder others before they murdered him). Needless to say, this was quite instructive for Mrs. B.

Family therapy produced some significant results with the B. family, but only after much intense effort by them and the therapist. Most noticeably, family members, after continued feedback and instruction, are much more aware of Ken's serious handicap. This has led to decreased expectations for him, which were agreed to and carried out in the problem-solving phase of treatment. His mother no longer pressures him into going nightclubbing with his sister; family members no longer argue with him regarding his religious beliefs and paranoid delusions; and Ken is allowed to sleep longer and withdraw from family conversations with impunity. Communication skills and problem-solving training have assisted Ken's mother in becoming less intrusive and overprotective. She no longer speaks for him at family meetings, lets him help with the housework, and has considered, although not yet followed through, on letting him take care of his own finances. Also, she is now able to talk about being "too close" to Ken, has begun to spend evenings out with old girlfriends, and has recently joined a gourmet club. In addition, the family reports fewer arguments between the parents. Finally, two unanticipated consequences have occurred for Ken's sister: she is now seeking a living arrangement outside of the household and has begun individual psychotherapy with a local psychologist.

Case 2: William V.

Most likely any therapist would feel a deep sense of accomplishment with the results obtained with the B. family. The following case, however, illustrates a less satisfying outcome. An argument could be developed that the pathology in this family case has merely shifted the advent of our program. However, it will also demonstrate that we have reached our goal of keeping the index patient out of the hospital.

William V. is a 20-year-old unemployed male who lives with his mother, father, and brother. William is the youngest of three children and has an older brother, Anthony, age 24, and an older sister, Marie, 25. Marie is a graduate student in theology at a West Coast college and lives away from home.

At the time of admission to the hospital the situation in William's home was no less than chaotic. His parents were arguing violently whenever they came together, his father was threatening divorce, whereas his mother attempted covertly to gain legal control over the family's financial holdings. The patient's brother, Anthony, was abusing amphetamines and PCP. William was speaking incoherently, hearing voices, and was unable to sleep.

A family assessment, using the Camberwell Family Interview, found Mrs. V. to be emotionally overinvolved with William. She required him to attend church services every morning and evening with her, drove him wherever he wanted to go, fearing that he would get into an accident if he drove himself, and dictated virtually all of his waking behaviors.

William had been transferred to our Veterans Administration medical center from a Navy regional medical center. He had been discharged to us on Navane, 5 mg b.i.d. and 10 mg at bedtime. After a brief trial of Prolixin the patient was placed on Mellaril, 100 mg in the morning and 300 mg before bedtime. Gradually, the patient was tapered to 100 mg in the morning and 200 mg at bedtime. Cogentin, 1 mg in the morning, was prescribed for side effects.

William's first attempt at participation in our intensive social skills program failed. He was removed from the group for a week after a serious increase in psychotic symptomatology. However, his second attempt was quite successful. He reached the goals of decreasing distracting leg movements, initiating more conversations with others, expressing himself more clearly in conversation, and worked effectively on his problem of becoming overinvolved with helping other patients while neglecting his own needs.

The outcome of family therapy was quite different. The sessions were a constant struggle for the family members and the treatment team alike. Virtually every session erupted into loud verbal confrontations between two or more family members, usually brought on by the father or mother accusing one another of causing William's illness or not carrying out their role as parent or spouse.

Written rules for appropriate conduct during the treatment sessions, a written contract of mutual commitment to keep William out of the hospital, and firm, task-oriented leadership behavior by the treatment team could not prevent the family from engaging in violent arguments and periodically refusing to participate during sessions.

During the psychoeducation module the parents frequently made cynical comments about the material (e.g., "He doesn't need that junk [referring to the medication]" or "I knew all this before, it doesn't help"). It was also clear that the communication skills training was ineffective, even though we provided this family with close to three times the number of sessions usually allotted in this module. Neither Mr. or Mrs. V. demonstrated consistent competence in any aspect of listening skills. Verbal communication between them was characterized by frequent interruptions, misidentification of each other's statements and feelings, and ineffective and distracting nonverbal communication (raising voices and making poor eye contact).

To complicate things even further, William's older brother, Anthony, presented the treatment team with a special problem. Anthony attended sessions regularly. He seemed quiet but vigilant and would participate in roleplays at the request of the therapy team. He was often accused by both parents, but especially by his mother, of being uncooperative about helping around the house, not looking for a job, and abusing drugs. Anthony vehemently denied all of these accusations. The therapy team was aware that Anthony seemed depressed and that he was probably abusing drugs. They also knew that Anthony was under the care of a local psychiatrist. However, William's psychotic behavior and the parents' volatile interaction were their first concerns. The day after William's discharge from the hospital, Anthony took a serious overdose of medication and was hospitalized for 3 months. His discharge diagnosis was schizophrenia. Anthony's behavior has not stabilized since his discharge, and he continues to have drug problems.

Despite all these difficulties, family members attended sessions regularly, and the patient has continued to improve since discharge. Subjective and quantitative clinical assessments show evidence that the patient is without positive symptoms of schizophrenia. Moreover, he has begun to socialize with peers, drive his own car, and attend a vocational training program 4 days a week. In addition, Mr. and Mrs.

V. have been able to keep their arguing to a minimum when in the presence of William. Further, both parents and the patient have recognized the need for continued medication, and medication compliance has been achieved with the patient.

Summary

We regard schizophrenia as a *open-ended hypothetical construct*. We feel that schizophrenia is multiply determined and multiply maintained. Our model for schizophrenia is the diathesis–stress model, which assumes that individuals inherit a predetermined degree of vulnerability that will make them more likely to demonstrate schizophrenic symptomatology. Whether the symptomatology is displayed is dependent upon environmental stress.

Our assessment program includes four major areas of measurement: (a) differential diagnosis and symptom measurement; (b) vulnerability or predisposition to schizophrenia; (c) life stress; and (d) moderating variables. To assist us in establishing a correct diagnosis, we use the Diagnostic Interview Schedule. The Diagnostic Interview Schedule is a highly structured interview that provides reliable and valid diagnoses for a variety of psychiatric disorders. In order to monitor the course of the disorder we use two rating scales: Brief Psychiatric Rating Scale and Target Symptom Ratings. Questions from the Present State Examination are used to collect information needed to rate each of the 21 dimensions on the Brief Psychiatric Rating Scale. Target Symptom Rating Scales are developed for individual patients by having their clinicians specify three schizophrenic symptoms that are characteristic of each patient.

Vulnerability is measured in a number of indirect ways. We try to determine, using a semistructured interview known as the FH-RDC, the existence of a family history positive for schizophrenia. A number of measures of our patients premorbid level of social adjustment are obtained, including the UCLA Social Attainment Survey, Phillip's Premorbid Adjustment Survey, and the Strauss-Carpenter Prognostic Scale.

Our primary measure of important life stressors is the Psychiatric Epidemiology Research Institute's Life Events Scale. We use several instruments to measure the amount of stress existing in a patient's family environment, including expressed emotion ratings based on the Camberwell Family Interview, affective style, problem-solving ability ratings derived from the Direct Family Interaction Test, and finally a measure of family knowledge regarding schizophrenia from the Family Knowledge Questionnaire. A number of moderating variables are also assessed, including the patient's socioeconomic status, social support network, and level of social competency.

Our inpatient unit is a moderately sized acute, general psychiatric unit, which treats a wide variety of psychiatric disorders. As a treatment unit it employs a biopsychosocial model, which recognizes that psychiatric disorders require attention to biological, psychological, and social factors. Unit structure and rules have been established such that they integrate both behavioral contingency systems and milieu principles of treatment. Step levels are employed on the unit, and patients are expected to progress through them as a means of preparation for discharge. At each step more is required from the patient, whereas more privileges are available. Each patient is assigned to a team and is a member of the patient government. Decisions such as who is assigned passes, advancement through step levels, and treatment care planning take place at both team and ward government meetings. Patients are regarded as active participants in their clinical care. We feel that the structure and philosophy of our inpatient unit are compatible with, and contribute to, the overall effectiveness of our two psychosocial programs for schizophrenia.

In one of our psychosocial programs (social and task-functional skills training), we focus on teaching patients how to cope with problematic social and life events. While in the other psychosocial program (behavioral family therapy), we teach skills to all of the family members with the intention of decreasing the amount of family stress.

Our social skills and task-functional skills training program is a response acquisition approach to treatment. The assumptive basis behind our skills program is that some minimal level of competency in social and task-functional situations is required for patients in order for them to function and remain in the community. Failure in these situations leads to interpersonal disharmony and psychological distress.

We explain to patients the diathesis–stress model of schizophrenia and underscore the importance of learning strategies for decreasing the stress level they experience. The intensive phase of our skills training program for our schizophrenic patients covers a period of 6 weeks. It is a group-based program with the group meeting twice a day (Monday through Friday) for 1 hour on each occasion. A training routine for each session follows a structured format including (a) a review of the previous session and the homework assignment issued at that session; (b) a didactic presentation of the day's lesson with its accompanying rationale; (c) videotape or live modeling of the major points of the lesson; (d) a discussion and some quizzing of the patients on the major points; (e) behavioral rehearsal and roleplaying; (f) both videotape and group members' feedback; (g) mastery of the lesson by repeated trials; and (h) practice assignments to promote transfer of learning.

We divide the contents of our skills program into three relatively arbitrary areas: (a) generic communication skills, which we feel have a wide range of applicability across situations (e.g., giving and receiving compliments, active listening skills, etc.); (b) general task-functional skills that are skills required in particular discrete situations (e.g., money management, use of leisure time, etc.); (c) individual task-functional skills that are skills required by some of our patients in particular types of situations (e.g., job-seeking and job-interviewing skills, etc.).

It should be noted that much more than discrete behavioral skills is taught as part of our skills program. Goals are established, social perception is taught, and cognitive assumptions and self-statements are labeled and modified. More than just discrete behaviors is taught. What is taught is the process of generating skillful behavior.

Our family program is based on the philosophy that families are major caregivers and should be perceived as allies in the treatment of schizophrenic patients. Our 12-session intensive program entails a family meeting weekly or twice a week and consists of three modules or components: (a) education (2 sessions); (b) communication (5 sessions); and (c) problem-solving (5 sessions). In the education model we try to inform families regarding what we know about schizophrenia and what we do not know about it. The diathesis–stress model of schizophrenia is presented to the family. The evidence for the genetic predisposition of schizophrenia is discussed. The role of neurotransmitters and the importance of neuroleptic medication are stressed. In addition, the schizophrenic patient is described as being very vulnerable to stress and that although the family did not cause the illness, it can protect the ill member by providing an interpersonal environment of low stress.

The communication skills training phase of our family program resembles our social skills training program. That is, the same training procedures and routines are used. Skills that are taught include listening skills, giving and receiving positive feedback, giving and receiving criticism, feeling talk, making a request, assertive behavior, and reciprocity of conversation. The problem-solving phase consists of six steps: (a) pinpoint and specify the problem; (b) develop several options or alternative responses; (c) evaluate each option in terms of its possible consequences; (d) choose option(s) that maximize(s) satisfaction and seem(s) reasonable; (e) plan out and implement that option (or those options) as a family; and (f) review the problem after the selected option has been implemented.

Our aftercare program is consistent with the intensive inpatient treatment. That is, the patient's skill trainer or family therapist also serves as therapist during this phase of the program. Aftercare visits are planned twice monthly for the first 2 months and then are faded to monthly visits thereafter. Unscheduled visits may be warranted and will be arranged as needed.

The chapter ends with two case illustrations. These cases are representative of our experience in treating our schizophrenic patients and illustrate the complexity in such treatment programs.

References

American Psychiatric Association. (1968). *Diagnostic and statistical manual of mental disorders* (2nd ed.). Washington, DC: Author.

American Psychiatric Association. (1980). *Diagnositic and statistical manual of mental disorders* (3rd ed.). Washington, DC: Author.

Anderson, C. (1983). A psychoeducational program for families of patients with schizophrenia. In W. R. McFarlane (Ed.), *Family therapy in schizophrenia* (pp. 99–116). New York: Guilford Press.

Andreasen, N. J. C., Endicott, J., Spitzer, R. L., & Winokur, G. (1974). The family history method using diagnostic criteria. *Archives of General Psychiatry, 34,* 1229–1235.

Anthony, W. A., Cohen, M. R., & Vitalo, R. (1978). The measurement of rehabilitation outcome. *Schizophrenia Bulletin, 4,* 365–383.

Atwood, N. (1983). Supportive group counseling for the relatives of schizophrenic patients. In W. A. McFarlane (Ed.), *Family therapy in schizophrenia* (pp. 189–205). New York: Guilford Press.

Brown, G. W., & Birley, J. L. T. (1968). Crises and life change and the onset of schizophrenia. *Journal of Health and Social Behavior, 9,* 203–214.

Brown, G. W., & Rutter, M. (1966). The measurement of family activities and relationships: A methodological study. *Human Relations, 19,* 241–263.

Brown, M. (1982). Maintenance and generalization issues in skills training with chronic schizophrenics. In J. P. Curran & P. M. Monti (Eds.), *Social skills training: A practical handbook for assessment and treatment* (pp. 90–116). New York: Guilford Press.

Curran, J. P. (1979). Pandora's box reopened? The assessment of social skills. *Journal of Behavioral Assessment, 1,* 55–71.

Curran, J. P. (1982). A procedure for the assessment of social skills: The simulated social interaction test. In J. P. Curran & P. M. Monti (Eds.), *Social skills training: A practical handbook for assessment and treatment.* New York: Guilford Press.

Day, R. (1981). Life events and schizophrenia: The "triggering" hypothesis. *Acta Psychiatrica Scandinavica, 26,* 97–126.

Doane, J. A., West, K. L., Goldstein, M. J., Rodnick, E. H., & Jones, J. E. (1981). Parental communication deviance and affective style. *Archives of General Psychiatry, 38,* 679–685.

Dohrenwend, B. S., Krasnoff, L., Askenasy, A. R., & Dohrenwend, B. P. (1978). Exemplification of a method for scaling life events: The PERI Life Events Scale. *Journal of Health and Social Behavior, 19,* 205–229.

Falloon, I. R. H., & Liberman, R. P. (1983). Behavioral family intervention in the management of chronic schizophrenia. In W. R. McFarlane (Ed.), *Family therapy in schizophrenia* (pp. 117–137). New York: Guilford Press.

Falloon, I. R. H., Boyd, J. G., McGill, C. W., Razani, J., Moss, H., & Gilderman, A. M. (1982). Family management in the prevention of exacerbation of schizophrenia. *The New England Journal of Medicine, 306,* 1437–1440.

Falloon, I. R. H., Doane, J. A., & Pederson, J. (in press). Family versus individual management in prevention of morbidity of schizophrenia: III. Family functioning. *Archives of General Psychiatry.*

Fischer, M., Harvald, B., & Hauge, M. A. (1969). Danish twin study of schizophrenia. *British Journal of Psychiatry, 115,* 981–990.

Gittelman-Klein, D. F. (1969). Premorbid asocial adjustment and prognosis in schizophrenia. *Journal of Psychiatric Research, 7,* 35–53.

Goldsmith, J. B., & McFall, R. M. (1975). Development and evaluation of an interpersonal skill training program for psychiatric inpatients. *Journal of Abnormal Psychology, 84,* 51–58.

Goldstein, M. J., Judd, L. J., Rodnick, E. J., & LaPolla, A. (1969). Psychophysiological and behavioral effects of phenothiazine administration in acute schizophrenics as a function of premorbid status. *Journal of Psychiatric Research, 6,* 271–287.

Goldstein, M. J., Rodnick, E. H., Evans, J. R., May, P. R. A., & Steinberg, M. R. (1975). Drug and family therapy in the aftercare of acute schizophrenics. *Archives of General Psychiatry, 35,* 1169–1175.

Gottesman, I. I., & Shields, J. (1972). *Schizophrenia and genetics: A twin study vantage point.* New York: Academic Press.

Hanson, D. R., Gottesman, I. I., & Meehl, P. E., (1977). Genetic theories and the validation of psychiatric diagnosis: Implications for the study of children of schizophrenics. *Journal of Abnormal Psychology, 86,* 575–588.

Harder, D. W., Gift, T. E., Strauss, J. S. Ritzler, B. A., & Kokes, R. F. (1981). Life events and two-year outcome in schizophrenia. *Journal of Consulting and Clinical Psychology, 49,* 619–626.

Harris, J. G. (1975). An abbreviated form of the Phillip Rating Scale of Premorbid Adjustment in Schizophrenia. *Journal of Abnormal Psychology, 84,* 129–137.

Hatfield, A. B. (1983). What families want of family therapist. In W. R. McFarlane (Ed.), *Family therapy in schizophrenia.* New York: Guilford Press.

Hawk, A. B., Carpenter, W. T., & Strauss, J. S. (1975). Diagnostic criteria and five-year outcome in schizophrenia: A report from the International Pilot Study of Schizophrenia. *Archives of General Psychiatry, 32,* 343–347.

Hedlund, J. L., & Vieweg, B. W. (1981). Structured psychiatric interviews: A comparative review. *Journal of Operational Psychiatry, 12,* 39–67.

Heston, L. L. (1966). Psychiatric disorders in foster home reared children of schizophrenic mothers. *British Journal of Psychiatry, 112,* 819–825.

Hogarty, G. E., Goldberg, S. C., Schooler, N. R., & the Collaborative Study Group. (1974). Drug and sociotherapy in the aftercare of schizophrenic patients: III. Adjustment of nonrelapsed patients. *Archives of General Psychiatry, 31,* 609–618.

Jacobsen, N. S., & Martin, B. (1976). Behavioral marriage therapy: Current status. *Psychological Bulletin, 83,* 540–556.

Kaplan, H. I. & Sadock, B. J. (1980) Neurophysiology of behavior. In H. I. Kaplan, A. M. Freedman, & B. J. Sadock (Eds.), *Comprehensive textbook of psychiatry* III. Baltimore: Williams & Wilkins.

Kendall, R. E. (1975). *The role of diagnosis in psychiatry.* London: Blackwell.

Kety, S. S., Rosenthal, D., Wender, P. H., Schulsinger, F., & Jacobsen, B. (1975). Mental illness in the biological and adoptive families of adopted individuals who have become schizophrenic: A preliminary report based on psychiatric interview. In R. R. Fieve, D. Rosenthal, & H. Brill (Eds.), *Genetic research in psychiatry.* Baltimore: John Hopkins University Press.

Kokes, R. F., Strauss, J. S., & Klorman, R. (1977). Premorbid adjustment in schizophrenia, Part II: Measuring premorbid adjustment, the instruments and their development. *Schizophrenia Bulletin, 3,* 186–213.

Kringlen, E. (1967, a). *Heredity and environment in the functional psychoses.* London: Heinemann.

Kringlen, E. (1967, b). Heredity and social factors in schizophrenic twins: An epidemiological-clinical study. In J. Roman (Ed.), *The origins of schizophrenia* (pp. 105–122). New York: Excerpta Medica Foundation.

Kringlen, E. (1968). An epidemiological-clinical twin study on schizophrenia. In D. Rosenthal & S. S. Kety (Eds.), *The transmission of schizophrenia* (pp. 49–64). New York: Pergamon.

Lin, N., Dean, A., & Ensel, W. M. (1981). Social support scales: A methodological note. *Schizophrenia Bulletin, 7,* 73–89.

Lowe, M. R., & Cautela, J. R. (1978). A self-report measure of social skill. *Behavior Therapy, 9,* 535–544.

May, P. R., & Simpson, G. M. (1980). Schizophrenia: Evaluation of treatment methods. In H. I. Kaplan, A. M. Freedman, & B. J. Sadock (Eds.), *Comprehensive textbook of psychiatry* III. Baltimore: Williams & Wilkins.

McFarlane, W. R. (Ed.). (1983). *Family therapy in schizophrenia.* New York: Guilford Press.

Meehl, P. E. (1972). Specific genetic etiology, psychodynamics, and therapeutic nihilism. *International Journal of Mental Health, 1,* 10–27.

Monti, P. M., Corriveau, D. C., & Curran, J. P. (1982). Social skills training for psychiatric patients: Treatment and outcome. In J. P. Curran & P. M. Monti (Eds.), *Social skills training: A practical handbook for assessment and treatment* (pp. 185–223). New York: Guilford Press.

Neale, J. M., & Oltmanns, T. J. (1980). *Schizophrenia.* New York: Wiley.

Neugebauer, R. (1983). Reliability of life-event interviews with outpatient schizophrenics. *Archives of General Psychiatry, 40,* 378–383.

Paul, G. L. (1969). Chronic mental patient: Current status—future directions. *Psychological Bulletin, 71,* 81–94.

Paul, G. L., & Lentz, R. J. (1977). *Psychosocial treatment of chronic mental patients: Milieu versus social-learning programs.* Cambridge: Harvard University Press.

Rainer, J. D. (1980). Genetics and psychiatry. In H. I. Kaplan, A. M. Freedman, & B. J. Sadock (Eds.), *Comprehensive textbook of psychiatry* III. Baltimore: Williams & Wilkins.

Robins, L. N., Helzer, J. E., Croughan, J., & Ratcliff, K. S. (1981). National Institute of Mental Health Diagnostic Interview Schedule: Its history, characteristics, and validity. *Archives of General Psychiatry, 38,* 381–389.

Rosenthal, D., Wender, P. H., Kety, S. S., Schulsinger, F., Welner, J., & Ostergaard, L. (1968). Schizophrenics' offspring reared in adoptive homes. In D. Rosenthal & S. S. Kety (Eds.), *The transmission of schizophrenia* (pp. 377–392). New York: Pergamon Press.

Rosenthal, D., Wender, P. H., Kety, S. S., Welner, J., & Schulsinger, F. (1971). The adopted away offspring of schizophrenics. *American Journal of Psychiatry, 128,* 307–311.

Singer, M. T., & Wynne, L. C. (1966). Communication styles in parents of normals, neurotics, and schizophrenics. *Psychiatric Research Reports, 20,* 25–38.

Stoffelmayr, B. E., Dillavou, D., & Hunter, J. E. (1983). Premorbid functioning and outcome in schizophrenia: A cumulative analysis. *Journal of Consulting and Clinical Psychology, 51,* 338–352.

Strauss, J. S., & Carpenter, W. T. (1972). The prediction of outcome in schizophrenia: I. Characteristics of outcome. *Archives of General Psychiatry, 27,* 739–746.

Strauss, J. S., & Carpenter, W. T. (1974). Characteristic symptoms and outcome in schizophrenia. *Archives of General Psychiatry, 30,* 429–434.

Trower, P. (1982). Toward a generative model of social skills: A critique and synthesis. In J. P. Curran & P. M. Monti (Eds.), *Social skills training: A practical handbook for assessment and treatment.* New York: Guilford Press.

Valone, K. (1983). *UCLA family assessment procedures.* Los Angeles: UCLA Family Project.

Valone, K., Norton, J. P., Goldstein, M. J., & Doane, J. A. (in press). Parental expressed emotion and affective style in an adolescent sample at risk for schizophrenia spectrum disorders. *Journal of Abnormal Psychology.*

Van Putten, T., & May, P. R. A. (1978). Akinetic depression in schizophrenia. *Archives of General Psychiatry, 35,* 1101–1107.

Vaughn, C. E., & Leff, J. P. (1976). The influence of family and social factors on the course of psychiatric illness: A comparison of schizophrenic and depressed neurotic patients. *British Journal of Psychiatry, 129,* 125–137.

Vaughn, C. E., Snyder, K. S., Freeman, W., Jones, S., Falloon, I. R. H., & Liberman, R. P. (1982). Family factors in schizophrenic relapse: A replication. *Schizophrenia Bulletin, 8,* 425–426.

Wender, P. H. (1974). Crossfostering: A research strategy for clarifying the role of genetic and experiential factors in the etiology of schizophrenia. *Archives of General Psychiatry, 30,* 121–128.

Zerbin-Rudin, E. (1972). Genetic research and the theory of schizophrenia. *International Journal of Mental Health, 1,* 42–62.

Zubin, J., & Steinhauer, S. (1982). How to break the logjam in schizophrenia: A look beyond genetics. *Journal of Nervous and Mental Disease, 169,* 477–492.

Outpatient Treatment of Schizophrenics
Social Skills and Problem-Solving Training

JEFFREY A. KELLY AND DANUTA M. LAMPARSKI

Introduction

In the United States, over 1% of the population carries a diagnosis of schizophrenia. Schizophrenics occupy one-third to one-half of all psychiatric hospital beds (Goodwin & Guze, 1979), and compared to other psychiatric patients, require longer inpatient treatment, show lower levels of adjustment following discharge, and return more frequently to the hospital.

The diagnosis of schizophrenia implies a distinct deterioration from previous levels of day-to-day functioning. It is characterized by a variety of behavioral excesses and deficits. There may be disruption in nearly all aspects of functioning including overt behavior, thought processes, affect, and perception. Schizophrenics may manifest bizarre, stereotypic motor behaviors such as rigidity, postures, and grimaces. Disordered thinking may be evident in loosening of associations, neologisms, and blocking. Delusions, usually involving persecution or control by an external agent, are commonly found. Affective responding tends to be expressionless (flat) or markedly inappropriate to the ongoing interpersonal context. Sensory faculties may also be affected, as evidenced by auditory, visual, olfactory, or haptic hallucinations.

To date, no single pathognomonic explanation of schizophrenia has been

---

JEFFREY A. KELLY and DANUTA M. LAMPARSKI • Department of Psychiatry, University of Mississippi Medical Center, 2500 North State Street, Jackson, Mississippi 39216.

established. The most widely accepted theories assume that some combination of organic and psychosocial factors account for the development of the disorder. Studies of risk rates in twins have shown higher rates of schizophrenia in identical as compared to nonidentical twins (Allen, Cohen, & Pollin, 1972; Fischer 1971; Gottesman & Shields, 1966), providing support for a genetic vulnerability, and current research focuses specifically on a neurotransmitter-biochemical basis for the disorder. Psychosocial factors usually postulated include (a) exposure to stress (defined in various ways such as adverse life events), along with (b) an inability to adequately cope with stressors.

In the past, the accepted treatment for schizophrenia was long-term institutionalization, often spanning a period of many years. However, extended hospitalization fosters what is known as the *institutional syndrome* (Barton, 1966; Gruenberg, 1967; Hansell & Bensen, 1971); as a result of the schizophrenic disease process, poor premorbid adjustment and dependence tolerated within the institutional milieu, patients become apathetic and appear unable to initiate goal-directed behavior. As the length of hospitalization increases, the likelihood of release from an institution decreases (Paul, 1969). In time, some patients actually prefer continued hospitalization over discharge (Wing, 1962).

Over the last two decades, however, the care of chronic schizophrenics has changed dramatically. More and more, community-based outpatient facilities, rather than long-term institutions, provide treatment to the chronically ill individual. A number of factors have contributed to this change, including the discovery of phenothiazines, the advent of community mental health centers, and legislation upholding the civil rights of psychiatric patients. Phenothiazines, which often control elements of overt psychosis including hallucinations, delusions, and agitation, revolutionized the treatment of schizophrenics. With the period of acute psychosis made more brief with medication, patients now tend to be discharged from hospitals relatively quickly. A series of court decisions upholding the rights of psychiatric patients for humane treatment have also facilitated outpatient treatment of schizophrenics. Lawmakers have increasingly invoked the "principle of the least restrictive alternative" in setting guidelines for patient care. Consequently, many state statutes (a) specify the circumstances under which an individual can be committed; (b) place limits on the length of time the courts can order inpatient or outpatient treatment; and (c) insist that courts examine alternatives to long-term hospitalization prior to commitment (Chambers, 1975).

Although biochemical intervention ameliorated many of the behavioral excesses of schizophrenics, such as hallucinations, delusions, and bizarre gestures, it did little to improve the quality of life of many patients. Adjustment still remains poor for many schizophrenics following discharge from the hospital. Some patients leave institutions for boarding houses or nursing homes where the institutional syndrome is perpetuated, whereas others exhibit interpersonal deficits and poor problem-solving skills that impair their quality of life. Medication often has little effect on the behavioral deficits and inadequate coping skills that preceded the disease, that contributed to its onset, or that remain even following the alleviation of overt psychotic behaviors. With the advent of community health centers and the recent movement toward deinstitutionalization, the primary focus in treatment of chronic schizophrenics has shifted from custodial care to rehabilitation and reintegration within the community. As a result, behavioral techniques designed to remediate the deficits of schizophrenic outpatients are now being developed.

Assessment Procedures

One of the major differences between schizophrenia and most other disorders involves the sheer diversity and pervasiveness of problems experienced by the schizophrenic individual. Persons with depressive disorders require, logically, treatment of their depression; individuals with anxiety disorders require treatment of anxiety. In each of these cases, intervention is targeted toward some set of fairly clear problem behaviors (depression or anxiety) whose presence essentially defines the presence of the disorder and whose absence signals that the disorder has been effectively treated.

In contrast, the schizophrenic individual often exhibits a wide range of impairments in effective functioning, and there is frequently no single problem behavior that can be isolated as the sole target for intervention. Some schizophrenic patients seen in outpatient settings exhibit extreme impoverishment of their social-interpersonal skills, whereas others are highly deficient in the skills needed to solve everyday living problems effectively. Some schizophrenic individuals exhibit excessive and frequent sensory or cognitive disturbances in the form of hallucinations or delusions. Others, characterized by insufficient behavioral activity or withdrawal, say and do very little. Many schizophrenics have severe problems in several of these areas. Our point here is that the diagnosis *per se* of an individual as *schizophrenic* provides relatively little information about the specific problems that the person is experiencing and about the type of behavioral treatment intervention that will be most useful for him or her. Clearly, the first step in behaviorally treating the schizophrenic individual seen in an outpatient setting is identifying those aspects of his or her behavior that will require treatment.

An assessment approach that seems well suited for identifying intervention targets for schizophrenic patients seen in outpatient settings involves evaluating an individual's competence in those skill areas necessary for effective, independent functioning in the community. If one can identify the skills critical to successful community living, it should be possible to teach those competencies to skill-deficient patients and thereby reduce their likelihood of needing rehospitalization. Moreover, within the community, schizophrenic individuals with well-refined skills for effective functioning should be able to achieve a better quality of life than persons who lack these competencies.

What Are "Community Living Skills?"

When treating a schizophrenic individual in an outpatient setting of some kind—be it a mental health center, a hospital outpatient clinic, or a similar facility—the therapist begins behavioral assessment by attempting to determine those skill deficits and/or behavior excesses that contribute to the person's difficulties in successful functioning. Although the problems and difficulties of schizophrenic individuals are just as diverse as the problems experienced by the rest of the population, several types of difficulties commonly found in patients with this disorder have received special attention in the behavior therapy literature.

Social Skill Deficits

Social skills refer to the interpersonal competencies needed to interact successfully with other people. Bellack and Hersen (1978) have observed that in spite of the many different theories about the causes of schizophrenia, one area of agreement among almost all clinicians is that schizophrenics exhibit deficits in their abilities to interact skillfully with others in social settings. In particular, such difficulties as extreme passivity and lack of assertiveness (Bellack & Hersen, 1978; Hersen & Bellack, 1976) and deficient conversational skills (Kelly, Urey, & Patterson, 1980; Urey, Laughlin, & Kelly, 1979) are problem areas for many schizophrenic individuals. Social skill deficits are often targeted for behavioral intervention with this clinical population because poor interpersonal competence can impair the individual's ability to establish relationships and social supports with others, can give the person the appearance of a "former psychiatric patient," and can otherwise interfere with normal community functioning.

Problem-Solving Skill Deficits

Successful independent living requires that one be able to recognize and appropriately solve everyday problems. Making decisions and arriving at workable solutions to problems that one encounters ("My car won't start; what should I do now?" "The SSI check is a week overdue and I'm out of money," or "My medication is gone and I don't remember my clinic doctor's name") are important competencies that many schizophrenic individuals lack. In some cases, problem-solving skill deficits may be traceable to having lived in "total care" institutions that promoted excessively dependent behavior. In other cases, poor problem-solving judgment seems to be a characteristic of the schizophrenic disorder itself. Regardless of its origins, the inability to identify and follow through on appropriate solutions to everyday problems is a competence deficit that, if present, merits treatment intervention by a therapist.

The treatment of social skill deficits and problem-solving skill difficulties are certainly not the only areas that can be addressed by behavior therapists working with schizophrenic outpatients. Behavioral techniques have also been successfully applied to many other problems encountered by schizophrenics. Moreover, the fact that an individual is schizophrenic does not preclude that person from having difficulties in other areas; schizophrenics can, and sometimes do, have such problems as substance abuse, anxiety, sexual dysfunction, depression, marital conflict, and other difficulties that can benefit from behavior therapy intervention. However, in the balance of this chapter, we will focus on the assessment and treatment of social and problem-solving skill deficits in schizophrenic outpatients. These deficits will be addressed in detail here because they represent problems experienced by a significant number of severely disturbed individuals and because relatively well-developed treatment techniques exist for each problem.

Assessment of Skill Deficits

In clinical outpatient practice, we are usually consulted by someone with a complaint of a problem for which she or he seeks treatment. Sometimes, schizophrenic outpatients do seek treatment for social or problem-solving skill inadequacies. In our experience, however, these kinds of problems often seem to be noticed more quickly by someone *other than* the client. For example, treatment of a schizophrenic's social skill problems is frequently originated because the therapist or someone else observes the extreme passivity, dullness, or idiosyncratic nature of the individual's social interactions. Identification of problem-solving skill deficits as an intervention target may occur, not because the client directly asks for help in this area but because the therapist sees evidence (such as inadequate handling of everyday problems) that treatment is needed. In such cases, it is important to explain carefully to the client why assessment and treatment are needed, what benefits will accrue from successful intervention (e.g., the client will learn skills needed to meet people more easily and come across better to others), and to interest the client in the planned intervention.

Assessment of a client's social and problem-solving skills always makes use of behavior sampling procedures. The purposes of behavior sampling are to objectively evaluate the client's current competence in the skill area and to pinpoint those specific aspects of his or her performance that will require intervention. We will now review how the clinician can construct behavior sample assessments of social and problem-solving skills.

Behavioral Assessment of Social Skill

Under the most ideal circumstances, a therapist might be able to follow a client about, carefully observing how that client behaves with others across a variety of everyday social interactions. The therapist could see how the individual actually handles situations that call for the expression of opinions, views, or disagreeing comments ("assertiveness"); how the client behaves in everyday conversations with others ("conversational skill"); how she or he handles conversational encounters with persons of the opposite sex ("heterosocial skill"); or how the person behaves even in very specialized social interactions, such as job interviews. If the therapist could observe the client's day-to-day social interactions firsthand, it would be possible to determine not only what *kinds* of interactions are troublesome, but also the specific social behaviors of the client in those situations.

It is not usually feasible for the therapist to conduct this sort of exhaustive, surreptitious, *in vivo* observation of client behavior. It is, however, possible to construct simulated or sample social interaction tasks and to evaluate client social skill in these simulations. If the social interaction tasks are sufficiently similar to the naturalistic interactions that cause difficulties for the client, performance in these tasks can provide useful information about the individual's skill and can help to target skill elements that will require treatment attention.

Roleplays are the most commonly used interaction tasks for assessing social skill. In roleplay assessments, a client is asked to interact with another person (typically a therapist confederate) and to behave just as she or he would if the roleplay situation were, in fact, real. The situations roleplayed depend on the type of skill being assessed. For example, to evaluate a client's skill in refusal assertiveness, the therapist might narrate the background for a situation in which someone is trying to take advantage of the client:

THERAPIST: In the group home where you live, your roommate plays her radio quite loudly, even very late at night. You are tired and want to sleep. She says to you:
ROLEPLAY PARTNER: I love this music, don't you?

The client then roleplays with the partner how she or he would handle the situation described in the vignette, and the therapist observes the skill quality of the client's responses. Ordinarily, a number of different scenes are roleplayed in a single assessment session.

Although roleplays are used to evaluate assertiveness, they can also be tailored to other kinds of social skills. For example, if a therapist wishes to assess a client's conversational skill, the client might be asked to converse with a partner for some period of time (e.g., 5 or 10 minutes). Depending on the purpose of the assessment, the client could be told merely to get to know the other person better or, alternatively, could be given a specific purpose for the conversation (e.g., to talk with the opposite-sex partner and conclude the conversation by asking for a date, if the therapist wishes to specifically assess heterosocial/date initiation skill). These procedures have been used to evaluate the social skill of chronic schizophrenics who have difficulties conversing appropriately with other people in the community (Kelly, 1982; Kelly *et al.*, 1980; Urey *et al.*, 1979). Roleplays have also been used to assess the job interview social skill of psychiatric patients completing vocational rehabilitation (Kelly, Laughlin, Claiborne, & Patterson, 1979). Here, a partner plays the part of a job interviewer, and the client plays the part of an applicant; the therapist, by observing how the client handles standard job interview questions, is able to determine whether the client will need social skills training in order to successfully compete for employment openings in the community.

Roleplay procedures, then, can be employed by the clinician to evaluate client social skill in a variety of areas; the type of roleplay situations used are determined by the type of skill that the therapist wishes to assess. Clearly, however, any roleplay assessments of social skill will be useful only if the client behaves in the roleplay much like she or he would in the same situation occurring *in vivo*. Because several studies (Bellack, Hersen, & Lamparski, 1979) have found that client behavior in assessment roleplays may not correspond to behavior in the natural environment, the therapist should take steps to ensure that roleplays yield valid data on client skill. We have found the following procedures to be useful in securing valid assessment information: *(a) Roleplayed situations should be relevant for the client being evaluated.* If the therapist learns, through interviews or direct observation of client behavior, that the individual encounters difficulties in a number of specific social situations, roleplay approximations of *those* situations should be developed for behavioral assessment purposes. Whenever possible, assessment roleplays should be tailored to the individual client, should reflect situations in which she or he has actual difficulty, and should be based on data obtained from careful interviews with the client or with persons who observe the client's social interaction problems. *(b) Extended roleplay interactions, rather than brief and structured roleplays, may yield a more comprehensive behavior sample.* Real-life social interactions are not always highly structured, predictable, and brief. In order to be realistic and comprehensive, role-played approximations of real-life interactions may also need to be extended inter-actions. Thus, if we wanted to evaluate client conversational or assertive skill, we might have a client interact with a roleplay partner who makes many different com-ments to the client, rather than offering just a single "prompt" or line to which the client responds. So much as possible, roleplays should closely simulate (in nar-rative backdrop, in partner comments, in duration, and in affective tone) the sit-uations that are actually troublesome for the client.

When the client engages in roleplay assessment interactions, it is necessary for the therapist to closely evaluate the quality of his or her performance. As we have noted elsewhere (Christoff & Kelly, in press; Kelly, 1982), the therapist seeks to determine what elements (or "components") set the client's behavior apart from an ideal, socially skilled handling of the situation(s) being roleplayed and, there-fore, what skill aspects will be the focus of intervention. At this point, the therapist should be asking questions such as these: Is my client handling the roleplayed sit-uation in the best possible manner? If not, what specific verbal, nonverbal, or sty-listic elements are problematic? If those elements were remediated during training, would the client then be seen as more socially skillful?

A detailed discussion of all the specific behavioral elements that comprise social skill is beyond the scope of this chapter. Readers might wish to consult a social skills training resource (cf. Bellack & Hersen, 1979; Kelly, 1982) for discus-sion, definitions, and rating procedures of behaviors that comprise social skill. However, therapists will generally examine three aspects of a client's handling of roleplayed situations. *Verbal skill components* refer to the verbal content of the indi-vidual's roleplayed performance. The therapist here considers whether the client is saying those things that are appropriate, socially skilled, and likely to lead to a favorable social outcome in the situation being enacted. *Nonverbal components* include such behaviors as eye contact, voice tone and clarity, posture, gestures, the presence or absence of smiles and appropriate affect, and so forth. *Interaction style* elements refer to the way in which the individual integrates, times, and paces behavior during the roleplay. As one example, in a roleplayed conversation, we would expect to find a client asking open-ended questions to the partner (a verbal element), doing so with warm, friendly affect if the situation was positive in nature (a nonverbal element), but asking questions in a reciprocal manner with the part-ner rather than "shotgunning" many unrelated questions repetitively (a stylistic skill aspect). In a later section of this chapter, we will present a case study that illustrates this rating procedure in more detail.

Because the clinical task of the therapist is to identify all of those verbal, nonverbal, and stylistic elements that keep a client's roleplay performance from being ideal, it is often useful to videotape (or, less preferrably, audiotape) all assessment roleplays. This affords two advantages: first, the therapist can review and study the client's performance from a recording to better pinpoint skill components that will need to be trained; and, second, recorded assessment roleplays can be compared with roleplays following treatment to pinpoint areas where change occurred.

To summarize, clinical assessment of social skills usually relies on behavior samples (roleplays) of the client's handling social interactions that appear to be problematic for him or her. The therapist's task is to carefully observe the performance of the client and identify any verbal, nonverbal, or stylistic elements that cause him or her to handle the enacted situations poorly. Those deficient elements will become the targets for subsequent social skills training.

Behavioral Assessment of Problem-Solving Skill

When a social skills training intervention is planned, we have seen that assessment focuses on the client's handling of social interactions. In the case of problem-solving skill deficits of schizophrenic outpatients, the therapist will again use a sample of the client's skill behavior to pinpoint problem-solving inadequacies and target them for later training.

D'Zurilla and Goldfried (1971), as well as Shure, Spivack and their colleagues (Platt & Spivack, 1972; Siegel & Spivack, 1976; Spivack & Shure, 1974) conceptualize effective problem-solving as a process consisting of several identifiable steps. They include the following components:

1. *Identification of a Situation as a Problem.* Some low-functioning individuals do not appear to effectively recognize situations as problematic and, therefore, as requiring a solution. Consequently, learning to discriminate problem from nonproblem situations is a basic initial step in developing solutions.
2. *Generating Multiple Possible Courses of Action.* A second step in effective problem solving is being able to identify a range of potential solutions. Sometimes termed *brainstorming,* this involves simply generating many (or all) possible courses of action without regard to the probable success of each.
3. *Evaluating courses of action* takes place after a range of potential solutions have been generated; here, each potential solution is evaluated in terms of its consequence (e.g., its likelihood of solving the problem), and the best course of action is selected.
4. *Implementing the best solution* is the final step of the problem-solving process. At this point, the individual follows through on the selected course of action or demonstrates that she or he has the skills to follow through on its implementation.

As we suggested earlier, the need to teach problem-solving skills to a schizophrenic outpatient is clinically evident when the person uses "bad judgment" or becomes overwhelmed and unable to decide how to handle certain life problems.

In order to assess the nature of a client's problem-solving deficits, it is helpful to construct scenarios of everyday problem situations that the client will need to handle effectively but presently deals with ineffectively. As one example, let us suppose that a schizophrenic outpatient requiring prescribed psychotropic medication repeatedly allows his or her medication supply to run out. When this occurs, the individual becomes psychotic and at risk for hospitalization. If we conceptualize this difficulty as due to a problem-solving deficit (e.g., not knowing what to do when the medication supply first becomes low), it is possible to develop a scenario to behaviorally test the client's problem-solving skill in the situation.

Platt and Spivack (1975) have described what they term *The Means–End Problem Solving* (MEPS) test for evaluating problem-solving skill. MEPS assessment scenarios begin with a description of the client in the problem situation and end with the problem resolved satisfactorily. The client is asked to tell what needs to happen (e.g., what she or he could do) to bring about that satisfactory conclusion. A MEPS-format scenario of the previously described problem could be constructed as follows:

> It has been 2 months since you got your medication prescription. You notice one morning that the vial has only a few tablets left inside it. You know that you must take your medicine every day. The way the story ends is with you again having a vial filled with your medication. Tell me exactly what you would need to do in order to bring about this end of the story.

The situations used to construct MEPS assessment scenarios can be derived from a variety of sources, including the client's self-reports of situations she or he finds difficult; reports made by "significant others" (family, group home supervisors, aftercare program staff) who see the client's community behavior firsthand; and by the therapist, who may simply wish to evaluate how well a client can handle problems likely to arise in everyday community living. Assessment could be of a single situation, with a single MEPS response evaluated and later trained. However, it is more comprehensive to develop a battery of different scenarios in order to tap the client's skill for handling a variety of problem situations.

Clients can be directed to provide their solutions to each problem vignette by writing how they would handle the situation, or they can verbally and orally describe the proposed solution. Although much of the research literature makes use of written solutions, we find it more feasible for low-functioning clients to give their solutions orally. The therapist, for each scenario, transcribes the client's full response or tape records it for later transcription.

Just as social skill roleplays are scrutinized by the therapist to determine the adequacy of the client's performance, the proposed solution to each MEPS scenario is also rated for the presence or absence of problem-solving skill elements. Although investigators differ somewhat in how they rate problem-solving vignettes, the following components are usually assessed in the client response to each vignette: (a) *number of steps,* defined as the number of different behavioral actions the person would take to bring about the end; "I would call my doctor" (1 step); "I would look up the clinic's phone number, call it, ask to speak to my doctor, and tell him I am almost out of medicine" (4 steps); (b) *number of obstacles,* with an obstacle being rated whenever the client mentions something that would thwart his or her plan and how he or she would overcome it; *(c) number of means,* which can be defined as the number of different *types* of strategies the client might follow to bring about the solution ("I'd call the drugstore first to see if they can refill the prescription. If they couldn't, I'd call the doctor" would be two means); and *(d) overall effectiveness,* which is a judgment, often made on a numeric scale (1 = poor to 5 = good), reflecting the overall success probability of the client's total solution.

In problem-solving research, investigators normally assign two scores to the client's response to each scenario; a first score reflects the sum of all steps, obstacles, and means included in the story, whereas a second score reflects the story's overall effectiveness judgment. Higher sum scores, accompanied by high effectiveness ratings, are taken to indicate problem-solving skill because the client would then be describing multiple pathways and many elaborated steps for problem resolution in each response. In clinical assessment of a client's skill, it is also useful to rate client responses quantitatively, counting all steps, means, obstacles, and assigning an overall effectiveness rating. By doing so, the therapist will be better able to identify the client's problem-solving deficits and will be able to quantitatively determine change as a result of later treatment.

Treatment Techniques

As we noted earlier in the chapter, both social competence and problem-solving competence can be conceptualized as "skills," or learned behaviors. The aim of training in these areas is to increase the client's behavioral repertoire for handling interpersonal situations (in social skills training) or the client's cognitive-behavioral problem resolution skills (in problem-solving training). Regardless of which type of intervention is planned, the same general principles guide treatment. These principles include *instruction, modeling, behavior rehearsal,* and *feedback/reinforcement/shaping.*

Early clinical research on social skills training attempted to determine which of these treatment elements is most crucial to skill acquisition. Although intervention based, for example, on the modeling of correct skill alone results in some improvement in the client's social skills (Edelstein & Eisler, 1976), it appears that the most potent clinical interventions incorporate all of these principles in training sessions (Kelly, 1982). Later in the chapter, we will present a clinical treatment case in some detail. For now, let us consider the general ways that treatment sessions are conducted in both social skills and problem-solving skills training interventions. Special treatment variations that are especially important when working with low-functioning persons will be stressed.

Social Skills Training Techniques

Following behavioral assessment of a client's social skills in the manner described in the previous section, the therapist should have a relatively clear idea of (a) the type of skill area where training is needed (e.g., assertiveness, conversational, heterosocial, job interview, or some other skill); and (b) the nature of the client's present verbal, nonverbal, and stylistic deficits, as observed in assessment roleplays. The deficits observed in the client's assessment interactions ordinarily become the specific targets for attention in training sessions.

Skills training with schizophrenic outpatients is usually conducted over a number of treatment sessions; depending on the pervasiveness of the client's social deficits and his or her speed in mastering new skills, intervention of 10 to 20 or more sessions may be needed (Kelly, 1982). In clinical interventions, the format of each training session is relatively constant, although the skill behaviors targeted for treatment do change over the course of the intervention. For example, with a conversationally deficient client, one set of sessions could be targeted toward helping the person learn to ask and answer conversational questions appropriately. Another set of sessions might cover those topics appropriate to converse about with other people. Then, when these verbal skills are mastered, attention in yet another set of sessions might be directed toward improving the client's affective tone (e.g., making eye contact, smiling, and "sounding" friendly and animated). Exactly how many different skill aspects (or "components") will be covered in an intervention depends on how many behavioral deficits were observed in the client's initial assessment roleplays. However, because skill aspects receive attention sequentially and cumulatively across the intervention, by the end of the training program the client should have improved in all aspects of conversational skill that had been deficient previously.

Each training session begins with the therapist introducing the skill aspect being covered that day, instructing the client in its use, and discussing with the client its rationale. Modeling the skill behavior for the client can take place if the therapist demonstrates examples of the skill behavior, "shows" the client how to exhibit the behavior, or plays a videotape of a skillful interaction with correct use of the skill modeled in the film. Next, an opportunity for client behavior rehearsal should be staged. Rehearsal usually consists of repeating roleplayed interactions similar to those used during the initial assessment phase (e.g., having the client roleplay a simulated conversation or some other interaction), but at this point asking the client to incorporate the trained skill behaviors in his or her performance. The therapist observes the client's roleplay and provides feedback, reinforcement, and corrective instruction in order to further shape the client's skill. Sessions focusing on a skill behavior continue until that aspect of the client's performance is no longer deficient; then, some other aspect of the social skill is targeted for treatment attention. As we noted, if the therapist accurately identifies all skill behaviors that had been deficient and if the intervention successfully treats each of them, the client should be capable of skillful roleplay interactions by the conclusion of treatment.

The training model described here is that usually employed in social skills training with low-functioning populations. However, there are several additional factors that must be taken into account if treatment is to be successful. These include (a) *training social style skills* and (b) *promoting skill generalization to the natural environment.*

Teaching Elements of Social Style

Traditionally, social skills interventions with lower functioning clients have relied on teaching discrete, "molecular" aspects of competence. For example, when confronted by an antagonist trying to take advantage of them, unassertive psychiatric patients might be taught to speak clearly, maintain eye contact, refuse the antagonist's unreasonable behavior, and request that the antagonist refrain from causing problems (Eisler, Miller, & Hersen, 1973). Conversationally deficient patients are often taught to engage in such behaviors as asking open-ended questions, talking about appropriate and socially acceptable topics of conversation, smiling, conveying warm affect, and so on (Kelly *et al.*, 1980).

Implicit here is the notion that if a client can be taught to do the "right things," she or he will come across to others as more skillful in social interactions. *Things* are traditionally defined as individual, discrete verbal and nonverbal social behaviors. However, handling a conversation skillfully (or being assertive, initiating dating interactions, or interviewing for a job) requies more than exhibiting correct verbal and nonverbal behaviors. It is also necessary to pace, style, and integrate them correctly if one is to appear socially skilled. For this reason, and as investigators like McFall (1982) have stressed, it is important that the therapist attend to more global aspects of a client's skill when practicing skill behaviors in the treatment setting. Among the questions of social style to which therapists should attend are the following: Is my client's overall social pacing smooth and approprate? Do topics of conversation relate smoothly with one another, or are there abrupt shifts in topics? Do nonverbal skills, such as affective tone or smiles, occur in temporal conjunction with the appropriate verbal comments of the client? Do my client's comments follow logically from the roleplay partner's comments? And, does my client's performance seem, globally and subjectively, skillful?

Perhaps more than high-functioning individuals, we have found that schizophrenic outpatients often lack the ability to smoothly integrate elements of social competence and to follow the often subtle "rules" governing social interaction skill (such as not smiling at the wrong points in a conversation, "shotgunning" questions during conversations, or failing to smoothly integrate their comments with those of the person with whom they are talking). To the extent that such stylistic idiosyncracies are observed, they also require attention in training.

Promoting Social Skills Generalization

Social skills training is usually conducted in a clinic setting of some kind but is intended to change the client's behavior during social interactions occurring in the natural environment. Therefore, a fundamental question of clinical importance is whether improvements shown during practice roleplays will actually generalize to the corresponding interactions in the "real" world. Unfortunately, most data seem to indicate that generalization will not occur unless it is specifically planned.

There are a number of steps that a therapist can take to help promote a client's *in vivo* use of trained social skills. These include attention to the following:

1. *Does the client have ample opportunities to practice newly trained social skills?* If the schizophrenic individual is socially isolated, it may be necessary to plan increased opportunities to interact with others socially in order for skills to be used.
2. *Can the client discriminate situations when it is appropriate to use newly learned skills?* Clients may require specific training that will assist them in identifying situations where they should (or should not) initiate conversations, be forcefully assertive, initiate dates, and so on.
3. *"Homework" assignments to practice skill use* in vivo *should be included in training.* Once a client has become proficient in a social skill area, explicit assignments to practice the skill can be made and reviewed.
4. *Efforts to reinforce skilled handling of problematic interactions should be included in the intervention.* The therapist can reinforce client reports of *in vivo* skill use. By making "significant others" in the client's environment (such as family members, roommates, or halfway house staff) aware of the areas covered in training, it may well be possible for them to also reinforce social skill improvement shown by the client.

Problem-Solving Training Techniques

Just as an intervention "package" of instruction—modeling, behavior rehearsal, and shaping—is used to improve a schizophrenic outpatient's social skills, the same treatment principles can be applied to problem-solving deficits. In social skills training, assessment roleplays are used to pinpoint the individual's social skill deficits and later serve as a vehicle for behavioral practice in training sessions. In problem-solving training, MEPS problem scenarios are used in analogous fashion.

It will be recalled that each assessment scenario is ordinarily scored by the therapist to determine the number of verbalized problem-solving steps described, obstacles overcome, and solution means employed as well as the overall judged effectiveness of the complete solution. When a client is deficient in any of these skill aspects, training attention is warranted. Once again, the number of training sessions that will be needed depends on the pervasiveness of the client's problem-solving skill deficits and his or her rate of skill improvement over time.

Initially, it is wise to spend session time discussing with the client when some situation in fact represents a problem that requires solution; some investigators (Siegel & Spivack, 1976) have noted that schizophrenics have difficulty discriminating situations as problematic. This can be accomplished by asking the client to describe, for each scenario used in the assessment, the consequences that would result if no steps were taken to solve the problem. The therapist may need to help the client see that she or he would suffer some loss, inconvenience, or negative outcome in each of the situations if action were not taken.

Problem-solving training itself begins by selecting one of the MEPS scenarios for intensive training attention. Earlier in this chapter, we used as a problem example a situation in which the patient is running low on his or her prescribed medication. The MEPS scenario targeted for initial training should be read aloud to the client, but now instruction in basic problem-solving is also introduced. For example, after presenting the scenario, the therapist might say:

> The best way to reach a solution to a problem is by thinking of *all* the different things you might do in the situation, regardless of how workable they seem to you. Don't just get locked into one solution. . . . Tell me a *number* of different things you might do to solve the problem of having your medication run low, even if some of them seem to be silly or extreme.

If the client is able to provide several different alternatives, she or he should be praised by the therapist. However, in our experience, many schizophrenics are not able to verbalize multiple solution strategies with instruction alone. Therapist modeling may also be needed.

The therapist can model the solution-generation phase of problem solving by doing the same task just asked of the patient. Thus, for a patient unable to verbalize solution means in the medication situation, the therapist could say:

> Let's see. The first thing I would do is call the clinic where I see my doctor. I'd look up the number in the phone book, call, and tell them that my prescription supply is running down. Another thing I could do is go to the drugstore where I got the prescription filled and see if they can refill it. I guess something else I could do is just let the medicine run out and get more whenever I go back to the clinic.

In this modeled response, the therapist is verbalizing several different solution means (calling the clinic, calling the pharmacy, or allowing the medication to run out) as well as several steps to accomplish them. When the client understands the notion of describing multiple solutions, she or he then practices responses to the same or some related scenario.

It is important for clients to elaborate the individual steps needed to accomplish each potential solution mean; otherwise, the individual might identify a correct goal (e.g., "I'd get more medication from my doctor") but not, in fact, know how to bring about that end. Consequently, the patient should be reminded and prompted to elaborate responses fully, explaining exactly how each would be implemented (e.g., "I'd get the phone book, look up the number of the mental health center, call it, and tell the doctor I was almost out of my medicine").

Effective problem solving requires more than just verbalizing all of the things one might do to handle the problematic situation; it is then necessary to anticipate the outcome of each potential solution and, from this outcome anticipation, select the one alternative that would best resolve the problem and be feasible to implement. The therapist can instruct and model this evaluation process as well.

> If I were to let my medicine run out and if I got more whenever I went to the clinic, I might get sick because I don't go there very often. That wouldn't be good. I could check at the pharmacy where I got the medicine, but I don't think I get refills of it without a prescription. So, the best solution is for me to call the doctor at the clinic right away and explain the situation to him.

Following one or more modeling exposures, the client should then attempt to evaluate all of the potential solutions to the problem presented in the training scenario. At this point, the therapist provides prompts, suggestions, and feedback until the client arrives at a feasible, effective solution to the problem. Two or three MEPS scenarios can usually be trained in a single session, and the training intervention continues until the individual can show skilled problem solving in all of the scenarios used in assessment.

Skill Generalization in Problem-Solving Training

Problem-solving treatment, at least as traditionally conducted, has been criticized because it alters only a client's verbalizations to scenarios presented in the training setting (Rubin, 1982). This criticism is warranted; unless the client is able to solve problems more effectively in day-to-day living, the clinical intervention has accomplished little. Just as it is necessary to explicitly plan for generalization in social skills training, similar attention is needed when conducting problem-solving skills treatment.

Several steps can be taken to promote *in vivo* skill use. First, all practice scenes should be salient for the individual and should represent situations that are, or will be, problematic for him or her. Second, clients should be questioned at each session about real-life problems they have encountered; these new situations should also form the basis for practice and training, and clients should be given explicit homework assignments to apply their new skills to real-life problems. The therapist can actively reinforce reports or other evidence of improved *in vivo* client problem-solving efforts. Finally, the therapist should be aware that knowing how to solve problems is one skill; having the behavioral repertoire to carry out the actual solutions is another competence (Krasner & Rubin, 1981). For that reason, it is wise to assess the person's behavioral skill for actually implementing a solution to a problem. This might entail having the client roleplay, with the therapist, an enactment of what she or he will say or do to implement a proposed problem solution.

Case Study

G. E. J. was a 24-year-old, white, unmarried male, currently living with his parents. He worked part-time and attended a mental health center aftercare program for approximately 6 months. During the past 6 years, he was hospitalized three times at a state institution with the diagnosis of Schizophrenia, Undifferentiated Type, Chronic (DSM-III, 295.92). His maintenance medication consisted of Haldol, 5 mg b.i.d., and Cogentin, 2 mg b.i.d. G. E. J. was referred for behavioral treatment by the staff in the aftercare program. Despite regular attendance in program activities, G. E. J. would not interact with the staff or other patients very often.

In the intake session, no bizarre behavior was evident. G. E. J. rarely looked at the interviewer, spoke very softly, and would answer questions with a few words, seldom elaborating. By his report, he took his medication as prescribed. He denied current delusions or hallucinations, homicidal and suicidal ideation, and any substance abuse. After the mental status, we conducted a more systematic assessment of his behavioral skills repertoire by having him engage in a 5-minute conversation with an unfamiliar person and roleplay a number of scenes requiring assertiveness.

Further information from the staff and his family corroborated our findings that G. E. J. demonstrated deficits in a variety of interpersonal situations. In addition to a lack of an appropriate conversational repertoire in social interactions, the staff noted that he appeared to be unassertive. The staff observed that another patient had borrowed money from G. E. J. and failed to return it, and other patients would cut in front of him in bus lines, resulting in his standing during the journey. His case worker reported that he complained of difficulties at home but did not appear to have skills for settling the problems.

In light of these difficulties, we decided to implement a two-phase program incorporating both behavioral skills training and a problem-solving approach to interpersonal conflicts. Because there are no research guidelines available for determining the sequencing of treatment, we reasoned that teaching the behavioral skills first would provide more immediate social reinforcement and require less time. Moreover, these skills could then be applied within the more complex training found in interpersonal problem solving.

After further assessment of G. E. J. and information gathering from the day program staff, we met with him to outline our treatment recommendations. We gave him a very simple, straightforward explanation of the treatment.

> From what the staff members say, you seem to have difficulty talking to people and knowing what to do when other people take advantage of you. We want to help you speak up more around others. So we have designed a program just for you that is divided into two parts. First, we will teach you how to carry on a conversation with the people you see in the aftercare program and with others. Then, we will show you ways to figure out what to do when you have a conflict or problem with someone. What do you think of this? Would you like to do this? We will be meeting three times a week for about a half hour.

Phase 1: Conversation Skills Training

Based on our observations of G. E. J. in assessment conversations, we selected five behaviors for this phase of the treatment. We targeted two nonverbal behaviors (eye contact and voice volume) and three verbal skills: asking information-gathering questions to the partner; expressing nondisparaging remarks about himself, his interests, and hobbies; and giving compliments to the partner indicating enjoyment of the conversation. These skills were selected because G. E. J. demonstrated a marked deficiency in them, and research has strongly linked these behaviors to overall ratings of social proficiency.

During the conversational skills training, the sessions were highly structured. We taught each behavior until G. E. J. had mastered it before introducing the next one. The nonverbal skills received attention before we taught more complex verbal skills. Each behavior was taught through modeling, discussion/coaching, behavior rehearsal, feedback and *in vivo* practice in the session. Sessions were organized with these components.

Target Skill Presented

At the start of each session, we defined the target skill and gave a rationale for using it in conversations. Here is a typical introduction:

> Today we are going to learn how to get people to talk more about themselves. Asking people questions about themselves and their interests is one of the best ways to get to know them. There are two ways you can ask for information—through open-ended questions and through closed questions. Open-ended questions need more than a *yes* or *no* for an answer. Closed questions can be answered with just one word. You can ask questions about a person's hobbies, interests, daily activities, or about his or her family and friends. Open-ended questions are usually best because they keep conversations flowing.

Target Skill Modeled by Therapist

It is important to provide many examples to counteract the schizophrenic's tendency toward concrete thinking. We contrasted "yes-no" questions, such as "Do you like to watch TV?", with open-ended questions such as "What do you like to do when you're not here in the aftercare program?" We pointed out why open-ended questions are better.

After discussing a number of positive and negative examples, we asked G. E. J. to identify the open-ended questions on a prepared handout. We reviewed each of the questions and had him explain why each was open or closed. We always praised him for correct identification. In anticipation of his next targeted skill (self-disclosing statements), we gradually began to ask him how he might answer particular questions.

Target Skill Rehearsal

After G. E. J.'s performance on the recognition task demonstrated that he understood the skill to be mastered, we asked him to generate questions that could be used with family members and the people he met in the aftercare program. Because he had considerable difficulty thinking up appropriate examples, we generated a number of strategies in order to assist him. First, we showed him pictures of familiar political and motion picture personalities and had him ask them questions about themselves, their work, and so forth. After he demonstrated some proficiency in this, we handed him a brief description of a fictitious individual and asked him to generate appropriate open-ended questions. We then pretended to be a fictitious person and engaged in a series of 5-minute conversations with G. E. J. We gave brief responses to his questions, so that he was responsible for most of the conversation. Following each interaction, we noted the number of open-ended questions asked and praised him for his performance.

Target Skill Practice with a Stranger

We then introduced an unfamiliar individual to G. E. J. (usually a secretary or health care worker) and left the room. Since one-way mirrors were not available in our setting, the 5-minute conversation was tape-recorded. Following the interaction, we asked the conversation partner to judge G. E. J.'s performance on all the behaviors he had learned to date as well as his overall level of skillfulness.

We also reviewed the tape prior to the next therapy session, noting the frequency of the targeted behaviors and the variety of questions. At the start of the next session, we played back parts of he tape during which G. E. J. showed mastery of the skill and praised him. The same format was followed in each conversational skill training session, and G. E. J. was encouraged to practice the new skills in his day-to-day life between sessions.

Phase 2: Social Problem Solving

The second phase of treatment focused on teaching the client strategies for handling interpersonal problems. Although we conceptualized problem solving according to the D'Zurilla and Goldfried (1971) model, a number of the exercises employed in this phase were adapted from Siegel and Spivack's (1976) training package for chronic schizophrenics.

General Orientation

The first two sessions of this phase were used as a general orientation to problem solving. We explained to G. E. J. why we felt this treatment would benefit him. We also stressed that although problems are unavoidable, there are ways of handling them effectively. Adapting situations from the Behavioral Assertiveness Test (BAT-R: Eisler, Hersen, Miller, & Blanchard, 1975) and the Conflict Resolution Inventory (McFall & Lillesand, 1971), we gave him many examples of common problems arising between people, especially ones where someone was taking advantage of another person. One such situation described to him was

> You have an acquaintance from the day hospital who is constantly borrowing dimes from you in order to buy Coke and candy, but he never pays you back. You don't want to give him any more money. After the next program activity he comes up to you and asks you for some change. Later, he leaves and you didn't give him the money. How did you reach that end of the story?

After each scene, we discussed what the problem might be. We also wanted to begin to make G. E. J. aware of what constitutes a problem. If he was unable to see any problem we continued to the next situation.

The second point we wished to convey to G. E. J. was that people tend to react first and think later about what they did. We stressed that this approach did not usually produce the best results. We told him that it would be better to say "stop and think" when he was faced with a problem, and this strategy was again illustrated with specific problem situation scenes. In presenting the cue *stop and think*, we stressed to G. E. J. that behaving passively is one solution to each problem, but it is probably not the best strategy for obtaining his goals.

We also discussed how to recognize that one is having a problem. We began by giving him an exercise designed to teach him how to better recognize emotions in other people. In it, he was presented with magazine pictures of people expressing a variety of emotions (such as anger, fear, sadness, etc.) and had him identify the emotion. We then read him some stories and asked him what kind of emotions the people in the stories may be experiencing. For example, we described a situation where someone lost their pet. The purpose of these exercises was to facilitate the recognition of emotions. These emotions could then be used as a cue to identifying potential interpersonal problems. During these exercises, we continuously reminded G. E. J. that his affective response should be used as a cue to utilize the problem-solving steps that he will be learning. At the end of this preparation for problem solving, we asked him to monitor situations where he felt upset during the next few days.

Conduct of Training Sessions

Using both scenes from the BAT-R and situations already known to be problematic for him (e.g., persons borrowing money or cutting in front of him on the bus), training then focused on G. E. J.'s skill in developing solutions to social problems. In each session, we trained problem-solving steps in two or three of the scenarios; in later sessions, the same training format was applied to still other scenarios, until G. E. J. was skilled in all of them.

At the start of each session, we read to the client a scenario describing one of the problem situations. Next, we asked G. E. J. to pause, think, and then tell us several different ways the situation could be handled. Because he had some trouble generating multiple alternatives, we would occasionally suggest, model, and prompt various means to him. As G. E. J. became more proficient, it was necessary to prompt him less often. We tried to have the client identify at least four different possible courses of action for each MEPS scenario.

In order to teach him to evaluate potential solutions, the client was then asked to verbally describe the probable outcome for each solution he had identified (e.g., whether it would be likely to achieve the story vignette's ending), whether it would be feasible for him to implement, what obstacles might be encountered, and how he would handle them. The therapist gave feedback on his comments as necessary. After he did this for each potential solution of a scene, G. E. J. was asked to select the best.

Because most of the problems encountered by G. E. J. involved social conflicts or others taking advantage of him, we then roleplayed with him the situation described in the MEPS scenario. For example, in one scene, the therapist played the part of the person attempting to panhandle money, whereas G. E. J. actually implemented, in the roleplay, the solution he had arrived at. This was done in order to determine that the client could actually perform behaviors he had earlier verbalized that were the correct ones to use in the situation. Feedback on his performance was provided, and G. E. J. was encouraged to handle the problem in that way in real life.

The problem-solving phase of G. E. J.'s treatment consisted of ten 45-minute sessions that trained 24 different problem scenes. Throughout treatment, the client monitored real-life problems he encountered between sessions; this was accomplished by asking him to keep a diary in which he briefly recorded any problem situations he encountered or any decisions he had to make. At the start of each session, we reviewed G. E. J.'s diary entries with him. For each problem situation that arose, G. E. J. was asked to go through, in the session, all of the problem-solving techniques we were training. We especially praised and encouraged the client for engaging in the problem-solving step process on his own, at home, between our sessions. By the conclusion of the treatment intervention, G. E. J. would routinely tell us how he stopped to think of many solution alternatives when confronted with a real-life problem, and he could verbalize how he chose the best solution.

Other Considerations

The therapist conducting either social or problem-solving skills training with schizophrenic patients (or, as illustrated in the case example, a combination of both forms of training) is attempting to improve the client's skill during practice simulations in the training setting. As the client acquires new skills, improvement will become evident in the quality of his or her performance in roleplays, MEPS scenarios, or so on. Clinically, this change can be detected by the presence of skill behaviors late in training that were not present during pretreatment assessment.

The larger question is whether, following intervention, the client really develops better social relationships, better personal problem-solving capabilities, and a better quality of life. As we suggested earlier, the therapist must encourage, assign, reinforce, and otherwise help the individual use newly trained skills in his or her day-to-day living to bring about this change. It is, in our opinion, unlikely that most severely disordered schizophrenics can be taught such effective social or problem-solving skill expertise so that they would be indistinguishable from high-functioning persons without emotional problems. Even after training, many schizophrenics tend to remain somewhat literal and concerete.

It is also important, from a clinical perspective, to integrate specific social or problem-solving skills training into a broad-based, comprehensive, and long-term intervention plan for the individual. Although skills training as described in this chapter can effectively address certain areas of deficit commonly observed in schizophrenic outpatients, it is not in itself a sufficient treatment for the many types of difficulties experienced by these patients. Consequently, the behavior therapist working with a schizophrenic outpatient should remain cognizant of the need for intervention in such additional areas as psychotropic medication compliance, especially for those patients whose psychotic behavior reappears without "maintenance" medication; the need for ongoing social support development, which can promote the patient's social adjustment in the community and reduce the likelihood of recidivism; vocational rehabilitation planning, if it is appropriate; and intervening with the patient's family members to assist them in dealing with the behavior of the patient. The latter point is especially important because family members who spend time daily with the schizophrenic individual are in a position to foster the development of his or her adaptive community living skills if they can be brought into treatment and instructed in proper methods of dealing with the patient.

The treatment of schizophrenic outpatients is neither quick nor easy. However, the seriousness of the disorder, the poor life quality experienced by so many schizophrenics, the range of problems associated with this disorder, and the continuing trend toward noninstitutional forms of treatment all require that behavior therapists become even more skilled in dealing with these patients in outpatient settings.

Summary

Schizophrenia is a severe disorder characterized by a variety of behavioral excesses and deficits. Although the overt psychosis of many schizophrenic patients is controllable through medication, behavior therapy techniques can be used to further enhance the community living adjustment of these individuals. In particular, interventions using social skills training procedures and/or training in problem-solving skills can foster the schizophrenic outpatient's ability to relate appropriately to others in the community, to function independently, and to solve everyday problems in a more effective manner. Following behavioral assessment of patient competence in simulated interactions, skills training procedures (including modeling, instruction, behavior rehearsal, and shaping) are used to teach new social or problem-solving competencies. Once the new skills are learned, additional and systematic efforts must be made to encourage their use in the natural environment. Although training in social and problem-solving skills is useful for many schizophrenic outpatients, it should be undertaken in the context of the broader, ongoing, and comprehensive treatment of the individual.

References

Allen, M. A., Cohen, S., & Pollin, W. (1972). Schizophrenia in veteran twins: A diagnostic review. *American Journal of Psychiatry, 128,* 939–945.

Barton, R. (1966). *Institutional neurosis.* Bristol: John Wright and Sons.

Bellack, A. S., & Hersen, M. (1978). Chronic psychiatric patients: Social skills training. In M. Hersen & A. S. Bellack (Eds.), *Behavior therapy in the psychiatric setting* (pp. 169–195). Baltimore: Williams & Wilkins.

Bellack, A. S., & Hersen, M. (1979). *Research and practice in social skills training.* New York: Plenum Press.

Bellack, A. S., Hersen, M., & Lamparski, D. A. (1979). Role-play tests for assessing social skills: Are they valid? *Journal of Consulting and Clinical Psychology, 47,* 335–342.

Chambers, D. L. (1975). Community-based treatment and the constitution: The principle of the least restrictive alternative. In L. I. Stein & M. A. Test (Eds.), *Alternatives to mental hospital treatment* (pp. 23–39). New York: Plenum Press.

Christoff, K. A., & Kelly, J. A. (in press). Social skills training with psychiatric patients. In L. L'Abate & M. Milan (Eds.), *Handbook of social skills training.* New York: Wiley.

D'Zurilla, T. J., & Goldfried, M. R. (1971). Problem solving and behavior modification. *Journal of Abnormal Psychology, 78,* 107–126.

Edelstein, B. A., & Eisler, R. M. (1976). Effects of modeling and modeling with instructions and feedback on the behavioral components of social skills. *Behavior Therapy, 7,* 382–389.

Eisler, R. M., Miller, P. M., & Hersen, M. (1973). Components of assertive behavior. *Journal of Clinical Psychology, 29,* 295–299.

Eisler, R. M., Hersen, M., Miller, P. M., & Blanchard, E. B. (1975). Situational determinants of assertive behavior. *Journal of Consulting and Clinical Psychology, 43,* 330–340.

Fischer, M. (1971). Psychoses in the offspring of schizophrenic twins and their normal co-twins. *British Journal of Psychiatry, 118,* 43–52.

Goodwin, D. W., & Guze, S. B. (1979). *Psychiatric diagnosis* (2nd ed.). New York: Oxford University Press.

Gottesman, I. I., & Shields, J. (1966). Contributions of twin studies to perspectives in schizophrenia. In B. A. Maher (Ed.), *Progress in experimental personality research* (Vol. 3) (pp. 1–80). New York: Academic Press.

Gruenberg, E. (1967). The social breakdown syndrome—Some origins. *American Journal of Psychiatry, 123,* 1481–1489.

Hansell, N., & Benson, M. L. (1971). Interrupting long-term patienthood: A cohort study. *Archives of General Psychiatry, 24,* 238–243.

Hersen, M., & Bellack, A. S. (1976). Social skills training for chronic psychiatric patients: Rationale, current findings, and future directions. *Comprehensive Psychiatry, 17,* 559–580.

Kelly, J. A. (1982). *Social skills training: A practical guide for interventions.* New York: Springer-Verlag.

Kelly, J. A., Laughlin, C., Claiborne, M., & Patterson, J. (1979). Group job interview training for unemployed psychiatric patients. *Behavior Therapy, 10,* 299–310.

Kelly, J. A., Urey, J. R., & Patterson, J. (1980). Improving the heterosocial conversation skills of male psychiatric patients through a small group training procedure. *Behavior Therapy, 11,* 179–188.

Kranser, L. R., & Rubin, K. H. (1981). Assessment of social problem-solving skills in young children. In T. Merluzzi & M. Genest (Eds.), *Cognitive assessment* (pp. 452–476). New York: Guilford Press.

McFall, R. M. (1982). A review and reformulation of the concept of social skills. *Behavioral Assessment, 4,* 1–33.

McFall, R. M., & Lillesand, D. B. (1971). Behavior rehearsal with modeling and coaching in assertion training. *Journal of Abnormal Psychology, 77,* 313–323.

Paul, G. L. (1979). Chronic mental patient: Current status, future directions. *Psychological Bulletin, 71,* 81–94.

Platt, J. J., & Spivack, G. (1972). Problem-solving thinking of psychiatric patients. *Journal of Consulting and Clinical Psychology, 30,* 148–151.

Platt, J. J., & Spivack, G. (1975). *Means–end problem-solving procedure (MEPS): Manual and tentative norms.* Philadelphia: Department of Mental Health Sciences, Hahnemann Medical College and Hospital.

Rubin, K. H. (1982). Social and social-cognitive developmental characteristics of young isolate, normal, and sociable children. In K. H. Rubin & H. S. Ross (Eds.), *Peer relationships and social skills in childhood* (pp. 353–369). New York: Springer-Verlag.

Siegel, J. M., & Spivack, G. (1976). Problem-solving therapy: The description of a new program for psychiatric patients. *Psychotherapy: Theory, Research, and Practice, 13,* 368–373.

Spivack, G., & Shure, M. B. (1974). *Social adjustment of young children: A cognitive approach to solving real-life problems.* San Francisco: Jossey-Bass.

Urey, J. R., Laughlin, C., & Kelly, J. A. (1979). Teaching heterosocial conversational skills to male psychiatric patients. *Journal of Behavior Therapy and Experimental Psychiatry, 10,* 323–328.

Wing, J. K. (1962). Institutionalism in mental hospitals. *British Journal of Clinical Psychology, 1,* 38–51.

Special Problems

VI

18

Unassertiveness

HAROLD E. SCHROEDER AND MARY JANE BLACK

Introduction

It is difficult to estimate the importance and prevalence of problems with *assertiveness* because the construct has been so variously and vaguely defined. For some it has meant standing up for one's rights. Wolpe and Lazarus (1966), for example, defined it as all socially acceptable expression of rights and feelings. In a similar vein, Alberti and Emmons (1974) defined assertiveness as acting in one's own best interests without anxiety or destroying the rights of others. In these definitions, the meaning of *socially acceptable* and *rights* is not clarified. For others, it has come to refer to any difficulty in social interactions. Either the aggressive or withdrawn person, in this context, may be understood as unassertive. Rich and Schroeder (1976) proposed a functional definition that could accommodate a wide variety of social skills:

> Assertive behavior is the skill to seek, maintain, or enhance reinforcement in an interpersonal situation through an expression of feelings or wants even when such expression risks loss of reinforcement or even punishment. (p. 1082)

Subsequent investigations based on this definition have revealed that assertiveness is not a unitary construct but is composed of several response classes. Bucell (1979) has empirically identified seven relatively distinct response classes that are consistent with the factor structure of various assertiveness inventories. These are the abilities to (a) refuse requests; (b) express unpopular opinions; (c) admit personal shortcomings; (d) accept compliments; (e) express positive feelings; (f) make behav-

HAROLD E. SCHROEDER • Department of Psychology, Kent State University, Kent, Ohio 44242.
MARY JANE BLACK • Department of Psychiatry, St. Luke's Hospital, Cleveland, Ohio 44104.

ior change requests; and (g) initiate and maintain conversations. Clinical experience supports Lazarus's (1973) position that training of one response class results in little transfer to another. Specific training appears necessary.

The first step, therefore, in dealing with "unassertiveness" is to identify the particular response class that is of concern. In this chapter, we have chosen to describe behavior therapy for training conversational behavior. Conversational skills may be viewed as typical of other social skills with respect to the kind of therapeutic techniques employed. Both the basic structure (discussed later) and the specific procedures (e.g., modeling, cognitive restructuring) for developing a social skill are similar across response classes. That is, modification techniques for developing, say, the ability to refuse unreasonable requests are similar to those involved with learning conversational behavior. Nevertheless, as noted earlier, it is crucial to identify the specific target behavior of interest and to address it separately from behaviors involved with another response class because little transfer across response classes can be assumed.

Though the importance of good conversational skill is perhaps obvious, clients are seldom referred specifically because of conversational deficits. Nevertheless, the research literature as well as clinical experience support the relevance and utility of teaching conversational skills to specific populations. The clinical usefulness of social skills training for psychiatric patients has been demonstrated in many investigations (e.g., Eisler, Blanchard, Fitts, & Williams, 1978; Hersen, Eisler, Miller, Johnson, & Pinkston, 1973; Hersen, Kazdin, Bellack, & Turner, 1979). The treatment rationale is based on the positive relationship between premorbid social competence and prognosis (Zigler & Phillips, 1961) and the corollary that posthospital adjustment is facilitated by increased levels of interpersonal skills (Hersen & Bellack, 1976).

Patients themselves have recognized their need for conversational skills. Goldsmith and McFall (1975) asked patients to identify specific interpersonal situations that were troublesome. Among the most "critical moments" mentioned within a variety of social circumstances (dating, making friends, being with people perceived as more intelligent or attractive) were initiating and terminating interactions, making personal disclosures, and handling conversational silences.

Depressed individuals are a population for whom training in conversational skills has potential usefulness. Lewinsohn (1975) takes the theoretical position that depression reflects a behavioral deficit; depressives fail to engage in the behavior required to maintain adequate social reinforcement. Based on the assumption that, as a group, depressives are either less socially skilled or are currently incapacitated in their use of social skills, conversational training gains rich possibilities. When a person's problems limit his or her ability to engage in potentially rewarding social interactions, training in conversational behavior may profitably be employed as an adjunct to other psychotherapy or a course of medication.

Given the contrast between opportunities for heterosocial interaction in a university setting and the reported discomfort and failure in such situations (Martinson & Zerface, 1970), college students have understandably become an appropriate target population for social skills training. The ability to initiate contacts and engage in conversations has been a central focus in the literature on dating behavior. Minimal and frequent daters can be discriminated according to their ability to initiate and continue conversations in heterosocial situations (Glasgow & Arkowitz, 1975; Twentyman & McFall, 1975; Williams & Ciminero, 1978).

The basic finding from approximately 5,000 responses to the Stanford Shyness Survey was that "shyness is common, widespread, and universal" (Zimbardo, 1977, p. 25). More than 80% of those questioned reported that they were shy at some point in their lives; over 40% considered themselves presently shy. With junior high school populations, the presently shy figure reached 60%. Of 2,482 American students 42% were presently shy; 60% reported shyness as a personal problem. Because Zimbardo does not attempt to define shyness, it is not known how respondents interpreted the construct for themselves. Nonetheless, these data are impressive in terms of personal distress. Although shyness cannot necessarily be construed as a conversational deficit *per se*, clinical experience indicates that problems with conversations are frequently observed and reported by clients who characterize themselves as *shy*.

In summary, it appears that conversational ability is among the more important of the response classes of assertiveness. However, because the problem may be embedded in other, more recognized syndromes, specific treatment may be overlooked. Careful analysis of the components of the presenting syndrome is necessary. Then, once a conversational deficit has been identified, specific training can proceed. As with other types of unassertiveness, training consists of four basic or generic elements (Rich & Schroeder, 1976): cognitive restructuring, response acquisition, response reproduction, and response shaping. The fifth element in Rich and Schroeder's classification—response transfer—is not elaborated extensively because, as will be seen, it is embedded within each of the other four elements through our emphasis on experimentation and practice in real-life situations.

Therapeutic Techniques

Cognitive Restructuring

Socially inhibited clients are usually resistant to the effort involved in developing conversational skills. In order to teach conversational response acquisition and reproduction with later shaping of these responses, initial resistance must be overcome. This resistance may be attacked through an analysis of specific conversational problems, direct confrontation of unrealistic expectations, anxiety management techniques, and training attention to conversational behavior.

Clients commonly have unrealistic expectations about how people become good conversationalists. They may think that it is a gift or talent, but only rarely do they see it as an acquired skill. Consequently, they may expect somehow to be *endowed* with the ability through therapy. They hope for initimate conversation, social ease, a date, or exciting interactions to happen immediately. If they do not develop immediate expertise they want to give up. Because such expectations make it difficult to continue generating behavior, it is important to modify these attitudes early in therapy and whenever they recur. Cognitive restructuring therefore occurs not only at the beginning of training but throughout the therapy process.

Cognitive restructuring, for us, typically begins with structuring the therapeutic process. First, clients are instructed how conversational behavior may be conceptualized as a skill that can be learned much like any other skill. We define conversations as mutual communications (rather than simply talking) that involve expression of thoughts and feelings and effective listening. The risks of social communication (e.g. being misunderstood, gaining fewer rewards than anticipated) are discussed. The therapeutic program is described as one designed to teach the components of this skill while maximizing the rewards and minimizing the risks of conversations. The process of learning a skill is then reviewed. Clients are reminded that learning is an active process that will involve not only developing an understanding of how and why to act in specific ways but also practice with the therapist and real-life experimentation.

A conversational analysis is then conducted. Difficulties with conversations may derive from behavioral, emotional, or cognitive problems. Some people have simply had inadequate or insufficient learning experiences to teach them to communicate effectively. These individuals have a true skill deficit. Others suffer from anxiety. Even though they may possess adequate skills, their anxiety prevents them from using the skills fully. Still others have irrational thoughts that create negative self-appraisals and overemphasize the risks of social interaction. All difficulties result in avoidance of conversational opportunities. We have found it helpful to use a self-rating scale to assign priorities to the three categories of problems so that specific therapeutic efforts may be better focused.

Unrealistic expectations are attacked with a rational-emotive approach. Four irrational ideas (Ellis, 1962) seem most common with conversationally deficient persons. These are (a) when the world or my behavior deals me an undesired consequence, it is awful, terrible, and unfair *(catastrophizing)*; (b) I must prove thoroughly competent, adequate, and achieving in order to consider myself a worthwhile person *(demand for perfection)*; (c) I must have love and approval from all the people I find significant, or else it is terrible and I am worthless *(fear of rejection)*; (d) the past is all important, and because something once influenced my life it has to keep determining my feelings and behavior today *(I can't change)*. Using Ellis's ABC conceptualization, in which activating events (A) and emotional consequences (C) are mediated by an individual's belief system (B), clients are trained to substitute more rational thoughts.

Anxiety management techniques are closely related to the rational-emotive procedures. However, we include two additional techniques beyond training in rational-emotive therapy coping procedures. Clients are taught relaxed breathing techniques as a tool for immediate use in threatening situations. Clients also practice covert rehearsal of satisfying encounters.

Finally, clients are encouraged to become conversationally minded. Using a checklist of specific questions about conversations (How do people start conversations? What do they find to talk about? How do people agree or disagree? What do people do that makes you want to talk to them? etc.), clients are asked to observe conversations during their normal routines. Directed attention to specific characteristics of conversations appears to have both desensitizing and instructional value.

Response Acquisition

Direct therapist instruction is a basic mode of response acquisition. Therapists may choose to teach a general strategy for conversational content (e.g. "Talk about something you know well") or a specific one ("Tell her about the movie you saw last night"). Obviously, regressed or very socially inadequate clients will require more specific instructions than will individuals who have the appropriate responses in their repertoires but are handicapped by shyness or who have difficulty with only one type of interaction.

Whether they are general or specific, instructions have numerous pitfalls. Even a basically competent client can have difficulty translating general instructions into discrete verbal behaviors; low-functioning individuals get lost and confused. If a client is able to translate one suggestion into a specific conversational gambit, the client often is unable to develop a second topic, and deadly silence results. This seems particularly true with highly anxious clients. Overly explicit instructions, on the other hand, train the client to expect that there is one, and only one, correct approach to an interaction. Rigidity and inflexibility are therefore encouraged, whereas naturalness and spontaneity are discouraged.

One of the most challenging tasks facing the therapist is how to provide direct instruction to facilitate social approach. Most clients can produce some kind of a response when addressed by another person; their greatest difficulties typically arise in their painful struggle to find something to say to initiate conversations. General instructions have the advantage of covering a range of conversational situations, but they rarely provide enough security to motivate a client to risk the awkwardness or rejection he or she fears may result from a conversational effort. Specific instructions directed toward particular types of interactional opportunities are usually necessary to create the structure clients require; yet they do have the limiting potential noted earlier.

We have devised a comprehensive strategy for clients that combines the best features of general and specific instructions while minimizing the disadvantages of each. We teach a *general* stimulus-response strategy that is applicable to any *specific* conversation. To develop conversational content, we take a two-step approach. First, we teach clients how to become better observers of people and situations. Because they are truly "self"-conscious, clients are usually so preoccupied with themselves that they fail to notice conversational stimuli within the social context itself, including salient aspects of their own and the other person's behaviors. When they do attempt to initiate a conversation, they tend to search almost randomly for a topic—any topic—to get started. If they are fortunate, they happen on one that is reasonable and can be discussed further; if not, they must begin another desperate search on the spot while in a state of increasing anxiety. In contrast, clients who are taught to utilize their own innate observational capacities are able to create conversations that flow naturally from their normal, everyday relationships to the world. Similarly, the second step in building conversations is to teach clients to pay attention to their own internal responses as sources of content. Reactions to environmental or conversational stimuli can be expressed as emotions, interest, curiosity, and the like. Relying on his or her *observations* and *reactions*, the client learns to become his or her own authority, resource, and instructor. How we systematize and structure the client's learning to become more aware of observations and reactions and then translate them into conversational behaviors is presented in the remainder of this chapter.

Engaging in this ongoing process of observation and reaction is especially critical for maintaining conversations once they have begun. It is noteworthy that difficulties at the maintaining stage of interactions are not limited to failure to speak. A common therapist error is to assume that because a client wants to become more socially involved, he or she is already socially aware. Deficits in timing and social perception are often major contributors to interpersonal dissatisfaction. Active listening, in the form of observations and reactions, focuses attention, increases interpersonal sensitivity, fosters continuity and relevant responses, and interferes with the development of anxiety.

A final limitation of instructions as a method of response acquisition is that instructions of any sort are easily forgotten. In medical psychology, researchers have documented that more than half of the instructions given by physicians are recalled erroneously. There is little to suggest that clients with psychological problems recall any better. Consequently, we have found it helpful to back up our instructions by concrete reminders such as written guidelines. For example, it is useful to provide clients with an observational checklist to remind them of observational cues.

The second major method used for response acquisition is modeling. Although modeling can be performed either live or with electronic techniques, the former is more common because most therapists lack access to expensive video equipment. Most empirical investigations of the benefits of modeling demonstrate a facilitative effect. An exception may be the case of learning very simple behaviors where direct instructions alone may be adequate. Because social conversations are extremely complex, modeling procedures here are particularly helpful. Through modeling, it is possible to focus on the interactional aspect of conversations and demonstrate responses to a constantly changing social stimulus situation. Modeling also has the advantage of illustrating nonverbal and paralinguistic components of conversations.

A major pitfall in the use of modeling, however, derives directly from its strength. So much complexity may be presented that the client is overwhelmed and fails to learn just as he or she has failed to learn through observation of conversations in daily life. It is important for the therapist to direct the client's attention to separate, defined components of conversations to reduce this complexity. For example, in the early stages of learning the observation-reaction procedure, the model may identify various observations available in the social situation. Later, emphasis may be directed to how an observation is turned into a conversation opener. Or, the model may demonstrate good eye contact, appropriate facial expression, and body language. Even here there is danger that the therapist may overwhelm the client with the therapist's own sophistication. Effective modeling requires a reflection of the client's baseline competency and specific, limited focus.

Another important consideration in orchestrating a model's behavior concerns the type of verbal behavior to be modeled. One of our goals is to avoid teaching a conversational script that provides only a rigid, limited, almost memorized conversational performance. We try to teach a strategy by modeling a variety of conversational statements. In the course of learning this strategy, clients often object to certain statements. Not all statements demonstrated by the model are acceptable to a particular client. Commonly a client may react with, "I couldn't say that." Such a response reflects the client's discomfort with certain conversational styles and should be taken seriously by the therapist. The goal is to help the client develop his or her own unique style of conversing that is genuine and emotionally comfortable. For example, an emotionally constricted client may have difficulty sharing feelings even after learning to observe and identify those feelings. Different interest (and lack of interest) patterns emerge with other clients. Such individuality should be noted and encouraged. The advantage of teaching a general strategy of *how* to make conversation is, of course, to encourage genuine and spontaneous (rather than scripted) conversations.

Response Reproduction

Response reproduction involves translating observations and reactions into verbalizations. This may be the most difficult part of the treatment program. Therapists who have dealt with highly inhibited clients will recognize how difficult it is merely to elicit behavior. The unassertive client has decided that *no* social behavior is less discomforting than failing at social interactions. A major therapeutic challenge, therefore, is to produce any behavior at all in a social world that the client perceives as filled with competent people likely to have little patience with the woeful efforts of the client.

Typically, the technique of behavioral rehearsal is used for response reproduction, either through roleplay or by homework assignments. Role playing has the advantage that it can be accomplished while the therapist observes. Direct evaluation of behavior, of course, provides rich opportunities for feedback. It also may hold less threat value than spontaneous encounters because it is done in the (relative) safety of the therapist's office. The chief disadvantage of roleplay is its artificiality. Clients generate little confidence for daily conversations through roleplay practice. Therefore, we tend to use roleplay as a means of documenting that clients have acquired specific responses rather than as a method of increasing ability to reproduce the responses.

Homework assignments require a client to engage in conversational behaviors in natural settings. Success in these settings instills confidence for further efforts. Because such assignments may become extremely difficult for clients, however, they must be structured carefully. Initially, it may be necessary simply to place the client in a conversational situation with no demand to talk. This can be done by asking the client to make observations first. Through active listening and observing, the client becomes increasingly aware of conversational opportunities, although performance demands remain low. With greater familiarity and comfort in natural conversational settings, the client becomes willing to assume more conversational responsibility. The danger of therapist error at this point involves underestimating the difficulty of homework assignments. Clients may express their willingness to carry out homework assignments because they may be highly motivated to improve or reluctant to disappoint the therapist. Clients also may not accurately evaluate their ability to perform when they are influenced by the persuasiveness of the therapist or the security of the therapeutic setting. In any event, the therapist cannot rely on the client's motivation to generate behavior. The homework tasks need to be structured carefully.

One method of structuring was mentioned earlier: performance demands may be reduced by simply requiring observations within the conversational setting. Following this, a graded, step-by-step skill-building structure can be used. Tasks move from the simple to the complex. Simple tasks might involve interactions with a person who is seen as providing little threat. This might be a stranger ("I'll never see him again so how I do doesn't matter") or an accepting friend. Or, simplicity could involve a more structured setting that might provide some obvious conversational cues. Still another way of creating a simple task is to limit the length of the conversation. Perhaps the most obvious method, however, is to avoid dealing with too many variables at one time.

For particularly inhibited clients, it may be necessary to deal directly with internal performance demands. Sometimes clients may be unable to carry out even simple homework assignments because they are convinced they will be unable to perform as competently as they think they must. With this behavioral paralysis, the therapist has little to work with. We have found that this evaluation anxiety can be reduced by creating a new cognitive set. Homework assignments may be discussed as "experiments" in which no specific performance level is anticipated or required. When the level of performance is made less crucial, the client's resistance is often reduced.

These early attempts at conversation are generally crude and awkward. This is probably due partly to the structure imposed by the homework assignments and partly to the lack of skill and the emotional involvement of the client. In any event, an important step has been taken because the client has now produced relevant behavior that can be refined and shaped. Additional components of conversation can now be added, and the client can be encouraged to move into more complex conversations.

Response Shaping

Because initial attempts to use our observation-reaction model are likely to be awkward and unsatisfactory to the client, refinement of these conversational efforts is necessary. Clients may find their observational skills insufficiently developed and lapse into silence. Or they may be so fearful of silence that they talk too much. Either reaction will limit the satisfaction a client receives from conversations and may renew the desire to withdraw from conversational efforts. At this point the therapist must be very encouraging and reinforcing. It is helpful to recall that we are working here with a behavioral deficit. Consequently, it is crucial to continue generating approach behavior, no matter how limited or crude. Effort should be reinforced at this point, not success. Only if conversational efforts continue can response shaping occur.

It is also helpful for therapists to address directly the sense of failure that many clients express at this time. Clients seem prone to accept unrealistic amounts of responsibility for conversational problems and to expect rapid, magical progress. They need to learn how to evaluate their experiences realistically. We have found it helpful to provide a structure for this evaluation. When clients are directed to examine the conversation according to specific guidelines, they are less likely to make global judgments that assume total personal failure. The same conversational analysis discussed earlier (under cognitive restructuring) can be used here. Clients are encouraged to examine behavioral, emotional, and cognitive difficulties in a particular conversation. When *specific* reasons for conversational difficulties have been identified, clients are not overwhelmed with failure and can be encouraged toward remedial action. They also have a guide to measure their improvement. Without a measure of special difficulties, any progress is likely to remain undetected, and the satisfying rewards of improvement are lost. Clients are also taught at this stage that not all failures are their fault. Because conversations are reciprocal social interactions, the behavior of the conversational partner is an important ingredient of satisfactory conversations. Experiences with conversations must be evaluated sensibly.

A major component of response shaping is the addition of paralinguistic and nonverbal behaviors to the techniques of developing conversational content. Nonverbal behaviors include appropriate facial expression, genuineness, good eye contact, and facilitative body language. A pleasant facial expression or smile will invite an approach by others. Later, facial expressions should reflect the content of the conversation. Clients are encouraged to recognize that genuineness is a highly appealing quality. Shy clients often attempt to cover their shyness with an artificial sophistication. They fail to learn that genuine expression of shyness is generally met with a helpful and welcoming attitude because most people have experienced timidity in some way. Reasonable eye contact is encouraged to show attention and interest. Finally, clients are sensitized to how body language can enhance or detract from verbal messages.

Paralinguistics are characterized on four dimensions, although different therapists may conceptualize in other ways. We emphasize a clear, pleasantly modulated voice, fluent speech, meaningful expressive language, and emphasis and inflection appropriate to the emotional qualities of a particular conversation. Nonverbal and paralinguistic behaviors are facilitated through roleplay, real-life behavioral rehearsal, and self-feedback. Roleplays may involve experience with several types of feelings as well as the mixed messages that result from inappropriate non-verbal and paralinguistic behaviors. Behavioral rehearsal of nonverbal behaviors may begin with simply smiling at a number of people and noting the reactions of the other people and oneself. Later, nonverbal and paralinguistic elements can be combined with actual conversations in real-life experimentation. Self-feedback is accomplished through a checklist of the specific nonverbal and paralinguistic elements.

A final major component of response shaping involves using the client's reactions within the conversational context. Recall that in our model, conversation consists of observations and reactions. Although satisfactory conversation may be produced simply by expressing observations, more sophisticated and stimulating conversation requires personal reactions. Because learning to express reactions is probably a distinct skill from expression of observations, it might be considered an aspect of response acquisition. We have included it with response shaping, however, because it involves much more refined techniques than the ones discussed earlier.

Clients are taught that reactions are simply natural responses to observations, i.e.,thoughts, and feelings about what is happening. Reactions that are commonly shared include curiosity, interest, and opinion. To express interest and curiosity, clients are taught to ask open questions. Again, modeling, roleplay, behavioral rehearsal through homework, and self-feedback are the tools used. The emphasis at this point is to encourage the client to be facilitative through open questions that express genuine interest. In addition, clients are taught to respond to questions with more than one word through sharing of personal reactions. Later, the client is encouraged to express personal opinions. Most clients will feel more threatened at this point, particularly if the opinions are thought to disagree with those of the conversational partner. Some cognitive restructuring may be necessary so the client may understand an opinion simply as a summary of one's experience at a particular time. As experience changes through additional information or perspective, opinion may change. At any given time, however, it is reasonable to expect only the opinion held at that time. Clients are trained to use *I* or other self-references to communicate personal responsibility for opinions and lack of demand that others share these opinions. They also are encouraged to practice ways of expressing differences of opinion.

An even more complex reaction involves expression of emotional reactions and responding empathically to the feelings of others. Using roleplay and behavioral rehearsal with self-feedback through a structured handout, clients may be taught to make their conversations more interesting and alive by expressing personal feelings. Often, clients need to be taught to be aware of their feelings and how to label them. Socially inhibited persons restrict not only sharing feelings but even awareness of them. With limited experience in expressing feelings, clients often develop invalid guidelines about communication of emotions. For example, some clients may assume close friends automatically understand feelings without specific verbal communication; others may reserve emotional expression for intimate relationships. Such beliefs can be modified when clients see the color and vitality that conversations develop when distinctive, individual emotional reactions are shared.

A related aspect of conversational training involves reacting to others' expressions of feeling with empathy. Here again, clients often do not appreciate the value of merely understanding and acknowledging how others feel. They may fear they will misunderstand how someone feels or think they must feel the same way as the other person in order to empathize. Whatever the restricting belief, it may be modified through instruction, roleplay practice, and behavioral rehearsal with self-feedback in a real-life situation.

Response Transfer

Although generalization of performance skills from the office (or laboratory) to everyday settings has often been a problem for behavioral programs, the issue is minimized with the present approach because of the routine use of practice in real-life situations. Nevertheless, it is helpful for a client to have a review of the way conversations have been conceptualized. Continuing to think of conversations as a series of observations and reactions will help the client to respond in novel situations and unusual interactions. Therefore, toward the end of training, we reinforce the distinctive use the client has made of the model. In addition, several special situations are chosen to illustrate how the model may be applied to problems frequently difficult for the unassertive person. These include joining a group already talking, introductions, expressing sympathy, talking with people who are "different," and reacting to silence. In each case, the client is taught to use the observation-reaction model. Finally, clients are taught to learn from experience. Because not all conversations are satisfying, clients must learn to evaluate their feedback in a realistic way. If they analyze both what they did wrong and what they did well, they will be less inclined to inhibit conversational behavior in the future.

An Illustrative Case Study

As indicated in the previous sections, treatment of the following client is based on a stimulus-response (observation-reaction) model that lends itself to integrated, progressive learning. Although other therapists may prefer an alternative organization of the behavioral techniques employed, we have found our training sequence to be a highly effective mode of skill building. A significant advantage of our structured approach is concurrent assessment of client behavior in the presence of the therapist and in real-life, extratherapy experiences. Training proceeds from very simple, time-limited conversations to more complex, open-ended interactions. Obviously, some conversational components will be easier than others for the individual client to master. The basics may have to be repeated to ensure that the client has a firm foundation on which to build additional skills. Because anxiety may be heightened as clients become more active in conversational situations, they need to be coached to use anxiety management techniques to maintain their efforts. Note that in the dialogue that follows the therapist consistently employs the terminology and concepts of the behavioral model to strengthen client confidence for real-life, unanticipated interactions.

This client is a 26-year-old, single male who is a graduate of a 2-year city college. He works in a large office. He enjoys reading and sports but rarely engages in the latter because of lack of companionship. He has been referred by a psychiatrist who diagnosed him as moderately depressed, mainly due to social isolation. The psychiatrist felt the client would benefit more from psychotherapy directed at his social maladjustment and generalized anger than from medication.

Even the person who claims almost complete isolation has some skills; the therapist must do a thorough behavioral analysis to assess the client's strengths and needs accurately. Self-reports completed by the client at home save in-session time. These include the range of current social interactions, anxiety-rating scales, and a checklist of cognitive factors that influence social behavior. The client's tape-recorded responses to sample situations are also useful. The therapist is reviewing the client's completed self-rating materials.

T: On your checklist you indicate that you can converse fairly well with people you have known for a while.
C: I think I do OK there, although it's hard for me to get a conversation started sometimes.
T: So starting a conversation can be a problem with people you know, but it's always more difficult with strangers.
C: I just don't know what to say. Even if I got invited to parties, I wouldn't go unless I were sure I would know everybody there; and then it still would be hard to speak up in a group.
T: Now we have at least two goals: talking with strangers and talking in a group. I see, too, that in these situations you have a great deal of anxiety and a lot of negative thoughts about how things will turn out for you.
C: Yes, I get really nervous, and I know I will embarrass myself. I don't know what to do about it. I'm really discouraged.

The therapist helps the client understand how his problems can be addressed effectively. Conversational behavior is conceptualized as a complex of skills that can be learned. Note that even a highly motivated client will repeatedly express resistance that must be countered realistically and anticipated if possible.

T: It is discouraging to feel that you are so limited socially. However, you have mentioned an important asset that you already have. Do you know what it is?
C: No, all I see are problems.
T: The fact that you can function well in some social situations is a real plus. That means you already have some skills; we can build on them. Tell me, do you drive a car?
C: Sure, but what does that have to do with conversations?
T: Conversational behavior is a set of skills, just like the skills involved in driving a car. Neither of us was born knowing how to drive; we had to learn to do it gradually through a series of experiences. It's the same way with conversations. We weren't born knowing how to converse with people; we learned to do it, step by step.
C: That's just the trouble. I don't think I ever learned much about conversations; people were very quiet at our house unless they were arguing. I know I can't talk with strangers. It's too scary.

T: Of course it is when you haven't worked up to it. Remember when you learned to drive? Your first time behind the wheel was probably a little scary, too. But you didn't start out in the middle of the freeway with no preparation. First, you worked on basic skills: you learned to find the accelerator and the brake and how to steer. You practiced these skills and then gradually applied them to different driving situations. You learned to go forward, to back up, turn corners, and travel on local streets. When you developed some confidence through practice, you used your basic skills to tackle heavier traffic and eventually the freeways. That's how we will work here: learning basic skills, refining them through practice, and applying them to a variety of circumstances. We'll start with very simple conversational situations and work step by step toward more complex ones.

C: I understand what you mean about driving, but what's my first basic skill for conversations?

T: I'll teach you an all-purpose strategy that you can rely on for almost any conversational situation you can imagine. We'll practice the strategy and then use it to find something to say to begin short conversations.

C: I'm getting nervous just thinking about talking with people I don't know.

Anxiety may arise from lack of skill or may prevent a client from utilizing perfectly adequately skills already in his or her behavioral repertoire. In either case, an effective approach to conversational problems includes anxiety management techniques. Similarly, cognitive restructuring is employed to counter negative thinking and expectations that also interfere with performance.

T: You've brought up a good point. In addition to skill problems, people have difficulty with conversations for other reasons. Anxiety is a big one. We're all a little anxious when we are trying something new. I see you noted on your checklist that your mouth gets dry and your heart pounds when you are nervous. I'll teach you some techniques to minimize anxiety so that you can devote your attention to conversations.

C: That's another thing. When I do get up my nerve to say something—even with my friends—people don't seem to pay much attention to me. I'm always going to be boring. No wonder people reject me.

T: You've just given me a good example of the third major reason why people have problems with conversations: negative thinking about themselves or their experiences. Anyone who expects to be boring or rejected will certainly be hesitant about getting into a conversation. We'll work together to change these negative thoughts that are getting in your way. I'll give you written materials to take home with you today to teach you techniques to manage anxiety and some exercises to help you begin to change your negative thinking.

C: This sure sounds like a lot of work.

The client is correct, and the therapist acknowledges this. Maintaining motivation throughout the learning of complex, anxiety-provoking new behaviors is a continuing problem. Self-reinforcement is an effective component of training so long as it is clearly tied to client efforts to follow through and not to absolute perfection or haphazard attempts.

T: It is going to take some effort on your part. Changing old behaviors and learning new ones does take work. Your main reward, of course, will be feeling more comfortable and being more effective in conversations and these experiences will lead to more rewards. However, we all need incentives to keep us going. It will be easier for you if you start now to plan some small rewards for the work you do on the assignments I give you and some bigger ones for what you do on your own.

The client's homework includes several written assignments to be completed prior to the next session. To facilitate cognitive behavior change, worksheets are provided to identify and then modify negative thoughts along the lines of Ellis's irrational belief model. Anxiety management techniques involve the client's formulation of rational coping statements, practice in breathing control, and positive imagery. As a personal focus for learning, the client chooses three "target persons" with whom he would like to initiate conversations. Some clients have difficulty selecting these people because they have not thought specifically enough about what they want to accomplish and with whom. At this point, however, at least one person should be chosen; others are added as the client's exposure to conversational situations becomes more common.

Any assignments given should be carefully followed up. This procedure mandates the client's involvement at the outset; as homework becomes more challenging, he or she has already established an active behavioral pattern of complying with therapist instructions. Completed assignments are reinforced by the therapist's verbal recognition of client effort. Incomplete assignments are discussed thoroughly. Some assignments are directed toward a behavioral analysis. A careful analysis may lead to the discovery that a client's problems are different from those initially stated, or other therapy issues may emerge. For example, some clients are chronically angry in response to intense family conflicts. They have learned to control others by passive-aggressive behaviors such as silence and withdrawal. Despite a wish for greater socialization outside their homes, *not* talking has acquired the greater reinforcement value. Issues such as this must be addressed by the therapist before reasonable social interactions can occur.

In the next session, the therapist describes the basic conversational strategy:

T: I told you last time that I would teach you an all-purpose, basic strategy for conversations.
C: I don't see how that's possible. Every situation is different.
T: That's right, it is; but our strategy takes care of that very easily. It has two parts: observation and reaction. "Observation" means information gathering—what we know, what we see, what we hear, and anything else we notice about the other person and the situation.
C: Give me an example.
T: OK, driving a car requires a series of observations and reactions. You observe a red traffic signal, and you react to it by stopping. Conversations can also be thought of as a series of observations and reactions. You "observe" someone smiling at you and saying "Hello." You "react" by smiling back and saying "Hi." You "observe" someone asking you a question; you "react" by answering it.
C: That makes sense, I guess, so long as the other person starts things off. But I still wouldn't know where to go from there.
T: That's what I'll begin to teach you today. We'll concentrate on starting a conversation with the observation part of the strategy. We'll work on your becoming more alert to your own observations so that you can use them as conversational cues to find something to say. Let's see what observations you can come up with about one of your target people. Who is first on your list?

C: Well, there's a woman at work I'd like to talk to, but I wouldn't know what to say.

T: Let's see what observations you have already been making.

C: None. I told you she is new at work. She started last month sometime.

T: Those are observations; they are what you have noticed about her. Since all of them are potential cues for conversation, I want you to write them down so that they easily become conversation—instant conversation. When you are referring to yourself, write *I;* when you are referring to the other person, write *you.* So for this first observation, write something like "You started working here last month" or "I understand you are new here."

C: All right, but I don't see how this will help me talk to her.

T: It will be clearer as you list more of your observations just how many cues you have for conversation with this woman. What else do you know about her?

C: Well, she always looks as if she has a lot of work to do. Oh, and once I saw her in the parking lot. She has a rack on her car for skis. She looks pretty athletic, come to think of it. Maybe she is interested in art, too. I saw her once at an art show at the shopping center.

T: Good. Write those observations, too.

The client's list includes observations about the person with whom he wishes to talk and those occurring in any shared situations or environments, no matter how remotely experienced. The client is encouraged to become more conversationally minded by being alerted to the multiplicity of cues available. Implicit in this process is covert rehearsal of "instant conversation"; in most cases his observations can be translated into relevant comments without further modification.

T: Now you have about 15 observations.

C: I didn't know I knew that much about her. I suppose I could say some of these instant conversation things to her, but I'm too shy to do it now. I probably can't ever do it.

The therapist allows the client to maintain his resistance on the basis of lack of readiness, not impossibility. He is reinforced for skill building, and his observation list is expanded to include interpersonal sensitivity.

T: It's understandable that you don't feel quite ready to approach her yet, but you have made a good start on instant conversation with her. You're quite a good observer. Let's see what we can do with another important class of observations, cues about feelings— the other person's emotional state, attitude, or what his or her experience seems like at a particular time.

C: I don't think I'm very good at that.

T: I expect you are better than you think. For example, if someone is frowning, what does that suggest to you?

C: That they're mad.

T: Yes, a frown can indicate anger. It can also suggest confusion, puzzlement, concentration, or something else, depending on what other circumstances you observe. Let's go back to the woman at your office. How did she look at you at the art show?

C: Well, she was buying a vase. I guess she was kind of excited . . . pleased; she carried it very carefully after she bought it.

T: Good for you. You noticed another kind of emotional cue: body language. How people sit, stand, gesture, and so forth can tell us a lot about their emotional experiences. The tone of people's voices or the emphasis they place on certain words are cues to feelings, as well. Now, since we can't be absolutely certain what another person's experience is really like, when you list your observations about feelings I want you to use words like

"You look . . ." or "You seem . . ." That way, when you begin to use them for instant conversation you will be suggesting, rather than insisting, how someone feels.

C: I don't know what you mean about "suggesting."

T: In most instances, people want to have their feelings recognized and acknowledged, but they don't like to be told what they are. So when we speak about another person's feelings from the perspective of our own observations, we want to make our remarks more of a gentle inquiry than a strong statement of fact. But let's not get too far ahead of ourselves; we'll be working more intensively later on how to talk with people. Let's finish your observation list and then discuss what you will work on between sessions.

Although the therapist is always preparing the client to involve himself in conversations, at this stage of training demand for this behavior is minimal. The objective here is to reinforce in-session learning with real-life practice. Increased social exposure is achieved in the process.

The therapist describes homework assignments as experiments, to "see what happens." For the next session the client is directed to make observations on three separate occasions and to record them in the manner discussed previously. To aid the less perceptive client in discriminating feelings, it is helpful to have him or her watch television for a half hour with the sound off and record emotions observed, using a descriptive word list provided by the therapist to build an emotional vocabulary.

Another form of resistance involves unassertive clients' isolation. They commonly reiterate that they are so inactive socially that they can think of no situations in which to make real-life observations.

C: Where can I do this? I told you, I only go to work.

T: There is no reason why you can't make one set of observations at your office. In fact that is a very good idea, since one of your goals is to talk with your woman acquaintance there. However, I think there are other good opportunities for practice that you are overlooking. How about today? Where else have you been with people?

The therapist helps the client to recognize that there are numerous opportunities for observation, and conversation, during the course of his ordinary daily activities (e.g., returning a book to the library, stopping at the drugstore, waiting in line, etc.). The therapist suggests that the client can take advantage of these opportunities to talk if he wishes.

T: I want you to use the kinds of situations you have mentioned to make your observations this week. Repeat your observations to yourself as you make them, so that if you decide to talk you'll be ready. Don't worry about awkwardness or what to say next; the other person is likely to help you out quite a bit. Remember, you are just doing experiments to see what happens. And don't forget to reward yourself for doing them.

Following real-life observational practice, the therapist begins to model and roleplay with the client.

T: You said that you almost spoke to the man standing in the cashier's line with you at the supermarket.

C: Yeah, we had to wait a long time. I was going to say something, but my throat was too dry.

T: You'll soon be feeling more at ease in these situations. Let's talk about your observations and see what you might have said.

C: Well, the store was really crowded. I've never seen so many people there at that time of day.

T: OK, good. What about the man next to you?

C: He was about my age. He had a nice-looking running suit on. Oh, and he had about 50 cans of dog food in his grocery cart. Amazing!

T: Was he grumpy looking?

C: Oh, no. A little tired looking, maybe. Actually, he smiled at me a couple of times and looked as if he might say something.

T: Good observation. That's a pretty positive sign he would be pleasant and receptive to a few words from you.

C: There still didn't seem to be anything for me to say.

T: That's where your observations come in. They make good instant conversation. You don't have to search for something to talk about; your observations of what was happening right there were the most logical place to start.

C: Well, maybe. What would you have said?

T: I think I might have gestured toward all that dog food and said: "If your dog eats that much I hope I don't meet him in the parking lot!"

C: Oh, gosh! I could never say anything like that. It's too pushy, too personal.

T: You're right. I would feel comfortable saying that, but if you're not, then you shouldn't consider it. Let's try something less personal, one of your observations about the situation.

Using the client's observations as the basis of roleplay, the therapist makes suggestions, keeping in mind the client's own personal style and comfort. The therapist continually emphasizes the generality of the observational strategy.

C: Hey, that was a good line. Let me write that down.

T: You can do that if you wish, but it may not be helpful at all in the future. We want to avoid writing "scripts" because, as you pointed out earlier, every situation is different and this comment may not fit in the next one. That's the advantage of making observations on the spot; they free you to be responsive to what is happening at the moment. They keep you aware of your conversational priorities.

C: What priorities?

T: Let's say you are meeting a friend. You can't wait to tell him about a great movie you saw. You're thinking about what you'll say about it, but when you see him the first thing you notice—observe—is that he really looks depressed. What would you say to him first?

C: Well, I'd want to know what was wrong. I'd say something like "You really look down."

T: Exactly. That's what you observed when you saw him; anything you might have rehearsed to open your conversation would not have been appropriate right then. You've done very well today, just using your observations in our roleplays.

C: We did OK, but our conversations didn't sound very real to me. You were helping me a lot by giving me openings to say more. People don't do that in the real world.

T: Most people will respond if you give them a chance. You're right though; the best way for you to appreciate what you can accomplish is to do some experiments to see what happens.

The client's homework, like all succeeding assignments, is designed to incorporate additional practice of previous learning and at least one new conversational component from the current session. Structured self-feedback material is provided. For the next session, this client is to make observations and to have three "instant conversations." He is instructed to choose situations that have natural time limits—for example, to say a few words to someone waiting with him at the copy machine in his office, so that content demands are low.

There are bound to be rough spots in the client's performance. The therapist helps the client evaluate experiments constructively and to make rational self-statements about unsuccessful experiences. Once some conversational behavior is generated, nonverbal and paralinguistic refinements are introduced.

T: We agree now that although one of your conversations did not go so well as you would have liked, two satisfying ones out of three is a pretty good average. It sounds as if you were feeling a little awkward, and that may have contributed to some of your difficulties. But you have to keep in mind that a conversation is a two-way street. Everything that happens is not all your responsibility. It sounds to me as if this person did not give you much to go on. If she had something else on her mind and just didn't feel like talking, you're not responsible for that.

C: Well, she did look sort of grouchy and spoke in a monotone. She really turned me off.

T: You've brought up something very important. So far we have been concentrating on conversational content, what is said. But, as you observed, there is more to conversation than just what we say. Another component is nonverbal behavior—facial expression, eye contact, body language, and other aspects of our appearance when we talk with someone. How we sound—the tone of our voices, the energy we put into a conversation—make a difference in how people react toward us. When all these aspects of our behavior are in tune, people feel at ease with us; mixed messages make others uncomfortable or confused.

C: What do you mean by "mixed messages"?

T: Let's do an experiment to show you what I mean. Imagine you are walking down the street and you see an old friend who has meant a great deal to you. You are surprised and delighted; you haven't seen this person for a long time. Pretend I am your friend. I want you to say "Hi" to me, but do it with your teeth clenched tightly together, like this. As you listen to yourself speak, be aware of the tension in your face. Now, go ahead.

C: Hi! Ugh, that sounded like a growl.

T: Exactly. A stern voice, a rigid facial expression, and a friendly word just don't add up to a consistent impression. They don't feel right together. That's what I mean about a mixed message. If I were your friend, I wouldn't know whether you were glad to see me or not. Now, I want you to try again, but this time smile and put some enthusiasm in your voice.

C: Hi!

T: That was much better. You made good eye contact and sounded glad to see me.

C: I felt different, but I don't know if I can remember everything at once. It's hard for me to look people in the eye all the time, too.

T: We'll do some more practice here, taking one thing at a time. I'll show you how to make eye contact without feeling you have to stare at people.

Self-feedback for experimentation now includes content, nonverbal behavior, and paralinguistics. Assignments are a short conversation, smiling at five people, and relating an interesting or meaningful experience with appropriate feeling to a friend or into a tape recorder.

The second part of the overall conversational strategy, awareness and expression of reactions, is introduced in subsequent sessions. Reactions are described to the client as natural responses to observations, that is, thoughts and feelings about what is perceived. Reactions include indications of curiosity or interest, asking for clarification, making associations to one's own experiences, self-disclosure, changing or expanding a topic of conversation, and sharing opinions. A separate session is usually devoted to expressing emotional reactions and responding to those of others (e.g., empathy). The emphasis is on the facilitative aspects of observations and reactions for maintaining conversations and the satisfactions of mutual, active participation. Each instructional component is followed by appropriate homework (e.g., asking open questions to express interest).

The client has reported on a lunchtime conversation with some co-workers in which he was participating actively until the discussion turned to a current movie. He had an opinion about the film that differed from the others' reactions. Fearing rejection (and somewhat angry), the client kept silent and dropped out of the conversation.

T: So you didn't inquire why the others thought the film was so good, and you didn't say why you didn't care for it.
C: I knew they would jump all over me if I did.
T: The way people in your family got so angry when somebody had a different idea.
C: Yeah. I don't want to go through that again!
T: You don't necessarily have to. You are still going to meet people from time to time who are defensive and hostile, but most people don't find differences of opinion so threatening if we express ourselves well. When you think about it, differences of opinion are just differences in experience, and it makes sense that no two experiences are exactly alike. If you show you respect other people's experiences and indicate respect for your own, you can have quite an interesting conversation.
C: Maybe, but how do I do that without just giving in and agreeing with them?
T: It's partly what you say and partly how you say it. For example, what was your reaction when you heard these people praising the movie?
C: Well, I wanted to know what they saw in it that was so great.
T: That's a very appropriate open question. Good for you. But you sounded a little hostile and challenging as you expressed your reaction. If you had been asking me, I would have felt that you were saying there was something wrong with my experience—that you were offended personally. Ask me again. Sound interested; you respect my opinion and would really like to hear it.
C: What was there about it that you liked?
T: Good! That was much better. I wouldn't be at all afraid to answer you. Now we have a conversation going. You have an opportunity to express your reactions to my experience and to the movie. When you do, make it clear that you are expressing an opinion; try to avoid sounding harsh or dogmatic. That can put a stop to a conversation.
C: Give me an example.
T: Well, if you thought the acting was poor, you could say something like "I was disappointed in the acting," and elaborate on that, rather than saying "The acting was lousy, period" in an angry tone. Let's choose a movie we have both seen and talk about our reactions to it. We'll pay particular attention to how we sound to one another so that we are encouraged to continue talking, rather than shutting the other person down.

Timing and active listening are critical aspects of refining conversational skills. Here the client is reporting on a conversation with a young woman who talked of her demanding job and long overtime hours without reward. The client responded by offering several practical solutions to the problems caused by this situation. The therapist helps him discriminate response deficits from social perception deficits.

T: How did she react to your suggestions?

C: I guess they weren't very good because she didn't seem interested in hearing about them. We didn't talk much after that. I must have sounded stupid.

T: Let's see if we can understand better what may have happened to learn something for the next time. Actually, I think the suggestions you made were quite sensible, but you may have missed something.

C: What do you mean?

T: What did you observe about this woman's feelings as she told you about her experience?

C: She sounded real upset.

T: How did you react to that observation?

C: I felt sorry for her, but I thought if I called attention to her feelings she might get more upset. So I just told her what I thought there was to do about her problem.

T: It might have worked out better for your conversation if you had timed your suggestions differently, saved them for later. Often when people talk about a problem, they are interested in solutions only after they have had a chance to talk a little about their feelings. Do you remember our discussion about empathy—putting yourself in someone else's emotional shoes for a minute to see what his or her experience might be like?

C: You mean what I would have been feeling if that had been my situation. I guess I would feel sort of unappreciated.

T: I think that's the kind of response she may have wanted from you—a reaction to her feelings—before she heard your suggestions.

C: I really messed up, didn't I.

T: How about saying something more rational to yourself. After all, a few weeks ago you wouldn't have been in this conversation at all.

C: I guess you're right. I did keep it going a while. It would have been better if I had been sharper, but it wasn't a disaster.

The preceding dialogue highlights only the major elements of the training process. More sophisticated components of expressiveness such as offering condolences or joining a conversation in progress can easily be accommodated with the conversational model. Occasionally, clients will discover they have had the requisite skills all along; the training process and homework have mainly served to provide the necessary expert endorsement and structure to allow them to perform with confidence. Although each client should be allowed to proceed at his or her own pace, to maintain continuity, the therapist should insist that the basic aspects of training be completed within 6 weeks. So long as behavior is being generated, special needs and difficulties can be addressed effectively.

Assessment of the client's progress is a multifaceted process. Structured homework assignments yield his or her own reports of conversational skill, satisfaction, and involvement. More formal quantitative and qualitative evaluation is achieved by a second administration of the pretreatment instruments and tape recordings. Because conversational problems generally represent only a portion of a client's overall difficulties, follow-up assessments can be accomplished in the ongoing therapeutic context.

Summary

Unassertiveness is a broad, generic term that may be applied to several types of social difficulties. Research has specified seven relatively distinct response classes. The response class that involves initiating and maintaining conversations was chosen for discussion because it appears to be a component of several important psychiatric syndromes. Although conversational difficulties are the cause of much subjective distress, they are seldom the reason for referral. More often, the therapist must identify the conversational problem as an important source of depression, social isolation, and so forth. Treatment should include the basic elements of all assertiveness training—cognitive restructuring, response acquisition, response reproduction, response shaping and response transfer. In our approach, each element has been addressed through an observation-reaction (stimulus-response) model of conversational behavior.

The power of the observation-reaction conversational strategy is its generalizability. Cross-situational, it is a model for initiating and maintaining conversations in a variety of social contexts. It facilitates the client's moving from superficial to more intimate relationships in which the ability to observe accurately and react with sensitivity are critical factors. The strategy is comprehensive, yet it preserves client uniqueness. Incorporated into a structured format, the strategy minimizes the typically vexing problems of response transfer from training to real-life experiences. What is being taught in therapy is the recognition of behaviors already employed in normal, everyday functioning. Training shapes these behaviors into specific skills for interactions that are a focal point of the social environment. Through feedback in natural settings, ecological validity of the client's skills is achieved.

Training in conversational skills has obvious, direct value. The ability to interact with others in a variety of situations and settings is personally enriching and effective behavior. However, there are indirect benefits as well. For example, depressed individuals commonly remain withdrawn and isolated in spite of available social opportunities. Gradual social exposure achieved through a structured conversational training process has the potential to produce reinforcing experiences that can contribute to improved mood and, in turn, motivate further constructive behaviors. Whatever the client's presenting problem, improved social competence has widespread implications for overall well-being, changes in affect, and other adjustive functions.

References

Alberti, R. E., & Emmons, M. L. (1974). *Your perfect right: A guide to assertive behavior.* San Luis Obispo, CA: Impact.

Bucell, M. (1979). *An empirically derived self-report inventory for the assessment of assertive behavior.* Unpublished doctoral dissertation, Kent State University.

Eisler, R. M., Blanchard, E. B., Fitts, H., & Williams, J. G. (1978). Social skill training with and without modeling for schizophrenic and non-psychotic hospitalized psychiatric patients. *Behavior Modification, 2,* 147–171.

Ellis, A. (1962). *Reason and emotion in psychotherapy.* New York: Lyle Stuart,

Glasgow, R., & Arkowitz, H. (1975). The behavioral assessment of male and female social competence in dyadic heterosexual interactions. *Behavior Therapy, 6,* 488–498.

Goldsmith, J. B., & McFall, R. M. (1975). Development and evaluation of an interpersonal-skill traning program for psychiatric inpatients. *Journal of Abnormal Psychology, 84,* 51–58.

Hersen, M., & Bellack, A. S. (1976). Social skills training for chronic psychiatric patients: Rationale, research findings, and future directions. *Comprehensive Psychiatry, 18,* 559–580.

Hersen, M., Eisler, R. J., Miller, P. M., Johnson, M. B., & Pinkston, S. G. (1973). Effects of practice, instructions, and modeling on components of assertive training. *Behaviour Research and Therapy, 11,* 443–451.

Hersen, M., Kazdin, A. E., Bellack, A. S., & Turner, S. M. (1979). Effects of live modeling, covert modeling, and rehearsal on assertiveness in psychiatric patients. *Behaviour Research and Therapy, 17,* 369–377.

Lazarus, A. A. (1973). On assertive behavior: A brief note. *Behavior Therapy, 4,* 697–699.

Lewinsohn, P. M. (1975). The behavioral study and treatment of depression. In M. Hersen, R. M. Eisler, & P. M. Miller (Eds.), *Progress in behavior modification* (Vol. 1) (pp. 19–64). New York: Academic Press.

Martinson, W. D., & Zerface, J. P. (1970). Comparisons of individual counseling and a social program with non-daters. *Journal of Counseling Psychology, 17,* 36–40.

Rich, A. R., & Schroeder, H. E. (1976). Research issues in assertiveness training. *Psychological Bulletin, 83,* 1081–1096.

Twentyman, C. T., & McFall, R. M. (1975). Behavioral training of social skills in shy males. *Journal of Consulting and Clinical Psychology, 43,* 384–395.

Williams, C. L., & Ciminero, A. R. (1978). Development and validation of a heterosocial skills inventory: The Survey of Heterosexual Interactions for Females. *Journal of Consulting and Clinical Psychology, 46,* 1547–1548.

Wolpe, J., & Lazarus, A. A. (1966). *Behavior therapy techniques.* New York: Pergamon.

Zigler, E., & Phillips, L. (1961). Social competence and outcome in psychiatric disorder. *Journal of Abnormal and Social Psychology, 63,* 264–271.

Zimbardo, P. G. (1977). *Shyness.* New York: Jove.

Sex Role Considerations for the Behavior Therapist

Patricia A. Resick

Introduction

When asked if I would write a chapter on behavior therapy with women I had a number of reactions. I was looking forward to the opportunity to integrate my reading, research, and therapy experience more formally. However, I had some concerns. Most of the other chapters in this book focus on problems rather than populations. Being a woman is not a problem. The way that women are treated is sometimes a problem. A chapter on behavior therapy with women also carries a connotation that the problems of women are outside the mainstream of behavior therapy. Franks and Rothblum (1983) have written:

> Too often, textbooks on issues affecting both sexes include a chapter or section on how the particular topic affects women. One is led to conclude then, that all preceding material must refer specifically to men. (pp. 262–263)

Therefore, I have decided not to write a chapter on behavior therapy for women but on sex role considerations for both genders. Sex role socialization is so ingrained in all of our upbringing that it is often easy to overlook and separate it out as an important facet of our learning histories.

This chapter is less clinical and more academic than the other chapters in this book because the appropriate behavioral techniques for the special problems of men and women are already found in the other problem-oriented chapters. The

PATRICIA A. RESICK • Department of Psychology, University of Missouri–St. Louis, St. Louis, Missouri 63121.

purpose of this chapter is to help the clinician consider how sex role socialization may affect the development of the particular problems that clients present with and to help the clinician determine targets for change. After general issues have been presented, two specific problems, depression and nonassertive behavior, will be considered as examples.

Sex Differences in Psychological Disorders

One of the questions that has received a fair amount of attention in the past decade is whether women suffer from more psychological problems than men (Dohrenwend & Dohrenwend, 1974; Goldman & Ravid, 1980; Gove & Tudor, 1973). After reviewing the body of research on the topic, Gove (1980) concluded that women have higher rates of "mental illness" than men. He also concluded that this was not an artifact based on differences in treatment seeking or clinician bias. He determined, however, that there were different rates, depending upon marital status. Married women have higher rates of mental illness, whereas single, widowed, and divorced women have comparable if not lower rates than men. Gove concluded that the marital role was probably responsible for this sex difference because modern housewives have less to contribute in our mechanized society than in the past, are more isolated, and have only one source of gratification and reinforcement (family), whereas men have two (family and work). He further pointed out that even when women occupy two roles by working, they typically hold less reinforcing positions (less prestigious and lower salaries) in the job market and have greater role strain, trying to perform most of the household chores and child rearing as well as the job.

Gove's conclusions regarding sex differences in mental illness have not gone unchallenged (Johnson, 1980). One of the major problems with Gove's review and conclusions is that his definition of mental illness is very narrow and includes only problems that involve personal discomfort and/or mental disorganization. By this definition he excludes all personality disorders, such as the antisocial personality, and the misuse of alcohol and drugs, which he contends causes more discomfort for society than the afflicted individual. Dohrenwend and Dohrenwend (1976) reported that men are more frequently diagnosed as having personality disorders, and the sex difference in alcohol use is well established (Johnson, 1982). If one were to examine "maladaptive behavior" rather than "mental illness," the sex differences in crime and aggression that result in incarceration for men, rather than treatment in a mental health facility, would surely alter the conclusion that women have more psychological problems.

Even disregarding prison populations, it appears that there is no sex difference in the usage of mental health facilities. In a study based on data compiled by the National Institute of Mental Health, Belle and Goldman (1980) and Belle (1980) found that overall, men and women utilize mental health facilities at equal rates, but the most frequent diagnosis for men is alcoholism, whereas for women it is depression. There were, however, no sex differences in schizophrenia. Ultimately, it is probably not as meaningful to determine if there is an overall sex difference in the rate of psychological disturbance as it is to identify differential patterns of maladjustment, and more importantly, to determine why these differences exist.

There appear to be sex differences in most of the disorders that behavior therapists treat (American Psychiatric Association, 1980); for instance depressed women outnumber men by as much as 2 or 3 to 1 (Silverman, 1968; Weissman & Klerman, 1977; Weissman & Myers, 1978), whereas men have greater problems with alcohol abuse than women at a ratio of about 5 to 1 (Efron, Keller, & Gurioli, 1974; Gomberg, 1974). Women exhibit more anxiety, phobias, and agoraphobia than men (Brehony, 1983; Fodor, 1974). Men have greater problems with anger, aggression, and antisocial behavior (Maccoby & Jacklin, 1974; Uniform Crime Reports, 1980). Women have more problems with eating disorders: obesity, anorexia, and bulimia (Metropolitan Life Insurance Co., 1960; Ross, 1977; U.S. Department of Health, Education, and Welfare, 1979). Men have greater problems with sexual deviations.

A logical source for these sex differences lies within sex role socialization. Boys and men are treated differently than girls and women. They are reinforced for different types of responses and develop different repertoires of coping strategies and maladaptive behaviors. Through vicarious learning, most men and women have imitated to at least some extent the stereotypes for each gender that are represented as the ideal in our cultural norms. Unfortunately, it appears that people may be in a double bind with regard to sex roles.

Men and women appear to be judged harshly when they deviate from behavior that is judged to be appropriate for their sex. In both analog studies and a retrospective survey of a child clinic's referrals, Feinblatt and Gold (1976) found that the child exhibiting behavior inappropriate to his or her sex was seen as more severely disturbed, as more in need of treatment, and as having a less successful future. In the clinic setting, they found that more boys than girls were referred for being emotional or passive and more girls than boys were referred for being defiant and verbally aggressive. Similar judgments were made of adults who deviated from the stereotypes in analog studies by Marecek (1974), Israel, Raskin, Libow, and Fravder (1978), and in a study of psychiatric hospitalization patterns (Rosenfield, 1982). It appears from these findings that children and adults who exhibit cross-gender behaviors are the targets of concern if not punishment. On the other hand, aspiring to the stereotypes may moderate the negative judgments of other people, but it may cause problems with effective functioning, particularly for women.

The Problem with Femininity

The frequently cited study by Broverman, Broverman, Clarkson, Rosenkrantz, and Vogel (1970) first illustrated the problem that women face when they behave in a stereotyped feminine manner. Characteristics that are deemed appropriate and desirable in adult women are not the characteristics judged desirable in a healthy adult. There have been a number of studies that have found that femininity is associated with poor psychological functioning.

In a series of studies conducted to validate the reformulation of sex role constructs into masculinity, femininity, androgyny, and undifferentiated roles, Bem and her associates found that feminine individuals showed behavioral deficits even in situations that called for nurturant responses (Bem, 1975; Bem & Lenney, 1976; Bem, Martyna, & Watson, 1976). LaTorre (1978) found that both feminine men and feminine women scored higher on the neuroticism scale of the Eysenck Personality Inventory than masculine or androgynous individuals of either gender. Femininity has been associated with lower self-esteem than masculinity and androgyny in several studies (Antill & Cunningham, 1979; Jones, Chernovetz, & Hansson, 1978; Kimlicka, Cross & Tarnai, 1983). In a series of studies, Jones et al. (1978) also found that femininity in men was associated with greater external locus of control and alcohol use than masculine men, whereas feminine women were more introverted than masculine women.

For women, then, it appears that there are negative consequences with either choice. If women behave in a masculine fashion (i.e., with instrumental behavior), they may develop greater competence and self-esteem. They will, however, risk more negative evaluations from others if they act in a manner that is typically viewed as masculine. Feminine behavior may not be as personally adaptive, but it may elicit greater social support.

In men, femininity is related to problems in personal adjustment as well as negative evaluations by others. The positive behaviors that are viewed as masculine lead to greater self-esteem and social reinforcement in men. It has been pointed out by Kelly, Caudill, Hathorn, and O'Brien (1977) that

It may be that masculine-typed behaviors carry a higher probability of socially reinforcing outcomes than feminine-typed behavior. It is also likely that the same masculine or feminine typed behavior will lead to differentially reinforced outcomes depending upon whether the person engaging in it is a man or a woman. (p. 1186)

In an analysis of ecological sources of dysfunction for women, Elaine Blechman (1980) has modified Radloff and Rae's (1979) two-factor sequential model to explain the etiology of depression. Their model first includes a susceptibility factor. Susceptibility to depression would result from a learning history of helpless behavior and negative cognitions. The second factor, precipitating conditions, are life problems and crises that require goal-oriented problem solving and persistent action. Blechman's third factor is a paternalistic social setting. She proposes that this factor may account for the sex differences observed in depression.

Paternalism is the setting under which all children are socialized. In adolescence and adulthood, however, paternalism toward women continues, whereas it ceases for men. Paternalism is a setting in which individuals can rely on others to take responsibility for their life problems. Such individuals are not given opportunities to develop effective instrumental skills or take risks and are not expected to cope with life's stressful events. Under such a system it is understandable why many women would not develop the instrumental skills that have been labeled *masculine*. Once women exhibit deficits in instrumental skills, they may self-select into paternalistic marriages or continue to live with their parents, therefore maintaining the problem. To substantiate this model, Blechman cites studies that illustrate paternalistic behavior, such as greater use of medication and number of therapy sessions given to depressed women than men (e.g., Stein, DelGaudio, & Ansley, 1976).

Other examples of how instrumental behavior in women is devalued or punished are readily found in the social psychological literature. There have been a number of studies that have looked at attributions for success and failure as well as performance evaluation by women and men. The typical paradigm in these studies is for participants to read vignettes or view artwork accompanied by a story about the artist and then rate the person who has been described. The variables that are manipulated are usually the gender of the person, the masculinity or femininity of the task, and whether the person is accomplished or still striving for success. Although there have been some conflicting findings regarding judgment in stereotyped or nonstereotyped fields (Goldberg, 1968; Kaschak, 1981; Mischel, 1974), overall, accomplishments are rated as greater when the subject of the vignette is a man rather than a woman (Feldman-Summers & Keisler, 1974; Goldberg, 1968; Kaschak, 1981; Pheterson, Kielser, & Goldberg, 1971). The exception is when women are clearly given an award for their accomplishments, they are viewed as equal to award-winning men (Kaschak, 1981; Pheterson *et al*, 1971). Unfortunately, in real life, acclamation and awards for performance are rare.

Using similar designs, researchers have also examined attributions of performance. It appears that when explaining successful performance, people tend to credit men with having more ability, whereas women are viewed as lucky (Deaux & Emswiller, 1974). When luck cannot be used as an explanation, men are assumed to possess more ability, whereas women's success is ascribed to either trying harder or having an easier task (Feather & Simon, 1975; Feldman-Summers & Kiesler, 1974).

In one study about award-winning college professors, Kaschak (1981) found that, although they were considered equally excellent, male professors were considered to be more powerful and effective. Female professors were considered to be more concerned and likable but only when teaching in feminine stereotyped fields (home economics and elementary education). It appears that attributions for success may be based on stereotypes of masculinity and femininity (instrumental versus affective) when given limited information about that person. Similarly, Feather and Simon (1975) found that both genders were viewed as more masculine if they succeeded and more feminine if they failed.

Self-attributions tend to follow a similar pattern. When given a choice between playing a game of skill or of chance, men tend to choose the game of skill, whereas women tend to choose the game of luck (Deaux, White, & Farris, 1975; Jones *et al.*, 1978). These men and women appear to be trying to maximize their probability of success and, because of their differential self-evaluations, they choose different means of doing so. Studies that ask subjects to predict how they will perform on a task usually find that men have a greater expectancy for success than women do, even when the actual outcome is the same (Brim, Glass, Neulinger, & Firestone, 1969; Crandall, 1969; Feather, 1969).

After the fact, men feel they have done better than women do even when the performance is the same. Men who do well attribute their success to ability, whereas women credit luck. At the same time, when women fail, they see it as a lack of ability, whereas men tend to externalize failure (Deaux, 1976; Dweck & Gilliard, 1975).

All in all, it appears as though women are shaped by a paternalistic society that expects very little of them and tends to discount or devalue women's accomplishments relative to those of men. Femininity is encouraged and differentially reinforced in women, who then may grow to believe that they are not as competent as they, in fact, may be. Such a situation is fertile ground for the development of depression and anxiety.

The Masculine Edict

Because the instrumentality that is associated with masculinity is probably more functional in terms of eliciting reinforcers than the affective responses labeled *feminine,* masculinity would appear to be clearly advantageous for men. Men do not face the double bind that women have of being viewed as neurotic if they behave in a feminine manner, but being viewed negatively and deviant if they behave in a masculine manner. Therefore, it appears that men have a clear path to instrumental success. Why, then, do men have greater rates of some disorders? Some of the reason may again be explained by differential shaping, and some of it may derive from extreme adherence to a rigid and narrow masculine role. On the one hand, men appear to receive greater recognition and reinforcement when they succeed, but what happens when they fail? In a competitive society, relatively few people are recognized as winners. Far more may be labeled or label themselves as *losers* or fall into the large middle range of performance. Although men may persist longer than women in the face of failure (Dweck & Gilliard, 1975), narrow definitions of masculinity eventually lead many men to be labeled (or to label themselves) as *unsuccessful.*

In the same way that women are devalued or disapproved of for success, there is evidence that men receive greater disapproval for failure than women and are viewed as less masculine (Deaux & Taynor, 1973; Feather & Simon, 1975). However, attribution for failure in women is that they do not have ability, whereas for men it is a lack of hard work (Feather & Simon, 1975). This pattern has also been seen in children and may help account for the fact that, given equal behavior, boys receive more behavioral criticism, and boys are more likely to persevere after failure, whereas girls are more likely to quit (Dweck & Bush, 1976). However, when expectancies and pressures to succeed do exceed ability, the boy or man may feel unsexed (Mead, 1949) and may need to compensate in some fashion.

One interesting study found that masculine sex-typed males reported being more aggressive and antisocial than they had several weeks earlier after listening to a tape that presented research findings of decreased masculinity in American college males. They did not increase their reports of prosocial masculine behavior. Androgynous men reported anxiety but responded by endorsing fewer masculine items. Men exposed to neutral or masculine validation tapes showed no such compensating responding (Babl, 1979). The author concluded that the results supported a social learning model of masculine compensation whereby highly sex-typed men reduced the anxiety that resulted from social comparison by means of an exaggerated display of masculinity. With such a model, rape and other acts of violence could be viewed as exaggerated masculine display and a means to reestablish power and dominance. Because holding one's liquor has traditionally been viewed as a sign of masculinity, increased alcohol use might also follow some threat to a man's identity.

At this point in time, our society appears to have developed an interesting new double standard. Although sex roles for women are becoming less confining and women are beginning to receive more reinforcement for behaving in an instrumental fashion, sex roles for men have not expanded much. On the one hand, it could be argued that there is no need for the male sex role to change. Masculinity as it has been measured is reinforced and functional. Masculine people have greater self-esteem than feminine people (Antill & Cunningham, 1979; Jones et al., 1978). On the other hand, the apparent one-sided advantages of masculinity may be at least partially a function of measurement and experimental design. Most of the scales that have been used recently in research to classify people as masculine, feminine, or androgynous are composed of only positively valued characteristics. It could be that some of the negative characteristics that are associated with masculinity are those that could prevent help-seeking or could lead to the development of particular problems that men develop at a greater rate than women. Some evidence supporting this has been provided by Holahan and Spence (1980) and Spence, Helmreich, and Holahan (1979).

Spence et al. (1979) extended the Personal Attributes Questionnaire (PAQ), a frequently used measure of sex role typing, to include scales measuring negative characteristics. The negative masculine scale included characteristics on which men score higher than women (arrogant, greedy, dictatorial, hostile, looks out only for self), whereas the undesirable femininity scale was divided into two sets of items, four of which indicate a lack of sense of self (spineless, gullible, servile, and subordinates self) and four of which represent verbally aggressive behavior (whiny, complaining, fussy, nags). In the first study, Spence et al. (1979) found that, in a university sample, self-reports of neurotic complaints and low self-esteem were primarily associated with low positive masculine scores and to a lesser degree to higher scores on the two negative feminine scales. Problem behaviors that were of an acting-out nature such as fighting, quarreling, or disciplinary problems were correlated with high negative masculine scores and negative feminine verbal behaviors to a lesser extent.

Holahan and Spence (1980) then compared a clinic population and another university sample. They found that neither group differed on socially desirable feminine traits for their gender, but clients scored lower on positive masculine traits and higher on negative masculine and the two negative feminine scales. Within the client group, depression and worry were negatively correlated with socially desirable masculinity, whereas a positive relationship occurred between anger and both negative masculinity and negative verbal femininity. These findings indicate that there may be aspects of behavior associated with masculinity that are socially undesirable and that they may be related to the more aggressive and anti-social behavioral disorders. In these studies, all subjects denied substance abuse, so the relationship between negative masculinity and substance abuse must remain on the speculative level pending further research.

David and Brannon (1976) have described four primary dimensions of the male sex role: (a) avoidance of all things feminine; (b) achievement, success, and competence; (c) toughness, confidence, and self-reliance; and (d) the aura of aggression, violence, and daring. Masculinity is so highly prized in our society that it appears it is not assumed present in all males but is something that must be established and proven regularly. Should a man begin to feel depressed or anxious, he would be violating all four of the dimensions of masculinity in the male sex role. Crying and expressions of emotion, particularly depression, are viewed as femi-nine. The depressed person feels like a failure, has diminished self-confidence, and may be more passive and withdrawn.

In order to maintain internal and external reinforcers as well as avoid social punishment, it might seem necessary to the depressed or anxious man to deny his problem and reestablish a feeling of self-reliance and masculinity. The results might be positive and prosocial, or negative and antisocial, depending upon the means by which he attempts to reestablish his control. Therapists working with men should not overlook the importance of sex roles as explanatory variables in the development and maintenance of psychological problems. Sex role conditioning may well be an important factor in the types and rates of disorders that are seen in women and men. Furthermore, within disorders, men and women may express problems differently, have a different course, benefit by different procedures, and have different outcomes because they, and society, have different standards for "normal" behavior for men and women.

Behavior Therapy and Sex Roles

While other therapies and theories are being revised to accomodate the onslaught of information and criticism that has emerged in the past decade regard-ing women and sex roles, behavior therapy has remained relatively unaffected.

Because behavioral theories and techniques are relatively value free, behavior therapists have congratulated themselves for being nonsexist (Lazarus, 1974), but have not examined these issues much further. Perhaps behaviorists have avoided dealing with sex role socialization because masculinity and femininity appear all too traitlike or because they appear to fall under the province of developmental and social psychologists. Only recently have behaviorists suggested that sex roles are conditioned interpersonal strategies that men and women have learned through differential reinforcement and modeling (Kelly, 1983). As such, sex roles have received far too little attention by behavior therapists and theorists. Too often, therapy procedures and theories have been developed about specific disorders that skirt the issue entirely. Male subjects are used when therapists illustrate the effectiveness of treatments for anger control, alcohol abuse, type A coronary-prone behavior, or minimal dating. Female subjects appear in research on depression, assertiveness, or anxiety management. Because one can avoid analyzing sex differences in outcome if only one gender is used in the research, many researchers may not consider that their goals for therapy, treatment procedures, and results may only apply to the gender they are studying. And, sex role behavior may be a more important variable than gender *per se*. Kelly (1983) has pointed out that although most men are masculine typed and most women are feminine typed, gender and sex roles are certainly not identical. It may be that we should be analyzing for sex role differences rather than gender differences in order to determine the influence of sex role socialization and modeling on the development of appropriate behavior and interpersonal competence.

Although the technology of behavior therapy is value free with regard to the roles of men and women, the selection of target behaviors cannot be value free and may well reflect the beliefs of the therapist as well as society. For example, there was a flurry of reaction to a case study by Rekers and Lovaas (1974) in which they modified the behavior of a 5-year-old boy with cross-gender behavior patterns. Target behaviors that were selected as desirable were (a) male dress (military and football garb); (b) masculine aggression; and (c) playing with designated male toys. Undesirable target behaviors were (a) dressing in girls' clothes; (b) maternal nurturance; (c) feminine behaviors such as playing with girls or dolls; and (d) female role play.

Critics of the study (Nordyke, Baer, Etzel, & LeBlanc, 1977; Winkler, 1977; Wolfe, 1979) objected to the treatment for a number of reasons. Among other things, they argued that Rekers and Lovaas were imposing their value judgment that the sex role status quo would bring the greatest happiness and adjustment, and they objected to the suppression of the child's nurturance and interaction with girls and dolls while reinforcing him for aggression. These critics suggested that the child's repertoire of appropriate prosocial masculine behaviors could have been expended without eliminating prosocial feminine behaviors.

Wolfe (1979) further argued that by labeling some behaviors as *feminine a priori*, and therefore inappropriate for a boy, the therapists may be suppressing behaviors that are the precursors of important adult skills (e.g., parenting and nurturance) or that could more appropriately be defined as avoidance patterns or skills deficits, such as problems in motor skills development. Although it is understandable that the therapists wished to spare the child from what they believed would be future pathology and rejection, the lack of clear research on the relationship between early childhood behaviors and adult pathology or sex roles leaves this area open to much value judgment and debate. It may be the case that problems in motor development in a male child receive a pejorative feminine label from others. Upon being labeled as a *sissy*, the child then labels himself as such and behaves accordingly. He may avoid male activities in which he has little reinforcement and gravitate to female activities and company (Hay, Barlow, & Hay, 1981). It is an unfortunate fact that in present society the male role is so rigid that anyone who deviates somewhat from the prescribed behavior may be the cause for concern or ridicule. Much less attention is given to girls who cross-dress and behave like tomboys.

In a study that was responsive to these issues, Hay *et al.* (1981) taught a 10-year-old boy to exhibit more masculine mannerisms (such as book carrying and arm gestures) through covert modeling, without punishing pretreatment sex-typed feminine behaviors, or reinforcing aggression. By defining and assessing masculinity and femininity as the gender differences that are observed in mannerisms, rather than a whole constellation of instrumental and affective behaviors, these researchers have taken a step away from trait theory and toward a functional analysis of sex role behavior. Perhaps *androgyny* could be viewed as a summary term for a person who exhibits a wide range of skills in a variety of situations. As such, androgyny, like masculinity or femininity, could be used to describe, not immutable traits but types of behaviors that are emitted with varying effectiveness by men and women.

Assessment of Sex Roles

Unfortunately, because masculinity, femininity, and androgyny usually have been correlated with adjective traits in past research (e.g., nurturant, aggressive, competent, emotional), there has been almost no behavioral assessment research to examine these concepts. We know how society responds to the labels *men, women, masculine,* and *feminine,* but little research has been conducted to determine if there are gender or sex role differences in component interpersonal and cognitive behaviors. One exception is in the study of assertiveness (the topic of assertiveness training will be given more attention later in the chapter).

Kelly, O'Brian, and Hosford (1981) conducted a study that assessed subjects' behaviors independently of their self-reports in an attempt to move toward construct validation of the new sex role formulations for androgyny, femininity, masculinity, and undifferentiated. Female and male undergraduates were given the Bem Sex Role Inventory and were then assigned to one of the four sex role categories. The subjects then participated in a behavior assessment study of commendatory and refusal assertion. Ratings were made of components that are frequently assessed in social skills and assertiveness research: latency and duration of response, loudness, affect, speech dysfluencies, and overall assertiveness. They found that for gender-consistent behavior, refusal scenes for men and commendatory scenes for women, there were no differences among sex role types; all women were equally complimentary and all men were able to refuse assertively. For the cross-gender situations, the findings differed somewhat. Androgynous women were more effective with refusal assertion than the other three sex role types. Androgynous, masculine, and feminine men differed from undifferentiated men on commendatory scenes, with androgynous men scoring the highest. Although the sample size was small, these findings do provide some evidence that androgyny is associated with effective and flexible interpersonal style.

Within the social psychological paradigms, Bem and her colleagues (Bem, 1975; Bem & Lenney, 1976; Bem *et al.*, 1976) have also conducted a series of construct validation studies using the Bem Sex Role Inventory, which examines behavioral situations. They found that sex-typed individuals avoided or were uncomfortable with cross-sex situations. Masculine-typed men showed less supportive, expressive, and playful behaviors across several situations. Feminine females failed to maintain independence in conformity situations. Androgynous people functioned better across the majority of situations. Taken together, their findings are that *androgyny* may indeed be a summary term for the person who possesses a range of flexible interpersonal skills. Both masculine and feminine people appear to have more skills deficits and rigidity in some situations.

Without considering sex roles *per se,* there is a body of literature within social psychology that has examined sex differences in nonverbal behaviors. Across both human and primate research, the use of personal space has been associated with dominance. There are also sex differences in eye contact, smiling, and a variety of vocal qualities such as amount, volume, intonation, and interruptions that may indicate a person's status in interactions (Frieze & Ramsey, 1976). Although most therapists are aware, at least informally, of these differences, and those who do assertiveness training often target these nonverbal behaviors, most researchers have not associated them with sex roles or interpersonal dominance. Further work is clearly warranted in the behavioral assessment of sex roles.

There are four frequently used self-report scales that have classified people into one of the four sex role categories. They are (a) The Bem Sex Role Inventory (Bem, 1974); (b) The Personal Attributes Questionnaire (Spence, Helmreich, & Stapp, 1974, 1975); (c) The PRF: ANDRO Scale from the Personality Research Form (Berzins, Welling, & Wetter, 1975); and (d) Independent Masculinity and Femininity Scales from the Adjective Check List (Heilbrun, 1976). A review of these scales and their psychometric properties has been published by Kelly and Worell (1977). It should be mentioned again that except for the revised PAQ (Spence *et al.*, 1979), these scales contain only positive components of sex typing. In addition to Spence *et al.*, Kelly *et al.* (1977) found that undesirable characteristics were differentially distributed across sex role types. Androgynous men endorsed the fewest and undifferentiated men endorsed the most undesirable characteristics. Feminine females are least likely to attribute negative masculine characteristics to themselves. Although most behavior therapists would not find the scales helpful except for research purposes, they may provide information about gender role orientation generally.

For specific client assessment and treatment planning, a functional analysis of the client's behavior within the context of his or her environment is desirable. Without an understanding of the context, the environmental supports, and pressures affecting the client, it will not be possible to determine if the problem is a skills deficit of the client, if the problem resides within the environment, or whether there is an interaction between the client's behavior and his or her environment that may be responsible. In addressing this point, Blechman (1980) cites the findings that women take more responsibility for failure and difficulties than may be warranted. Without further investigation, therapists may misattribute the cause of the difficulties based on the female client's self-report.

In addition to observation of clients' behaviors and skills levels in several situations, a careful interview may elicit important cognitions regarding how clients view their behavior in light of current sex roles. Questions about the type of behavior that was expected of them and reinforced by their parents may point out areas of role conflict and perceptions of failure. Cognitive restructuring or rational emotive therapy (RET) may be warranted when the therapist finds that there are no skills deficits but unrealistic expectations or feelings of inefficacy that are causing the distress. Role conflict and overload may be assessed by having clients monitor their activities. For example, although society may be more accepting of women in the workplace, many women are single parents or still carry the bulk of child care and housework responsibilities after work and on the weekends. Such role strain may contribute to depression, anxiety, and physiological symptoms of stress. Self-monitoring may provide valuable information to the therapist as well as point out areas that should be targetted for change. Assertion training and marital negotiation could be implemented to distribute a more equitable workload among family members, and task analysis may result in more efficient use of time. And finally, an examination of standards for tasks may help pinpoint priorities. Many women feel that they *must* do some activities or tasks, not because it is important or enjoyable to them, but because they fear that others may judge them as poor wives or mothers if they do not do them. For example, RET may prove beneficial in helping a working woman to let go of exceedingly high standards for housework that she had been taught.

In conclusion, interviews, self-monitoring, and behavioral observation should focus on learned sex roles as well as the presenting symptomatology of clients. Therapists should look for skills deficits, a rigid or limited range of skills, as well as environmental pressures to behave in only a narrow or extreme sex-typed manner. Expectations and standards regarding sex roles may also play an important role in the development of maladaptive behavior. In their effort to avoid being feminine, men may opt for self-medication (alcohol and drug abuse) rather than seeking help or expressing doubts and emotions, a sign of femininity (i.e., weakness), and women may confuse positive with negative masculinity and believe that to be assertive is to be aggressive, domineering, and self-centered. Such cognitions and beliefs should be explored in therapy as well as assessment.

Sex Roles and Maladaptive Behavior: The Case of Depression

It was mentioned earlier in the chapter that sex role typing has been implicated in the development of depression in women (Blechman, 1980; Rothblum, 1983). Although some researchers have cited hormones as at least a partial explanation for the sex differences in depression (Weissman, 1980), sex roles are probably a better explanation. The effects of sex role socialization can be incorporated within any of the major behavioral theories of depression. Blechman's (1980) three-factor social ecology model of adjustment can be used to explain sex differences in depression and is also compatible with the cognitive and learning theories of depression. Paternalism sets the environmental conditions for women to learn a helpless stance. They may then find that reinforcers or punishers in their lives are not contingent upon their responses (Lewinsohn, 1974; Seligman, 1975). The socialization of self-defeating evaluation and cognitions in women was illustrated earlier in the chapter. When women are taught to believe that their accomplishments are due to luck rather than skill, they may perceive that there is little connection between their responses and reinforcers. Status inequality in marriage, in the form of differential salaries for women, and the prevalence of violence (rape, incest, and spouse abuse) further enhance the perception of inadequacy and helplessness. Perhaps some of the cognitive theories (Beck, 1967; Rehm, 1977) should begin to incorporate sex role socialization as a precursor to depressive cognitions and the "kernel of truth" that is then overgeneralized. The success of self-control therapy (Fuchs & Rehm, 1977; Rehm, Fuchs, Roth, Kornblith, & Romano, 1979) may be due to the relearning of patterns of self-evaluation and self-reinforcement. Rehm *et al.* (1979) also found that assertiveness training was beneficial for many women.

Another explanation for at least some of the sex differences in depression has emerged recently. Warren (1983) examined the literature on depression regarding men. She has proposed that men have an intolerance for depression because the depressive experience is incompatible with the male sex role. Several studies support this contention. Depressed people of both genders have been rated more feminine than masculine (Hammen & Peters, 1978). In another study, Hammen and Peters (1977) found that depression elicited more rejection of men than women, and the sex difference in rejection of depression was more pronounced than for anxiety or flat affect-detached responses. They also found that depressed men were more likely to be perceived as impaired in role functioning than depressed women.

These studies indicate that there would be good reason for men to hide their depression from others. Although there has been no direct research that men deny and avoid depression, Kessler, Brown, and Broman (1981) found that men were less likely than women to perceive and report that they had a problem. In a study of sex differences in the expression of depressive responses on the Beck Depression Inventory, men appeared to be more stoic. They are less able to cry, have greater social withdrawal, and have a greater sense of failure. They appeared to express depression more somatically with weight loss, sleep disturbance, and somatic preoccupation. Padesky and Hammen (1981) also found greater aggression and tension among depressed men. It has also been suggested that some depressed men are identified as alcoholic but are not diagnosed as depressed (Rothblum, 1983; Weissman, 1980). More research on this proposition is necessary.

Warren (1983) has speculated that if men, in fact, are intolerant of depression, there are probably both positive and negative consequences. On one hand, their short-term coping responses are probably adaptive in that men are more likely to cope with depression with active responses such as keeping busy and engaging in enjoyable activities—responses that therapists are likely to encourage (Funabiki, Bologna, Pepping, & Fitzgerald, 1980). On the other hand, if men tend to withdraw and deny depression, interpersonal relationships, particularly marital relationships, may be strained. Also, they may not make important life changes if they do not acknowledge having problems.

Therapists should be aware that depression is a possibility even when male clients do not label themselves as such and do not behave like depressed women. When men said that they would not use the term *depressed,* Warren (1983) asked them what words they would use. Their choices were *bored, tired, disappointed, overworked, dissatisfied, stressed,* and so forth. Once appropriate diagnosis is made, the therapist will need to shape self-disclosure slowly and will need to discuss the limiting aspects of rigid sex roles with the client, perhaps confronting his irrational fears of losing his masculinity. Treatment of depression within this context could then proceed.

The Question of Assertion

The assertion training literature is rather lopsided. Ostensibly, assertion training can be used to help either passive or aggressive people become more appropriately assertive. It also can be used, depending upon one's definition of assertiveness, to teach positive assertion skills such as giving and receiving compliments, praise, empathy, self-disclosure, and social initiation skills (initiating conversations and asking for dates) as well as negative assertive behavior such as refusing unreasonable requests, expressing dissatisfaction, or requesting a change in behavior (Kelly, Frederiksen, Fitts, & Phillips, 1978; Warren & Gilner, 1978). Assertion training can be used with men as well as women.

However, an inspection of the literature leaves one with the impression that, except for minimal dating college males, assertion training is usually for women and particularly emphasizes negative assertion. This lopsidedness probably reflects who and why people seek out therapy.

A question that has been examined in the past few years is how people react to assertive behavior in men and women. The question carries important clues as to why some people might not be assertive. If a person anticipates punishment in response to assertion, she or he may suppress assertive responses. In fact, there is some evidence that, overall, assertive people have been rated as more competent and effective than nonassertive people, but they are also viewed as unsympathetic, hostile, and less likeable (Hull & Schroeder, 1979; Keane, St. Lawrence, Himadi, Graves, & Kelly, 1983; Kelly, St. Lawrence, Bradlyn, Himadi, Graves, & Keane, 1982; Woolfolk & Dever, 1979).

Thus far, the question of differential perception of assertion in men and women has been mixed. Kelly, Kern, Kirkley, Patterson, and Keane (1980) found that assertion by women resulted in more negative evaluations than by men.

Although all assertive models were rated higher on achievement but less likeable than nonassertive models, assertive women were viewed as significantly less attractive, less likeable, and lower on ability and competence than assertive male models by both male and female subjects. Lao, Upchurch, Corwin, and Grassnickle (1975) found similar sex differences in perception.

However, several other studies have not found differences in perception by the sex of the communicator (Gormally, 1982; Woolfolk & Dever, 1979) or the sex of the observer (Hull & Schroeder, 1979). Although more research is certainly needed to determine whether or not there are differences in perception of assertiveness in women and men, it may be that situational factors and the type of assertiveness being exhibited are important variables.

Gormally (1982) found that whether the subjects were listening to taped interactions or were actively involved in the interaction affected their perception of the confederate. The objective raters who just listened to the interaction rated the assertive confederate higher than the passive confederate on admiration, appropriateness, and enjoyment in working together, whereas the participants involved in the interactions rated the passive confederate higher than the assertive confederate on these same three variables.

St. Lawrence, Cutts, Tisdelle, Hansen, and Irish (1983) have proposed and investigated whether negative perceptions of assertion only occur with negative assertion or whether positive assertion may moderate perceptions. In their study, male and female participants observed videotapes of male and female confederates behaving assertively or unassertively in four refusal scenes, four commendatory scenes, or a combination of both refusal and commendatory scenes. Overall, as with previous research, assertive models were evaluated higher than nonassertive models on 10 competence variables, such as intelligent, socially skilled, and tactful, but were evaluated unfavorably on the 11 friendliness variables, such as considerate, open minded, sympathetic, kind, and warm. There also were main effects for the gender of the model in that female models were viewed as kinder, more agreeable and attractive, but less appropriate, truthful, and socially skilled than identically behaving male models.

With regard to the type of situation and behavior, St. Lawrence *et al.* (1983) found that in refusal situations assertive models were described as competent but strikingly unlikeable. However, in commendatory or mixed scenes, assertive models were viewed as both competent and likeable. Unassertive models in commendatory scenes were described as neither competent nor likable. Apparently, the presence of commendatory assertion moderates the negative impact of negative assertion. The gender of the model appeared to be much less important than the type of assertiveness being observed. Perhaps the harsh judgments on assertive people in past research are primarily due to the fact the subjects were only observing assertive models in negative, refusal-type situations. Clearly, perception of assertion is a complex reaction that requires more research to untangle.

Perceptions of masculinity and femininity may also play a role in a person's willingness to behave assertively. Hess, Bridgewater, Bornstein, and Sweeney (1980) conducted a study in which male and female subjects listened to "typical male," "typical female," or "ambiguous" tape-recorded assertive responses. The subjects then completed the Bem Sex Role Inventory and the Rathus Assertiveness Scale, as if they were the person on the tape. It was found that female subjects rated the actors more assertive, aggressive, and masculine across voice types and type of assertion (positive or negative). All subjects viewed actors in negative assertion scenes as more assertive, aggressive, and masculine, whereas feminine characteristics were ascribed to actors in positive situations. There also were differences in perception depending upon vocal characteristics. When the tape was easily identifiable as male or female, ratings of assertiveness were sex typed. When the voice was ambiguous, the subjects responded, depending upon assertion content (positive or negative). The authors concluded that because people are likely to be judged as feminine or masculine depending upon the type of assertion they exhibit, clinicians may encounter resistance teaching women expression of negative feelings and men the expression of positive feelings.

These findings receive support from the literature on sex differences in assertion. Although men have scored higher on assertion inventories than women in a number of studies, Hollandsworth and Wall (1977) found that there were sex differences in both directions on some of the component skills of assertiveness. They gave the College Self Expression Scale to four different samples of men and women. They considered items to represent sex differences if they were significantly different for two or more samples. There were no differences on any of the samples for 22 of 48 items. Twelve items met the criterion, of which 9 were found more frequently among women. Most of the items associated with men concerned negative assertion, particularly with employers. They were also more likely to initiate conversations and speak up in discussions. Women, on the other hand, were more likely to engage in commendatory assertion and express anger to parents than men.

The implications of this research are that sex roles should be considered in assertion training with men and women. Because commendatory, positive assertion may moderate the negative evaluations that can occur with refusal assertion, positive assertion should be taught first (St. Lawrence *et al.*, 1983). Fears of appearing too masculine or feminine should be addressed in the context of behavioral rehearsal or cognitive restructuring. Finally, mixed gender groups may be advantageous so that participants may observe positive and negative assertion in both genders and be able to practice with both. Stebbins, Kelly, Tolor, and Power (1977) found that both sexes were more likely to assert themselves with same-sex confederates. Mixed gender groups would allow for maximum rehearsal and feedback.

Case Study: Assertion Training with Rape Victims

The following transcript was selected for inclusion here because it illustrates some of the sex role implications that arise during the course of behavior therapy. Eight women were seen for six 2-hour sessions of assertion training. All had been raped at least 3 months previously. This assertion training was adapted from Lange and Jakubowski (1976). Therapy included a behavioral explanation of the development and maintenance of fear. The group members were taught to distinguish the components of assertive, nonassertive, and aggressive behaviors through exercises. They discussed personal rights and then were presented Ellis's ABC model of rational thinking. After two sessions of working on cognitive blocks to assertiveness, therapy then focused on modeling and rehearsal of assertive skills. The clients were taught covert as well as overt rehearsal.

This segment of the transcript was recorded during the fourth session. Although three of the group members spoke during this segment, the focus of this particular part of the session was on Margie, a single, 30-year-old woman who was employed as an administrative assistant for a local company.

Margie had never received any counseling or therapy prior to the rape and had never had particular problems with fear or depression. She was raped in her flat 2 years prior to this group by a man who had stolen her purse the day before. He let himself in with the keys he had stolen, and Margie awakened as he restrained her. After being forced to fellate him after being raped vaginally, she managed to throw him off and scream for help. Her roommate, who had been sleeping in another room, came into the room and in the confusion, the man fled, although Margie was trying to stop him. During the assault, Margie was terrified he would kill her. The assailant came back to the house on several other occasions but the police were unable to apprehend him. In the months that followed, Margie became depressed and developed fears of going out alone, of talking to strangers, or answering the phone at night. These problems continued for 2 years until she entered therapy.

During the first few sessions, Margie talked about how she had blamed herself for not changing the locks on her flat faster or doing something more to stop the rape. She focused on her "mistakes" and was finding it more difficult to interact with people than she had before the rape.

At the beginning of the fourth session we reviewed the material we had introduced the previous week, the ABC (event/belief/consequence) of rational emotive therapy. After explaining how the B statement could be changed to produce different consequences, we had the clients imagine scenes in which they changed their interpretation of the situation. Most of the group members reported having a different emotional reaction to their imagined situation, once they had changed their self-statements about it. We then had the clients discuss their self-monitoring of situations they had encountered that week. Margie volunteered to begin.

MARGIE: I had a problem with changing my feelings. I just . . . I thought of the things that were so stupid, that just drive me nuts. You know it's those tiny, itty, bitty little things, like, one of my roommates and I got into this argument because she wouldn't put more water in the chili. I wound up losing the argument. I always lose the argument and I figure, okay so she's stronger than I am. She always wins the argument. Then I started thinking, well that's stupid, that's really irrational. It doesn't make her a better person or a stronger person. And then, when it got down to "what do you tell yourself on such occasions in the future," I thought "she's gonna burn the chili if she doesn't add water the way I told her to," which is what happened. And some of the stupid little things just seem to aggravate me much more than the big things do.

CLIFF (therapist): What stupid little thing about that was the B statement?

MARGIE: She's stronger than I am. She always wins the argument.

CLIFF: She always?

MARGIE: Always!

CLIFF: Okay, well first of all let's deal with that, because that is an example of one of the faulty thinking patterns. *Always?* [*laughter*] Okay, just wanted to point that out. What other kind of B statement is there? "She's stronger than I am, *always,* and she always . . ."

MARGIE: "wins."

PATTI (therapist): I guess I want to take it back one further though. Why did you give up? If you knew she was going to burn it, why did you let her burn it?

MARGIE: Because . . . you can't win with her.

CLIFF: That's it. Now instead of saying "you," say "I" and see what that sounds like.

MARGIE: I can't win with her.

CLIFF: The two words, "I can't."

PATTI: What horrible thing would have happened if you'd continued?

MARGIE: She would have dumped the chili on the floor or something stupid like that.

PATTI: So in this case she controls you with her bad temper.

MARGIE: Yes, oh real good, yes. She sure does.

PAM: You're intimidated by their temper. I mean, even if it's not directed, you know she wouldn't have punched you out, but you're still intimidated by her anger.

PATTI: Okay, so you say, "Her anger is just a horrible thing and I can't tolerate it. And I'll do anything not to get her angry."

MARGIE: Yeah.

PAM: It's better to burn the chili than fight with her. It's better to let her do anything she wants, because she's such a pain in the ass.

CLIFF: I think it's important though to get back to the focus on yourself and what you're saying about yourself. And that is "I can't win with her." "I can't beat her." "I am weaker than she is." It's those kinds of things that you're not saying to yourself explicitly. You've got the focus on her. "*She's* stronger than I am. She always wins." In learning to be more assertive, you've got to put the focus back on yourself. And instead of saying "I can't," sometimes it's helpful to start off by saying "I won't." What would that sound like to you? "I can't win with her." What if you said "I won't win with her."

MARGIE: No matter what I say, she's gonna go ahead and do whatever she wants to do, but it's not going to be anything on my part. It's just gonna be—she's the way she is.

CLIFF: Do you see what you just did? Margie, what did you just do?

MARGIE: I have no idea.

CLIFF: What did she do?

SALLY: She brought it back to "you."

CLIFF: That's right; she shifted the focus right back to her roommate, didn't she?

SALLY: Do you think it has a lot to do with grammar?

PATTI: It's how she's viewing the situation.

CLIFF: Where her energy is, is on "her" rather than inside on "I." Okay? Did you ever hear Muhammad Ali say anything about him or he? He said "*I'm* the greatest," right? All of the *I* statements. That's a self-affirmation kind of statement. And you build yourself up that way rather than practicing building her up. The more you practice building her up in your mind, the more she grows. You're covertly rehearsing her being stronger than you.

PAM: You mean we're kind of making that person more of a monster than she is.

PATTI: Margie says she always gets away with it. It's because she's always allowed to get away with it and she always gets reinforced for getting away with it. Of course she's going to continue; it works.

MARGIE: But, I don't know how to stop it. I always figure, go ahead and give in, because it's so much easier that way.

PATTI: But, how do you feel about yourself? Let's bring it back to you. How do you feel about yourself when you keep giving in?

MARGIE: Stupid. Pushed around.

PATTI: Okay, that's the first place to start. What would you like? Instead of putting all the focus on what she is, what would you like?

MARGIE: I would like for her to listen to me and put water in the chili. I mean it's like paste or dough or something. I mean it's just . . .

CLIFF: Could you see yourself being assertive? I'd like for you to try this on. I want you to use your imagination right now. Okay? And to picture yourself as strong as she is. I want you to picture yourself looking her straight in the eye and saying firmly, "I'm going to put more water in the chili so it won't burn" or "I think you should put more water in the chili." Can you picture yourself doing that?

MARGIE: Yeah, I did something like that yesterday.

CLIFF: With the use of I language? "I want you to put more water in the chili." How does it look when you do that?

PAM: [*Interrupting*] Did it work?

MARGIE: It was a totally different situation. It was another situation that happened yesterday, and I just jumped all over her and said, "I don't ever want you to do anything like than again" and "you just upset me so much, you know, you scared me half to death." And she felt really badly about it. And I felt badly for making her feel bad.

PATTI: Your immediate reaction was guilt, then.

MARGIE: Uh huh.

CLIFF: You can't win.

MARGIE: I can't.

PATTI: You're not letting yourself win.

MARGIE: I know.

PATTI: Well, that doesn't have a whole lot to do with other poeple, does it? Because you won't let yourself win.

MARGIE: I guess I do put the emphasis on other people. That way I can't be blamed for anything.

PATTI: That would be horrible if you got blamed, wouldn't it?

MARGIE: Catastrophe.

CLIFF: It also prevents you from taking credit for anything.

MARGIE: [*Nods head*].

PATTI: That's the bad side of it.

MARGIE: Not being responsible for anything.

PATTI: That may be what this is about too. You just talked 10 minutes ago about not wanting to make decisions, because you're so scared of making mistakes. It sounds like it's a very similiar situation. "I don't want to argue with her." The excuse is "I don't want to argue with her because she's gonna do that and that would be a catastrophe." It sounds like an excuse. "I don't want to do it because . . . I'm afraid." You know you could have put the water in the chili and it could have come out runny [*sigh of horror*]. Oh, my God, that would be far worse than burning it, wouldn't it?

MARGIE: Yes, probably.

PATTI: See it's you and what you're saying to yourself and how you're interpreting the situation.

MARGIE: I guess that's why I'm so apprehensive about all this assertiveness because I keep thinking, "Oh I don't think this is gonna work . . . I don't think this is gonna work."

PATTI: Are you sure you're saying "I don't think this is" . . . or "I'm scared it won't?"

CLIFF: Or "I don't want this to work"?

MARGIE: Well, like I had this imaginary conversation with one of the guys at work. He's a vice-president. And it went along just beautifully and then at the end I thought, "If this does not work, I can blame it on my assertiveness class" [*laughter*]. And I thought, "Now that's poor reasoning." [*more laughter*] You know, if I get fired, I can just say "Well, you know, I'm in a therapy group."

PATTI: It's all my fault [*laughter*].

CLIFF: Okay, that's a self-responsibility issue, which is the very foundation for assertiveness to be self-responsible.

PATTI: It is pretty scary being responsible.

MARGIE: I think I used to be.

CLIFF: Before you got raped?

MARGIE: I think so.

CLIFF: But since you were responsible for the rape in your own mind because you failed to change the locks fast enough, you lost confidence in your decisions and your judgment of people, and although you know now that you weren't responsible for the rape, you still don't trust your judgment.

PATTI: You've been saying, "I was responsible for this big mistake and I'm scared of making other big mistakes." What that's doing though, is if you're not responsible, you don't have control. Do you? The good part of having responsibility is having control. In a sense, you're continuing to let everything else and everybody control you. That may work and it may not. You may be stuck with somebody who takes advantage of that—like your roommate.

MARGIE: Yeah, I think that's been happening.

SALLY: One thing though. Our being leary of taking responsibility and being assertive is something that's a common denominator to most women—I mean of my generation. I may be the oldest one here, but you know, I was taught to transfer everything, to males in particular. I was just to grow up and get married and clean house and have kids. It has nothing to do with being assertive or going after something I wanted or any of that. I was just sort of wishy-washy. Go through life and always say yes. Do what you're told. You know, that kind of thing.

PATTI: It got pretty scary when the world started changing.

SALLY: It went a little overboard in some directions.

PATTI: People started talking about new ideas and there was no way to fit that into the way you were.

CLIFF; What went along with that was that the man was responsible . . .

SALLY: Right.

CLIFF: . . . for your well-being.

PATTI: And you have to trust that he's going to be kind and considerate and loving and wonderful and that all men are going to do that. Unfortunately, there are some men out there who are not kind and considerate and responsible and wonderful. And there are some women out there who aren't always going to look after our welfare. It's a tough thing to move and step out from that a little bit and take control and responsibility. But, that means starting to look at these situations instead of "She did that," saying "Hold it—what's my role in this?"

MARGIE: Well, I think that one thing that has helped, is I'm able to look at these situations and say "This is ridiculous. This is stupid." Now it's a matter of actually doing something to change it.

PAM: At least, if you're not doing it, at least you're acknowledging what you should do.

PATTI: That's the first step.

MARGIE: I can see myself doing that at least.

CLIFF: OK, with one minor correction. Not what you *should* be doing, what you *could* be doing. There's a big difference, because you can just shift from one *should* to another *should* and you're still in trouble. If you don't do what you *should* do, then you're going to blame yourself and feel guilty.

PATTI: Let's do some role playing of the chili situation. Who would like to play Margie's roommate?

This transcript illustrates a number of the points that were discussed in this chapter. Margie was so concerned about the reactions of others that she was willing to sacrifice her own opinions and rights. She backed off and remained silent and then resented the other person for bullying her. Although the precipitating event for her helplessness and turning over responsibility to others was her sexual assault 2 years before, she was probably susceptible to this type of reaction from years of sex role conditioning. Sally, another group member, pointed out that many women are taught to defer to men. Such paternalism encourages a lack of assertion and giving up control.

It is not so unusual to see women become more "stereotypically feminine" after sexual assault. Rather than being angry at the rapist, most women blame themselves for their assaults (Janoff-Bulman, 1979). Because women tend to engage in self-blame, this is not surprising. Furthermore, rape victims tend to be blamed for their assaults by society, so victims may be reflecting what they have been taught. Margie's solution to making a "big mistake" and being raped again was to refrain from making decisions in the future. This pattern had generalized to many areas of her life. Although she was unhappy with her interpersonal relationships and felt bad about herself, she was afraid of taking responsibility and risking negative consequences from others. Pam, another group member who was feeling intimidated and controlled by her husband, echoed Margie's concerns.

Women's role in society came up several times during therapy. The difference between what women had been taught and led to expect as children versus how the world actually functions leaves some women depressed, confused, or angry. When women are raised in a paternalistic society, they expect that other people will look after their well-being. Rape, spouse abuse, and divorce can be shattering experiences for women not just because of the immediate trauma but also because society often withdraws support and aid at a time when it is needed most. Women are often left disillusioned and bitter at a system that failed them and wonder what they could have done to deserve such treatment.

The focus of this therapy and the value of assertion training is on self-control and teaching women to move from feeling helpless to relying on themselves for change. Behavioral rehearsal, feedback, and reinforcement are important techniques to use to help clients try out new skills or to confront feared consequences. In the case of rape victims, other efficacy-increasing techniques, such as stress inoculation to control fear reactions, is helpful (Resick, Jordan, Marhoefer-Dvorak, Kotsis, Hodgdon, & Girelli, 1983).

General Considerations for Behavioral Therapists

Because therapists are more educated, may be more liberal than most of their clients, and are surrounded with colleagues and friends who share similar views, they tend to subscribe less rigidly to sex roles than their clients. By definition, male therapists have moved away from traditional masculinity by their professional acceptance of help seeking, emotions, and self-disclosure.

Although such role flexibility serves as an excellent model for clients, therapists may lose touch with the extent to which rigid and limiting sex roles are entrenched in society. Therapists may allow clients' irrational or erroneous beliefs concerning the sexes to pass by without challenging them as they would other irrational beliefs.

Early in the chapter, sex roles were implicated in the development of frequently seen psychological disorders. In addition to the use of standard behavioral techniques, therapists should consider how modification of sex roles could be incorporated into their therapy. Specific skills training for behavioral deficits may be required (e.g., shaping and reinforcing women to initiate conversations). Occasionally, the problem may be one of failure to discriminate stimuli. For instance, because emotions are considered generally unacceptable for men, some men have difficulty discriminating anger from fear, sadness, or embarrassment. Angry self-statements can lead to very different behavioral responses than other interpretations and subsequent self-statements.

Clients may have skills they are suppressing because they do not believe that they are appropriate for their gender. Discussion of these issues and having clients experiment with new or infrequent responses may help them determine if their behavior, in fact, elicits punishment, or if feared consequences are unfounded. Self-reinforcement may also prove to be more potent than the mild disapproval of others if it is encouraged by the therapist. Finally, clients may be taught to modify their environment and their significant others, to accept more flexible sex roles through assertive social skills, shaping, and discrimination training.

References

American Psychiatric Association (1980). *Diagnostic and statistical manual of mental disorders (3rd ed.).* Washington, DC: Author.

Antill, J. K., & Cunningham, J. D. (1979). Self-esteem as a function of masculinity in both sexes. *Journal of Consulting and Clinical Psychology, 47,* 783–785.

Babl, J. D. (1979). Compensatory masculine responding as a function of sex role. *Journal of Consulting and Clinical Psychology, 47,* 252–257.

Beck, A. T. (1967). *Depression: Causes and treatment.* Philadelphia: University of Pennsylvania Press.

Belle, P. (1980). Who uses mental health facilities? In M. Guttentag, S. Salasin, & D. Belle (Eds.), *The mental health of women.* New York: Academic Press.

Belle, D., & Goldman, N. (1980). Patterns of diagnoses received by men and women. In M. Guttentag, S. Salasin, & D. Belle (Eds.), *The mental health of women.* New York: Academic Press.

Bem, S. L. (1974). The measurement of psychological androgyny. *Journal of Consulting and Clinical Psychology, 47,* 155–162.

Bem, S. L. (1975). Sex role adaptability: One consequence of psychological androgyny. *Journal of Personality and Social Psychology, 31,* 634–643.

Bem, S. L., & Lenney, E. (1976). Sex typing and the avoidance of cross-sex behavior. *Journal of Personality and Social Psychology, 33,* 48–54.

Bem, S. L., Martyna, W., & Watson, C. (1976). Sex typing and androgyny: Further explorations of the expressive domain. *Journal of Personality and Social Psychology, 34,* 1016–1023.

Berzins, J. I., Welling, M. A., & Wetter, R. E. (1975). *The PRF ANDRO Scale user's manual.* Unpublished material, University of Kentucky. (Available from J. I. Berzins, Department of Psychology, University of Kentucky, Lexington, Kentucky 40506.)

Blechman, E. A. (1980). Ecological sources of dysfunction in women: Issues and implications for clinical behavior therapy. *Clinical Behavior Therapy Review, 2,* 3–18.

Brehony, K. A. (1983). Women and agoraphobia: A case for the etiological significance of the feminine sex role stereotype. In V. Franks & E. D. Rothblum (Eds.), *The stereotyping of women: Its effects on mental health.* New York: Springer.

Brim, Jr., O. G., Glass, D. C., Neulinger, J., & Firestone, I. J. (1969). *American beliefs and attitudes about intelligence.* New York: Russell Sage.

Broverman, I. K., Broverman, D. M., Clarkson, F. E., Rozenkrantz, P. S., & Vogel, S. R. (1970). Sex role stereotypes and clinical judgments of mental health. *Journal of Consulting and Clinical Psychology, 34,* 1–7.

Crandall, V. C. (1969). Sex differences in expectancy of intellectual and academic reinforcement. In C. P. Smith (Ed.), *Achievement-related motives in children.* New York: Russell Sage.

David, D. S., & Brannon, R. (Eds.). (1976). *The forty-nine percent majority: The male sex role.* Reading, MA: Addison-Wesley.

Deaux, K. (1976). *The behavior of women and men.* Monterey, CA: Brooks/Cole.

Deaux, K., & Emswiller, T. (1974). Explanations of successful performance on sex-linked tasks: What is skill for the male is luck for the female. *Journal of Personality and Social Psychology, 29,* 80–85.

Deaux, K., & Taynor, J. (1973). Evaluation of male and female ability: Bias works two ways. *Psychological Reports, 32,* 261–262.

Deaux, K., White, L., & Farris, E. (1975). Skill versus luck: Field and laboratory studies of male and female preferences. *Journal of Personality and Social Psychology, 32,* 629–636.

Dohrenwend, B. P., & Dohrenwend, B. S. (1974). Social and cultural influences on psychopathology. *Annual Review of Psychology, 25,* 417–452.

Dohrenwend, B., & Dohrenwend, B. (1976). Sex differences and psychiatric disorders. *American Journal of Sociology, 81,* 1447–1454.

Dweck, C. S., & Bush, E. S. (1976). Sex differences in learned helplessness: I. Differential debilitation with peer and adult evaluations. *Developmental Psychology, 12,* 147–156.

Dweck, C. S., & Gilliard, D. (1975). Expectancy statements as determinants of reactions to failure: Sex differences in persistence and expectancy chance. *Journal of Personality and Social Psychology, 32,* 1077–1084.

Efron, V., Keller, M., & Gurioli, C. (1974). *Statistics on consumption of alcohol and alcoholism.* New Brunswick, NJ: Rutgers Center of Alcohol Studies.

Feather, N. T. (1969). Attribution of responsibility and valence of success and failure in relation to initial confidence and task performance. *Journal of Personality and Social Psychology, 13,* 129–144.

Feather, N. T. & Simon, J. G. (1975). Reactions to male and female success and failure in sex-linked occupations: Impressions of personality causal attributions and perceived likelihood of different consequences. *Journal of Personality and Social Psychology, 31,* 20–31.

Feinblatt, J. A., & Gold, A. R. (1976). Sex roles and the psychiatric referral process. *Sex Roles, 2,* 109–122.

Feldman-Summers, S., & Keisler, S. B. (1974). Those who are number two try harder: The effect of sex on attributions of causality. *Journal of Personality and Social Psychology, 30,* 846–855.

Fodor, I. G. (1974). The phobic syndrome in women: Implications for treatment. In V. Franks & V. Burtle (Eds.), *Women in therapy: New psychotherapies for a changing society.* New York: Brunner/Mazel.

Franks, V. & Rothman, E. D. (1983). Concluding comments, criticism, and caution: Consistent conservatism or constructive change? In V. Franks & E. D. Rothbaum (Eds.). *The stereotyping of women: Its effects on mental health* (pp. 259–270). New York: Springer.

Fuchs, C. Z., & Rehm, L. P. (1977). A self-control behavior therapy program for depression. *Journal of Consulting and Clinical Psychology, 45,* 206–215.

Funabiki, D., Bologna, N. C., Pepping, M., & Fitzgerald, K. C. (1980). Revisiting sex differences in the expression of depression. *Journal of Abnormal Psychology, 89,* 194–202.

Goldberg, P. A. (1968, April). Are women prejudiced against women? *Transaction,* pp. 28–30.

Goldman, N., & Ravid, R. (1980). Community surveys: Sex differences in mental illness. In M. Guttentag, S. Salasin, & D. Belle (Eds.), *The mental health of women.* New York: Academic Press

Gomberg, E. S. (1974). Women and alcoholism. In V. Franks & V. Burtle (Eds.), *Women in therapy: Psychotherapies for a changing society.* New York: Brunner/Mazel.

Gormally, J. (1982). Evaluation of assertiveness: Effects on gender, rater involvement, and level of assertiveness. *Behavior Therapy, 13,* 219–225.

Gove, W. R. (1980). Mental illness and psychiatric treatment among women. *Psychology of Women Quarterly, 4,* 345–362.

Gove, W. R., & Tudor, J. (1973). Adult sex roles and mental illness. *American Journal of Sociology, 78,* 812–835.

Hammen, C. L., & Peters, S. D. (1977). Differential responses to male and female depressive reactions. *Journal of Consulting and Clinical Psychology, 45,* 994–1001.

Hammen, C. L., & Peters, S. D. (1978). Interpersonal consequences of depression: Responses to men and women enacting a depressed role. *Journal of Abnormal Psychology, 87,* 322–332.

Hay, W. M., Barlow, D. H., & Hay, L. R. (1981). Treatment of stereotypic cross-gender motor behavior using covert modeling in a boy with gender identity confusion. *Journal of Consulting and Clinical Psychology, 49,* 388–394.

Heilbrun, A. B., Jr. (1976). Measurement of masculine and feminine sex role identities as independent dimensions. *Journal of Consulting and Clinical Psychology, 44,* 183–190.

Hess, E. P., Bridgwater, C. A., Bornstein, P. H., & Sweeney, T. M. (1980). Situational determinants in the perception of assertiveness: Gender-related influences. *Behavior Therapy, 11,* 49–58.

Holahan, C. K., & Spence, J. T. (1980). Desirable and undesirable masculine and feminine traits in counseling clients and unselected students. *Journal of Consulting and Clinical Psychology, 48,* 300–302.

Hollandsworth, J. G., & Wall, K. E. (1977). Sex differences in assertive behavior: An empirical investigation. *Journal of Counseling Psychology, 24,* 217–222.

Hull, D. B., & Schroeder, H. E. (1979). Some interpersonal effects of assertion, nonassertion, and aggression. *Behavior Therapy, 10,* 20–28.

Israel, A. C., Raskin, P. A., Libow, J. A., & Pravder, M. D. (1978). Gender and sex-role appropriateness: Bias in the judgment of disturbed behavior. *Sex Roles, 4,* 399–414.

Janoff-Bulman, R. (1979). Characterological versus behavioral self-blame: Inquiries into depression and rape. *Journal of Personality and Social Psychology, 37,* 1798–1809.

Johnson, M. (1980). Mental illness and psychiatric treatment among women: A response. *Psychology of Women Quarterly, 4,* 363–371.

Johnson, P. B. (1982). Sex differences, women's roles, and alcohol use: Preliminary national data. *Journal of Social Issues, 38,* 93–116.

Jones, H. J., Chernovetz, M. E. O'C., & Hansson, R. O. (1978). The enigma of androgyny: Differential implications for males and females? *Journal of Consulting and Clinical Psychology, 46,* 298–313.

Kaschak, E. (1981). Another look at sex bias in students' evaluations of professors: Do winners get the recognition that they have been given? *Psychology of Women Quarterly, 5,* 767–772.

Keane, T. M., St. Lawrence, J. S., Himadi, W. G., Graves, K. A., & Kelly, J. A. (1983). Blacks' perception of assertive behavior: An empirical evaluation. *Behavior Modification, 7,* 97–111.

Kelly, J. A. (1983). Sex role stereotypes and mental health: Conceptual models in the 1970s and issues for the 1980s. In V. Franks & E. D. Rothblum (Eds.), *The stereotyping of women: Its effects on mental health.* New York: Springer.

Kelly, J. A., & Worrel, J. (1977). New formulations of sex and androgyny: A critical review. *Journal of Consulting and Clinical Psychology, 45,* 1101–1115.

Kelly, J. A., Caudill, M. S., Hathorn, S., & O'Brien, C. G. (1977). Socially undesirable sex-correlated characteristics: Implications for androgyny and adjustment. *Journal of Consulting and Clinical Psychology, 45,* 1185–1186.

Kelly, J. A., Kern, J. M., Kirkley, B. G., Patterson, J. N., & Keane, T. M. (1980). Reactions to assertive versus unassertive behavior: Differential effects for males and females and implications for assertiveness training. *Behavior Therapy, 11,* 670–682.

Kelly, J. A., O'Brien, C. G., & Hosford, R. (1981) Sex roles and social skills considerations for interpersonal adjustment. *Psychology of Women Quarterly, 5,* 758–766.

Kelly, J. A., St. Lawrence, J. S., Bradlyn, A. S., Himadi, W. G., Graves, K. A., & Keane, T. M. (1982). Interpersonal reactions to assertive and unassertive styles when handling social conflict situations. *Journal of Behavior Therapy and Experimental Psychiatry, 13,* 33–40.

Kelly, N. A., Frederiksen, L. W., Fitts, H., & Phillips, J. (1978). Training and generalization of commendatory assertiveness: A controlled single subject experiment. *Journal of Behavior Therapy and Experimental Psychiatry, 9,* 17–21.

Kessler, R. C., Brown, R. L., & Broman, C. L. (1981). Sex differences in psychiatric help-seeking: Evidence from four large-scale surveys. *Journal of Health and Social Behavior, 22,* 49–64.

Kimlicka, T., Cross, H., & Tarnai, J. (1983). A comparison of androgynous, feminine, masculine, and undifferentiated women on self-esteem, body satisfaction, and sexual satisfaction. *Psychology of Women Quarterly, 7,* 291–294.

Lange, A. J., & Jakubowski, P. (1976). *Responsible assertive behavior: Cognitive behavioral procedures for trainers.* Champaign, IL: Research Press.

Lao, R. C., Upchurch, W. H., Corwin, B. J., & Grassnickle, W. F. (1975). Biased attitudes towards females as indicated by ratings of intelligence and likeability. *Psychological Reports, 37,* 1315–1320.

LaTorre, R. A. (1978). Gender role and psychological adjustment. *Archives of Sexual Behavior, 7,* 88–96.

Lazarus, A. A. (1974). Women in behavior therapy. In V. Franks & V. Burtle (Eds.), *Women in therapy: New psychotherapies for a changing society.* New York: Brunner/Mazel.

Lewinsohn, P. M. (1974). Clinical and theoretical aspects of depression. In K. S. Calhoun, H. E. Adams, & K. M. Mitchell (Eds.), *Innovative treatment methods in psychopathology.* New York: Wiley.

Maccoby, E. E., & Jacklin, C. N. (1974). *The psychology of sex differences.* Stanford, CA: Stanford University Press.

Marecek, J. (1974). *When stereotypes hurt: Responses to dependent and aggressive communications.* Paper presented at Eastern Psychological Association Meeting.

Marecek, J., Kravetz, D., & Finn, S. (1979). Comparison of women who enter feminist therapy and women who enter traditional therapy. *Journal of Consulting and Clinical Psychology, 47,* 734–742.

Mead, M. (1949). *Male and female.* New York: Morrow.

Metropolitan Life Insurance Company. (1960). Frequency of Overweight. *Statistical Bulletin Metropolitan Life Insurance Company, 41,* 4–7.

Mischel, H. (1974). Sex bias in evaluation of professional achievements. *Journal of Educational Psychology, 66,* 157–166.

Nordyke, N. S., Baer, D. M., Etzel, B. C., & LeBlanc, J. M. (1977). Implications of the stereotyping and modification of sex role. *Journal of Applied Behavior Analysis, 10,* 553–557.

Padesky, C. A., & Hammen, C. L. (1981). Sex differences in depressive symptom expression and help-seeking among college students. *Sex Roles, 7,* 309–320.

Pheterson, G. I., Kiesler, S. B., & Goldberg, P. A. (1971). Evaluation of the performance of women as a function of their sex, achievement, and personal history. *Journal of Personality and Social Psychology, 19,* 114–118.

Radloff, L. A., & Rae, D. S. (1979). Susceptibility and precipitating factors in depression: Sex differences and similarities. *Journal of Abnormal Psychology, 88,* 174–181.

Rehm, L. P. (1977). A self-control model of depression. *Behavior Therapy, 8,* 787–804.

Rehm, L. P., Fuchs, C. Z., Roth, D. M., Kornblith, S. J., & Romano, J. M. (1979). A comparison of self-control and assertion skills treatment of depression. *Behavior Therapy, 10,* 429–442.

Rekers, G. A., & Lovaas, O. I. (1974). Behavioral treatment of deviant sex role behaviors in a male child. *Journal of Applied Behavior Analysis, 7,* 173–190.

Resick, P. A., Jordan, C. G., Marhoefer-Dvorak, S., Kotsis, C. C., Hodgon, M. J., & Girelli, S. A. (1983, December). *A comparison of three types of group therapy for sexual assault victims.* Paper presented at the World Congress on Behavior Therapy, 17th Annual Association for the Advancement of Behavior Therapy, Washington, DC.

Rosenfield, S. (1982). Sex roles and societal reactions to mental illness: The labeling of "deviant" deviance. *Journal of Health and Social Behavior, 23,* 18–24.

Ross, J. L. (1977). Anorexia nervosa: An overview. *Bulletin of the Menninger Clinic, 41,* 418–436.

Rothblum, E. D. (1983). Sex-role stereotypes and depression in women. In V. Franks & E. D. Rothblum (Eds.), *The stereotyping of women: Its effects on mental health.* New York: Springer.

St. Lawrence, J. S., Cutts, T. F., Tisdelle, D. A., Hansen, D. J., & Irish, J. D. (1983). *Situational context: Effects on perception of assertive and unassertive behavior.* Submitted for publication, University of Mississippi.

Seligman, M. E. P. (1975). *Helplessness: On depression, development, and death.* San Francisco: W. H. Freeman.

Silverman, C. (1968). *The epidemiology of depression.* Baltimore: Johns Hopkins Press.

Spence, J. T., Helmreich, R., & Stapp, J. (1975). Ratings of self and peers on sex-role attributes and their relation to self-esteem and conceptions of masculinity and femininity. *Journal of Personality and Social Psychology, 32,* 29–39.

Spence, J. T., Helmreich, R. L., & Holahan, C. K. (1979). Negative and positive components of psychological masculinity and femininity and their relationship to self-reports of neurotic and acting-out behaviors. *Journal of Personality and Social Psychology, 37,* 1673–1682.

Stebbins, C. A., Kelly, B. R., Tolor, A., & Power, M. E. (1977). Sex differences in assertiveness in college students. *The Journal of Psychology, 95,* 309–315.

Stein, L. S., DelGaudio, A. C., & Ansley, M. Y. (1976). A comparison of female and male neurotic depressives. *Journal of Clinical Psychology, 32,* 19–21.

Uniform Crime Reports. Federal Bureau of investigation, U.S. Department of Justice. (1980). Washington, DC: U.S. Government Printing Office.

United States Department of Health, Education, & Welfare. (1979, November). *Obesity in America.* Washington, DC: NIH Publication No. 79–359.

Warren, L. W. (1983). Male intolerance of depression: A review with implications for psychotherapy. *Clinical Psychology Review, 3,* 147–156.

Warren, N. J., & Gilner, F. H. (1978). Measurement of positive assertive behaviors: The behavioral test of tenderness expression. *Behavior Therapy, 9,* 178–184.

Weissman, M. M. (1980). Depression. In A. M. Brodsky & R. T. Hare-Mustin (Eds.), *Psychotherapy: An assessment of research and practice.* New York: Guilford Press.

Weissman, M. M., & Klerman, G. L. (1977). Sex differences and the epidemiology of depression. *Archives of General Psychiatry, 34,* 98–111.

Weissman, M. M., & Myers, J. K. (1978). Affective disorders in a United States community: The use of research diagnostic criteria in an epidemiological survey. *Archives of General Psychiatry, 34,* 1304–1311.

Winkler, R. C. (1977). What types of sex-role behavior should behavior modifiers promote? *Journal of Applied Behavior Analysis, 10,* 549–552.

Wolfe, B. E. (1979). Behavioral treatment of childhood gender disorders: A conceptual and empirical critique. *Behavior Modification, 3,* 550–575.

Woolfolk, R. L., & Dever, S. (1979). Perceptions of assertion: Am empirical analysis. *Behavior Therapy, 10,* 404–411.

Work and Study Problems

C. STEVEN RICHARDS

Introduction

This chapter has a how-to emphasis. Examples of how therapists might help adults with work and study problems are the material of this chapter. Readers wishing traditional literature reviews of this area should consult the references noted next. Useful review and discussion articles include the following: Allen (1980); Cianni-Surridge and Horan (1983); Dahlstrom (1983); Dayton (1981); Fitzgerald and Crites (1980); Fretz (1981); Fretz and Leong (1982); Holland, Magoon, and Spokane (1981); Kirschenbaum and Perri (1982); Krumboltz, Scherba, Hamel, and Mitchell (1982); Richards (1981); and Tryon (1980).

Work Problems

There are few things more stressful than wanting a job and not having one. Being out of work—and sometimes out of hope—is so important, widespread, and depressing that most adults in an industrialized society have at least experienced it vicariously: they know people who are unemployed; they have seen vivid television documentaries of the problem; they are bombarded with distressing newspaper accounts of unemployment, underemployment, bad employment, and so on. This section will focus on one facet of this problem—young adults looking for their first full-time job. The assessment of success here is obvious: a good, stable job that leaves both the employer and employee satisfied.

C. STEVEN RICHARDS • Department of Psychology, College of Arts and Sciences, Syracuse University, Syracuse, New York 13210.

Techniques

The first task facing our hypothetical client is for him or her to decide what sort of job he or she wants and what he or she can realistically expect. This may be facilitated by looking through lists of job descriptions available in most libraries and career planning and placement centers. Then some solitary thought is needed. Finally, our client may benefit from some open-ended discussions with workers in the chosen area and with career counselors.

The next step for our client is to develop a résumé that is centered on his or her career choice. A sample résumé is presented in Figure 1. Notice that it is short and to the point. It is centered around Ms. Smith's career goal, which is clearly stated at the beginning of the résumé. In a few seconds, a prospective employer can ascertain Ms. Smith's education, experience, and goal.

A frequent error of clients in this stage is to pad their résumé. A discussion about this with their counselor might go as follows:

T: This draft of your résumé seems very long. I wonder if some of the material you have included here is really necessary? I doubt that employers are interested in your hobbies and volunteer work, and this information may distract them from the important part-time jobs you've held.

C: Yes, well, it seems like I haven't done that much, and I want to impress employers with my résumé. Besides, I'm proud of my hobbies and volunteer work.

T: Indeed, you should be. But employers are more likely to read your résumé if it is short and to the point. And they are more likely to hire someone who demonstrates an ability to be clear and relevant. One way to demonstrate this is by having a focused résumé like I'm suggesting. Why don't we try revising this draft now?

C: Okay.

Jill C. Smith
1390 Overhill Rd., Apt. 9G
Columbia, MO 65201
(314) 446-5424

CAREER GOAL:	To assume progressively more responsible newspaper positions in the fields of local news or science journalism. Willing to relocate and travel.
EDUCATION:	BJ 6/83 University of Missouri Columbia, MO Field: Journalism, GPA: 3.22
EXPERIENCE:	Four years of part-time experience as an assistant reporter on a local newspaper. Responsible for research and first drafts of local news stories and science news articles. Substantial didactic and applied course work in journalism.
WORK HISTORY:	Assistant Reporter, *Columbia Daily Times*, Columbia, MO (9/79–present; 10hr/wk). Responsible for initiation, writing, and occasional editing of local news stories. Secretary, *Columbia Daily Times*, Columbia, MO (9/78–8/79; 10 hr/wk). Responsible for standard secretarial duties in the editor's office. Counselor, YWCA Summer Camp, Branson, MO (6/78–8/78; 40 hr/wk). Responsible for a cabin of 12 10-year-old girls.
HONORS:	Graduated cum laude, University of Missouri, Columbia, MO (6/83).
REFERENCES:	Available on request.

Figure 1. A sample résumé.

Once a polished résumé is completed, the next step is for our client to develop an appropriate cover letter. A sample cover letter is presented in Figure 2. Notice that this is not a form letter. Rather, it is tailored specifically to the job in question. Such letters should be nicely typed, error free, and revised in alignment with each job opening. The cover letter should get the employer interested—hopefully, he or she will continue on and study the résumé.

A common issue here is time. It takes some time (and some sweat) to type up a personalized cover letter for every job application. Clients are often hesitant to do this. A conversation about this matter with our client might go as follows:

C: I tried doing a personalized cover letter for each job application, and it is a pain in the neck. It's a lot easier to use a form letter, "To Whom It May Concern . . ." and so on.
T: Yes, it's easier, but will it work? You need to present your most favorable impression to prospective employers, and a form letter won't do it. Furthermore, many employers get

---

1390 Overhill Rd., Apt. 9G
Columbia, MO 65201
(314) 446-5424

October 11, 1985

Mr. James J. Morgan
Editor, City Desk
Kansas City Tribune
614 N. Main St.
Kansas City, MO 64121

Dear Mr. Morgan:

I would like to apply for the position of reporter, City Desk, *Kansas City Tribune.*
Associate Dean William O. Johnson of the University of Missouri—Columbia School of Journalism called this position opening to my attention, and he thought that my experience and ability dovetailed nicely with the qualifications listed in your position advertisement.

For several years I have worked part-time as an assistant reporter at the *Columbia Daily Times.* This has often included major responsibility for the initiation and writing of local news stories. While pursuing a bachelor's degree in journalism at the University of Missouri—Columbia, much of my didactic and applied course work has focused on local news reporting—the sort of background and training you are looking for. I have also had secretarial experience in the editor's office of the *Columbia Daily Times.* Finally, I have experience and interests in the field of science journalism.

These latter experiences evidence another quality that you seek: breadth. The enclosed résumé further details my professional training and experience in a newspaper setting.

I will be in Kansas City next week and would appreciate the opportunity to discuss your job opening and how my background fits your needs. I will call your secretary in the next few days to see if I can arrange an interview.

Thank you for considering my application.

Sincerely,

Jill C. Smith

Enclosure

Figure 2. A sample cover letter.

turned off by form letters and may not even look at your résumé if it is accompanied by a "To Whom It May Concern . . ." letter.

C: I suppose so. But personalized letters are hard and time consuming.

T: Well, once you get the hang of them they won't be very hard—they may even be fun and challenging at times. They don't need to be long; they just need to be accurate and personalized. True, they may take a little more time, but the reward is a good job. Let's go through this sample cover letter, talk about it, and then you can write out a practice one here and we'll talk about that.

C: All right; but it still seems like a lot of work.

The next big step for our client is the interview. A sample job interview guide is presented in Figure 3. This guide emphasizes style over substance. In a perfect world this would probably not need to be the case. But, alas, this is not a perfect world: style is the key to successful job interviewing.

Also notice that many of these interview tips should make things easier for the job applicant. For instance, it is not only better to tell the truth, it is easier. Because

---

JOB INTERVIEW TIPS

BEFORE THE INTERVIEW

1. Look sharp. Wear clean, neat clothing appropriate for the job. Shower, shave, and gargle right before the interview.
2. Be enthusiastic. Show excitement about the job. Plan to state your career goals and have some relevant questions. Stress what you can do for the employer, not vice versa.
3. Be prepared. Rehearse your answers to questions the employer is likely to ask.
4. Be reliable. Plan to show up 15 minutes early for each interview. If you must be late, call the employer and forewarn them—explain why and apologize.

DURING THE INTERVIEW

1. Be enthusiastic. Look the employer in the eye, smile, and ask relevant questions. Tell him or her you want the job. Explain how you can help the company.
2. Keep cool. Do not get emotional, aggressive, or rude.
3. Be honest. Tell the truth. If you do not know the answer, say so.
4. Be conservative. Do not stress salary and vacations. Wait for them to bring these issues up—and they will.
5. Be polite. Begin and end the interview by thanking the employer for the opportunity to meet with him or her. Be friendly, optimistic, and courteous.

AFTER THE INTERVIEW

1. Send a note. When you get home, send the employer a short note of thanks. Include any answers you were unable to give during the interview.
2. Be philosophical. Successful job interviewing is like successful politics: it requires a thick skin, a short memory, and a sense of humor.
3. Be enthusiastic. Remind the employer that you want the job. In your note mention that you will call the employer for his or her decision after an agreed-upon interval. Stress what you can do for them, not what they can do for you.

Figure 3. A sample job interview guide.

this interview guide focuses on stylistic issues, it lends itself well to role playing. An example follows:

T: You mentioned that your last job interview was pretty rough—lots of difficult and stressful questions from the employer.

C: I'll say! She threw lots of hard questions at me. Often I didn't know the answer, or at least I didn't know a good answer. I got a bit emotional and rude. I later apologized, but the damage was done.

T: Why don't we roleplay that part of the interview—you roleplaying the interviewer with the tough questions and me roleplaying the job applicant. Okay?

C: Fine. Well, Mr. Richards, I'm disappointed in the amount of relevant experience you have for this job.

T: True, I don't have a lot of directly relevant experience yet, but I'm eager to learn and I think I could pick up the basics quickly. Furthermore, much of my education and previous work experiences dovetail nicely with the demands of your position opening. For instance, my education in journalism and my experiences solving problems for the editor of the *Columbia Daily Times* mesh well with your needs.

C: Okay. But there remains the problem of style. We need someone who is very poised and articulate. Frankly, Mr. Richards, you seem a bit nervous.

T: I am a bit nervous! That's because I want this job very much. However, my references will vouch for the fact that I'm usually poised and articulate. And given that there is an excellent job at stake here, I think I've been reasonably poised and articulate during this interview.

C: Okay. What would you want for a starting salary?

T: Salary is negotiable. I prefer that you name what you think is an appropriate starting salary, and then we can discuss that.

After talking with our client about the content of this roleplay, we could switch roles, and the client could try fielding the tough questions. Then we would discuss the latter roleplays and continue in this back-and-forth learning situation until the client reached an appropriate skill level. Notice that when the therapist roleplayed a job applicant he was honest but not self-deprecating, positive but not a braggart, and polite but not obsequious.

Our client's final step is to start applying for jobs. The key here is to *keep trying!* Because this is hard to do, self-monitoring—and the self-evaluation and self-consequation that it entails—is a useful technique. Self-monitoring involves systematic self-observation followed by self-recording of those observations. A sample self-monitoring form is presented in Figure 4. Notice that the form is concrete: it deals with things that can be seen and counted. Likewise, it sets goals that are concrete. The comparison of goals with self-monitored behavior allows our client ample opportunity for self-evaluation and self-consequation. Also notice that the form includes behaviors that our client wants to increase (e.g., number of résumés mailed per week) and decrease (e.g., number of mistakes made per interview).

A common issue here is unrealistic goals: clients underestimate the number of applications needed to get an interview, and they underestimate the number of interviews needed to get a job. Our client might discuss this with us as follows:

C: I've been doing some thinking about my job application strategy. I figure I'll apply for 10 jobs. This should yield at least a half dozen job interviews and probably four or five job offers.

T: I think you are underestimating how hard it is to land a job these days. A more realistic rule of thumb is that a person needs five applications to generate one interview, and a person needs five interviews to generate one offer. Furthermore, you may not like your first couple of job offers. So, you can see why career counselors often say that the key to getting a good job is to keep trying! Self-monitoring is useful in this regard because it gives you information about how much you are trying, and it—hopefully—gives you some positive feedback for these efforts while you are waiting for the long-term reward: a good job.

C: That sounds good, but self-monitoring is a pain in the neck. I don't like doing it, especially when I have been goofing off and haven't got much effort to record on the form. Wouldn't I do better to spend the time needed to fill out the self-monitoring form on doing more job applications instead?

T: No. Self-monitoring is the only easy way for you to keep a reliable record of what you are doing. Besides, it only takes a few seconds each day. If you haven't been doing much, then the self-monitoring records will make you feel guilty and prod you into doing more. Once you start doing more, the self-monitoring records will make you feel good and will help you persist, even if it takes months for a good job offer to come along. . . . Well, what do you think?

C: I don't know. You talk a good game. But I still don't like self-monitoring. Your points about the number of job applications and interviews needed to land a good job are hard to argue with, I guess, given the job statistics you've shown me. I suppose I'll start applying for more jobs. I'll plan on having to go through lots of interviews—some of which will probably be stressful as all get out—just to hopefully land a good job within a few months. Damn! This is hard and depressing! But . . . I just don't like self-monitoring. I don't think I am going to do it.

This last example also illustrates the proverbial difficulty of therapy: clients often do not do what their therapists want them to. This is just as problematic for

Name: Susan A. Jones				Date of first Monday: 10/11/85		
Goals: 10 résumés & cover letters mailed/week; 10 follow-up phone calls/week; 2 interviews/week; 2 postinterview thank you notes & phone calls/week; less mistakes per interview each week; 1 job offer/month (.25/week).						
MONDAY DATE	Résumés	Calls	Interviews	Notes	Mistakes*	Offers
10/11/85	7	5	0	0	0	0
10/18/85	8	6	1	1	5	0
10/25/85	10	7	0	0	0	0
11/1/85	11	9	2	2	4	0
11/8/85	10	8	3	2	4	1
11/15/85	12	9	2	2	3	0
11/22/85	8	7	1	0	2	0
11/29/85	12	9	3	3	1	1
12/6/85	12	10	4	4	1	1
12/13/85	10	10	4	4	0	1†
Weekly Average:	10	8	2	1.8	2	.3

Figure 4. A sample Self-Monitoring Form I. *Examples of mistakes should be discussed and roleplayed with the therapist. †This job offer was accepted.

a behavioral self-control technique like self-monitoring as for any other technique or therapeutic strategy. Literature reviews of self-monitoring sometimes gloss over this compliance problem or ignore it. Such an approach, however, mainly demonstrates that the author spends much more time writing literature reviews than working with clients. The compliance problem is pervasive and difficult. Therapists may have to use all the cognitive (e.g., explaining), behavioral (e.g., rewarding), and relationship (e.g., trusting) factors at their disposal to effectively grapple with this problem.

Final Comments

Specific groups of individuals may be confronted with work-related problems that are beyond the scope of this chapter. For instance, female, minority, handicapped, adolescent, reentry, and elderly workers may encounter employment problems that are related to their group membership. However, these individuals will also have to deal with the issues focused on in this chapter: job application skills and persistence. Behavioral techniques such as role playing and self-monitoring should prove as useful for them as for anyone else.

The key for getting a job is persistence. Behavioral techniques like self-monitoring and self-consequation are particularly useful in this regard. They are not, of course, panaceas. There are no panaceas for work problems. Even if our client does eventually land a great job, the search process can be incredibly frustrating and depressing. Work problems are not so easy that they will just succumb to the onslaught of techniques; they also require good therapists—with a sympathetic ear, a gentle tongue, and a patient hand.

Study Problems

Problems with studying frequently concern college students, and they have proven more refractory to treatment than one might intuitively suspect. The first thing a behavior modifier learns is that behavior is hard to modify! Nevertheless, behavioral interventions for this problem—particularly self-control interventions—have been extensively researched, and many of the results are promising. Self-control techniques, with their emphasis on clients gradually learning to become their own therapists and teachers, are appealing here for two reasons: they often work, and they are practical. With 12 million students in institutions of higher education and a few thousand professional therapists available at such institutions, the students have no choice but to learn to become their own therapists and teachers. Therapists can still give them a helpful push, of course, and illustrations of this push will form the rest of the chapter. This section will focus on the two major study problems: how students study and how much they study. The assessment of success here is obvious: a substantial, consistent improvement in grades that leaves both the student and significant others satisfied.

The first task facing our hypothetical client is for him or her to find out what he or she is doing, particularly how much he or she is studying. Self-monitoring lends itself well to this task. A sample self-monitoring form is presented in Figure 5. This is a good form to start with: it gives the student detailed and precise information about his or her study efforts for a week; yet it is still focused and simple. It also is concrete; it deals with behaviors that can be seen and counted. Students are usually chagrined to learn that they are studying much less than they thought. A discussion with their counselor might go as follows:

T: From your self-monitoring records for last week I see that you set a goal of 25 hours studied, but you actually studied 11 hours. What do you think of this?

C: I was surprised! I was also sort of . . . well, sort of guilty and upset. I thought I was studying a lot more than that. Studying is hard! I really don't like it much. But I do want to do well in school. I was sort of angered by these records, but I guess I need them. I wish I was studying more.

T: These self-monitoring records may help you do that. And as you study more you will start finding that the records make you pleased rather than angry. But let's pick a more modest goal for next week—say 15 hours studied—and then gradually go up from there. I think it would be helpful for you to self-monitor with this form next week and shoot for a goal of 15 hours studied. Does that sound okay?

C: Well, I'd rather try to change all at once, but perhaps this gradual approach is better. It is also more realistic, I suppose. I'll try it.

The next step for our client is to shift to a form of self-monitoring that is easier and that affords a better long-range perspective. Such a form is illustrated in Figure 6. Our client only needs to self-record one number per day, yet he or she can gain a weekly and semester overview of his or her study efforts. As our client progresses through therapy, the self-monitoring procedures should progress with him

Name: C. Steven Johnson		Date Of Monday: 9/16/85
Goal for total hours studied per week: 32*		

DAY	Hours studied in hardest course*	Hours studied in easiest course*	Hours studied in all courses*
Monday	2	0	3
Tuesday	0	1	4
Wednesday	1	0	3
Thursday	2	1	5
Friday	1	0	2
Saturday	3	0	4
Sunday	1	1	6
TOTALS	10	3	27

Figure 5. A sample Self-Monitoring Form II. *Does not include lectures.

or her. Self-monitoring should adapt to his or her changing needs, and it should become easier. Initially, the client needs a brief period of intensive self-monitoring that provides lots of information (cf. Figure 5). Then he or she needs an easier form that provides less information per day, but more information over the long haul (cf. Figure 6). Then, he or she needs a still easier form that may even be crude and aperiodic but that will nevertheless provide some useful information while being nearly effortless (cf. Figure 7).

Therapists often make self-monitoring too complex and ask their clients to continue it for too long. If a client comes in with a presenting problem of not working enough, then starting them off with a Herculean self-monitoring assignment is not the most auspicious way to begin therapy.

An issue that often arises in the context of Figure 6 is a large discrepancy between the client's weekly goal for hours studied and the reality of what will be needed for a substantial grade improvement. Because poor grades have usually precipitated the client's request for professional help, he or she already may have experienced the triumph of reality over wishful thinking. A brief, tense discussion sometimes follows.

C: I've got 16 credits, and I figure I need to study about 8 hours a week for that.

Name: Joseph S. Peterson   Date of first Monday: 8/26/85

Goal for total hours studied per week: 30*

MONDAY DATE	Mon.	Tues.	Wed.	Thur.	Fri.	Sat.	Sun.	Totals*
				Hours studied in all courses*				
8/26/85	1	4	5	2	2	0	8	22
9/2/85	3	4	4	3	3	0	7	24
9/9/85	4	3	4	5	2	1	7	26
9/16/85	3	4	5	6	0	0	8	26
9/23/85	6	2	3	4	3	2	7	27
9/30/85	5	5	1	3	3	3	8	28
10/7/85	1	4	5	4	1	0	9	24
10/14/85	3	3	4	3	3	0	7	23
10/21/85	6	5	6	7	1	1	6	32
10/28/85	4	3	4	2	3	0	7	23
11/4/85	6	2	3	4	2	2	6	25
11/11/85	8	9	3	2	3	0	8	33
11/18/85	7	6	2	1	3	2	9	30
11/25/85	5	4	1	0	0	0	0	10
12/2/85	7	8	5	6	4	4	9	43
12/9/85	9	9	2	7	6	8	9	50
							Average weekly total:	28

Figure 6. A sample Self-Monitoring Form III. *Does not include lectures.

T: What?! The usual rule of thumb is 2 hours of studying for every hour of credit. You've flip-flopped that. . . . What was your GPA last semester?
C: 1.8.
T: I think you need to study more.
C: I suppose.

The final self-monitoring step for our client is exemplified in Figure 7. This form of self-monitoring is so easy and intuitively appealing that some college students develop it on their own, without professional help. But despite its ease, it gets the job done. This form of self-monitoring gives a useful overview of the pattern and amount of studying during a semester. An issue that may come up here is the distribution of effort: students forget their introductory psychology lecture on the advantages of spaced practice over massed practice, and they try to clump all of their studying into a couple of days.

C: I like to leave my weekends open for social activities, and Mondays and Fridays are busy days, so I think I'll try to study a total of 20 hours each week—10 hours on Tuesdays and 10 hours on Wednesdays.
T: That would make Tuesdays and Wednesdays a grueling experience! It would be more efficient—and a lot more pleasant—to distribute that 20 hours of studying over four weekdays, say Tuesday through Friday. This schedule would still leave your weekends open for socializing and Mondays open for recuperating. What do you think?
C: I understand the advantages of the study schedule that you are suggesting, but somehow it still sounds easier to get all of my studying done on two weekdays.

Name: Ann K. McDonald   Date of first Monday: 8/26/85
Goal for number of scheduled study periods completed per week: 5
Schedule: Study Monday, Wednesday, and Friday mornings in the UMC main library;
          Study Tuesday and Thursday afternoons in the UMC Medical Center library; and Study Sunday afternoons and evenings in the dormitory study hall.

Date Mon.	Mon.	Tues.	Wed.	Thur.	Fri.	Sun.	Totals
			Study periods completed (Xs)				
8/26	X	X	X		X		4
9/2	X	X	X	X	X		5
9/9		X	X	X		X	4
9/16	X	X	X	X	X		5
9/23	X		X	X	X		4
9/30	X	X	X	X	X	X	6
10/7	X		X		X		3
10/14	X	X	X	X	X		5
10/21	X		X	X	X		4
10/28	X	X	X	X	X	X	6
11/4		X	X		X		3
11/11	X	X	X		X		4
11/18	X		X		X		3
11/25	X	X	X	X	X	X	6
							M = 4.4

Figure 7. A sample Self-Monitoring Form IV.

T: Have you ever been able to do that?
C: No. . . . Okay. Okay. I guess that spreading the study time out over more days is more realistic.

At some point, of course, our client not only needs to address how much he or she studies, but how. This is where Figure 8 comes in.

This figure summarizes standard study skills advice. Good advice is like a good résumé: it is short and to the point. A crucial discussion that often comes up in this

---

WHERE TO STUDY

1. Make your study environment work for you by scheduling regular times and places to study. Be realistic: plan several study periods per week in appropriate places and self-monitor how well you are sticking to your plan.
2. Study in places where you will not be distracted (e.g., reading rooms in the UMC main library). It is particularly important to avoid interpersonal distractions (e.g., a setting where friends will come over and strike up a conversation with you while you are studying).

HOW TO READ TEXTBOOKS

1. Use the SQ3R method when reading your course assignments:

   SURVEY the chapter first.
   QUESTION yourself about the survey
   READ to find the answers to your questions.
   RECITE the answers to your questions
   REVIEW the main points of the chapter last.
2. Underline one to five key sentences per textbook page. Consistently underlining less or more than this may indicate that you are being too exclusive or inclusive in what you consider important. Review the underlined material after you complete each chapter and before you take each exam.

WHAT YOU DO IN LECTURES

1. First and foremost, go to as many lectures as possible. If you must miss a lecture, then make arrangements to copy a classmate's notes.
2. Take lots of notes. If in doubt, always take more notes, not less. Record all assignments in your notes, and if you have a question—ask it!

WHAT YOU DO IN TESTS

1. Before the test: prepare early, not just the night before. Know what kind of test (multiple choice, essay, etc). will be given and what material it will cover. Be on time for the test.
2. During the test: read the instructions, questions, and all of the potential answers very carefully, even if you suspect that you know the correct answer right away. Leave the hard questions and come back to them after you have finished the rest of the test. Keep track of the time and try to pace yourself so that you will have at least 3 minutes of ``free time'' at the end of the test.

WHAT YOU THINK OF THIS ADVICE

Study skills suggestions are like rules of etiquette: we can all think of a successful person who breaks them but that does not mean that the rules have no value.

Figure 8. A sample study skills summary.

context is where to study. In particular, students usually have trouble finding study environments where they can avoid interpersonal distractions. This is an important, but difficult, aspect of stimulus control that they need to wrestle with.

C: I have a lot of trouble concentrating. When I study in my dorm room it seems that there is always someone who wants to come in and talk for a few minutes. The total time taken up by this may not be that great, but the interruptions really interfere with my concentration—I don't get much done and I have trouble learning the material. I've tried putting "Do not Disturb" signs on the door and asking people to come back later when they interrupt me, but they ignore the signs and they get angry when I say I can't talk because I'm studying. I don't want to lose my friends or be perceived as a jerk. I don't know what to do.

T: Is there some alternative place where you could study that would be less likely to have these interpersonal distractions? For instance, would it be possible for you to do some of your studying at the UMC library?

C: The UMC library is the pits! They ought to just knock that thing down and start from scratch.

T: I don't think that is going to happen. You would not be bothered by interpersonal distractions if you studied at a carrel there. What do you say?

C: You have got to be kidding! I hate libraries. Besides, I usually study at night and it is dangerous to be walking around campus alone at night.

T: You've got a good point there. Could you get a friend to walk over to the library with you?

C: Probably. But I'm not going to study at the library! I like my dorm room—I'll just continue studying there and try to make the best of it.

This last example illustrates a common problem with stimulus control: it is difficult to get clients to use it. But the therapist should try, try, and try again. All of the other help and techniques that we provide to our client will rain on barren soil if the client continues to study in an environment with frequent interpersonal distractions.

Our client's final step is to become her or his own counselor. Behavioral problem solving fits in well here. Problem solving is a systematic strategy for recognizing, assessing, and coping with personal problems. A typical problem-solving model is illustrated in Figure 9. This is a self-control technique in full bloom, with the client learning all facets of becoming her or his own counselor. Not surprisingly, this technique is harder to teach and learn than most self-control procedures, and it may be best to reserve it for the capstone of a treatment program or for a maintenance strategy. Indeed, what better maintenance strategy is there than clients learning to be their own counselors when they no longer have recourse to professional ones? Furthermore, problem-solving techniques dovetail nicely with the college student's need to address an ever-changing array of academic difficulties and to do so over long periods of time.

A frequent mistake that clients make with problem solving is to use vague, abstract definitions of their problem rather than specific, concrete definitions. Because a good definition is half the solution to most problems, this needs to be addressed:

T: How would you define your study problem?
C: I'm in a funk.

PROBLEM-SOLVING INSTRUCTIONS

Introduction. Problems involving study habits and academic situations can vary considerably as you go through college. Hence, to be a successful student you need to learn a strategy for coping with new and novel school problems as they arise. It is not enough to learn a specific solution to a current specific study problem because that specific solution is unlikely to work for new and different study problems that will probably come up later on. The problem-solving strategy outlined here is an effective procedure for recognizing, assessing, and coping with personal study problems.

Problem-Solving Model. The problem-solving model outlined here has five steps: (a) general orientation or "set"; (b) problem definition and formulation; (c) generation of alternatives; (d) decision making; and (e) verification. These five steps are defined next, and examples relevant to study problems are given for each step.

1. *General Orientation or "Set"*—This means that you need to recognize that a problem exists and that you should try to cope with it. Problems are a normal aspect of living, but to deal with them effectively you cannot act impulsively and you cannot give up. When a new problem develops or an old problem flares up, you should actively cope with the situation in a systematic fashion. *Example:* "Something is wrong with my studying. I can cope with this problem, but I need to carefully determine what is wrong and develop a specific solution for it."

2. *Problem Definition and Formulation*—This means that you need to define the problem concretely and classify relevant information, issues, and goals. This step is crucial and, indeed, there is an old saying that "defining the problem is half the solution." Your definitions should be concrete and specific rather than abstract and general. Include plenty of details (events, situations, circumstances, feelings, etc.) in your definitions. Try to separate relevant from irrelevant details. Help from others is often useful during this step. *Example:* "I am not studying enough. I am currently studying 15 hours a week, and to do well I need to study 25 hours a week. I need to figure out how I can get myself to regularly study 10 hours more a week."

3. *Generation of Alternatives*—This means that you need to list the potential solutions or strategies for your problem. List several potential solutions before you try to evaluate or judge them; thinking of many alternative solutions increases the likelihood that you will come up with a good one. You may need to develop both specific and general solutions, but you will always need specific solutions for the problem at hand. *Example:* "I could stop going out on weekends. Three nights a week I could continue to study until 3 A.M. I could gradually increase the number of daytime hours I study each weekday by two (and keep track via self-monitoring) but continue to go out on weekends. I could study in the library more and my dorm room less, so that I am less tempted to stop studying and goof off with my friends. I could get up an hour before breakfast (7 A.M.) everyday and study then."

4. *Decision Making*—This means that you need to pick the best solution or strategy described in the previous step. Try to anticipate the likely consequences of each of the alternative solutions you listed. Think of the personal and social consequences and the short- and long-term consequences. Sometimes the best solution is a combination of some of your alternatives. Frequently, "perfect" solutions do not exist, and the best possible or "lesser-of-evils" solution should be adopted. *Example:* "From the alternatives I have listed, I think the best solution is to gradually study 2 more hours each weekday and study in the library more but continue to go out on weekends."

5. *Verification*—This means that you need to try out the chosen strategy and see if it works. Give the solution a fair chance—try it several times. It may take practice and several trials for you to make the solution effective. Keep track (preferably in writing) of how well your solution worked. Have a concrete, specific definition of success so that you can reliably tell how well your solution worked (defining the criterion for success in terms of something you can see and count is the best way to do this). If the solution you chose does not work, then recycle to Steps 2 or 3 and try, try again! *Example:* "I will try out the strategy I chose. If in a few weeks my self-monitoring records show that I am studying 25 hours a week, then my strategy has worked; if I am still at 15 hours studied a week, then I need to recycle to the generation-of-alternatives step and try again."

Figure 9. A sample problem-solving handout.

T: That's pretty abstract. I don't know what you mean. Try to be more specific and concrete.

C: I don't like school. All but one of my classes bore me to tears.

T: That's better. It would be even clearer if you could define your problem in terms of things someone could see and count. For instance, classes can be seen and counted. Which ones do you like and dislike?

C: I love my English 26 course! It's an advanced writing class; we primarily write short stories. I've done a lot of fictional and nonfictional writing—sort of as a hobby—since junior high school. I really like it, and I'm very good at it! I hate all of my other courses: Chemical Engineering 114, Inorganic Chemistry 60, Physics 211, and Intermediate Calculus 170. I'm a chemical engineering major and these are all required for my major. I hate this stuff. My dad—who is an electrical engineer—says over and over to "get an engineering degree so you can get a job!" I'm passing the courses okay, but I'm unhappy. Life can be a bummer!

T: Hold it! Your last statement was vague again. But the other things you said were very concrete and helpful. We're making good progress here. Let's continue to work on a definition of your study problem in terms of what you are, and are not, majoring in. Does this make sense?

C: Yes.

It is usually helpful to roleplay each of the five steps in Figure 9 with the client, alternating roles back and forth, until it is clear that the client understands and appreciates the problem-solving model.

Summary

As was the case with work problems, there are specific groups of individuals who may be confronted with study-related problems that are beyond the scope of this chapter. Female, minority, handicapped, military veteran, reentry, and elderly college students, for example, may encounter study problems that are related to their group membership. Space and topic constraints also do not allow for the discussion of some potentially relevant issues such as test anxiety, peer relationships, and match ups of certain types of students to certain types of institutions. Nevertheless, these students will have to cope with the issues focused on here: how they study and how much they study. The study skills advice and behavioral self-control techniques illustrated in this chapter could be very helpful to them.

Certainly for many students with study problems, the key to improvement is to *study more*. But, alas, this is hard to do. Some students find that increasing their study behavior is a relentlessly difficult task. Self-control techniques help. Good therapists help. A cavalier attitude, however, does not help: anyone who underestimates the tenacity of study problems will wrench defeat from the jaws of victory.

References

Allen, G. T. (1980). The behavioral treatment of test anxiety: Therapeutic innovations and emerging conceptual challenges. In M. Hersen, R. M. Eisler, & P. M. Miller (Eds.), *Progress in behavior modification* (Vol. 9, pp. 81–123). New York: Academic Press.

Cianni-Surridge, M., & Horan, J. J. (1983). On the wisdom of assertive job-seeking behavior. *Journal of Counseling Psychology, 30,* 209–214.

Dahlstrom, H. (1983). *Job hunting handbook.* Franklin, MA: Dahlstrom.

Dayton, C. W. (1981). The young person's job search: Insights from a study. *Journal of Counseling Psychology, 28,* 321–333.

Fitzgerald, L. F., & Crites, J. O. (1980). Toward a career psychology of women: What do we know? What do we need to know? *Journal of Counseling Psychology, 27,* 44–62.

Fretz, B. R. (1981). Evaluating the effectiveness of career interventions. *Journal of Counseling Psychology, 28,* 77–90.

Fretz, B. R., & Leong, F. T. L. (1982). Vocational behavior and career development, 1981: A review. *Journal of Vocational Behavior, 21,* 123–163.

Holland, J. L., Magoon, T. M., & Spokane, A. R. (1981) Counseling psychology: Career interventions, research, and theory. *Annual Review of Psychology, 32,* 279–305.

Kirschenbaum, D. S., & Perri, M. G. (1982). Improving academic competence in adults: A review of recent research. *Journal of Counseling Psychology, 29,* 76–94.

Krumboltz, J. D., Scherba, D. S., Hamel, D. A., & Mitchell, L. K. (1982). Effect of training in rational decision making on the quality of simulated career decisions. *Journal of Counseling Psychology, 29,* 618–625.

Richards, C. S. (1981). Improving college students' study behaviors through self-control techniques: A brief review. *Behavioral Counseling Quarterly, 1,* 159–175.

Tryon, G. S. (1980). The measurement and treatment of test anxiety. *Review of Educational Research, 50,* 343–372.

Aging

ROGER L. PATTERSON AND JAMES R. MOON

Introduction

Older people are subject to almost all the problems that younger people may have, and younger people may have most of the problems that older people may have. Therefore, all the techniques of behavior therapy are potentially applicable to older as well as younger people. Yet, there is merit to attending especially to an elderly group in a book such as this. Much of this merit derives from the fact that the typical elderly person in need of behavioral intervention may present quite differently to the therapist than does the typical younger person; and those therapists not knowledgeable specifically about working with the elderly may find themselves at a loss as to the best way to proceed. In this chapter we will present the differences a behavioral therapist will typically encounter between elderly and nonelderly clients. Next, we will describe the process whereby events related to "old age" can produce problems. Then we will present the behavioral approach developed at the Florida Mental Health Institute to help the elderly client overcome these problems. Finally, we will present two case studies that illustrate the application of the behavioral approach to two problems commonly encountered by the elderly.

The first difference encountered is in defining and assessing the problems for which intervention is desired. A simple self-report of problem definition as gathered in a few sessions is not easy to obtain and may well be insufficient when it is obtained. Furthermore, factors affecting the elderly are many, and they are com-

ROGER L. PATTERSON • Director, Geriatric Rehabilitation Project (116B), Veterans Administration Medical Center, Tuskegee, Alabama 36083.   JAMES R. MOON • Department of Aging Programs, Florida Mental Health Institute, The University of South Florida, Tampa, Florida 33612.

plexly related. Both the assessment and the interventions will probably have to take into account several variables affecting the behavior.

Two major classes of factors that must be considered are physiologically based problems and environmentally based problems. Physiologically based problems include illness and may also include developmental changes, such as a variety of sensory changes and a decrease in response speed. With regard to illnesses, more than 40% of the elderly people beyond the age of 65 have some limitations of their activities caused by chronic diseases, such as arthritis or hypertension (Kalish, 1975). Some illnesses may have psychological impact by direct effects of the disease on cognitive functioning. Illnesses may also produce indirect effects by producing distracting chronic pain or by restricting the mobility of the individual and thus limiting the individual's exposure to environmental cues, prompts, and reinforcers. Even more indirectly, illnesses may cause the victim to perceive of himself or herself as being a less powerful, less effective person.

The dementias are illnesses that deserve special attention because they may produce profound direct effects on all functions. The reader is probably most familiar with the Primary Degenerative Dementia that is usually caused by Alzheimer's disease and causes gradual but steadily decreasing losses of intellectual functioning, usually over a period of years. This latter disease is currently untreatable, though some types of interventions may help to alleviate its effects (Yeasavage, Westphal, & Rush, 1981).

Multi-infarct Dementia is a second type of dementia that is produced by a series of arterial hemorrhages in the brain. This disease may progress in a sequence of rather sudden losses of functioning. Some recovery may occur after each loss. Medical treatments aimed at improving the functioning of the cardiovascular system may help to prevent such strokes.

Sensory losses are frequently found in elderly persons. More than 40% of the elderly between the ages of 60 to 89 report hearing loss (Maurer, 1976). A variety of visual impairments is also frequent (Gordon, 1974). Changes in taste and smell may also occur, though these are less well documented (Carroll, 1978). Perhaps it is obvious that changes in vision and hearing may make communication and continued mobility more difficult. It may be less obvious that any sensory deficit may serve to weaken many behaviors by reducing *both* the effectiveness and frequency of occurrence of many prompts and reinforcers.

Like the physiologically based changes, changes in the environment of the elderly person are often of considerable consequence. The issue of psychosocial losses is often discussed in gerontology. Retirement and/or the end of the active parenting role may produce important losses. For most people retirement produces an economic loss as well as the loss of numerous relationships and a certain status in life. Also lost are the important routine and organized activities required for work and many social arrangements. Retirement may present no important problems for most people, but the potential for problems is present. Any clinician working with retired people will likely soon confront some retirement-related difficulties. Many of these difficulties are related to the rather massive loss of prompts and reinforcers that retirement represents. Probably, most nonretired adults organize their lives around their own employment and/or that of their spouses. The number and potency of antecedents and consequences (economic as well as social) that the workplace offers to promote competent, organized prosocial behavior is large. If these are terminated and no adequate system exists to continue to replace prompts and reinforcers for desirable behaviors, then great and often undesirable behavioral changes are to be predicted.

Other kinds of psychosocial losses that are frequent for the elderly are the partial or complete losses of interaction with spouses, friends, relatives, and social organizations. Such losses may be caused by death, illness, loss of mobility, or simply by relocation. These losses, if not replaced somehow, may produce important decreases in cues for desirable behaviors as well as social reinforcement for maintaining important desirable behaviors.

A final type of environmentally based problem that may exist only in certain environments has been demonstrated by Baltes and her associates (Baltes, Burgess, & Stewart, 1980). These authors made systematic observations of the behavior of residents and staff in a nursing home and found that the staff often either actively or passively discouraged residents from exhibiting social and self-care skills.

The reader must by now have recognized that many of the factors described here carry the risk of producing less competent behavior on the part of an elderly person and thus causing problems. Before discussing this matter further, however, it is necessary to reiterate that most elderly people probably never experience severe problems from most of the factors discussed. It is true that most people may never experience dementia and most people may adapt well to retirement. Although most may experience some losses, such as sensory deficits and losses in reaction time and strength, these losses may not be experienced as distinguishable problems in living.

In clinical practice, however, it is extremely likely that the clinician working with the elderly will see people who are experiencing problems that are related to the preceding factors in rather complex ways. It is necessary that the clinician be aware of the possible operation of such variables in every case. As will be discussed later, the assessments need to be adequate to detect or discount the operation of the variety of physiological and/or environmental conditions that may account for particular problems. Likewise, an awareness of these conditions is needed in order to develop suitable interventions. This does not mean that the behavioral practitioner must be qualified to obtain all the needed information firsthand. For example, few behavior therapists practice general or internal medicine so as to be able to ascertain directly the existence or nature of many physical conditions. In most cases, it does mean that the practitioner must be able to obtain from some source the relevant information regarding such conditions and their impact on behavior.

Description of the Disorders

Major reasons for referral are often a lowered level of self-care accompanied by poor social functioning. The clients will often be unhappy, if not clinically depressed, and tend to blame their problems on physical illness and/or other people who are said to mistreat them. There is very little if any awareness of psychological problems. Anxiety may often be present and recognized by clinicians; however, elderly clients often refer to anxiety as "nerve problems," which are thought of as a physical defect. There is very little awareness that elderly clients can do anything to improve their lives.

With cases such as this, relatives, friends, and even many professionals may have a perception of the client's problems, which is similar to that of the client. That is, the affected person may be seen as merely suffering from the problems of "old age" that are basically physical in nature. Thus "old age" is not a problem; rather, the lowered level of self-care and poor social function are the problems. The task of the behavioral clinician is therefore to identify and address the multiple sources that combine to produce these problems. In this way the behavioral clinician utilizes his or her training to help the client. The concern of well-meaning but unenlightened potentially helpful people may be with humoring the old person by treating him or her rather childishly. The only types of meaningful assistance may be those of providing goods and personal assistance with specific tasks. Although some forms of the provision of goods and personal services may be useful or even necessary, they may be given in such a way so as to serve to increase dependence, lower positive self-attribution, and further degrade competent behavior. Thus, many would-be helpers may actually become part of the problem by maintaining helpless and hopeless concepts and helpless behaviors, rather than assisting the older person to maximize his or her competency and self-respect.

Assessment

The multiplicity of problems that might affect the behavior of an elderly person is something that may not often confront the therapist accustomed to working with most younger adults. Indeed, most therapists not working with the elderly may be accustomed to looking only at well-defined problems rather than a more global assessment of the person and his or her situation in life. After all, when one is afraid of flying in airplanes, a global assessment is not really required. However, for the reasons just discussed, a multifaceted assessment of environmental/social factors and medical/physiological problems is needed to develop adequate interventions for the elderly. The assessment process and techniques described here is an example of such a comprehensive assessment. It was developed by the Residential Aging Program (RAP) of the Florida Mental Health Institute over a period of 8 years. Treatment interventions described later also took place in RAP. (An earlier version of this program and its evaluation has been described extensively by Patterson, Dupree, Eberly, Jackson, O'Sullivan, Penner, & Dee-Kelley, 1982.)

RAP uses a number of standard assessments both for the initial assessment and for measures of progress. These are of several types; they serve several different purposes and are described next.

One of the first assessments administered is the Functional Assessment Inventory (FAI). The FAI is a structured interview technique developed by Pfeiffer, Johnson, and Chiofolo (1981) to reliably and validly assess an elderly client's assets and deficits in five important areas. The areas assessed are social resources, economic resources, mental health, physical health, and activities of daily living (ADL) abilities. The FAI as such is primarily a self-report technique, although it contains provisions to obtain data from an informant if the client is judged to be an unreliable source. The FAI is useful in that it provides a structured and standardized interview technique that elicits valuable information about a client in a variety of areas.

The FAI contains a brief and useful mental status examination, the Short Portable Mental Status Questionnaire (SPMSQ) (Pfeiffer, 1975). The SPMSQ consists of 10 simple questions regarding time, place, and person. Validity data have been supplied by Pfeiffer (1975) that show that persons missing more than 4 questions are probably suffering from dementia of some type.

Two behavior-rating scales are completed by the staff in order to obtain global and relatively comprehensive descriptions of problems and areas of competence. In the residential setting, both of these are completed by the direct-care staff on the evening shift. One of these scales, the Missouri Inpatient Behavior Scale (MIBS) (Sletten & Ullett, 1972; Missouri Psychiatric Institute, n.d.) was designed to measure a great variety of behaviors considered to be psychiatric symptoms. These behavioral ratings on 90 items were grouped together based upon factor analyses and rational considerations to form 11 subscales. Seven of these relate to problem areas, and 4 are competency related. The seven problem scales include Hostility, Excitement, Anxious Depression, Regression, Paranoid Thinking, Confused Communication, and Withdrawal. The competency-related scales include Social Competence, Work Competence, Personal Competence, and Activity (appropriate). Each of these scales measures what the title suggests. The MIBS is useful for identifying particular broad areas of problem behavior. Based upon such identification, more specific observations may be made to identify target behaviors for intervention. The MIBS also measures changes in behavior over time.

A second useful behavior rating scale is the Community Adjustment Potential Scale (CAPS) of the Discharge Readiness Inventory (Hogarty & Ulrich, 1972). The CAPS was designed to predict postdischarge adjustment. It contains 30 items generally pertaining to personal and social competencies that are needed in community life. The CAPS provides a very useful summary of the general ability of the client to lead a normal community life.

Three self-report inventories are included to measure three problem areas that are frequently found among elderly persons but that require self-report. These three measure anxiety, depression, and personal well-being (life satisfaction). Although the behavior rating scales can measure overtly observable behaviors related to anxiety and depression, we feel that self-report is a crucial element of these problems. The rating scales measure behaviors rather grossly. Personal well-being can probably be measured only by self-report.

The anxiety measure is a special form of the State-Trait Anxiety Scale for children (STAIC) (Spielberger, Edwards, Lushene, Montouri, & Platzek, 1973), vali-

578
CHAPTER 21

dated for use on mentally ill elderly by Patterson, O'Sullivan, and Spielberger (1980). The reason that a special validation was done is that the adult form of this scale proved difficult for many elderly persons to complete. The children's form is much easier to use and appeared to provide similar information. However, specific validity data were needed to assure the appropriateness of the latter scale. Anxiety may be a major problem for many elderly (Kalish, 1977; Kuhlen, 1959). Therefore this variable should be assessed.

The Beck Depression Inventory (BDI) (Beck, 1979) is used as the self-report measure of depression. It contains 21 items. Each item consists of four statements of which the client is to select at least one. Depression is widely noted to be a frequently found problem among the elderly. Therefore, an assessment of this type is made on all RAP clients.

Life satisfaction or subjective well-being is one of the more frequently discussed concepts in the gerontological literature. RAP assumes as one of its therapeutic objectives the improvement of life satisfaction. The Life-Satisfaction Index (LSI) (Neugarten, Havighurst, & Tobin, 1961) is the oldest scale used for this purpose and has been repeatedly demonstrated to be quite useful (Larson, 1978). Therefore, RAP includes the LSI as a standard assessment.

Much of the effort of RAP is devoted to assessing and remediating specific deficits in the behavior of the elderly clients. Deficits are often found in the ability of these individuals to care for themselves, their environment, and their belongings. Such self-care activities are often called *activities of daily living* or ADL (Katz, Ford, Moskowitz, Jackson, & Jaffe, 1963). Other areas of deficits are more social in nature. The old person may have a low rate of social interaction or may try to relate ineffectively or inappropriately. Some clients do not know significant personal information, such as their location, the names of their doctor and therapist, and so forth. Others may have difficulty finding their way around. RAP employs assessments to identify and interventions to remediate all these problems.

Several of the behavior-rating scales described here do include measures of ADL, social behaviors, and personal competence, but these measures are usually too global to describe target behavior or to provide sufficient information as to the effectiveness of specific interventions. For these reasons, other measures have been developed. These are called *modular assessments* because they are used directly in conjunction with training modules designed to overcome these deficits. Patterson *et al.* (1982) and Patterson, Penner, Eberly, and Harrell (1983) report reliability and validity data on most of the modular assessments.

Modular assesssments developed to measure ADL were divided into three levels. ADL I measures personal hygiene. Upon admission, each client is observed according to a standard protocol once each week to determine if his or her grooming is acceptable. Areas assessed include oral hygiene, bathing, hair care, face care (shaving or cosmetics), clothing cleanliness and appearance, and nail care. If deficiencies are noted, then further assessment of the client's ability to perform the activities needed to correct the particular grooming deficit(s) is performed. These assessments are basically task analyses; for example, "Obtain oral hygiene materials"; "Applies toothpaste to brush," and the like. The clients are asked to perform the tasks while being observed to determine whether they can do so independently, with verbal assistance, with modeling, with occasional physical assistance, or if they require complete physical assistance.

ADL II is concerned with the client's ability to take care of laundering needs, choose meals, care for own room and bath, and use the telephone correctly. The clients are observed to see if they can perform these chores independently and correctly.

The ADL III assessment concerns budgeting time and money, community resources, meal planning and preparation, and housekeeping. It is an interview in which clients are asked four questions within each area to determine if they have sufficient knowledge regarding these areas.

Two social skills assessments are used. One is a time sample of how frequently the clients are observed to converse appropriately when seated in a group and directed to converse. A second assessment is devoted to measuring the client's ability to utilize verbal and nonverbal behaviors appropriately in order to communicate effectively. This Communications Assessment consists of a rating scale on which ratings of several behaviors are made based upon observation of a roleplay. The behaviors rated include (a) content (what was said); (b) speech volume; (c) voice quality; (d) facial expression (including eye contact) (e) hand gestures; and (f) body position. A seventh rating is a global rating of all aspects of the performance. All ratings are made on a scale of 1 to 6 with 1 indicating inappropriate behavior or complete absence of behavior, and 6 indicating a completely correct performance that was delivered with a high degree of emphasis and enthusiasm. The two roleplay situations used for the assessment are one that calls for the expressions of pleasure and/or gratitude to another person, and another that calls for the appropriate expressions of displeasure combined with a request that another person correct an undesirable situation.

An assessment known as Memory Development (MD) (Bernstein & Dvorkin, 1978) is included to identify needs of clients in the area of personal orientation. Two parts to this assessment, as routinely used, are Personal Information (PIT) and Spatial Orientation (SO). PIT assesses the clients' abilities to supply on demand their name, address, telephone number, the name of a person who can speak responsibly for them, and the name of their therapist. SO assesses the clients' abilities to find, from the day room, the way to their room, the bathroom, the kitchen, the telephone, and the cafeteria. Clients are asked to demonstrate that they can do this while being observed.

In addition to the aforementioned rather structured assessments, it is necessary to obtain information about any idiosyncratic problem behaviors that a client may exhibit. Desired information includes a description of the behavior, the apparent antecedents, the immediate natural consequences, when and where the behavior occurred, and the information about others present. Frequency counts of the behaviors are also needed. In order to gather this information routinely, a Behavior Analysis Form (BAF) has been developed and made available to all staff at all times (see Patterson *et al.*, 1982). This form is divided into three sections: antecedents, behavior, and consequences; and it contains labeled space for all information described previously.

Other critical assessments are less formally structured than those cited before and are more traditional in nature. However, these latter assessments are critical to working with most elderly clients having more than minor problems. These include the social history, the physical examination, and the psychiatric evaluation. The physical and psychiatric evaluations become the basis of formal diagnosis and any medical treatments. These latter three assessments require no particular areas of expertise in behavior therapy and will not be elaborated upon further here. Rather, it will be shown how data from these nonbehavioral sources are integrated with information from the behavioral assessments described previously in order to finally determine the list of problems that should be addressed for any client. Thus, the behavioral practitioner can combine and integrate data from various sources to produce a thorough conceptualization of the problem and a behaviorally based treatment plan.

As a device for achieving this integration and also for assuring that no relevant problem area is overlooked, RAP uses a standard set of topics that identify 10 areas of potential problems. This set of topics is first addressed in the social history. The social worker is asked to get whatever information that can be obtained from the elderly client or from collateral sources regarding all these topics. As is explained next, this historical information is then integrated with the information from all of the other assessments in order to define specific problems for which intervention is required. The standard list of the 10 problem areas along with information utilized in examining each will be presented next.

Social Support System

The extent and quality of a client's social network is a very important factor to consider when evaluating a client's previous level of functioning and when planning his or her placement for long-term community readjustment. As part of the assessment of the client's social support system, his or her marital status and marital history are determined by the interviewer. Additionally, the client's current living arrangements are evaluated. Finally, the client's previous and current involvements in social clubs, organizations, and other support groups are determined.

Economic Resources

When the interviewer determines the client's economic resources, several different areas are examined. The client's educational history is taken as well as the client's vocational history. His or her current economic resources are evaluated in terms of income (Social Security, pension, vocational income, etc.), expenses, and other assets such as real estate, insurance policies, investment income, and the like.

Legal Problems

The client's current legal status is ascertained, and any current or pending legal actions are assessed. When necessary, the client is provided with referrals for legal assistance.

The client is asked to list or report current problems that he or she would like to solve during treatment. No restrictions are placed upon the types or amount of problems the client lists. Additionally, the client is given the opportunity to specify his or her treatment goals. The client's self-defined problems and goals then become an integral part of his or her treatment plan.

Mental Health History

During the social history interview, the client's psychiatric history is determined. The client's previous psychiatric hospitalizations, the length of stay, the precipitating circumstances, and the outcome of the hospitalizations are determined insofar as possible. The client is also interviewed about current problem(s), any hallucinatory or delusional experiences, and the precipitating circumstances. The interviewer determines the client's current level of suicidal or homicidal ideation and any previous suicidal or homicidal behaviors. The interviewer inquires into any substance abuse problems currently experienced by the client, including alcohol consumption, nicotine and caffeine intake, and the use of prescription and non-prescription drugs. Finally, various assessment scores are integrated into this section. These assessment scores are the SPMSQ score, which gives a general index of cognitive impairment (Pfeiffer, 1975); the BDI score (Beck, 1979), which provides a self-report of depression; the special form of the STAIC (Patterson & Jackson, 1980), which gives a self-report of anxiety; and the MIBS and CAPS scores, which give objectively obtained data on a number of different adaptive and maladaptive behaviors. Although these scores are first reviewed in this section, information from them is often used to indicate progress in overcoming skill deficits.

Maladaptive Behaviors

The kinds of behaviors that have caused problems for the client in the past are determined by the social history. Also, any problem behaviors observed by the staff (BAFs) are included. These include behaviors such as excessive isolation, agitation, confusion, lack of appetite, sleep disturbance, and the like.

Physical Health Status

The information gathered by the social history interviewer is combined with the information gathered by the medical staff to provide a comprehensive understanding of the client's physical health status and the limitations that may be placed upon him or her by poor physical health. In addition, the medical staff provides an explanation of the client's current medications and the probable effects of these medications upon behavior.

Social/Leisure Activities

Clients are asked to report leisure and avocational interests and activities in order to provide information regarding their utilization of unstructured time.

Additionally, clients' use of unstructured time since admission to the program as reported by routine staff observation is evaluated.

Placement Issues

The client's most recent placement is ascertained. In addition, the interviewer determines the client's most desired placement and the most likely placement upon discharge. Placement is considered with respect to the client's level of independent functioning, income, and the likelihood of continued community placement. Independent living and adult congregate living facilities (boarding homes and foster placements) with appropriate mental and physical health follow-up are the most frequent placements. Placements to more restrictive facilities such as state hospitals, crisis centers, or nursing facilities are discouraged unless absolutely necessary.

Summary

Thus, the standard problem list organizes a complex series of data into 10 functional units. The treatment staff reviews information relevant to each of the 10 sections to determine where problems exist and discusses the most appropriate treatment modality within the context of the program.

Behavioral Intervention Techniques

Very few behavior therapy techniques have been developed for use with the variety of problems of the elderly discussed here. The basic approach used in much of the literature on behavioral treatment of the elderly has been to concentrate only on extreme deficits of institutionalized groups or individuals (Patterson & Jackson, 1980). Most published studies have succeeded in establishing that the behavior of such elderly people is indeed modifiable, a point that had apparently been in doubt by many. However, almost none of these studies went beyond the point of such demonstrations in order to develop programs that could produce an important overall therapeutic impact on the subjects' lives.

An exception to the type of approach described previously was the program described in the book by Patterson *et al.* (1982). These authors developed a broad-scale behavioral treatment program that, when combined with medical and social approaches, succeeded in producing global behavioral changes in elderly people. Furthermore, important therapeutic outcomes were demonstrated. Elderly people treated in this program included not only those in mental institutions but also those still living in the community.

The behavior therapy techniques used by Patterson *et al.* concentrated on structured training groups (modules), which taught ADL, social skills, and other personal skills. These modules were complemented by behavioral interventions designed to alter idiosyncratic behaviors of specific individuals that the modules did not address.

Although apparently successful, it was noted by Patterson and his associates, during the course of the study, that many improvements could be made in the treatment modules. Also, persons treated by the program, depressed people in particular, could probably benefit from cognitive behavioral approaches similar to those developed by Beck and his associates (Beck, Rush, Shaw, & Emery, 1979).

The basis of the entire treatment program was a milieu that sought to provide social reinforcement and verbal feedback for accomplishments at every opportunity. Social reinforcement was often paired with tokens, which could be exchanged for goods, such as grooming items (cosmetics, clothing, etc.), snacks, and a few privileges. The program went well beyond the usual token economy, however, in that much of each client's day was occupied by highly structured training modules, each with its own assessment. The names of these modules were the same as those already presented in the section on assessments.

ADL Training

In the ADL I and II training, the clients met in groups if this was appropriate, and obtained or were presented with the objects or devices (nail clippers, telephones, washing machines) necessary to accomplish a particular ADL task. Brief instructions and modeling regarding the task was then presented. Clients were then asked to perform. Appropriate attempts at performing the task were reinforced according to the techniques of shaping and chaining. Additional verbal and/or nonverbal prompts and physical assistance was given only when needed. For example, a client might soak her toenails in warm soapy water preparatory to trimming them but then require assistance with using the clippers until she learned to use them.

In ADL III training, more typical classroom methods were used. The clients met in groups and were supplied with notebooks in which they were required to record information useful to them. Teaching was mainly by discussion of topics related to the target areas. ADL III was like ADL I and II, in that the emphasis was on a brief presentation by the leader with much of the training time being devoted to reinforcing responses by all the clients. Discussions were supplemented by actual practice in locating bus routes, identifying community resources, buying and preparing food, and so forth.

Social Skills Training

Teaching effective communication of pleasure and displeasure (Communications Training) required that all clients roleplay the expected behaviors and/or practice giving accurate positive feedback during each session. Clients were seated in a semicircle, with the roleplay occurring in the center. The group leader gave very explicit instructions to the role players and the other group members regarding the scene to be enacted (e.g., your neighbor cut your hedge for you and you want to express your gratitude). The group leader also made sure that all members understood the behaviors to be rated. Reinforcement was given both for improved performance and accurate positive feedback.

Conversation training occurred in a day-room area with chairs arranged facing each other in groups of four. Clients were instructed to converse appropriately. Observers time sampled the conversation and reinforced appropriate conversers on a variable interval schedule, averaging one reinforcement every 5 minutes.

Self-Esteem Training

Clients found to have low levels of personal well-being, as measured by the LSI, have been found to benefit from a training module called *self-esteem training*. Clients meet in groups to learn to recognize and claim positive characteristics of themselves. As with other modules, the leader has the task of prompting group members to make appropriate positive statements regarding themselves, and the leader must also reinforce properly such statements where they occur. As part of the process, the group members are also taught to socially reinforce other group members for such statements. All negative self-references are placed on extinction by being ignored.

Memory Development (MD)

Consistent with the MD assessment, two skills areas are taught in the MD training module: (a) any deficits in personal information (PIT); and (b) any deficits in the ability to locate the designated areas (SO). PIT training is accomplished by using reinforced practice of prompted verbal responding and mnemonics. As with other modules, the skillful fading of prompts is required. In this case, prompting may be done by giving the client several possible responses and requiring him or her to repeat the corrected one, or supplying part of the correct answer. Mnemonics used include semantically relating the new information to old memories ("The address is 30th Street, just like 30 days has September") making rhymes, and others.

SO training is accomplished by backward chaining. Clients are led to the furthest point from which they can find the location. They are then reinforced for reaching the destination. The distance from the location is then increased on subsequent trials. MD training is conducted individually three times daily until it is no longer required, or until it becomes apparent that it will not work.

Cognitive Therapy for Depression

The interview of the depressed client reveals the manner in which he or she thinks about the self, the environment, and the future. Typically, the client's thoughts will be distorted in any one of several characteristic fashions. Beck *et al.* (1979) identify five types of cognitive distortions: arbitrary inferences, selective abstractions, overgeneralizations, magnifications or minimizations, and inexact labeling. Additionally, these depressive distortions tend to be automatic, involuntary, plausible, and persistent.

The elderly client must be given a rationale for therapy. The rationale should be as complex as the client's intellectual abilities will allow (e.g., from "This will be a time for you to tell me what's on your mind" to "We will identify your depressive self-statements and help you change their maladaptive characteristics"). Clients are then informed that thoughts or cognititions can influence the way they behave and "feel." When the client accepts the rationale, the therapist engages his or her cooperation in self-monitoring of depressive cognitions.

The client's willingness and ability to detect automatic depressive cognitions is essential for successful cognitive intervention. As the client identifies the distorted depressive cognitions, the therapist clarifies and then corrects the distortions. The therapist continues to correct the cognitive distortions until the client begins the process of self-correction. This process is accomplished via fading of therapist correction while simultaneously rewarding (through verbal reinforcement) the client's self-correction.

As the client becomes more adept at self-correction of distortions, the therapist intervenes in a new fashion to encourage him or her to increase the amount of positive cognitions and pleasurable behaviors. When necessary, the client will be required to keep a daily log of cognitions (positive and negative) and "feeling states."

Finally, a technique described by Meichenbaum (1977) is utilized to *inoculate* the client to future depressive stressors. After the depressive episode has remitted, the client is encouraged to prepare for future depressive episodes by describing what could cause future depressions and what he or she could do to prevent or alleviate such depressions. The client is encouraged to verbalize prevention techniques, such as regularly taking antidepressant medications and regularly engaging in pleasurable behaviors. Also, the client is encouraged to identify the signals of depression, for example, feeling "blue," loss of appetite and libido, and sleep disturbances. Lastly, the client is encouraged to identify the cognitive techniques he or she would employ to overcome the depression.

These techniques illustrate a comprehensive cognitively based psychotherapeutic intervention strategy for depression that has been useful in supplementing the other behavioral techniques illustrated in this chapter. In the elderly client who has sustained multiple sensory, behavioral, and social losses, individual psychotherapeutic techniques cannot begin to singlehandedly modify depression. However, for many elderly clients, individual psychotherapy is a useful and necessary adjunctive treatment that may help to minimize and foreshorten the client's psychological discomfort.

Summary

The RAP treatment staff administers these modular treatments and collects the data on a client's progress. The case manager periodically summarizes all of the behavioral treatment data. Similarly, the medical staff periodically summarizes medical and psychiatric treatment data, the psychologist summarizes cognitive therapy treatment data, and the social worker summarizes additional social history information. This information is presented for evaluation to the treatment team consisting of a behaviorally oriented psychologist, head nurse, unit director, social worker, psychiatrist, rehabilitation therapist, case manager supervisor, and case manager.

Thus, the treatment team periodically reviews the initial and progress assessments as the client continues through treatment and adjusts the treatment to the needs of the client. In this way the treatment team integrates information from 10 discrete areas of consideration on a continuing basis to help insure appropriate skill acquisition, which will generalize and be maintained after the client leaves treatment.

The process just described will now be illustrated with two case studies. These two cases represent two major diagnostic categories found among the elderly with mental health problems. These are depression in the case of Mrs. A., and organic brain syndrome as illustrated by the case of Mrs. C.

The Case of Mrs. A.

Social History and Treatment Development

As noted, all sources of information are presented to the treatment team for evaluation and planning. The initial treatment meeting is designed to review the social history, assessment data, and other data for the purpose of developing an initial treatment plan. Obviously, all data may not be present at the initial treatment meeting, and thus additions to the treatment plan may occur throughout treatment.

Background

Mrs. A. was a 77-year-old white female admitted to the program with a diagnosis of Major Affective Disorder–Unipolar, Recurrent. Mrs. A. was born in Georgia, where she resided until approximately 7 months ago when she moved to Florida. Mrs. A.'s husband of 60 years died approximately 1 year ago, and since his death she had progressively deteriorated by becoming increasingly depressed, irritable, and restless. She moved to Florida to live near her son and daughter-in-law, who are her primary sources of social support. Although Mrs. A. lived in her own apartment, she was extremely dependent upon her son and daughter-in-law who lived across town. She would frequently telephone and gasp, "Come get me, I'm dying!" Obviously, this behavior alarmed the son and daughter-in-law who would rush to the aid of Mrs. A., thus reinforcing her behavior. Upon entry to Mrs. A.'s apartment, they would find her tearful and complaining of loneliness but otherwise in good health.

Mrs. A. was an outpatient at a local community mental health center (CMHC) for approximately 5 months prior to admission and was taking antidepressant medication during this time. Because noticeable improvement was not forthcoming, Mrs. A., her children, and her CMHC therapist referred her to our facility for inpatient treatment.

Social Support Problems

Mrs. A.'s background information was reviewed. In addition to the aforementioned background information it was also found that prior to admission the client was living in an apartment complex designed specifically to promote social interaction among its elderly residents. Thus, the treatment team decided that the client had available social support systems in her apartment complex, and also in her son and daughter-in-law. However, it was clear that she relied too heavily upon her son and daughter-in-law and not heavily enough upon the resources in the apartment complex. The treatment team recommended behavioral counseling sessions with the client and her children to decrease such dependency. Also, the team recommended increased development of the resources available at the apartment complex. As the client neared discharge she was required to spend an increased amount of time on weekend passes developing social contacts at the apartment. The client was rewarded for her efforts by visits from the son and daughter-in-law.

Economic Problems

The client had a fifth grade education but had a long history of employment in her home town in Georgia. The client's income was primarily from Social Security benefits. She had a modest savings account and was also helped financially by her children. Mrs. A. was not judged to have financial problems.

Legal Problems

Mrs. A. had no legal problems. She was voluntarily admitted and was legally competent.

Self-Defined Problems

Mrs. A. identified her problem as "the move to Florida." She wished to move back to Georgia. The treatment team decided to explore the possibility of having the client return to Georgia. The client's children were willing to assist her in this effort if she became "less dependent and depressed."

Mental Health Problems

The client reported recurrent depressive episodes since she was 35 years old following a hysterectomy. These episodes often resulted in brief inpatient hospitalizations. The depression apparently remitted subsequent to the hospitalization and the use of antidepressant medications. Mrs. A. was currently not judged to be an active suicidal/homicidal risk. There was no evidence for substance abuse, nor was there evidence for psychotic behaviors of hallucinations or delusions. Mrs. A. showed no cognitive deficits on the SPMSQ and was judged to be well oriented. She was experiencing severe depression with some somatization. Her thoughts consisted of ruminations of being alone, being afraid, having no future, and thoughts of her deceased husband. Vegetative signs of depression, including sleep and appetite disturbances, weight loss, constipation, and loss of libido were not found. The team recommended evaluation by the clinical psychologist for consideration of individual cognitive modification therapy.

Maladaptive Behavior Problems

The client adjusted well to the inpatient routine, and no maladaptive behaviors were noted. Therefore, the team recommended no special treatment with regard to maladaptive behavior.

Physical Health Problems

The client was in good physical health with minor chronic physical conditions that were under medical control and did not significantly affect the client's activities. She had a significant hearing loss that was partially compensated by the use of hearing aids.

Social/Leisure Problems

The client could not identify any social/lesiure activities and was not observed to actively utilize her unstructured time on the unit. Therefore, the team decided to place her in the social/leisure activites module where crafts, table games, and other types of socialization are prompted and reinforced.

Skills Deficits Problems

Initial assessments indicated that Mrs. A. was deficient in several kinds of behaviors and skills. The MIBS behavior ratings showed her to be anxious, depressed, and socially withdrawn. Furthermore, she was lacking in work, social, and personal competences. Her general activity level was also very low. The CAPS showed that her general level of adjustment was at the inpatient rather than a community level of functioning. The STAIC confirmed that she was quite anxious. Her Life Satisfaction score was quite low. Within specific skills areas, her communication lacked effectiveness and appeared rather apathetic, primarily because she failed to use hand gestures and body movements appropriately. Within the area of daily living skills, she had good personal hygiene and intermediate level skills such as care of clothing and use of the telephone (ADL I and II). However, she was lacking in independent living skills, including budgeting, housekeeping, use of community resources, and meal preparation (ADL III). Her medication-taking skills were poor, and she expressed considerable anxiety about being able to learn about her medication and to learn to take it properly.

Based upon these assessments, the client was immediately entered into communications training and all available leisure activities. Although observation of her frequency of conversation found that participation was adequate, she was also scheduled to participate in the conversation group because this is an activity that is incompatible with depression and withdrawal. She was not entered into ADL III training or self-esteem training immediately because these groups were full. Neither did she begin medication training the first month because it was thought that her medication might be varied during this period.

Placement Problems

The client expressed great dissastifaction with her current placement. The team decided to help her and her family to explore the possibilities of returning to independent or semiindependent living in her hometown of Georgia.

Month 1

Mental Health Problems

The client was entered into individual cognitive behavior therapy for depression. The individual therapy began with an interview and consisted of identifying the client's depressive cognitive behavior. The client's cognitions centered around beliefs that she was weak, dependent, and helpless without her husband, John. A few lines of typical therapeutic interaction follow:

C: You know Doctor I just can't go on without John.
T: John meant a lot to you.
C: John did everything for me; he was so good [*cries*].
T: You did things for John, too. Like cooking and cleaning, and washing clothes.
C: But that's what I was supposed to do.
T: So you can still do these things.
C: I can't. I just can't. I don't have the strength. Doctor, my husband would be so angry to see the fix that I'm in. It'd break his heart.
T: That means if he'd see you active and happy and doing things more, he'd be happy . . . not angry and broken hearted.
C: I guess so, but I can't do it any more.
T: You've always been a strong, independent woman. And your reward was seeing John's happiness. Maybe when you begin to feel so weak and helpless, you could at least remember the times when you were so strong and independent and you could also remember how happy John felt. Then you felt happy because John was happy.
C: I don't know.

This excerpt depicts the therapist correcting various cognitive distortions. This excerpt also demonstrates the process of rewarding one thought, "I'm strong," with another, "That would make John happy."

The first month of twice-weekly therapy sessions focused on the development of a relationship with the psychologist. The client was not accustomed to talking about problems in cognitive or "psychological" terms; therefore, the initial task was to shift the focus from physiological complaints ("I feel shaky and hot") to more psychological complaints ("I feel anxious and scared"). This task was accomplished by simply representing physical complaints in psychological terms. For example:

C: I'm just shaking so badly. I'm just so hot and shaky. Do you reckon I'd die?
T: You look pretty anxious about something. I wonder why you're so scared.

The client also engaged in various cognitive distortions common to depression (Beck *et al.,* 1979). These included arbitary inferences made by drawing to a conclusion with no evidence, selective abstraction made by focusing on details of context, overgeneralizations made by drawing general conclusions based upon a single incident, and magnification or catastrophizing. For example:

"I'm no good." (arbitrary inference)
"The apartment is so small I can't stand it." (overgeneralization)
"I can't stand it anymore." (magnification)
"I'm useless without John." (selective abstraction)
"I can't cook, I can't clean, I can't do anything." (overgeneralization)

These distortions were corrected as they occurred. More realistic verbalizations were reinforced with approval by the therapist.

Maladaptive Behavior Problems

Approximately 15 instances of self-isolation and withdrawal behavior were noted (through BAF summaries) during the month. In addition to the formal observations, the hourly rounds indicated that the client spent a high percentage (85%) of her waking time engaged in solitary activities. Informal observations of the client further suggested that she was somewhat withdrawn and reclusive.

Thus, a treatment plan was developed to prompt the client to engage in prosocial activities when she was observed to be engaging in solitary activities. The client was reinforced with social praise from the staff.

Physical Health Problems

The client's hearing was evaluated by the unit's physician, and hearing aids were prescribed. In addition, she was started on a high dosage of tetracyclic antidepressants to actively combat the depression.

Skill-Deficit Problems

Mrs. A. showed progress on several of her assessments completed at the end of the first month. On the MIBS, the Anxious-Depression score had dropped dramatically to a normal level. Withdrawal improved moderately but remained an obvious problem. The competence scores showed very little or no improvement. The CAP score improved considerably to a level intermediate between the inpatient and discharge level. The STAIC score decreased somewhat, showing a moderate improvement in anxiety.

In the training activities, communication improved to a point that Mrs. A. was scoring at an acceptable level on all items. Life-satisfaction, however, improved only slightly. (She had not yet entered self-esteem training.) She was reassessed on ADL III at this time, and she scored lower than on the previous assessment. Training in this area had also not yet begun.

In the other structural activities, she attended and participated minimally. She began ADL III and medication training at the beginning of the second month.

Placement Problems

The clinical psychologist met with the client and her son and daughter-in-law to explain the program, to answer the concerns of all of them, and to establish and develop the necessary information on which to base future discussions of placement.

Month 2

During the second month of treatment, the client showed continued improvement. The greatest improvement was with respect to depression.

Mental Health Problems

The client continued in twice-daily individual therapy sessions. During the second month of individual therapy she began to verbalize several new concerns, including her feelings of anger toward the husband (for dying and leaving her alone) and anger at the son and daughter-in-law for "insisting" that she move from Georgia to Florida. The client also repeatedly asked: "Do you think I'll ever be well again?" An excerpt from a typical session follows:

C: Do you think I'm losing my mind?
T: What do you think?
C: Sometimes I wonder, Doctor. I'm so angry about being here in Florida. If I could just get back to Georgia.
T: What's stopping you from heading back to Georgia?
C: Well, I think Bobby and Marion [*son and daughter-in-law*] think I'll get upset again. Maybe I would, I don't know. This is an awful fix I'm in.
T: When you say those things to yourself like "How awful things are" you help to keep yourself unhappy.
C: I know.
T: So, getting back to what you said, do you think that if you get to feeling better Bobby and Marion might be more willing to get you back to Georgia?
C: I don't know. I guess they would help me.
T: Then that's all the more reason to get better, isn't it? By getting better you can think to yourself, "This is helping to get me home to Georgia."

In this excerpt, a useful reinforcing thought, *helping to get me home to Georgia,* and its usage is illustrated. Also, the modification of a maximization cognitive distortion ("an awful fix") is demonstrated.

At various times during a session, the client might venture into the topic of anger and/or sadness experienced over the husband's death. During these ventures the therapist shifted into a more client-centered/reflective mode. It was thought that by neither encouraging nor discouraging these expressions, the client was afforded the opportunity to desensitize herself to the hurtful reality of the husband's death.

Maladaptive Behavior Problems

The client began to interact more with the staff and clients during the second month. However, there were frequent reports of complaints, insults to other clients, swearing, and refusing to participate in several activities. The complaining and refusing were placed on extinction by instructing the staff to ignore them. The insults were dealt with by prompting the client to apologize as a form of restitution. Otherwise, the initial plan remained in effect.

Physical Health Problems

The client continued on a high dose of antidepressants. She decided to defer the purchase of new hearing aids.

Skill-Deficit Problems

By the end of the second month, the MIBS scores on the competency areas and/or activity level were high. The anxious-depression score remained quite low, and the withdrawal score improved enough to indicate that this problem had been practically eliminated. The CAPS scored improved slightly, and the score on the anxiety scale fell to a very low level. Life-satisfaction continued a slight decline; however, she had not yet begun self-esteem training, which addresses this problem. She continued to perform well in communications and reasonably well in leisure activities and conversation. ADL III training was still not begun. In spite of her anxieties about her medications, she learned very quickly their names, dosages, and reasons for application. She was now ready to start getting out her own medicines from the pharmacy cart but expressed much anxiety over being able to do this.

Placement Problems

The client and family met once during the month to discuss treatment progress and to discuss a return to Georgia. The client and family agreed to pursue a return to Georgia as long as the client showed improvement. Also, the concept of a gradual return to the Florida apartment as an "interim" placement was introduced.

Month 3

The third month was a "turning point" in treatment. It also marked the halfway point for the client in the program. She began to show noticeable improvement on various indexes.

Mental Health Problems

The client continued in twice-weekly individual psychotherapy sessions. She made the necessary cognitive changes for more adaptive functioning. Specifically, she showed a reduction in the number of cognitive distortions associated with depression.

Behavioral chaining techniques were utilized to facilitate the adoption of another reinforcing and adaptive cognition. Its development is depicted in the following excerpt:

C: You know, Doctor, I just can't wait to get back to Georgia. That's what I've needed all along.

T: I can sense your excitement. But I'm not sure that you'll be able to leave here and go straight to Georgia.

C: Oh, I've got to, I just couldn't stand going back to that closed in apartment [*in Florida*].
T: It might be unpleasant but I think you could "stand" it; especially if it were the final stepping stone to Georgia.
C: It would be hard to leave here and go straight to Georgia I guess. Somebody would have to pack up my things, at the very least.
T: So you see that returning to your apartment here in Florida is the last link in a struggle you've worked so hard to overcome. When you get to your apartment you can think, "I'm almost there."

Thus, the groundwork was in place upon which to build two additional ideas. First, the client was encouraged to think of a gradual return to the Florida apartment and, second, she was encouraged to think of returning to Georgia for a "trial visit." The "trial visits" to both the Florida apartment and her Georgia home allowed for flexibility in the treatment plan and afforded the client a chance to desensitize herself to the anxiety/depression cognitions provoked by the thought of returning to the Florida apartment.

Incidentally, the client's verbalizations about John decreased during the month. Her appetite, sleeping pattern, and activity level all showed improvement. No maladaptive behaviors were observed.

Skill-Deficit Problems

All clinical scores on the MIBS remained low, with the exception of the remaining small elevation on withdrawal. The CAPS again continued to show steady improvement to the point that this score reached the level acceptable for discharge. On the self-report instruments, there was an indication of a small increase on anxiety, but life satisfaction improved markedly for the first time.

In the training modules, she maintained all the gains previously attained. In addition, she improved on housekeeping in ADL III and was now taking her medications very comfortably.

Placement Problems

The client's son and daughter-in-law met three times with her and the psychologist to discuss the treatment plan. Initially, the children were reluctant to help their mother consider a return to Georgia. Nonetheless, they understood the value of this and agree that if she were able to overcome helplessness and depression there would be no reason why she could not return to Georgia. The client's children were also informed about operant conditioning processes. They learned that by rushing to their mother's aid at her every call perpetuated the very problem they were attempting to extinguish. Additionally, the children were instructed to vigorously dispute cognitive distortions when they heard them made by the client. Thus, the children began to become important therapeutic allies rather than therapeutic liabilities.

Month 4

The client continued to show programmatic improvement during Month 4 of treatment. She began to prepare for discharge during this month, and this increased stress appeared to influence her anxious/depressive verbalizations.

Mental Health Problems

There were no increases observed in the client's cognitive distortions. However, she reported slight increases in feelings of depression, sleep disturbances, and appetite disturbances. The client also reported anxiety about going home on weekend passes in preparation for discharge. She reported, however, that most of her "sad" thoughts and feelings occurred at mealtime and at bedtime when she would think of John. The client was instructed that it was permissible to think of John at any time except mealtimes and bedtimes to disrupt the chain of stimuli that elicited thoughts about him. She began to actively search out other clients to share her mealtimes and made modest changes in her bedtime routines. The client was instructed to change her cognitions about John by substituting cognitions centered around plans for the next day.

No significant maladaptive behaviors were noted during the month except for one report of the client's crying and complaining of being depressed. Her antidepressant medication was increased slightly to help combat the depression while discharge planning proceeded.

Skill-Deficit Problems

Scores on the MIBS competence scales remained at a very high level, whereas the scores relating to problem behaviors remained low. However, there still was an indication of some small problem with withdrawal. The CAPS score continued to improve. The anxiety score increased some, but remained moderate. Life-satisfaction continued to improve. Communications scores and participation in structured activities remained good. Scores on housekeeping continued to improve, but no improvement was noted in the other advanced ADL areas. She continued taking her medication confidently and without errors.

Placement Problems

A fortunate coincidence occurred during the initial weekend passes taken by the client, in that her children took a vacation away from the area. Despite bitter protests by the client that she would "die" if left alone in her apartment without the children nearby, weekend passes were encouraged. The first weekend pass was for 4 hours, the next was for 8 hours, the third was for approximately 12 hours including an overnight stay, and so on until the client was able to stay in her apartment for the entire weekend. During the first three weekend passes her children were out of town on vacation and thus were unavailable to reinforce her dependency. As predicted, she managed each of these passes without incident and seemed to be very pleased and surprised with her ability to tolerate the return to the apartment. During the fourth weekend visit, the client again complained bitterly, insisting that she could not survive the weekend. Not coincidentally, this was the first weekend pass issued since the return of the children. Thus, arrangements were made to work actively with the son and daughter-in-law during the last month of treatment.

The client was discharged at the end of the fifth month of treatment. She had spent nearly 6 months in the hospital completing the various assessments and treatment.

Mental Health Problems

The individual sessions during this month consisted of three therapeutic tasks. First, the client's weekend passes were evaluated, and the next weekend pass was planned. Second, the client engaged in termination from the therapeutic relationship. As is typical in termination, the client began to express anger toward the therapist and sadness at the thought of leaving. She was very reluctant to say goodbye to the other clients. Nonetheless, she was prompted to engage in telling the clients goodbye and to share with them her accomplishments while in treatment. Third, the client was prepared to continue her treatment on an outpatient basis.

Skill-Deficit Problems

The MIBS Problem Behavior scores all remained low at this time, although the small elevation on withdrawal remained. The competency scores remained high, and anxiety remained low. The CAPS score also remained high. Life-satisfaction remained at the level of the previous month, which was much improved. In ADL, she improved on community resources, meals, and housekeeping. She did not improve on budgeting, principally because she insisted that her son take care of several tasks and therefore she refused to learn.

Placement Problems

The client began to verbalize her doubt that a return to Georgia was in her best interest. She seemed to realistically wonder whether returning to Georgia would only bring back painful memories. She did, however, continue to plan a visit to Georgia. Her children met with the psychologist to review the client's treatment. It was reiterated to them that they should be extremely cautious about reinforcing the client's dependency. They were offered strategies to help reinforce the client's independence. For example, the children were to put all "catastrophic" phone calls ("I'm dying") on extinction by saying, "You should call an ambulance," and by hanging up. Pleasant conversations were to continue until complaining occurred, at which point the conversation was to be terminated. Additionally, visits to the client were to occur anytime she engaged in a new activity (e.g., making a new friend, going to an apartment residents' meeting, etc.). Otherwise, visits would occur at the rate of once every two weeks. Finally, the client was permitted to visit the children at any time if she drove herself. Prior to admission the client was very reluctant to resume driving her automobile and to learn the roadways of Florida. Thus, she was encouraged to resume this activity.

Although systematic and objective follow-up assessment is not a regular part of this program, informal follow-up data through telephone interviews with the client and the son and daughter-in-law were available.

Follow-Up

Six Weeks

The client decided to stop taking antidepressant medication because she was "doing too well." The children were not aware of this fact. The client had made an extremely good adjustment for approximately 2 weeks, then decided that she could stop her medication. She reported that she began to withdraw progressively during the next 3 weeks. True to form, the children began to respond more and more to the client's complaints and initiated a request to the psychologist for help. The psychologist recommended that the client visit a psychiatrist for refilling the antidepressant medication prescription. Also, the client was encouraged to seek out regular psychotherapeutic interventions. The family was reminded of the adverse effects of reinforcing the client's dependency.

Six Months

The client had maintained her community adjustment. She had not begun individual therapy but continued to take antidepressant medication. Although she complained that nothing had changed, she had made many new friends at the apartment complex and was involved in many activities there. She drove her automobile sporadically, mostly to the grocery store and to her children's residence. The relationship between the client and her children had stablilized somewhere between the extreme dependency exhibited prior to hospitalization and complete independence she had exhibited prior to her husband's death. The client had not yet initiated a visit to Georgia.

The preceding case illustrates the assessment and treatment of a common presenting problem in the elderly client (i.e., depression). The following case presentation illustrates another common presenting problem: dementia. The treatment program illustrated next relies heavily upon the structured modular assessments and treatments. No cognitive therapy was required; thus therapist–client dialogue is noticeably absent. To avoid redundancy, this case will not be presented on a month-by-month basis, but rather specific problem areas will be addressed in summary fashion.

The Case of Mrs. C.

Mrs. C. was a 69-year-old white widowed female referred to the program with a diagnosis of primary degenerative dementia, senile onset with delirium. The client also had Parkinson's disease. The onset of the client's problem was gradual and apparently accelerated subsequent to the death of her husband of 48 years. Her first psychiatric hospitalization occurred 1 month prior to admission to our program. Previous to the psychiatric hospitalization the client became very anxious, experienced memory problems, and feared that people were trying to break into her home. She was described as being confused and as having auditory and visual hallucinations.

Mrs. C. had a very supportive family and was part of a European ethnic community; thus, her social support system was excellent. The client's Parkinson's disease was under medical control, and she was in good physical health otherwise.

Her presenting problem of dementia required careful assessment to rule out depression, because the two diagnoses are often confused in elderly clients (Libow, 1977). Because nearly all elderly patients will have experienced significant losses of one sort or another, the potential for depression is quite high. Mrs. C. was evaluated by the clinical psychologist via a clinical interview. The interview and assessment data suggested a mild degree of depression due to the loss of the spouse, but the primary problems appeared to be due to dementia and the resulting loss of previously acquired behavioral skills.

Thus, the treatment team decided to focus the client's treatment on the reacquisition of memory and ADL skills, and the development of the client's communication skills and self-esteem skills. The total length of treatment was 6 months.

Memory Training

Spatial Orientation

The client was not found to be deficient in spatial orientation upon initial assessment. She continued to show no spatial orientation deficiencies throughout the 6 months of treatment.

Personal Information

The client was initially found to be deficient in personal information skills, but within 3 months of training her performance was at maximum levels and was maintained until discharge. Thus, she was able to reacquire and maintain basis memory skills.

ADL (Independent Living Skills)

Budgeting

The client maintained her budgetary skills at a moderate level throughout the 6 months of training. She was not judged to be capable of independent budgeting at the time of discharge, and thus the team recommended that she seek assistance from family members when writing checks, paying bills, and balancing her checkbook.

Community Resources

Initially the client was extremely deficient in her ability to utilize community resources. By the end of training she had improved considerably but was not judged to be capable of independent procurement of community resources.

Meals

Initially, the client was assessed as having good meal selection and preparation skills. She maintained these skills throughout training.

Housekeeping

Initially, the client was assessed as having moderate housekeeping skills. However, she gradually improved in this area throughout training. At the time of discharge, she was judged to have adequate independent housekeeping skills.

Summary of ADL Training

The client had no deficiences in personal grooming skills, use of telephone, and simple housekeeping and meal selection skills (ADL I and II). She did, however, evince deficiencies in more complex ADL skills. At the time of discharge, the client was not judged to be capable of completely independent functioning. She had difficulties in the areas of budgeting and obtaining community resources and was in need of assistance in these areas.

Communication Training

The focus of communication training was on all of the six discrete skills: content, loudness, feeling quality, hand gestures, facial expressions, and body position. The client was trained to communicate both pleasure and displeasure. Initially, she was assessed as having relative good pleasure communication skills and relatively poor displeasure communication skills.

After the third month of training the client was at, or near, the maximum levels in all skill areas of training in both the pleasure and displeasure roleplayed assessments. She was able to maintain these communication skills throughout the remaining 3 months of her treatment.

Self-Esteem Training

The client entered into self-esteem training during the final 3 months of her treatment. She was assessed with the LSI and with respect to the actual number of positive self-statements that she made during training sessions. During training, the client's life satisfaction scores increased from 10 to 17, which represented a significant increase in overall life satisfaction. Similarly, her positive verbalizations increased from an average of 5 per session at the beginning of training to as high as 13 per session near the end of training. This, too, represented a significant change in the client's behavior with respect to her self-esteem.

Other Areas of Training

In addition to the training areas discussed previously, the client's use of her unstructured time and her abilities to know the names and dosages of her medications were monitored. Throughout the course of treatment, use of her unstructured time was judged to be outstanding. She engaged in a wide variety of activties, including appropriate solitary (sewing, art work, etc.) and prosocial (conversation, table-game playing, etc.) activities. By the time of discharge, the client's knowledge of her medications was also judged to be excellent and her ability to take her medicines correctly was rarely, if ever, a problem.

Summary of the Case of Mrs. C.

The client entered into the program after a long and gradual deterioration of her independent living skills and increasing confusion, disorientation, and delirium. Although she had defined anxiety as a major problem, no significant evidence could be found for either anxiety or depression. The client's STAIC and BDI scores remained within normal limits throughout her treatment. In addition, MIBS subscales indicated no problems with withdrawal, anxious depression, or any other maladaptive behaviors. The MIBS competence subscales showed gradual improvement over the course of treatment.

The treatment for this client focused primarily upon the reacquisition of previous skills and abilities. The retraining accomplished over the 6 months of treatment resulted in the client's being able to return to independent community living while requiring occasional assistance. Her assessment scores reflected the results of the retraining.

Approximately 1 month before discharge, the client decided to move to the New England area to live with her son and daughter-in-law. They were very pleased to have her live with them. This arrangement appeared to be an ideal placement for the client because she would be in a supportive environment but could function relatively independently.

Follow-Up

A 3-month telephone follow-up revealed that the client continued to maintain the skills she had reacquired. She and the daughter-in-law were interviewed, and both gave convergent descriptions of the client's behavior. At follow-up the client reported no significant memory problems and was engaging in daily exercise doing regular housekeeping activities, caring for her granddaughter, socializing with neighbors, taking her medications, and attending follow-up mental and physical health appointments. No recurrence of the confusion or delirium was reported.

Summary

A treatment program for the hospitalized elderly has been described in some detail. Although an outpatient therapist may not be able to provide the type of comprehensive treatment described herein, it is hoped that the outpatient therapist will have increased awareness of all the facets involved in the treatment of the elderly. Furthermore, the assessment and decision process has been described in some detail to illustrate how behaviorally based clinical psychology can operate in the "real world" of treatment. As described, a thorough objective assessment is essential for treatment selection and evaluation. Finally, the actual application of treatment has been described through two case illustrations to allow the clinician to see how treatment decisions are carried through and applied to the client and are then systematically and objectively evaluated.

References

Baltes, M. M, Burgess, R. L., & Stewart, R. B. (1980). Independence and dependence in nursing home residents: An operant ecological study. *International Journal of Behavioral Development, 3,* 489–500.

Beck, A. T. (1979). *Cognitive therapy and emotional disorders.* New York: New American Library.

Beck, A. T., Rush, A. J., Shaw, B. F., & Emery, G. *Cognitive therapy of depression.* New York: Guilford Press, 1979.

Carroll, K. (Ed.). (1978). *Human development in aging: Compensating for sensory loss.* Minneapolis: The Ebenezer Center for Aging and Human Development.

Gordon, D. M. (1974). Eye problems of the aged. In A. B. Chinn (Ed.), *Working with older people* (Vol. IV). *Clinical aspects of aging.* Washington DC: U.S. Department of Health and Human Services.

Hogarty, G. E., & Ulrich, R. (1972). The discharge readiness inventory. *Archives of General Psychiatry, 26,* 414–426.

Kalish, R. A. (1975). *Late adulthood: Perspectives in human development.* Monterey, CA: Brooks/Cole.

Kalish, R. A. (1977). *The later years.* Belmont, CA: Wadsworth.

Katz, S., Ford, A. B., Moskowitz, R. W., Jackson, B. A., & Jaffe, M. W. (1963). Studies of illness in the aged. The index of ADL, a standardized measure of biological and psychosocial function. *Journal of the American Medical Association, 185,* 914–919.

Kuhlen, R. G. (1959). Aging and life adjustment. In J. E. Birren (Ed.), *Handbook of aging and the individual.* Chicago: University of Chicago Press.

Larson, R. (1978). Thirty years of research on the subjective well-being of older Americans. *Journal of Gerontology, 33,* 109–129.

Libow, L. S. (1977). Senile dementia and "pseudo-senility": Clinical diagnosis. M. C. Eisdorfer & R. O. Friedel (Eds.), *Cognitive and emotional disturbances in the elderly.* Chicago: Year Book Medical Publishers.

Maurer, J. F. (1976). Auditory impairment and aging. In B. Jacobs (Ed.), *Working with the impaired elderly.* Washington DC: The National Council on Aging.

Meichenbaum, D. (1977). *Cognitive behavior modification: An integrative approach.* New York: Plenum Press.

Missouri Psychiatric Institute. (n.d.). *Missouri Inpatient Behavior Scale (MIBS).* St. Louis: Author.

Neugarten, B., Havighurst, R., & Tobin, S. (1961). The measurement of life satisfaction. *Journal of Gerontology, 16,* 134–143.

Patterson, R. L., & Jackson, G. M. (1980). Behavioral approaches to gerontology. In L. Michelson, M. Hersen, & S. M. Turner (Eds.), *Future perspectives in behavior therapy* (pp. 206–241). New York: Plenum Press.

Patterson, R. L., O'Sullivan, M. J., & Spielberger, C. D. (1980). Measurement of state and trait anxiety in elderly mental health clients. *Journal of Behavioral Assessment, 2,* 89–97.

Patterson, R. L., Dupree, L. W., Eberly, D. A., Jackson, G. W., O'Sullivan, M. J., Penner, L. A., & Dee-Kelley, C. (1982). *Overcoming deficits of aging: A behavioral approach.* New York: Plenum Press.

Patterson, R. L., Penner, L. A., Eberly, D. A., & Harrell, T. L. (1983). Behavioral assessments of intellectual competence, communication skills and personal hygiene skills of elderly persons. *Behavioral Assessment, 5,* 207–218.

Pfeiffer, E. (1975). A short portable mental status questionnaire for the assessment of organic brain deficits in elderly patients. *Journal of the American Geriatric Society, 23,* 433–436.

Pfeiffer, E., Johnson, T. M. & Chiofolo, R. C. (1981). Functional assessment of elderly subjects in four service settings. *Journal of the American Geriatric Society, 29,* 433–437.

Sletten, I. W., & Ullett, G. A. (1972). The present status of automation in a state psychiatric system. *Psychiatric Annals, 2,* 77–80.

Spielberger, C. D., Edwards, C. D., Lushene, R. E., Montouri, J., & Platzek, D. (1973). *STAIC: Preliminary Manual for the State-Trait Anxiety Inventory for Children.* Palo Alto, CA: Consulting Psychologists Press.

Yeasavage, J. A., Westphal, J., & Rush, L. (1981). Senile dementia: Combined pharmacologic and psychologic treatment. *Journal of the American Geriatric Society, 24,* 164–170.

Anger and Violent Behavior

PHILIP H. BORNSTEIN, CHARLES E. WEISSER, AND
BERNARD J. BALLEWEG

Introduction

Violence has produced an endless chronology of human suffering. Throughout history, society has witnessed a seemingly endless array of wars, assassinations, murders, rapes, acts of terrorism, and forms of domestic violence. On a national scale, there is a growing awareness that aggression is a problem of epidemic proportions. Research on domestic violence, for example, has indicated that approximately 3.3 million American wives and over a quarter of a million husbands receive severe beatings from their spouses (Steinmetz, 1977). Other studies have shown that 1.5 million children are abused each year (Fontana, 1973), and 2,000 die annually as a result of injuries inflicted by their parents (Kempe, 1976). Moreover, national surveys have indicated that one out of every four women will be raped sometime during their lives (Russell & Miller, 1979). Cumulatively, these findings leave little doubt that violence is currently one of the most pervasive problems existent in contemporary society.

Given the magnitude of the problem, mental health professionals have devoted relatively little effort to the development and empirical validation of effective treatment strategies for the control of anger and aggression. Although there are probably a variety of explanations for this neglect, the initial inertia may have been engendered by early psychoanalytic (Freud, 1922) and ethological (Lorenz, 1966) theories, which portrayed aggression as an immutable, instinctual phenomenon. In contrast, more recently formulated social learning models (e.g., Bandura,

PHILIP H. BORNSTEIN, CHARLES E. WEISSER, and BERNARD J. BALLEWEG • Department of Psychology, University of Montana, Missoula, Montana 59812.

1973) conceive of violence as a learned response, acquired and modified in much the same manner as prosocial behavior. Briefly, social learning theory posits that aggressive behaviors are acquired both through instrumental and vicarious learning experiences. Once learned, violence is maintained through environmental (e.g., social approval), vicarious (i.e., seeing others receive positive consequences for aggression), and self-reinforcement consequences (i.e., internal cognitive appraisals regarding the appropriateness of violent behavior). In addition, the expression of violent behavior is facilitated by emotional arousal that reduces cognitive controls and environmental stimuli that have been repeatedly associated with prior aggressive episodes.

Social learning theory has stimulated the development of a variety of behavioral and cognitive-behavioral interventions that have proven useful in the control of violence across a variety of settings (Bornstein, Hamilton, & McFall, 1981; Fehrenbach & Thelen, 1982). The purpose of this chapter is to describe those treatment procedures in a manner that will be of utility to clinicians working with violent clients. Thus, the chapter presents the following: (a) a description of behavioral strategies used to assess violence; (b) a review of primary behavioral treatment approaches for the control of violence; and (c) a case presentation detailing the application of behavioral procedures in actual clinical practice. Throughout this exposition, the terms *violence* and *aggression* will be used interchangeably. Consistent with Baron's (1977) operational definition of aggression, both terms will designate any form of behavior that is intentionally directed toward the goal of harming or injuring another human being who is motivated to avoid such treatment. Consequently, the primary focus of this chapter will be on the management of overt harmful behaviors. Nevertheless, information pertaining to the assessment and treatment of maladaptive anger, an inferred internal state, is integrated into the discussion because anger arousal is central to the instigation of aggressive behavior (Novaco, 1975).

The Assessment of Aggressive Behavior

The assessment of human aggression is still in its relative infancy, continuing to pose a number of methodological and ethical problems (Bornstein *et al.*, 1981). As violent behavior is socially undesirable, measures of aggression tend to be reactive. Estimates of the frequency and/or severity of aggressive behavior therefore may be highly inaccurate. Moreover, social desirability response biases must be taken into consideration. Although unobtrusive measures may circumvent some difficulties in this area, the ethics of such practices have limited their utility. Nevertheless, a number of behavioral assessment strategies do yield data that can be helpful in the planning and evaluation of treatment. These include (a) self-report inventories; (b) behavior interviews; (c) self-monitoring techniques; (d) behavioral observations; and (e) physiological recordings. Data pooled from these sources can provide a comprehensive picture of violence as a target behavior. Such multimodal assessment can further aid in conceptualizing the interactive influence of stimulus conditions, internal states (i.e., emotional arousal and cognitive appraisals), and environmental consequences in control of a client's violent behavior.

Self-Report Inventories

A variety of self-report inventories for assessing anger and aggression have been published (e.g., Buss & Durkee, 1957; Evans & Strangeland, 1971; Novaco, 1975; Zaks & Walters, 1959; Zelin, Adler, & Myerson, 1972). Unfortunately, most of these measures have limited reliability and/or validity and are subject to social desirability response biases (Biaggo, 1980; Biaggio, Supplee, & Curtis, 1981; Edmunds & Kendrick, 1980). Despite their psychometric limitations, however, self-report inventories can be used as initial screening instruments. In so doing, they are apt to yield information about the range of situations that precipitate violence and the types of behaviors that clients typically exhibit under such circumstances.

Two of the most frequently used pencil-and-paper measures of anger and aggression are the Buss-Durkee Hostility Inventory (Buss & Durkee, 1957) and the Novaco Anger Inventory (Novaco, 1975). The Buss-Durkee Inventory is a logically derived instrument consisting of 75 true-false items, designed to tap eight modes of hostility expression: assault, verbal hostility, indirect hostility, irritability, negativism, resentment, suspicion, and guilt. For example, one "assault" item reads, "If I have to resort to physical violence to defend my rights, I will," whereas a sample "irritability" item reads, "I often feel like a powder keg ready to explode." The Buss-Durkee Inventory can provide the clinician with an initial index of the manner in which the client typically expresses his or her anger. Unfortunately, it does not provide a wide sampling of situations typically eliciting anger and/or hostile responses.

In contrast, the Novaco Anger Inventory was explicitly designed to assess anger reactions across a broad range of stimulus conditions. The instrument is comprised of 80 potentially provocative situations that clients rate, according to the degree of anger they would experience if the incident actually occurred. Each incident is rated on a 5-point Likert scale, and item scores are summed to yield a total index of the client's overall tendency toward anger arousal. The resultant total score can be used as a pre-post measure of treatment efficacy. In addition, the ratings on individual scale items can be examined to obtain a rough index of the types of situations that are most likely to incite anger and aggression. Those incidents can then be discussed in more detail in a subsequent behavioral interview.

The Behavioral Interview

The behavioral interview serves to augment self-report inventories by developing a more complete index of the frequency, intensity, and duration of violent impulses and a more detailed analysis of the factors that precipitate and maintain agressive responding. The clinician should ask questions pertaining to (a) the environmental situations in which the client exhibits violent behavior; (b) the internal cognitive and emotional states influencing the expression of violence; (c) the types of aggressive behaviors exhibited; and (d) the consequences or responses to violence.

The analysis of environmental stimulus conditions should identify the settings (e.g., home, work, school) and types of people, (e.g., parents, spouses, siblings, friends, strangers) that incite anger and aggression. In addition, forms of provocation (e.g., verbal threats, insults, unjust actions, frustrations) that elicit aggression should be identified. Finally, it is important to assess the degree to which the client's violence is related to the consumption of alcohol and drugs, as concurrent treatment for substance abuse may be suggested.

The assesssment of internal cognitive and emotional states entails an analysis of feelings, perceptions, expectations, and self-statements that lead to anger and aggression. This process can be facilitated by having the client close his or her eyes and describe a prior violent incident as if it were happening in the present, while providing a running commentary of thoughts and feelings as they occur. The clinician should watch for inflammatory cognitions such as unrealistic expectations of oneself or others and provocative self-statements (e.g., "Here she goes again, the same old b.s.!"; "I'll tell the idiot where he can stick it"). In addition, the presence of anxiety, anger, and/or guilt occurring prior to, during, and after the angry episodes should be noted. Data gained from the assessment of thoughts and feelings can be used to select treatments that are targeted at specific cognitive (e.g., self-instruction training) and/or emotional (e.g., systematic desensitization, relaxation training) components of the aggressive response pattern.

The analysis of violent behaviors should detail the person's overt responses (e.g., insults, threats, physical abuse, pushing) to a variety of stimulus conditions. In making this analysis, it is important to determine if the client has used lethal instruments such as guns and knives in previous violent episodes, and if he or she is currently an imminent threat to the safety of others. It is also important to identify adaptive behaviors within the client's repertoire. For example, the presence of appropriate assertive behaviors should be assessed to determine if the person has the social skills needed to respond to provocations in a constructive manner.

Finally, the behavioral interview should provide an analysis of positive and negative consequences associated with the client's aggressive behavior. Of primary importance are the reinforcement contingencies that may be maintaining the violent behavior, such as social attention, acquiescent responses from victims, release of personal tension, and the like.

Self-Monitoring Techniques

Self-monitoring procedures have also been employed in the assessment of anger and aggression (Nomellini & Katz, 1983; Novaco, 1975; Rahaim, Lefebvre, & Jenkins, 1980). These techniques are advantageous in that they (a) aid clients in becoming aware of their anger arousal and aggressive reactions; (b) provide valuable clinical material that can be used throughout the course of treatment; (c) serve to identify the specific stimulus situations that precipitate anger; and (d) allow for the collection of continuous assessment data throughout baseline and treatment conditions (Bornstein, Hamilton, & Bornstein, in press).

In the typical self-monitoring paradigm, the client is asked to keep a dairy of all instances of anger arousal. Either small notebooks or more formal self-monitoring forms, such as the Dimensions of Anger Reactions Scale (Novaco, 1977a), can be used for recording purposes. Clients are instructed to provide a description of each provocative event, note how they responded to the situation, and detail the consequences of their response. In addition, anger intensity ratings can be provided on a Likert scale ranging from "no anger" to "rage."

Self-monitoring can begin immediately after intake and continue throughout treatment. In introducing the diary, it is important to emphasize its role in the planning/evaluation of treatment and to stress the need for obtaining valid and accurate information. The aggression diary can be reviewed at the onset of each therapy session to assess therapeutic progress and stimulate discussion of unresolved problematic situations.

Behavioral Observations

Behavioral observational techniques are invaluable components of an assessment package as they potentially may yield *direct* indexes of a client's aggressive behavior. Current observational assessment approaches include (a) in-home observations of parent–child interactions; (b) behavioral observations in institutional settings; and (c) analog, roleplay evaluations.

Observations in the Home

Home-based observational procedures have been used by a variety of investigators to assess problematic parent–child interactions associated with child abuse and neglect (Crozier & Katz, 1979; Denicola & Sandler, 1980; Nomellini & Katz, 1983; Sandler, Van Dercar, & Milhoan, 1978). Most of these authors employed some variant of the Patterson Coding System (Patterson, Ray, Shaw, & Cobb, 1969) as the primary assessment procedure. The Patterson Coding System is comprised of 29 behavioral categories that assess both positive (e.g., expressions of praise or approval, laughing, talking, positive physical behavior) and aversive (e.g., teasing, yelling, negative commands, physical contact intended to inflict pain) behaviors. The occurrence/nonoccurence of each response category is scored during each of 90 consecutive 20-second intervals that comprise the typical half-hour observational session. An overall "aversive behavior score" and a "positive behavior score" is then computed by calculating the percentage of intervals in which aversive and positive behaviors occurred during each of the observational sessions. These percentages can be graphed across sessions as a means of providing a continuous assessment of treatment efficacy. In addition, each of the 29 behavioral categories can be examined independently to determine specific parental response deficits and excesses targeted for change.

Typically, two to four home observation sessions are scheduled per week throughout baseline and treatment conditions. Although the times of the sessions may be varied, observations certainly should occur during periods when the highest level of conflict has been reported to occur. Throughout each observation period, family members are instructed to remain in the same room but are generally encouraged to engage in their normal interactional patterns.

Observations in Institutional Settings

Direct observational procedures have also been used extensively in the assessment of aggressive behaviors in institutional settings (e.g., Bornstein, Rychtarik, McFall, Bridgwater, Guthrie, & Anton, 1980; Martin & Foxx, 1973; Matson & Stevens, 1977, 1978; Novaco, 1977b; Sumner, Meuser, Hsu, & Morales, 1974). In the typical assessment paradigm, problematic violent behaviors are identified and operationally defined. Staff members are then trained to monitor targeted behaviors via frequency charts or behaviorally specific rating forms. To allow reliability checks, at least two staff members monitor target behaviors simultaneously during a portion of all observation intervals. In one investigation, Bornstein, Rychtarik, McFall, Bridgwater, Guthrie, and Anton (1980) evaluated the efficacy of a positively based treatment procedure by having correctional officers record the frequency of inmate offenses on daily report cards. Each card listed 12 behaviorally specific offenses (e.g., abusive remarks, property damage, fighting, threats to bodily harm). The occurrence/nonoccurrence of each behavior was scored by one correctional officer designated as the primary observer. In addition, a second officer independently recorded offenses on 25% of all observation intervals to provide covert reliability checks. Using a multiple-baseline design, the total number of offenses exhibited daily by each of four inmates was then graphed throughout baseline and treatment phases.

Other investigators have unobtrusively observed the behavior of institutionalized patients in contrived situations (Frederiksen & Rainwater, 1979; Frederiksen, Jenkins, Foy, & Eisler, 1976). For example, Frederiksen *et al.* (1976) used contrived observational assessments to evaluate the generalization of a social skills training program designed to modify abusive verbal outbursts in two adult psychiatric patients. Following treatment, these investigators unobtrusively reproduced two on-ward situations in which each client had previously exhibited abusive behavior. In addition, both patients were exposed to one provocation they had never before encountered. Trained observers rated patient responses to each of these encounters by recording the occurrence/nonoccurrence of irrelevant comments (e.g., commenting about the weather when requesting repayment of a debt), hostile remarks (e.g., "Go to hell!"), inappropriate demands (e.g., "Move, or I'll throw you off the bus!"), and appropriate requests (e.g., "Please move, I have to sit down"). Further, observers assigned a global social skills rating to on-ward situations using a 5-point scale ranging from "very skillful" to "very unskillful."

Although a myriad of idiosyncratically derived observational strategies for assessing aggressive behavior have been devised, few investigators have attended to uncontrolled sources of bias and error in their data collection process (i.e., training of observers, expectation biases, reactivity of the observational process, consensual observer drift, etc.). Thus, behavior therapists who elect to use observational procedures must be cognizant of these potentially distorting influences and take steps to minimize their occurrence (see Kent & Foster, 1977).

Analog Observational Measures

Direct, *in vivo* recording of behavior has long been considered the hallmark of behavioral assessment. Although such strategies may provide excellent means for deriving valid information about client functioning, naturalistic observation is sometimes neither cost-effective nor practically feasible. As a result, alternative analog procedures have been developed for use in laboratory or contrived clinic situations (Hersen & Bellack, 1977). Although the validity of analog techniques does not appear to be optimal (Bellack, Hersen, & Turner, 1978; Bellack, Hersen, & Lamparski, 1979), they can provide clinicians with an objective, data-based index of target behavior occurrence.

Analog procedures have been used by a number of investigators to assess aggressive behavior (e.g., Foy, Eisler, & Pinkston, 1975; Frederiksen *et al.*, 1976; Kirchner, Kennedy, & Draguns, 1979; Matson & Stevens, 1978; Moon & Eisler, 1983; Rahaim *et al.*, 1980). The majority of these authors hypothesized that assaultive behavior resulted from deficiences in social competence. Consequently, maladaptive aggression was treated through assertiveness and social skills training approaches.

The analog assessment of social skills deficits is obtained through a behavioral analysis of the client's roleplay responses to either standardized interpersonal scenes or personally relevant conflict situations. The original (Eisler, Miller, & Hersen, 1973) and revised (Eisler, Hersen, Miller, & Blanchard, 1975) Behavioral Assertiveness Tests are excellent examples of standardized roleplay assessment procedures. Both instruments are comprised of a series of standard interpersonal situations that require assertive responses from the subject. Each vignette is read by a narrator and followed with a prompting statement delivered by a role model.

NARRATOR: You come home late one night, and your wife demands an explanation of why you are so late. As soon as you begin to explain, she interrupts you and starts screaming about how inconsiderate you are.
ROLE MODEL PROMPT: I don't care what happened. You are the most inconsiderate person in the world for making me worry about you.

For research purposes, clients' responses to each of these situations are videotaped and rated with respect to specific undesirable (e.g., hostile or irrelevant statements, threats, interruptions, compliance with unreasonable demands) and desirable (e.g., assertive requests, eye contact, appropriate affect, adequate speech volume) social behaviors. However, in less methodologically rigorous clinical situations, clients' responses can be examined more informally to identify specific social skills deficits that may subsequently be targeted for change.

Roleplay assessments can also be individually tailored to maximize their relevance with regard to the client's presenting complaint. Specifically, data generated from the aforementioned self-report sources can be used to identify situations that typically arouse anger and/or aggression. Those situations can then be reenacted in roleplay interactions. For example, Rahaim *et al.* (1980) reconstructed the following situation in the assessment of a police officer who sought treatment for maladaptive verbal and physically aggressive outbursts on the job:

> You see a person go through a red light. You pull him over, and he complains that the light was yellow and not red. He says, "What, are you blind?"

As in the standardized roleplay assessments, the client was asked to respond to the prompt as if he were actually in the situation.

The therapist can also use a series of predetermined stimulus lines that are designed to be increasingly provocative (e.g., Kirchner *et al.*, 1979; Novaco, 1975). To illustrate, Kirchner *et al.* (1979) used the following sequence of statements to recreate a conflict situation in which the client was an employee working on a new job with a critical boss:

> (1) That order you filled yesterday was all fouled up. Stupid mistakes like that cost us money. Try to get yourself together, will you? (2) Your job isn't so complicated that you should be having all this trouble with it. (3) Look, I hired you because I thought I wouldn't have to lead you through every detail of your job. (4) If you are too lazy or thick headed to figure out your job on your own, you won't have a job here for long.

This multiple stimulus format can be used to develop the provocative situation more completely than the single-prompt procedure. By generating higher levels of arousal, more typical of real-life conflict situations, greater external validity may be achieved.

In constructing roleplay assessments, it is important to tap a diversity of potentially provocative incidents as a means of developing a comprehensive situational analysis of the client's social skills deficits. Furthermore, via the incorporation of roleplay tasks not used in the training process, generalization of behavior to novel situations can also be assessed.

Physiological Measures

Behavior therapists have rarely used physiological measures in the assessment of anger and aggression. However, several investigators (Frederiksen & Rainwater, 1979; Moon & Eisler, 1983; Novaco, 1975) have used physiological indexes of arousal such as pulse rate, systolic and diastolic blood pressure, and/or galvanic skin responses to assess emotional reactivity during laboratory roleplay provocations. In the typical laboratory procedure, subjects are first seated and are asked to remain quiescent for a short adaptation period. Baseline physiological measures are then obtained via blood pressure cuffs and skin electrodes. Reactivity to the assessment procedures is reduced by taking several baseline measures and by monitoring the client's physiological responses to neutral roleplay scenes prior to introducing provocative situations. Clients are then asked to roleplay a provocative interpersonal encounter with an experimenter, and physiological readings are taken when the interaction is completed. Mean changes in physiological indexes taken before and after each roleplay are then computed. To assess treatment efficacy, these mean changes are compared with mean changes in arousal to the same provocation scenes administered after treatment.

Psychophysiological measures of anger and aggression are clearly in a formative stage of development and continue to present a number of methodological, practical, and interpretive problems (Edmunds & Kendrick, 1980; Kallman & Feuerstein, 1977; Novaco, 1975). Until these obstacles are overcome through further research, it is unlikely that physiological assessments will enjoy widespread use in the selection and evaluation of treatments for aggression.

The Treatment of Aggressive Behavior

Although numerous therapies for violent adults have been proposed, many have not undergone close experimental scrutiny. Catharsis, group therapy, traditional insight-oriented therapy, hypnosis, chemotherapy, electroconvulsive shock, and psychodrama have all been suggested at one time or another (Hartogs & Artzt, 1970; Maughs, 1961; Warren & Kurleycheck, 1981). Clearly, the most frequently studied treatments, however, are those programs utilizing operant techniques, systematic desensitization, interpersonal skills acquisition, and cognitive-behavioral procedures. Although these will be reviewed next, space limitations do not permit descriptions that allow for an explicit "how-to-do-it" exposition.

Operant Interventions

Operant techniques have primarily been used in the treatment of institutional violence. These interventions are based on the belief that violent behaviors can be reduced by removing rewarding consequences. In addition, most clinicians pragmatically attempt to strengthen appropriate or prosocial behaviors.

Extinction

Extinction refers to the process of eliminating behavior by the withdrawal of reinforcing conditions. Extinction was successfully used by Martin and Foxx (1973) to reduce the assaultive behaviors of a mentally retarded institutionalized female. During the treatment phase, staff members were trained to ignore assaultive occurrences. Although decreases in frequency did occur, results did not generalize to others not taking part in the study. Of some note, Bandura (1973) suggests that extinction may be feasible only for mild forms of aggression and, as indicated, should be accompanied by the reinforcement of incompatible prosocial responses.

Time-Out

Time-out from positive reinforcement involves the elimination of rewarding consequences as well as the removal of all other potentially rewarding stimuli that are present. Because extinction may initially increase the occurrence of violent behavior and often requires a longer time period to become effective (Ferster &

Skinner, 1957), time-out procedures are often preferable to extinction. Foxx, Foxx, Jones, and Kiely (1980) succeeded in markedly reducing the violent behavior of a psychoticlike retarded adult through the use of a 24-hour time-out period in combination with relaxation procedures. However, although time-out is preferable to extinction, a number of limitations do exist. First, time-out also should be used in conjunction with strengthening of adaptive social behavior. Second, there are no clear guidelines that delineate the optimal duration of time-out. Third, time-out is a negatively oriented procedure. Consequently, it offers a more "restrictive" form of control than other positively based techniques.

Differential Reinforcement of Other Behavior

The development of incentives for nonviolence or prosocial behavior has been considered of paramount importance to the control of aggression (Berkowitz, 1962; Buss, 1961). Differential reinforcement of other (DRO) behavior refers to the presentation of reward when violent behavior has not been exhibited for a specified period of time. A combination of time-out and differential reinforcement of nonviolent behavior was found to be successful in the reduction of violent behavior in two mentally retarded, hospitalized adults (Bostow & Bailey, 1969) and a 29-year-old male mental patient (Edwards, 1974). Bornstein, Rychtarik, McFall, Bridgwater, Guthrie, and Anton (1980) also significantly reduced the violent behavior of four male prisoners. Using a modified DRO procedure, correctional officers were taught to monitor inmate offenses with reinforcement administered contingently upon reduction of observed inmate offenses.

The Combined Use of Reinforcement and Punishment

The use of physical punishment alone has received little attention in the aggression literature. In fact, it has been suggested that physical punishment may model injurious behavior, arouse counteraggression, or be so lacking in acceptability as to preclude its effective implementation (Fehrenbach & Thelen, 1982). Bandura (1973) and Baron (1977) have proposed that the following conditions should be met before applying severe forms of punishment: (a) milder forms of treatment have proven unsuccessful in reducing the patient's violent behavior; (b) alternative adaptive social responses are available; (c) the patient is knowledgeable of the specific behaviors being punished; (d) the intent of the punishing agent is perceived as helping rather than being vindictive or self-serving; and (e) the punishment is administered immediately and consistently following an offense.

When physical punishment is used, greater success is achieved with the concomitant reinforcement of alternative socially adaptive behaviors (Azrin & Holtz, 1966). Ludwig, Marx, Hill, and Browning (1969) eliminated the physically and verbally assaultive behavior of a hospitalized schizophrenic woman through the combined use of contingent electric shock for violent behavior and positive rewards for adaptive responses.

Response cost (loss of reinforcement contingent upon the emission of some inappropriate behavior) has also been used to control violence. Incidents of physical abuse by chronic schizophrenics were shown to be modifiable by the withdrawal of tokens (fines) for aggressive behavior (Winkler, 1970). Keltner and Gordon (1976) rewarded violent prisoners with ⅛-day sentence reductions for each 24-hour period in which aggressive behavior was absent. A response-cost strategy was simultaneously implemented in which any incidence of violence resulted in a loss of all earnings occurring during a 30-day interval. Results indicated significant reductions in violent behavior from pretreatment assessment.

Overcorrection

Positive practice overcorrection (OC) requires a client to rehearse incompatible, prosocial behaviors contingent upon the occurrence of some inappropriate violent behavior (Ollendick & Matson, 1978). Overcorrection was developed by Azrin and his colleagues (Foxx & Azrin, 1972) to circumscribe some of the problems with traditional forms of punishment. Such a procedure has been employed successfully by Klinge, Thrusher, and Myers (1975) with institutionalized, chronic schizophrenics and by Webster and Azrin (1973) with profoundly retarded adults. In both studies, the OC consisted of bed rest relaxation contingent upon violent behavior. Webster and Azrin (1973) had found previous applications of time-out to be ineffective. Moreover, OC was preferred by staff over both time-out and sedative medication.

Positive practice OC is often used in conjunction with restitutional OC. In restitutional OC, the offender is required to correct the damage that results from his or her violent behavior. Foxx and Azrin (1972) successfully treated a profoundly retarded adult by requiring her to engage in 30 minutes of restitutional activity (providing medical assistance to the victim, apologizing, etc.) following each aggressive incident. The OC procedure followed previously unsuccessful trials of time-out, positive reinforcement for prosocial behavior, and social disapproval for aggressive behavior. Sumner *et al.* (1974) have also successfully utilized OC procedures (30 minutes of apologizing plus restoration of physical damage) with aggressive adult patients.

In conclusion, operant interventions do appear to have success in the reduction of violent behaviors in institutional settings. However, research in the area is fraught with methodological difficulties, and a number of questions remain unanswered. Maintenance of treatment effects following termination as well as treatment generalization to extratherapeutic settings has largely been ignored. Questions still remain as to the comparative effectiveness of different treatments, the isolation of essential therapeutic components, and the interaction of important subject variables with different treatment modalities. Important ethical and legal questions are also brought into play with the use of punishment, seclusion techniques, and the withholding of reinforcement (see Kazdin, 1978). For a more detailed review of methodological concerns as well as ideas for future research, the reader is referred to Bornstein *et al.* (1981).

Systematic Desensitization

Bandura (1973) has suggested that events perceived as aversive produce a general state of emotional arousal that facilitates violent behavior in certain individuals. Based on the assumption that relaxation can serve as an incompatible response to states of arousal, Von Benken (1977) has suggested that systematic densensitization (SD) be utilized in the treatment of aggression. A number of case studies (Evans, 1971; Herrell, 1971; Saunders, 1978) have offered support for this hypothesis by successfully using SD to reduce violent behavior. In each instance, the clients were trained in relaxation and subsequently exposed via imagination to a hierarchy of anger-inducing events. Smith (1973) did find SD unsuccessful in the treatment of a female with lifelong problems in the control of anger. However, when humor replaced relaxation as the competing response, the aggressive behavior was successfully eliminated.

Although the results of case studies offer support for the use of SD in the treatment of anger arousal and violent behavior, controlled experimental investigations have not yielded results quite as promising. The use of SD in the treatment of anger arousal had been investigated in a number of outcome studies (Evans, Hearn, & Saklofske, 1973; Hearn & Evans, 1972; O'Donnell & Worell, 1973; Rimm, de Groot, Boord, Herman, & Dillow, 1971; Von Benken, 1977). In general, the overall effects of SD have not differed significantly from those of control conditions. However, studies have suffered from a number of methodological flaws. Assessment was typically limited, comparison groups of equivalent credibility were not utilized, subjects were selected only on the basis of self-report, and follow-up assessment was generally ignored. More research will clearly be needed in this area.

Interpersonal Skills Acquisition Approaches

Assertion and Social Skills Training

Proponents of social learning theory have suggested that violent behavior is the result of poorly developed social skills. Bandura (1973) has suggested that aggressive behavior continues to be performed because a person has failed to learn more acceptable ways of handling the demands of interpersonal relations, such as the appropriate expression of anger. Several studies (Reid, Taplin, & Lorber, 1980; Toch, 1969) have reliably demonstrated an association between violent behavior and deficiencies in social skills. Proponents of this model postulate that as anger increases, the behavioral inhibition of anger also increases until a "critical state" is reached, at which time the individual "explodes" (Rimm & Masters, 1974). Therefore, training in assertiveness (Hersen & Bellack, 1976) or social skills (Goldsmith & McFall, 1975) is recommended as a means of teaching the client to express anger appropriately and thus reduce violent behavior.

Various programs exist for training the violent client in interpersonal skills, but all generally involve various combinations of instructions, modeling, behavioral rehearsal, and feedback. Typical of such programs is the work of Frederiksen, Eisler, and their colleagues (Eisler, Frederiksen, & Peterson, 1978; Foy *et al.*, 1975; Frederiksen & Eisler, 1977; Frederiksen & Rainwater, 1979; Frederick *et al.*, 1976). All of these programs essentially involve five sequentially ordered steps.

Step 1: Rationale. It is important for the therapist to first convince his or her client that it is advantageous to stand up for one's rights and express one's feelings in an assertive but not aggressive manner. The therapist should emphasize to the client that talking through interpersonal difficulties is not indicative of cowardice. It may be pointed out to the client that violence may have been an effective way of handling problems in the past (e.g., childhood, adolescence) but that that no longer is the case. In fact, violent behavior is only apt to result in further problems, confinement, or institutionalization.

Step 2: Instructions. Next, clients are provided with a description of the particular target behaviors to be taught along with a rationale for their use (e.g., "Direct eye contact makes you appear more confident"). The target behaviors are organized along a hierarchy of difficulty. Examples of these target behaviors include eye contact, posture, gesturing, appropriate facial mannerisms and affect, directness, refusal of inappropriate requests, and generation of alternative behaviors.

Step 3: Modeling. The therapist elicits from the client a number of situations that have previously elicited violent behavior (e.g., "I come home after working overtime, and my wife accuses me of spending all my time at the tavern"). The therapist then models appropriate responses to each of the situations, while instructing the client to pay attention to a particular targeted response. The use of a videotape is helpful here so that the client may view the modeled behavior several times while observing different response characteristics.

Step 4: Behavioral Rehearsal. After the client has viewed the therapist modeling appropriate assertive responses, he or she is then asked to roleplay the scene. It is helpful to have a cotherapist at this point who can stand behind the client and provide appropriate prompts if necessary. The prompts are gradually faded until the client is able to respond in a nonaggressive manner without help from the therapist.

Step 5: Feedback. The therapist gives immediate verbal feedback regarding the client's performance on the roleplayed scene. Although positive aspects of the client's performance are emphasized, deficiencies are also discussed. The client is asked to repeat a scene until all deficiences are corrected.

Social skills and assertion training have been successfully employed in the reduction of anger arousal and violent behavior with a number of different client populations. Analog studies with college students have demonstrated an increase in assertive behavior, with a corresponding decrease in self-reported anger-provoking incidents (Lehman-Olson, 1975; Moon & Eisler, 1983; Rimm, Hill, Brown, & Stuart, 1974). However, generalization to actual clinical settings still remains limited.

Gregg (1977) compared group assertion training to discussion group controls in the treatment of aggressive prison inmates. Those receiving assertion training showed significantly greater improvement on the Buss-Durkee Inventory and during on-ward aggressive provocations. However, the effects of both time and setting generalization were not determined.

A number of studies have utilized multiple-baseline designs to evaluate assertiveness and social skills training with aggressive psychiatric inpatients (Eisler, Hersen, & Miller, 1974; Foy *et al.*, 1975; Frederiksen *et al.*, 1976; Matson & Stephens, 1978; Turner, Hersen, & Bellack, 1978). The results of these studies, taken collectively, indicate a significant reduction in aggressive behavior concomitant with a marked increase in socially appropriate alternative responses during roleplayed interactions. In addition, the effects of treatment were found to generalize across settings, situations, and time, although reductions in aggressive behavior in the natural environment were documented only by anecdotal reports.

Rahaim *et al.* (1980) reported upon a social skills training program with an adult outpatient who complained of frequent bouts of violent behavior. The client demonstrated a marked increase in socially appropriate assertive responses during roleplays as well as a significant reduction in self-reported anger on the Dimensions of Anger Reactions Scale (Novaco, 1975). However, the lack of generalization across settings, nonbehavioral indexes of aggression, and methodological problems inherent in case study research limit generalizability of the findings.

In conclusion, studies employing social skills and assertion training have demonstrated positive results in reducing aggressive behavior although increasing appropriate interpersonal behavior. Little evidence has been provided, however, that demonstrates that these effects generalize to a reduction in violent behavior in the natural environment or that the effects are maintained over an extended period of time. Greater attention needs to be paid to *in vivo* application of these procedures rather than limiting practice to circumscribed roleplay situations. Significant others should also be brought in to enhance treatment gains and to learn to reinforce assertive behavior in the natural environment. Follow-up booster sessions can also be made part of the treatment program. Furthermore, research is needed to determine whether social skills training in combination with other more cognitively based procedures would be more effective than social skills training alone. And, finally, too little attention has been paid to clients' motivation as a mediating variable in acquisition and performance. For example, if a male client views an increase in assertive verbal skills as a decrease in masculinity, he may be unlikely to implement the skills he has learned. A thorough assessment of the client's cognitions regarding these issues as well as training in self-administered reinforcement for successfully employing the skills to cope with provocation appears necessary.

Cognitive-Behavioral/Coping Skills Approaches

Novaco (1975) has proposed that aggressive behavior is often the result of anger arousal. Anger arousal is seen as an emotional response to provocation that is determined by three variables: (a) cognitive variables, such as appraisals, attributions, expectations, and self-statements; (b) somatic-affective variables, such as tension, agitation and ill-humor; and (c) behavioral variables, such as withdrawal and antagonism. Novaco's (1976a) treatment program, which attempts to intervene on all three levels, places particular emphasis on the modification of maladaptive cognitions. The approach, entitled stress innoculation, involves three basic steps or phases.

Phase 1: Cognitive Preparation

Clients are educated regarding the functions and causes of anger. A thorough assessment of the client's anger control problem is completed. The determinants of anger arousal are pinpointed, with particular emphasis on (a) external events (e.g., those people and situations that most often and most easily arouse anger); (b) internal factors (e.g., what does the client say to himself or herself when provocations occur?; how does the body feel during the early stages of provocation?); and (c) behavioral factors (i.e., how does the client respond when provoked?). Clients are educated about their personal anger patterns, and a treatment rationale is provided. The construction of an anger diary is assigned as homework, and initial instruction is given in anger management via coping strategies.

Phase 2: Skill Acquisition and Rehearsal

Cognitively, the client is taught to modify the irrational expectations and appraisals that lead to anger arousal. Clients are taught to use self-instruction to (a) prepare for provocation (e.g., "Remember, I know how to control my anger"); (b) cope with provocation (e.g., "Calm down, take a deep breath, it's not worth getting mad about this"); and (c) reflect upon the provocation (e.g., "Forget about it now. I can be proud of myself for not getting angry"). Affectively, the client is taught relaxation skills and is encouraged to maintain a sense of humor. Behaviorally, the client is encouraged to recognize the arousal of anger and to then either communicate that anger in a nonhostile form or use it to energize problem-solving action.

Phase 3: Application Practice

The client is asked to practice the skills he or she has learned, first imaginally and then in roleplay situations. The situations are constructed from a hierarchy of anger experiences based upon the client's previously recorded anger diary. During application, the client is asked to sharpen his or her anger management skills by beginning with the mildest hierarchy item and progressing to the most anger arousing.

Novaco (1976b) evaluated the effects of such a program upon anger arousal in 34 people with anger control problems. Both the separate and combined effects of cognitive self-instruction and relaxation training were compared to an attention-control condition. As predicted, subjects in the combined treatment experienced the greatest reduction in anger on most self-report and physiological measures of arousal. Subjects in the self-instruction-alone condition improved less than those in the combined condition, but they still demonstrated significant reductions in anger arousal when compared to the control condition. The relaxation condition differed from the control condition only on self-report of anger during imaginally produced provocations. It should be noted that Konečni (1976) has suggested that the study could have been improved through the use of follow-up assessments and unobtrusive measures of anger and aggression in the natural environment.

Further support for the use of cognitive-behavioral interventions in the regulation of anger arousal has been provided by numerous other investigators (Crain, 1978; Frederiksen & Rainwater, 1979; Harvey, Karan, Bhargara, & Morehouse, 1978; Moon & Eisler, 1983; Novaco, 1977b). Although the results of these studies, taken collectively, demonstrate the successful regulation of anger arousal by cognitive-behavioral interventions, a number of methodological problems limit their generalizability. The Novaco (1977b), Frederiksen and Rainwater (1979), and Harvey *et al.* (1978) studies failed to provide adequate experimental controls, whereas generalizations of the Crain (1978) and Moon and Eisler (1983) findings are limited by the selection of subjects on the basis of self-report criteria alone.

LeCroy (1980) extended the use of stress innoculation to the treatment of spouse abuse. He reported two cases studies in which abusive males were treated with a self-instructional training program. In both cases, the frequency and intensity of self-reported anger outbursts were significantly reduced at both posttreatment and follow-up. However, the case report nature does not allow for the demonstration of functional control.

The use of cognitive behavioral procedures has also been extended to the treatment of child abuse. Nomellini and Katz (1983) employed stress inoculation training to help abusive parents control their angry impulses. A multiple-baseline design across three families was utilized. Upon instigation of the stress inoculation program, parents showed significant reductions in aversive behavior, along with decreases in angry urges and overall proneness to provocation. These changes were maintained at follow-up, which ranged from 2 to 6 months. However, it should be noted that reductions in aversive parent behavior were not accompanied by increases in positive parental behaviors unless treatment was supplemented with training in child management skills.

Another potential strategy for reducing anger arousal that combines both cognitive and behavioral elements is the problem-solving approach of D'Zurilla and Goldfried (1971). Clients are trained to define their anger problem precisely, generate as many solutions as possible, and implement and evaluate the best available alternative. Moon and Eisler (1983) employed such an approach with college students selected because of problems with anger arousal. Subjects achieved a marked reduction in anger-provoking cognitions as well as an increase in assertive/socially skilled behaviors. Unfortunately, the clinical significance of the study is undermined by the sole use of self-report selection criteria, lack of specific behavioral indexes of anger/aggression, and failure to obtain follow-up data.

Case Report

The following is a series of case reports evaluated by means of a multiple-baseline design across behaviors. All subjects were institutionalized at the time of treatment and had been referred for therapy as a result of their interpersonal skills deficits within the area of anger and aggressive disturbances.

Subjects

Subject 1 was a 25-year-old Caucasian male convicted of rape and child molestation. During his 2-year institutionalization, Subject 1 had been involved in a wide variety of institutional rule violations (e.g., attempted escape, numerous attacks upon hospital staff, etc.). His history revealed episodic periods of violence with subjective loss of control. The subject was desirous of treatment, although he was aware that therapy *per se* would probably have little effect upon his indeterminate sentence.

Subject 2 was a 38-year-old male Caucasian who had been hospitalized for 10 years. This subject had an extensive juvenile record including repeated threats of bodily harm and use of weapons (knives, scissors, razor blades, etc.). Within the hospital, Subject 2 had an extremely poor adjustment record. He perceived the world as an extremely hostile, dangerous place and continually expressed the notion that he must "counterattack" lest others take advantage of him.

Subject 3 was a married 45-year-old Caucasian male. This subject also had received an indeterminate sentence, primarily because of his repeated aggressive behavior directed toward his spouse. Outbursts were typically verbal in nature followed by physical attack and occurred both during intoxicated and nonintoxicated states. Prior to hospitalization, some 6 years earlier the subject had achieved a marginally successful adjustment (i.e., regularly employed, some community involvement, etc.). However, as a result of familial problems, Subject 3 had lost his job, severely damaged the marital relationship, and experienced considerable legal difficulties. Within the hospital, he was extremely belligerent and hostile and had on numerous occasions flatly refused all offers of therapeutic assistance.

Laboratory Assessment and Target Behaviors

Four scenes depicting commonly encountered anger-eliciting interactions were modified from Novaco (1975) and Frederiksen and Eisler (1977) and used for roleplay assessment purposes (scene themes included an automobile incident, an argument, a grocery encounter, and roommate sleep disturbance). Immediately following each baseline or training session, subjects were escorted to an experimental laboratory where videotape apparatus allowed for unobtrusive recording of responses to roleplayed situations. Because all assessment scenes involved interaction and/or provocation by a male, a male role model was used throughout the assessment program. Based upon retrospective ratings of baseline videotapes, the following target behaviors were selected for modification:

1. *Number of words spoken.* Total number of words (i.e., utterances found in standard modern dictionaries) used in responding to prompts.
2. *Response latency.* Length of time (in seconds) from termination of prompt to initiation of subject response.
3. *Enunciation.* Scored on a 5-point scale (1 = poor enunciation; 5 = excellent enunciation). Ratings reflected both intelligibility of response and crispness of vowel–consonant speech forms.
4. *Loudness.* Rated on a 5-point scale (1 = inappropriate levels; 5 = appropriate levels). Judges' ratings were based upon standard conversational levels of speech.
5. *Inappropriate hand movement.* Seconds of inappropriate hand movement (e.g., clenched fist, pointing finger, etc.) divided by corresponding scene response duration.

6. *Eye contact.* Length of time during which the subject looked directly at the role model divided by corresponding scene duration.
7. *Intonation.* Scored on a 5-point scale (1 = inappropriate; 5 = appropriate) based upon pitch and voice quality characteristics (e.g., deep raspy, smooth, nervous, etc.).
8. *Rate of speech.* Speech rate ratios were computed by calculating number of words spoken divided by corresponding speech duration.
9. *Requests.* Verbal behavior indicative of an attempt toward adequate coping; subjects' request must be reasonable and appropriate to the situation; scoring was on an all-or-none basis (1 = reasonable request; 0 = unreasonable or no request).
10. *Verbal content.* Demonstration of nonangry, nonaggressive verbal behavior; raters were most attentive to threats, hostile verbal remarks, foul language, and commanding behaviors; scored on a 5-point scale (1 = angry/aggressive verbal content; 5 = firm yet reasonable/nonaggressive content).

Ward Ratings

Each subject's angry/aggressive behavior was monitored daily, across both baseline and treatment phases, on their respective wards. Specifically, six classes of behavior were observed. These included

1. *Abusive language.* Directing to another person, any word, remark, or phrase that is insulting or severely critical; this included foul language and cursing but not colloquial expressions.
2. *Refusing written/verbal orders.* Subject ignores or refuses to comply with a direct order given to him by a staff member with authority over his domain (e.g., living quarters, work placement, library, etc.).
3. *Threats.* Threatening another person with bodily harm; subject directs remarks, words, or phrases to others that are physically threatening to them, their family, or friends.
4. *Fights.* Physically fighting with another person; subject physically attacks another person and initiates or participates in aggressive contact.
5. *Property destruction.* Subject intentionally damages or destroys property belonging to himself, others, or the institution.
6. *Interference with staff.* Subject verbally or physically interferes with staff members in the performance of routine duties when such interference distracts or delays staff members from said duties.

Because hospital staff were quite familiar with subjects' behavior and the preceding categories of aggressive behavior, observational training was mimimal (i.e., one group session of less than 2 hours' duration). Observations were conducted on a continuous and daily basis from approximately 8 A.M. to 9 P.M. by one male nurse designated as the primary observer. Covert reliability checks (Taplin & Reid, 1973) by a second staff member occurred across 25% of all observational periods.

This was accomplished on those days when both observers were on shift throughout the length of the day. When this occurred, staff members independently recorded subjects' behavior with regard to the six categories of assessment listed previously and simply recorded whether the behavior had, in fact, occurred during the scheduled period of observation. Any such occurrence resulted in the scoring of an aggressive offense. Point-by-point comparisons were made, and agreements were scored when both observers recorded a *yes* or a *no* for the same behavior. Reliability for each aggressive behavior was calculated by dividing the number of agreements by the number of agreements plus disagreements for a given subject and multiplying by 100.

Procedure and Treatment

A multiple-baseline design (Bornstein, Bach, Friman, & Lyons, 1980) across target behaviors was employed as a means of assessing the effects of treatment.

Baseline

The length of baseline was dependent upon the sequence of target behavior intervention. In all cases, however, a minimum of a 3-week baseline was provided across all subjects and all behaviors. The major purpose of the baseline phase was to (a) educate subjects regarding the nature of anger and aggression (e.g., causes, functions, consequences, etc.; see Novaco, 1975); (b) identify persons and/or situations that trigger anger (i.e., collect information relevant to cognitive [e.g., self-statements], physiological [e.g., increased heart rate], and behavioral [e.g., physical attack] components; and (c) instruct in the general *concepts* of anger management (i.e., teaching that highly problematic, threatening situations can be handled via

Table 1. Anger Diary

Time and date	Place	Anger incident	Thoughts	Sensations	Actions	Degree of anger arousal 1–7	Degree of anger management 1–7

personally effective coping strategies). The preceding elements of the baseline phase were implemented in the following manner:

1. Session 1—Education (a); Identification (b)
2. Session 2—Identification (b)
3. Session 3—Identification (b); Instruction (c)

Education and instruction elements were presented as a discussion lecture based upon the earlier work of Novaco (1975). Identification, however, was implemented by means of a self-monitored anger diary. In fact, a primary dependent used throughout the course of the investigation was derived from the anger diary. This was the Weekly Anger Totals. This score was the 7-day sum of Anger Arousal (1 [low] − 7 [high]) × Anger Management (1 [good] − 7 [poor]) scales.

Treatment

Individual therapy sessions were begun during the fourth contact session with target behaviors introduced sequentially and cumulatively over the course of an 8-week treatment program (Hersen & Bellack, 1976). Training was conducted by the senior author and utilized three primary components. Because anger has been conceived of as a tripartite construct having physiological, cognitive, and behavioral components (Novaco, 1975), intervention focused upon each of these components across all treatment sessions. This was accomplished as follows:

Physiological Component. One way in which arousal can be reduced is through relaxation training. However, rather than viewing relaxation as a procedure applied by some external agent, it was instead presented as a self-control, cue-conditioned technique (Goldfried, 1971). Thus, subjects spent the first 15 minutes of each session practicing procedures in tension and anxiety reduction by utilizing personally effective coping strategies. This was clearly explained as a skill that one acquires and subsequently applies on his or her own.

Cognitive Component. This component included three major procedures. First, the subject was informed that anger-arousing situations were not personal affronts or threats. Rather, they are to be interpreted simply as difficult situations that demand a problem-solving orientation. As such, the crucial question becomes, "What can I do to resolve this present problem?" Subjects were taught to answer this question in discrete behavioral terms such that the response could be easily translated into actions. Second, subjects were trained in cognitive self-instruction (Bornstein & Quevillon, 1976). In the present program, self-instruction was applied at various stages of the provocation sequence: (a) preparatory to provocation; (b) during provocation; (c) as a means of coping with arousal; and (d) at the close of the conflict situation (see Table 2). The goal here was that private speech would function as an instructional cue to guide the subject's thoughts, feelings, and behaviors toward more effective coping strategies. Third, subjects were instructed in consequence clarification. Here, the following questions were raised: "What is it that I have typically done in this situation?" "What have been the effects?" "What else could I do?" And, "What is likely to be the effect of that action?"

Behavioral Component. Using scenes derived from the baseline identification of problematic situations, subjects were given the opportunity to rehearse physiological, cognitive, and behavioral components of anger/aggression control. One situation was used per treatment session with the following sequence implemented for each of the roleplay interactions: (a) subject was reminded to concentrate on physiological, cognitive, and target specific behavioral components (behavioral components [eye contact, intonation, etc.] were added every other week); (b) subject listened to a description of the problem as presented by the experimenter; (c) the experimenter then roleplayed the situation serving in the role of confederate; (d) subject response was given; (e) the response was evaluated first by the subject; (f) corrective feedback and verbal reinforcement was provided by the experimenter; (g) more adaptive responding was then modeled by the experimenter; (h) a discussion was held reemphasizing physiological, cognitive, and behavioral components and the means by which these can be integrated into effective response strategies; (i) rehearsal was repeated until a more effective response was delivered by the subject. At the conclusion of the roleplay sequence, the subject was thanked for his participation and then transferred from the therapy room to the laboratory for purposes of weekly assessment.

Follow-Up. Two months following the termination of treatment, all dependent measures (i.e., roleplay assessments, ward ratings, and anger diary ratings) were readministered for a 1-week period.

Table 2. Self-Instructions for the Regulation of Anger

Preparing for a provocation
  This could be a rough situation, but I know how to deal with it.
  I can work out a plan to handle this. Easy does it.
  Remember, stick to the issues and don't take it personally.
  There won't be any need for an argument. I know what to do.
Impact and confrontation
  As long as I keep my cool, I'm in control of the situation.
  You don't need to prove yourself. Don't make more out of this than you have to.
  There is no point in getting mad. Think of what you have to do.
  Look for positive and don't jump to conclusions.
Coping with arousal
  My muscles are getting tight. Relax and slow things down.
  Time to take a deep breath. Let's take the issue point-by-point.
  My anger is a signal of what I need to do. Time for problem solving.
  He probably wants me to get angry, but I'm going to deal with it constructively.
Subsequent reflection
Conflict unresolved:
  Forget about the aggravation. Thinking about it only makes you upset.
  Try to shake it off. Don't let it interfere with your job.
  Remember relaxation. It's a lot better than anger.
  Don't take it personally. It's probably not so serious.
Conflict resolved:
  I handled that one pretty well. That's doing a good job.
  My pride can get me into trouble, but I'm doing better at this all the time.
  I actually got through that without getting angry.

Social Validation

Scenes and responses from roleplay laboratory assessment Sessions 1, 2, 3 (baseline) and 10, 11, 12 (final two sessions of treatment plus follow-up) were arranged and played in random order to a group of three volunteer raters who had agreed to judge subjects' level of anger/aggression. Before viewing the tapes, judges were instructed to evaluate overall competence in anger-eliciting situations using a 7-point (1 = poor; 7 = excellent) bipolar semantic differential scale (Osgood, Suci, & Tannenbaum, 1957). In addition, judges were asked not to base ratings on direct comparisons between subjects, to rate independently of one another, and to avoid being influenced by subjects' age, appearance, and so forth.

Results

Two judges independently rated roleplay videotapes for all subjects across baseline, treatment, and follow-up sessions. Results indicated Pearson Product-Moment reliability coefficients ranged from .81 to .98 across all target behaviors. In addition, percentage agreement and exact agreement on Likert-scale ratings and ratio reliabilities (defined as +5% agreement criterion) were all within acceptable levels (range = .80 to .99). Ratings of ward behavior similarly achieved high levels of interobserver agreement. Interobserver reliability scores across all six ward behaviors ranged from .86 to .96.

The results of treatment are quite clear. These can best be represented by examining changes across baseline treatment and follow-up phases for each subject individually. Subject 1 showed improvement on all roleplay dependent measures. The number of words spoken and speech latency increased fourfold (speech latency may be particularly important because it is indicative of pensive rather than impulsive cognitive strategies). Ratings of enunciation and verbal content similarly improved from a mean of 1.25 to 1.4, respectively, to treatment levels of 3.25 and 3.5. All behaviors continued to show further, although slight, improvement at follow-up. Ward ratings for Subject 1 indicated 32 aggressive incidents per week at baseline, 12.6 during treatment, and 10 per week at follow-up. Self-reported anger totals were highly correspondent with these findings.

Subject 2's results were quite similar to those previously mentioned. Ratings of appropriate loudness and verbal content more than doubled from baseline through treatment. Inappropriate hand movement decreased more than tenfold, and eye contact increased five times its baseline rate. All these gains were maintained at follow-up. Ward ratings decreased from 28 incidents per week at baseline to 8 per week during treatment, and only 4 at follow-up. In addition, Subject 2 indicated substantial improvement in the self-report of arousal and management of anger outside of the treatment setting.

Subject 3 also showed improvement across all targeted behaviors. Intonation doubled, the rate of speech was cut in half (perhaps again demonstrating a tendency toward nonimpulsive thought), and verbal content ratings reached a "perfect score" of 5 by the time of follow-up. Moreover, anger-eliciting roleplays generated requests for behavior change on every occurrence. Finally, ward ratings and self-monitored anger totals were in high correspondence and clearly indicative of substantial progress.

A few further points are worthy of some comment. First, all behaviors targeted for change showed improvement as a result of treatment. Second, changes were clearly maintained over the course of the 2-month follow-up period. Third, in almost all instances, improvement was quite dramatic and corresponded with the introduction of treatment for each targeted behavior. Fourth, baselines appeared to be highly independent and not influenced by prior treatments. Lastly, decreases in aggressive behavior on the ward were noted across all six categories of offensive behavior.

Social Validation

The mean ratings by judges for overall anger control across all three subjects was Sessions 1, 2, 3 = 1.64; Sessions 10, 11, 12 = 5.72 (indicative of substantial improvement). A Kendall coefficient of concordance (W) was employed to determine the extent of interjudge agreement regarding overall anger control (Siegel, 1956). This was accomplished by rank ordering each judge's semantic differential scores from the six sessions evaluated. A resulting W of 29.60 was obtained ($p <$ .001), indicating extremely high agreement among judges with regard to overall anger control.

Discussion of Case Report

The results of the present case report indicate clear behavioral improvement for all subjects across all behaviors. The success of the program is further augmented by a demonstration of discrete behavioral gains in the laboratory as well as obvious and documented behavioral improvements on the ward. Moreover, the ward behaviors monitored (i.e., abusive language, threats, etc.) were *not* the direct focus of the therapeutic program. Thus, it would appear that subjects had developed nonaggressive interpersonal styles rather than idiosyncratic responses to selected problem situations.

Worthy of some mention is the clear maintenance of behavioral improvement at 2-month follow-up and the rather strong evidence provided by the social validation methodology. Unfortunately, however, the experimental design utilized does not provide information regarding the active components of treatment. As a consequence, future research must address this particular question. In addition, further definition of nonaggressive competence is required. Certainly, if we knew the exact specifications of a competent, nonaggressive response, the training of such behaviors and cognitive styles would be greatly facilitated. As one might presume, the behavior-analytic model of Goldfried and D'Zurilla (1969) might be quite useful in this respect.

Summary

This chapter began with an introduction to the pervasiveness and devastation of aggressive behavior. In attempting to study violence, we first concentrated on a formal assessment of its occurrence. This included a discussion of self-report inventories, behavioral interviews, self-monitoring techniques, direct observations, and physiological measures. In detailing available treatment techniques, we concentrated on operant procedures, systematic desensitization, interpersonal-skills acquisition methods, and cognitive-behavioral coping skills approaches. Our chapter concluded with a rather elaborate case presentation formally evaluated via a multiple-baseline design.

References

Azrin, N. H., & Holtz, W. C. (1966). Punishment. In W. K. Honig (Ed.), *Operant behavior: Areas of research and application* (pp. 380–447). New York: Appleton.

Bandura, A. (1973). *Aggression: A social learning analysis.* Englewood Cliffs, NJ: Prentice-Hall.

Baron, R. A. (1977). *Human aggression.* New York: Plenum Press.

Bellack, A. S., Hersen, M., & Turner, S. M. (1978). Role play tests for assessing social skills: Are they valid? *Behavior Therapy, 9,* 448–461.

Bellack, A. S., Hersen, M., & Lamparski, D. (1979). Role-play tests for assessing social skills: Are they valid? Are they useful? *Journal of Consulting and Clinical Psychology, 47,* 335–342.

Berkowitz, L. (1962). *Aggression: A social psychological analysis.* New York: McGraw-Hill.

Biaggio, M. K. (1980). The assessment of anger arousal. *Journal of Personality Assessment, 44,* 289–298.

Biaggio, M. K., Supplee, K., & Curtis, N. (1981). Reliability and validity of four anger scales. *Journal of Personality Assessment, 45,* 639–648.

Bornstein, P. H., & Quevillon, R. P. (1976). The effects of a self-instructional package on overactive pre-school boys. *Journal of Applied Behavior Analysis, 9,* 179–188.

Bornstein, P. H., Bach, P. J., Friman, P. C., & Lyons, P. D. (1980). Application of a social skills training program in the modification of interpersonal deficits among retarded adults: A clinical replication. *Journal of Applied Behavior Analysis, 12,* 171–176.

Bornstein, P. H., Rychtarik, R. G., McFall, M. E., Bridgwater, C. A., Guthrie, L., & Anton, B. (1980). Behaviorally-specific report cards and self-determined reinforcements: A multiple baseline analysis of inmate offenses. *Behavior Modification, 4,* 71–81.

Bornstein, P. H., Hamilton, S. B., & McFall, M. E. (1981). Adult aggression: Assessment and modification via behavioral intervention strategies. In M. Hersen, R. M. Eisler, & P. M. Miller (Eds.), *Progress in behavior modification* (pp. 299–350). New York: Academic Press.

Bornstein, P. H., Hamilton, S. B., & Bornstein, M. T. (in press). Self-monitoring procedures. In A. Ciminero, K. Calhoun, & H. Adams (Eds.), *Handbook of behavioral assessment.* New York: Wiley.

Bostow, D. E., & Bailey, J. B. (1969). Modification of severe disruptive and aggressive behavior using brief timeout and reinforcement procedures. *Journal of Applied Behavior Analysis, 2,* 31–37.

Buss, A. H. (1961). *The psychology of aggression.* New York: Wiley.

Buss, A. H., & Durkee, A. (1957). An inventory for assessing different kinds of hostility. *Journal of Consulting Psychology, 21,* 343–349.

Crain, D. R. (1978). Awareness and modification of anger problems (Doctoral dissertation, University of California, Los Angeles, 1977). *Dissertation Abstracts International, 38,* 3870B. (University Microfilms No. 77–30, 897)

Crozier, J., & Katz, R. C. (1979). Social learning treatment of child abuse. *Journal of Behavior Therapy and Experimental Psychiatry, 10,* 213–220.

Denicola, J., & Sandler, J. (1980). Training abusive parents in child management and self-control skills. *Behavior Therapy, 11,* 263–270.

D'Zurilla, T. J., & Goldfried, M. R. (1971). Problem solving and behavior modification. *Journal of Abnormal Psychology, 78,* 107–126.

Edmunds, G., & Kendrick, D. C. (1980). *The measurement of human aggressiveness.* West Sussex, England: Ellis Harwood.

Eisler, R. M., Miller, P. M., & Hersen, M. (1973). Components of assertive behavior. *Journal of Clinical Psychology, 29,* 295–299.

Eisler, R. M., Hersen, M., & Miller, P. M. (1974). Shaping components of assertive behavior with instructions and feedback. *American Journal of Psychiatry, 131,* 1344–1347.

Eisler, R. M., Hersen, M., Miller, P. M., & Blanchard, E. B. (1975). Situational determinants of assertive behavior. *Journal of Consulting and Clinical Psychology, 43,* 330–340.

Eisler, R. M., Frederiksen, L. W., & Peterson, G. L. (1978). The relationship of cognitive variables to the expression of assertiveness. *Behavior Therapy, 9,* 419–427.

Evans, D. R. (1971). Specific aggression, arousal, and reciprocal inhibition therapy. *Western Psychologist, 1,* 125–130.

Evans, D. R., & Strangeland, M. (1971). Development of the reaction inventory to measure anger. *Psychological Reports, 29,* 412–414.

Evans, D. R., Hearn, M. T., & Saklofske, P. (1973). Anger, arousal, and systematic desensitization. *Psychological Reports, 32,* 625–626.

Fehrenbach, P. A., & Thelen, M. H. (1982). Behavioral approaches to the treatment of aggressive disorders. *Behavior Modification, 6,* 465–497.

Ferster, C. B., & Skinner, B. F. (1957). *Schedules of reinforcement.* New York: Appleton-Century.

Foxx, R. M., & Azrin, N. H. (1972). Restitution: A method of eliminating aggressive-disruptive behaviors of retarded and brain damaged patients. *Behaviour Research and Therapy, 10,* 15–27.

Foxx, C. L., Foxx, R. M., Jones, J. R., & Kiely, D. (1980). Twenty-four hour social isolation: A program for reducing the aggressive behavior of a psychoticlike retarded adult. *Behavior Modification, 4,* 130–144.

Foy, D. W., Eisler, R. M., & Pinkston, S. (1975). Modeled assertion in a case of explosive rages. *Journal of Behavior Therapy and Experimental Psychiatry, 6,* 135–137.

Frederiksen, L. W., & Eisler, R. M. (1977). The control of explosive behavior: A skill development approach. In D. Upper (Ed.), *Perspectives in behavior therapy* (pp. 127–138). Kalamazoo, MI: Behaviordelia.

Frederiksen, L. W., & Rainwater, N. (1979, March). *Explosive behavior: A skill development approach to treatment.* Paper presented at the 11th Annual Banff International Conference on Behavior Modification, Banff, Canada.

Frederiksen, L. W., Jenkins, J. O., Foy, D. W., & Eisler, R. M. (1976). Social-skills training to modify abusive verbal outbursts in adults. *Journal of Applied Behavior Analysis, 9,* 117–125.

Freud, S. (1922). *Beyond the pleasure principle.* London: International Psychoanalytic Press.

Goldfried, M. R. (1971). Systematic desensitization as training in self-control. *Journal of Consulting and Clinical Psychology, 37,* 228–234.

Goldfried, M. R., & D'Zurilla, T. J. (1969). A behavioral-analytic model for assessing competence. In C. D. Spielberger (Ed.), *Current topics in clinical and community psychology* (pp. 151–196). New York: Academic Press.

Goldsmith, J. G., & McFall, R. M. (1975). Development and evaluation of an interpersonal skill-training program for psychiatric inpatients. *Journal of Abnormal Psychology, 84,* 51–58.

Gregg, R. E. (1977). Passivity, assertion, and aggression: Assertive training with two types of institutionalized criminal offenders (Doctoral dissertation, The University of Texas Health Science Center at Dallas, 1976). *Dissertation Abstracts International, 37,* 4139B–4140B. (University Microfilms No. 77-2, 582)

Hartogs, R., & Artzt, E. (1970). *Violence: Causes and solutions.* New York: Dell.

Harvey, J. R., Karan, O. C., Bhargara, D., & Morehouse, N. (1978). Relaxation training and cognitive behavioral procedures to reduce violent temper outbursts in a moderately retarded woman. *Journal of Behavior Therapy and Experimental Psychiatry, 9,* 347–351.

Hearn, M. T., & Evans, D. R. (1972). Anger and reciprocal inhibition therapy. *Psychological Reports, 30,* 943–948.

Herrell, J. M. (1971). Use of systematic desensitization to eliminate inappropriate anger. *Proceedings of the 79th Annual Convention of the American Psychological Association.* Washington, DC: American Psychological Association.

Hersen, M., & Bellack, A. S. (1976). A multiple-baseline of social skills training in chronic schizophrenics. *Journal of Applied Behavior Analysis, 9,* 239–245.

Hersen, M., & Bellack, A. S. (1977). Assessment of social skills. In A. R. Ciminero, K. S. Calhoun, & H. E. Adams (Eds.), *Handbook of behavioral assessment* (pp. 509–554). New York: Wiley.

Kallman, W. M., & Feuerstein, M. (1977). Psychophysiological procedures. In A. R. Ciminero, K. S. Calhoun, & H. E. Adams (Eds.), *Handbook of behavioral assessment* (pp. 329–364). New York: Wiley.

Kazdin, A. E. (1978). The application of operant techniques in treatment, rehabilitation and education. In S. L. Garfield & A. E. Bergin (Eds.), *Handbook of psychotherapy and behavior change: An empirical analysis* (pp. 549–555). New York: Wiley.

Keltner, A. A., & Gordon, A. (1976). The functional analysis of a reinforcer in a prison population. *Corrective and Social Psychiatry and Journal of Behavior Technology, Methods and Therapy, 22,* 42–44.

Kempe, C. (1976). Approaches to preventing child abuse. *American Journal of Childhood Disease, 30,* 941–947.

Kent, R. W., & Foster, S. L. (1977). Direct observational procedures: Methodological issues in naturalistic settings. In A. R. Ciminero, K. S. Calhoun, & H. E. Adams (Eds.), *Handbook of behavioral assessment* (pp. 279–328). New York: Wiley.

Kirchner, E. P., Kennedy, R. E., & Draguns, J. G. (1979). Assertion and aggression in adult offenders. *Behavior Therapy, 10,* 452–471.

Klinge, V., Thrusher, P., & Myers, S. (1975). Use of bed-rest overcorrection in a chronic schizophrenic. *Journal of Behavior Therapy and Experimental Psychiatry, 6,* 69–73.

Konečni, V. J. (1976). Good news for angry people. *Contemporary Psychology, 21,* 397–398.

LeCroy, C. W. (1980, November). *Self-instructional anger control for the treatment of wife abuse.* Paper presented at the 14th Annual Convention of the Association for Advancement of Behavior Therapy, New York.

Lehman-Olson, P. (1975). Cognitive-behavioral approaches to the reduction of anger and aggression (Doctoral dissertation, Oklahoma State University, 1974). *Dissertation Abstracts International, 35,* 5118B–5119B. (University Microfilms No. 75-8, 822)

Lorenz, K. (1966). *On aggression.* New York: Harcourt.

Ludwig, A. M., Marx, A. J., Hill, P. A., & Browning, R. M. (1969). The control of behavior through faradic shock. *Journal of Nervous and Mental Disease, 148,* 624–637.

Martin, P. L., & Foxx, R. M. (1973). Victim control of the aggression of an institutionalized retardate. *Journal of Behavior Therapy and Experimental Psychiatry, 4,* 161–165.

Matson, J. L., & Stephens, R. M. (1977). Overcorrection of aggressive behavior in a chronic psychiatric patient. *Behavior Modification, 1,* 559–564.

Matson, J. L., & Stephens, R. M. (1978). Increasing appropriate behavior of explosive chronic psychiatric patients with a social-skills training package. *Behavior Modification, 2,* 61–76.

Maughs, S. B. (1961). Current concepts of psychopathology. *Archives of Criminal Psychodynamics, 4,* 550–557.

Moon, J. R., & Eisler, R. M. (1983). Anger control: An experimental comparison of three behavioral treatments. *Behavior Therapy, 14,* 493–505.

Nomellini, S., & Katz, R. C. (1983). Effects of anger control training on abusive parents. *Cognitive Therapy and Research, 7,* 57–68.

Novaco, R. W. (1975). *Anger control: The development and evaluation of an experimental treatment.* Lexington, MA: Lexington Books.

Novaco, R. W. (1976a). *Anger and coping with provocation: An instructional manual.* Unpublished manuscript, University of California, Irvine.

Novaco, R. W. (1976b). Treatment of chronic anger through cognitive and relaxation controls. *Journal of Consulting and Clinical Psychology, 44,* 681.

Novaco, R. W. (1977a). A stress inoculation approach to anger management in the training of law enforcement officers. *American Journal of Community Psychology, 5,* 327–346.

Novaco, R. W. (1977b). Stress inoculation: A cognitive therapy for anger and its application to a case of depression. *Journal of Consulting and Clinical Psychology, 45,* 600–608.

O'Donnell, C. R., & Worell, L. (1973). Motor and cognitive relaxation in the desensitization of anger. *Behaviour Research and Therapy, 11,* 473–481.

Ollendick, T. H., & Matson, J. L. (1978). Overcorrection: An overview. *Behavior Therapy, 9,* 830–842.

Osgood, C. E., Suci, G. J., & Tannenbaum, P. H. (1957). *Measurement of meaning.* Urbana: University of Illinois Press.

Patterson, G. R., Ray, R. S., Shaw, D. A., & Cobb, T. A. (1969). *A manual for coding of family interaction.* New York: Microfiche Publications.

Rahaim, S., Lefebvre, C., & Jenkins, J. O. (1980). The effects of social skills training on behavioral and cognitive components of anger management. *Journal of Behavior Therapy and Experimental Psychiatry, 11,* 308.

Reid, J. B., Taplin, P. S., & Lorber, R. A. (1981). A social interactional approach to the treatment of abusive families. In R. Stuart (Ed.), *Violent behavior: Social learning approaches to prediction, management, and treatment.* New York: Brunner/Mazel.

Rimm, D. C., & Masters, J. C. (1974). *Behavior therapy: Techniques and empirical findings.* New York: Academic Press.

Rimm, D. C., de Groot, J. C., Boord, P., Herman, J., & Dillow, P. V. (1971). Systematic desensitization of an anger response. *Behaviour Research and Therapy, 9,* 273–280.

Rimm, D. C., Hill, G. A., Brown, N. N., & Stuart, J. E. (1974). Group-assertiveness training in treatment of expression of inappropriate anger. *Psychological Reports, 34,* 791–798.

Russell, D. E. H., & Miller, D. L. (1979). *The prevalence of rape and sexual assault.* (Final Rep. NIMH Grant RO1-MH-28960.)

Saunders, R. W. (1978). Systematic desensitization in the treatment of child abuse. *American Journal of Psychiatry, 135,* 483–484.

Sandler, J., Van Dercar, C., & Milhoan, M. (1978). Training of child abusers in the use of positive reinforcement practices. *Behaviour Research and Therapy, 16,* 169–175.

Siegel, S. (1956). *Nonparametric statistics for the behavioral sciences.* New York: McGraw-Hill.

Smith, R. E. (1973). The use of humor in the counterconditioning of anger responses: A case study. *Behavior Therapy, 4,* 576–580.

Steinmetz, S. K. (1977). *The cycle of violence: Assertive, aggressive, and abusive family interaction.* New York: Praeger.

Sumner, J. G., Meuser, S. T., Hsu, L., & Morales, R. G. (1974). Overcorrection treatment for radical reduction of aggressive-disruptive behavior in institutionalized mental patients. *Psychological Reports, 35,* 655–662.

Taplin, P. S., & Reid, J. B. (1973). Effects of instructional set and experimenter influence on observer reliability. *Child Development, 44,* 547–554.

Toch, H. (1969). *Violent men.* Chicago: Aldine.

Turner, S. M., Hersen, M., & Bellack, A. S. (1978). Social skills training to teach prosocial behaviors in an organically impaired and retarded patient. *Journal of Behavior Therapy and Experimental Psychiatry, 9,* 253–258.

Von Benken, E. A. (1977). Clinical reduction of anger and aggression by systematic desensitization: The relation of anger to fear (Doctoral dissertation, University of Cincinnati, 1977). *Dissertation Abstracts International, 38,* 2388B–2389B. (University Microfilms No. 77-23, 079)

Warren, R., & Kurleycheck, R. (1981). Treatment of maladaptive anger and aggression: Catharsis vs. behavior therapy. *Corrective and Social Psychiatry, 27,* 135–137.

Webster, D. R., & Azrin, N. H. (1973). Required relaxation: A method of inhibiting agitative-disruptive behavior of retardates. *Behaviour Research and Therapy, 11,* 67–78.

Winkler, R. C. (1970). Management of chronic psychiatric patients by a token reinforcement system. *Journal of Applied Behavior Analysis, 3,* 47–55.

Zaks, M. S., & Walters, R. H. (1959). First steps in the construction of a scale for the measurement of aggression. *Journal of Psychology, 47,* 199–208.

Zelin, M. L., Alder, G., & Myerson, P. G. (1972). Anger self-report: An objective questionnaire for the measurement of aggression. *Journal of Consulting and Clinical Psychology, 39,* 340.

23

Sexual Deviation

JACK S. ANNON AND CRAIG H. ROBINSON

Introduction

There are few, if any, areas of human behavior in American culture that can generate as much concern, controversy, and confusion as that of sexual deviation. It should be emphasized here at the outset that the cultural context is an important factor in that many behaviors that are labeled *deviant* in the United States would not be so labeled if they occurred in other countries. What further adds to the confusion is that there is virtually no agreed upon criteria as to what constitutes *deviant*. For example, statistical definitions would simply look at the various frequencies of human sexual behaviors and then make mention of how far the behavior falls from the norm. Legal definitions, which tend to vary considerably from one state to the other, focus on the behavior if it falls outside the boundaries of the law, and the frequency of occurrence would have little relationship to this definition. Psychiatric definitions tend to be related to the theoretical perspectives of the individual defining *deviant,* and would have little apparent relationship to statistical or legal ones. There also tend to be social definitions of deviant behavior, and even within the same country (i.e., United States) there can be significant variability from one social milieu to the next as to what constitutes deviant sexual behavior. In this chapter, we will not try to define the term *deviant,* as it is assumed that the vast majority of readers would agree that the behavior of the rapist and attempted murderer we have chosen as a treatment example would be considered as deviant. For purposes of clarifying the reasons for various treatment decisions

JACK S. ANNON and CRAIG H. ROBINSON • The Royal Queen Emma, Suite 604, 222 South Vineyard Street, Honolulu, Hawaii 96813.

discussed later, some attention should be given to how we tend to conceptualize and categorize sexual behaviors commonly referred to as deviant.

Classification

There are a number of classification systems that have been proposed by behaviorally oriented clinicians (Eysenck & Rachman, 1965; Lester, 1975; Staats & Staats, 1963). Although each has certain advantages and disadvantages, human sexual behavior does not categorize easily. Ullmann and Krasner (1975) note that one possible reason for the difficulty in categorizing behavior is that the same act may be performed for different reasons, due to different antecedent conditioning. They further note that because the same person typically engages in a variety of behaviors, it is very difficult to place a given behavior in mutually exclusive categories. Also, as soon as a behavioral pattern is labeled, the emotional connotation associated with the label further confuses the picture. Annon and Robinson (1980a) have discussed at length the difficulties associated with labeling a person's sexual behavior, not the least of which is that labeling sexual problems or behaviors does not dictate treatment. They have referenced over a hundred labels for what are commonly assumed to be possible sexual disorders. The authors' ROBI description–classification scheme (response, object, behavior, and identity) is presented in detail elsewhere (Annon & Robinson, 1980a) and will only be briefly mentioned here.

Most sexual problems we are aware of seem to fall within one of the four categories noted before. The category *response* includes all of the problems that are commonly referred to as dysfunctions with sexual response, such as desire, arousal, and orgasm concerns. Problems involving sexual response usually are experienced as problems by an individual and his or her partner, and concerns in this area would not typically be labeled as *deviant.*

The second category is *object* or *object choice,* and it refers to animate or inanimate objects that an individual interacts with in some sexual manner. Problems in this area may be viewed differently by various segments of a given society or culture. However, it is not the behavior *per se* that the individual does that leads to problems as much as the issue of with whom or what they do it that leads to societal and/or legal sanctions. For example, animate object choice would be an adult who sexually fondles children or animals; and inanimate object choice would involve objects such as leather, shoes, feces, and so forth.

The third category, *behavior,* refers to the type of sexual behaviors that an individual engages in for the purpose of facilitating or generating sexual arousal. In this category the concern is not so much with whom or what the individual interacts but rather the *way* the person goes about interacting with the "object" for purposes of sexual gratification. The sexual aggressiveness displayed by the rapist would fall in this category, as would sexually touching strangers, or a person's exhibiting himself or herself. The fourth category involves problems of sexual *identity,* such as gender and body image, and will not be dealt with further here. How this type of categorization system relates to various treatment options will be clarified later.

Although assessment for the purpose of treatment of sexual deviations has been going on for many years, it is our firm opinion that the prognosis for lasting behavior change will probably depend upon the type of therapy that the person enters into. For example, one approach to treatment is the *indirect* or *dynamic* viewpoint, which defines such behavior as "symptomatic" of possible or assumed underlying conflicts. Therapy is aimed at attempts to provide the person with insight into these conflicts, with the hope that this will then resolve the symptomatic behavior. Although these approaches are occasionally successful, they are not generally effective and are gradually being supplemented by more *direct* approaches, such as those based upon a *psychological learning model.* This viewpoint holds that, in the absence of endocrinological or genetic abnormalities, the person is only sexual, and the direction of this biologically based potential is determined mainly by learning and cultural influences. In other words, the person's behavior is viewed as the result of learned behaviors that follow the general psychological principles of learning.

From this view it follows that the extinction or change of such behavior may be achieved by the direct application of appropriate procedures derived from such learning principles. Although there is no guarantee of success for either approach, there is much accumulating evidence that a direct approach has a higher probability of leading to more change in the problem behavior of concern.

The learning approach to assessment and therapy derives its theoretical constructs from psychological learning theory and bases its therapeutic procedures on experimentally established principles of learning. The basic assumption underlying this system is that "neurotic" or other maladaptive behaviors are acquired or *learned,* and therefore are as subject to the normal laws of learning as are "non-neurotic," adapative behaviors.

Learning is defined in a broad sense as a relatively permanent change in behavior that occurs as a result of experience, and excludes any behavior that results from direct intervention in the functioning of the nervous system or for maturation. In its early formulations, *behavior* referred only to overt behavior that could be observed and/or measured by another. Today, many learning-oriented clinicians have moved away from what is seen by them as a limitation in working exclusively with overt behaviors and now deal with covert behaviors such as cognitions and feelings as well. It is typically assumed that these behaviors all follow the same basic principles of learning.

Experience is generally defined as behavior that is acquired or changed by one and/or two, and/or possibly three methods. Each method is generally assumed to be based on what is called a basic learning principle. One principle is *classical conditioning,* first formulated by Ivan Pavlov who demonstrated the ringing of a bell immediately followed by the presentation of meat could eventually result in a dog salivating to the sound of the bell alone. This type of conditioning is seen as involuntary, and it has been demonstrated that many human emotional and sexual responses are acquired through such learning (this point has particular relevance for the sexual arousal conditioning that appears to take place with most sexual offenders).

The second basic principle is *operant conditioning,* most clearly described by B. F. Skinner who demonstrated that when an animal demonstrating a certain random voluntary behavior was consistently and immediately rewarded with a food pellet, the animal's demonstrations of that behavior increased accordingly. For some time these two principles were applied only in the animal laboratory; many theoretical questions were asked and empirically answered.

Gradually it was found that both these principles appeared to apply equally to human learning as well. The amassed body of data on learning theory was then re-examined in relation to human behavior. Through the use of the experimental methods of science it soon became apparent that psychological learning theory was directly relevant to human behavior. The clinical treatment of complex human problems through the application of appropriate learning based procedures was thus begun.

Many consider a third principle of learning to be the process of *vicarious learning.* This is a broad term that covers any learning process whereby the person changes or acquires a behavior as a result of observing the behavior of another person, either directly, or through the use of films, videotapes, or the reading of books or magazines.

As may be seen from a reading of the other chapters in this book, there are now numerous therapeutic assessment and treatment procedures based upon psychological learning principles, and some of these procedures have considerable empirical evidence as to their efficacy, whereas others are of too recent origin to have accumulated such experimental verification.

Initially, learning principles were used after the fact to explain various processes used in other therapy systems. However, this transition stage then gave way to the prior use of learning concepts in assessment and treatment, and the systematic application of these concepts to achieve a particular behavior goal selected at the start of treatment. In earlier days some felt that a learning approach was effective only with clearly defined problems such as unitary phobias (even though prior to a learning approach, phobias were widely known as difficult to treat from within any other orientation). However, in recent years the psychological learning approach has been greatly expanded and although there are many areas that need to be explored and researched, much information now exists showing the successful extension of learning principles to the treatment of a wide range of complex human problems.

More directly relevant to the assessment and treatment of sexual deviations, these learning principles have also been applied in this area as well (e.g., the work of the present authors in the late 1960s and early 1970s) (see Annon, 1971a, 1971b, 1972; Robinson, 1974, 1975). Pioneers in this area, such as Abel, Barlow, Blanchard, and Guild (1975), have also pointed out that treatment for people such as rapists has typically not been available, and in the few programs that do exist, it has been lengthy, lasting at least 2 years. Also, recidivism rates after simple incarceration are alarmingly high (e.g., 35% depending upon the program and length of follow-up). Part of the difficulty results from the past lack of objective measures of a person's "urge" to approach children sexually, to rape, or exhibit, or secretly view others, and so forth, and thus evaluation of such people has traditionally rested with the subjective clinical impressions of therapists.

As Abel and his associates have long pointed out, the measurement of a person's sexual arousal has awaited the development of a physiologic measure specific for sexual arousal, a stimulus specific to the sexual behavior of concern to present to such persons while measuring their arousal and an experimental design that would tease out the different components of the person's sexual arousal pattern.

Since the mid-1970s a number of clinicians and laboratories have begun to evaluate the arousal patterns of such persons by the use of the penile transducer. This technique involves the male's wearing a small circumferential penile transducer while being presented with a variety of sexual materials. These stimuli may be presented by videotaped or filmed scenes, by asking the person to fantasize sexual scenes or to listen to audiotaped descriptions of sexual scenes. During any one presentation, the person's degree of erection response to the sexual material can be calibrated as a percentage of his full erection. It has been found that this calibration is the most accurate measure because this is the only physiologic variable in males that occurs exclusively during sexual arousal and not through other emotional states.

For females, a photoplethysmographic vaginal probe has also been developed that serves as a photoelectric transducer for measuring the changes in the optical density of vaginal walls. Increased relative pulse pressure and increased pooling of blood in the vagina thus become a means for recording changes in sexual arousal while being presented with different sexual materials.

With the development of measurement studies with cooperative patients, we can currently separate rapists from nonrapists on the basis of their penile responses to rape versus nonrape cues (e.g., see Abel & Blanchard, 1976). Because this measurement capability is now available, it becomes more appropriate to treat this group of people who formerly were excluded from traditional therapy.

Abel, internationally recognized as a leader in this field, along with his coworkers (Abel, Barlow, Blanchard, & Mavissakalian, 1974), has also found that audiotaped descriptions of sexual activities are more useful than slides or movies for generating arousal to individualized complex sexual stimuli such as in the case of rape, or child molestation, or exhibiting, or viewing.

However, this method of measurement is not completely free of distortion because, by control of attention and fantasies, the person being measured is able to gain some degree of control over his sexual arousal to the stimuli presented. Therefore, measurements to determine the erotic aspects of a person's arousal must include instructions that he become as aroused as possible to some stimuli, whereas at other times he is instructed to suppress his sexual arousal by any mental means. By varying these instructional sets, it is possible to determine not only the extent to which the person becomes aroused to various stimuli but also his ability to suppress his arousal in an attempt to falsify the objective recording of his erection response. The mean difference between his arousal under these two conditions is an objective measure of his ability to inhibit sexual arousal. A large body of research now exists regarding the physiologic diagnosis of the sexual offender, and such research has shown that the offender is apparently able to maintain arousal to, say, "rape" cues months to years after the actual offense, and such an "internal" response may then eventually elicit "overt" behavior. Once such a response is learned, probably through classical conditioning, the response will be maintained until a new response is learned in its place through similar principles, such as masturbatory conditioning (see Annon, 1971a, 1973d).

For example, we were asked to provide an assessment and treatment program for an institutionalized sex offender who had been convicted of multiple rapes. This offender's life history illustrated how such arousal responses may be learned. The offender had begun masturbating in his early teens with random fantasies. At some point, he randomly thought of his mother and the satisfaction he would feel if he could dominate her for a change and tie her up. He incorporated such a fantasy into his masturbation. Also at this time, he came across a photo of a popular actress, and to enhance the sexual arousal of the photo he drew ropes binding her. Up to his late teens, these were his main fantasies during masturbation, offering many trials of a "classical conditioning" nature (so that the thought or sight of such binding or force "involuntarily" elicited arousal feelings due to the conditioning). In his late teens he began to interact with girls, and his fantasies changed to intercourse. However, at age 25 or 26, when separated from his wife, he began to have fantasies again of girls being bound and during masturbation would imagine forcedly taking their clothes off. He subsequently engaged in his first actual rape. Here, operant principles come into play. There were no immediate negative consequences to this behavior. He continued to use such a fantasy with masturbation, and he continued to bind and rape women, which also provided fresh fantasy material for masturbation. The continued interplay of masturbation fantasy and no adverse consequences to his overt actions of rape eventually ended with his capture, conviction, and institutionalization. At the time of completion of our initial assessment, the offender was continuing to masturbate daily to such fantasies; and even though he had been incarcerated over 2 years, he still showed almost three times more arousal to aggressive rape cues than to mutually consenting sexual cues. It was our prediction that regardless of the time that he continued to spend in general milieu treatment and group therapy, if he were to be released in the future he would most probably start to rape again even though he "cognitively" did not wish to or intend to do so. A more detailed description of this particular person's assessment and treatment may be found under the case study section.

Support for our findings is also supplied by Quinsey (personal communication, 1982), who reports about a child molester who had been institutionalized for 10 years and who had received 5 years of traditional group therapy, yet still showed a 98% mean erection to fantasies of sexual contact with children.

Finally, even stronger support for this viewpoint is supplied by Abel *et al.* (1975), who have written about a patient who had forced himself on a 3-year-old child 23 years prior to his evaluation by them. Since his arrest, all but 1 year had been spent in psychiatric hospitals, and he denied actual contact with children prior to his evaluation. In spite of this lack of contact, he maintained a 98% mean erection to descriptions of mutually enjoyable sex with a child, and a 65% mean erection to descriptions of raping a child.

All this data strongly suggests that a subject's simple removal from society without specific treatment for arousal to such cues does not significantly affect arousal to these stimuli, even after months or years of incarceration.

The usual approach to measuring arousal is to take the relative arousal of a person, say to "rape" or "child" stimuli, and divide the measure by the person's arousal to mutually consenting adult stimuli. This then becomes an *index* for diagnosing a rapist or one who sexually approaches children, and so forth. Abel proposes that with rape cues an index of .8 or less is to be considered normal, whereas an index of .9 or higher may be considered that of a rapist. This index then not only becomes an objective measure for diagnosis but also serves as a means for testing the effectiveness of various forms of therapy; and, most importantly, it may also become an objective measure to predict future behavior.

For example, Quinsey and his associates (Quinsey, Chaplin, & Carrigan, 1980) have reported the indexes of 30 child molesters who were tested in prison, subsequently released, and then followed up an average of 2 years later. Twenty-four of them did not recommit child molestation, and the mean of their indexes was 0.5. Six others did recommit child molestation, and their mean indexes prior to release (but following treatment) was 1.81, which is a significant difference between the two. This indicates that it may be possible to predict those offenders with the highest likelihood of recommission of their acts in spite of their having received treatment. Research into this prediction area is just beginning, but for the first time it looks as if we may now have some objective data upon which to base predictions instead of the usual subjective impression of the therapist.

It should also be kept in mind that learning a new response to inappropriate sexual stimuli is only one aspect of an overall treatment program. These programs have many components designed to effect cognitive, emotional, and overt behavioral changes, including the possible generation or development of mutually consenting heterosexual arousal, the learning of cognitive controls to prevent overt behavior chains and increase impulse control, the development of heterosocial skills, vocational planning as well as other areas. Hartung (1983) has conducted a comprehensive review of the literature on the treatment of sex offenders, and he also has pointed out that such offenders commonly present with problems in seven specific areas: aggressiveness, drug use, inappropriate sexual arousal, relationship self-esteem, sociosexual skills, sensitivity to others, and appropriate sexual arousal. He hypothesizes that effective treatment for each area assessed as problematic will prevent sexual recidivism. He also advises three special conditions as required for effective treatment; namely mandatory attendance for involuntary patients, an empathic treatment atmosphere, and provision for external means to monitor and maintain new behavior during and following treatment, such as family, spouse, group, and the like.

We concur with Hartung's findings, and we also believe that it is important in the initial assessment for the therapist to consider these problem areas from within three areas of functioning (i.e., cognitive, affective, and behavioral) and not to stress only one, or, one over the other, but to consider each in turn and their possible interaction.

For example, one important area is certainly the affective, and analysis could suggest which behaviors offer the highest degree of arousal at present and which is appropriate or not appropriate to future behavior in a legally acceptable manner. On the other hand, cognitive controls can also be utilized as well as behavioral training in heterosocial areas. Initial analysis, such as that described by Annon (1971a, 1973d, 1975a), should offer a plan for the simultaneous consideration of the full range of circumstances that might be related to the person's behavior, allow for the ordering of priorities for intervention, provide guidance for the timing of multiple interventions, and foster the development of appropriate procedures based upon theoretical analysis.

Individualized Assessment

With the intention of offering a possible psychological-learning-based model for the assessment and treatment of sexual deviations, we will now briefly describe our individualized approach to such assessment and treatment.

In the initial assessment, we utilize a wide range of assessment materials and procedures, including clinical interviews; interviews with spouse, family, relatives, and victims, as appropriate; past public and private records; police reports; previous test results; forms; inventories; tests; films; slides; audiotapes; objective arousal measurement; self-monitoring records; and so forth. This evaluation of the individuals' personal knowledge, feelings, and skills not only pertains to their understanding of themselves and their behavior but to their gender role area, the social-interpersonal area and the educational-vocational area as well.

Initial assessment usually begins with the administration of a battery of forms, inventories, and tests that the person individually fills out. These are then carefully studied, scored, analyzed, and finally discussed with the person privately. Typically, assessment may begin with the administration of the Life History Questionnaire (Annon, 1973c) and the Behavior Assessment Form (Annon, 1973a). To assess what is negative for the person and to develop situations for possible use in covert and/or overt conditioning, the Composite Fear Inventory (Annon, 1973b) is used. The Reinforcement Survey Schedule (Cautela & Kastenbaum, 1967) is similarly used to delineate the positives in the individual's life and to also provide material for possible covert and overt conditioning procedures.

In the social/interpersonal area, the self-report Social Performance Survey schedule (Lowe & Cautela, 1978) is used to screen for behaviors that comprise the person's social performance. In addition, the Heterosocial Skills Behavior Checklist for Males (Barlow, Abel, Blanchard, Bristow, & Young, 1977) may also be used to ascertain the person's overt interpersonal social performance in three areas: voice (loudness, pitch, inflection), form of conversation (initiation, follow-up, flow, interest), and affect (facial, eye contact, laughter).

In the sexual area, the person's fears and pleasures are assessed by use of the

Sexual Fear Inventory (Annon, 1975b) and the Sexual Pleasure Inventory (Annon, 1975d). This information usually offers cues and situations where possible attitudinal changes may be helpful in order to lead to mutually satisfactory adult sexual behavior that is not in violation of the law. If the person has, or had, a partner, then sexual attitudes concerning sexual behaviors with his or her partner are assessed by use of the Heterosexual Attitude Scale (Robinson & Annon, 1975a), whereas the presence and frequency of actual sexual behaviors with a partner are assessed by use of the Heterosexual Behavior Inventory (Robinson & Annon, 1975b). The person's knowledge of sexual anatomy, function, and vocabulary is tested by use of the Sex Knowledge Inventory, Form Y (McHugh, 1976), whereas broad sexual knowledge in general is tested by use of the Sex Knowledge Inventory, Form X (McHugh, 1979). Finally, an extended sexual history is obtained by clinical interview within the framework provided by the Sexual History Form (Annon, 1975c).

The final important area of initial assessment focus is directed to the person's sexual arousal response to various stimuli that have the potential of eliciting unwanted and/or illegal overt behaviors. Baseline data are collected by use of a penile tumescence monitor of the person's sexual responses to audiotaped descriptions of sexual behavior created from the assessment material. These data cover mutually consenting sexual relationships and the behavior of concern (e.g., exhibiting, viewing, rubbing, rape, child molestation behaviors, etc.; see Annon & Robinson, 1980a, for the wide range of behaviors that may be of concern here). The data gathered then may be used in four ways.

First, an attempt is made to clarify the most erotic cues that elicit arousal responses so as not to rely entirely on what the person may report verbally as most arousing (often people themselves do not fully realize exactly what the specific cues are to which they are responding). For example, people who exhibit themselves often do so from automobiles; noting arousal responses to descriptions of their entry into their cars is quite common. If this is not taken into account when designing a treatment program, they may find themselves experiencing unexplained "urges" every time they enter their car. Additionally, similar patterns have been noted in rapists who use cars in a systematic pattern connected with their rape behavior, such as in the case study to be described. Most often, these persons have no awareness of such responses. The data can be carefully reviewed for such cues, and, from them, subsequent tapes may be created emphasizing these cues in greater detail. Content not associated with increasing erection can be eliminated. This second generation of tapes is usually found to produce even greater arousal responses than the original set (see Abel & Blanchard, 1976).

Second, these measurements may uncover, or discover, unacknowledged or unknown arousal responses to unwanted or illegal behaviors not obtained by any other assessment material. For example, one of us recently assessed a person seeking assistance for exhibiting behaviors. He had never been arrested for such behaviors and said that he very much wanted to "get the behavior under control" before he was arrested. In the process of assessment, he listened to taped descriptions of rape behavior along with exhibiting behaviors, and not only did he attain Exhibition Indices of .98 and .81 but he also showed Rape Indices of .83 and .91, even though he never admitted to such behaviors or that he was aware of his arousal to such behaviors. This aspect of arousal was also incorporated into the overall treatment program as well. Had it not been, it is possible that this person might slowly approximate himself into such overt behaviors and move from exhibiting to rape— even though most people who exhibit themselves typically stay within that behavior pattern.

Another example is a case in which both authors were involved. The patient had a long history of exhibiting behavior and arrests and was referred by his attorney and the court for a comprehensive assessment and treatment program outline. In the process of assessing his responses to his exhibiting behaviors to young children, he was also assessed on his arousal responses to child molestation behaviors. Although he showed an Exhibiting Index of 1.1, he also showed a Child Molestation Index of 1.4, again indicating the possibility that this behavior could extend beyond the presenting behavior of interest.

Third, the tapes can also be used as assessment probes during treatment, to see what effect various interventions are having. Finally, the tapes can be used to obtain pre- and posttreatment indexes of the person's response for possible prediction purposes for the future (see Quinsey *et al.,* 1980).

In addition to these individualized tapes, we have also entered into a mutual clinical research exchange project with Abel and his colleagues who have derived a complete set of 2 minute standardized audiotape assessment tapes of adult rape and child molestation cues. These tapes also contrast mutually consenting adult sexual relationships with varying adult and/or child sexual relationships employing verbal coercion or physical coercion of varying degrees. These tapes may also be used either in initial assessment or as measures of generalization of effects of treatment.

Based on the initial data collected, an individualized treatment program is then carefully formulated (see Annon, 1971a, 1975a, for the use of various forms, inventories, and other data analysis to create such treatment programs). Treatment is usually then focused on interventions in the three major areas of functioning (the cognitive-thinking area, the affective-emotional area, and the overt-behavioral area), which have been mentioned previously.

Treatment Procedures and Techniques

It is our strong opinion that it is very important for the person to be fully informed of the rationale for the given treatment program and what is intended at each point. Particularly stressed is the importance of individuals' own responsibility for their behaviors and that there will be no "magical" thing "done" to them that would ensure lasting change—only the increased probability of lasting change as they assume more and more control of their behavior. This means that they must be aware of what they have learned and how they have learned in the past so that they can then recognize and learn to use alternative methods open to them. As mentioned before, there are no guarantees of success. However, with objective measurement and the use of coordinated selected interventions, it is our firm belief that the prognosis for lasting behavior change has a much higher probability of being achieved than under the typical *indirect* treatment program, one that is standardized for all persons, or simple time-limited institutionalization alone.

Cognitive-Thinking Phase

This phase usually involves going over the information gathered with the person, offering possible explanations of how the person might have acquired behavior patterns through the principles of learning, and providing specific examples from the person's past, pointing out how the principles seem to apply.

The person is then instructed on how behavior chains are learned. For example, this means breaking down a behavior sequence of concern (exhibiting, rape, child molestation, etc.) into units such as those proposed by Marshall (1973): thinking about engaging in the behavior; preparation prior to engaging in the behavior; approaching the person; commencing the behavior; engaging in the behavior itself; completion of the behavior; and subsequent thoughts, feelings, and actions after completing the behavior. Awareness of these chains and what elicits them is the first step in gaining some control over the behavior. Then, cognitive methods of interventions can be learned to break such sequences: for example, *thought stopping* and *impulse control procedures*. Finally, alternative procedures such as *redirection of attention* and *chain breaking* may be taught.

Another important area here is the person's information and skills in the heterosexual and heterosocial areas. Based on the original research in the use of vicarious learning in the treatment of sexual problems conducted by one of us (Robinson, 1974, 1975a, 1975b, 1976, 1977), we have subsequently demonstrated that a wide range of social and sexual behaviors can be appropriately learned through the use of such modeling and vicarious learning principles (see Annon & Robinson, 1978, 1981b, 1981d). The patient may be given directly relevant books, pamphlets, and brochures to read (e.g., in the sexual area in response to low scores obtained on the sexual knowledge inventories; in assertiveness training, in response to data obtained on the social performance assessment devices, etc.), or slides, films, and videotapes specifically designed for the individual's particular concern (see Annon & Robinson, 1980a, 1981b, 1981d).

The patient may also be further supplied with methods for short- and long-range goal setting and for setting current and future priorities. Vocational assessment and possible assistance are also provided. Some persons may also be taught a number of cognitive procedures to counteract possible depressive episodes that are often present in this population at this time (e.g., increasing positive thoughts, avoidance control of negative word usage, etc.). Finally, patients may be started in learning communication skills to assist them in being more direct and open with spouses, or friends—instead of the usual case where persons tell no one of their behavior of concern and often attempt to stop their behaviors by themselves with ineffective methods.

Affective-Emotional Area

Often the first focus in this area is directed toward assisting the patients in becoming aware of the distinction between thinking and feelings; learning to recognize and label their own emotions; and eventually learning to express these feelings to others (recognizing choice and appropriateness, of course)—all in relation to their past behaviors as well as their current behaviors.

One of the most important areas of focus here is the person's sexual arousal responses to various stimuli that have the potential of eliciting unwanted and/or overt behaviors. Masturbatory conditioning (see Annon, 1973d, 1975a) is often used at this stage in the hope of building up arousal to mutually cooperative adult cues and fantasies and to stop reinforcement of the unwanted fantasies that may lead to the behavior of concern.

Systematic desensitization or *overt desensitization* may also be used with some persons who show negative feelings connected with the very behaviors that they wish to learn. An example might be a molester of small girls who has strong negative feelings connected with the pubic hair and full breasts of adult females (see Annon, 1971a, 1975a, for such a case and the treatment used).

Usually, after the acquisition of appropriate fantasy and arousal has been achieved, some form of covert or overt aversion therapy (see Abel & Blanchard, 1976; Annon, 1973d, 1975a; Marshall, 1973) or satiation therapy (see Abel & Annon, 1982; Marshall, 1979) and shaping of new responses (see Annon, 1973d, 1975a) may be instituted. Then objective tumescence monitoring is again carried out to see the relative effectiveness of such procedures.

The Overt-Behavioral Area

Based upon the assessment data, various assertive and heterosocial skills programs may be devised for the person. Attention is paid to how often positive social behaviors are performed as well as negative social behaviors are not being performed. Often volunteers from the community may be utilized at this point in assisting the patient in acquiring the particular skills that are lacking. Here also vicarious learning and modeling principles may again be used. Assistance in acquiring marketable job skills is also another major area of attention in this phase. For persons with partners, it is often important to see if communication skills training is appropriate to increase the probability of communication with significant others leading to maintaining or creating more meaningful relationships.

Quite often there may also be a lack of mutually satisfying sexual interaction with a partner, either due to lack of knowledge, skills, or some emotional difficulties. However, there are now numerous interventions that can be made to improve the person's sexual satisfaction in these areas (see Annon, 1976a, 1976b, 1981; Annon & Robinson, 1980a, 1980b, 1981a, 1981c). Throughout treatment, contin-

ual tumescence probe measurement is important to assess the functional relation- 643
ships of the various therapeutic interventions.

SEXUAL DEVIATION

Problems and Limitations in Assessment and Treatment

There are inherent difficulties with some of the assessment materials that then contribute toward the ineffectiveness of some of the treatment procedures. For example, all forms and inventories are self-reporting devices, and if the person chooses to withhold factual information, the forms and inventories will not pick it up. An example encountered by us was a military person who had been accused of numerous counts of child molestation off base. The person was a mature and well-respected enlisted man who was about to retire and who had achieved a very respected and successful military career up to that point. He denied the allegations emphatically and agreed to be examined by any professional person selected by his or the opposing lawyers. He also underwent a polygraph examination that was equivocal and could not be scored. He then saw two psychologists and three psychiatrists, and they all concluded that he might best fit the category of *Schizoid Personality Disorder,* but that there was *no* foundation for the charges against him.

Finally, as a last buttress to his defense, he was referred for a final comprehensive assessment by us. Robinson conducted a detailed assessment utilizing all of the previous military and medical records, reports, and his responses to the complete battery assessment described previously. Robinson came to basically the same conclusion as had the previous professionals, and the patient was then transferred to Annon for an assessment of his arousal patterns to adults and children. It was assumed that the resulting data would be the final clinching argument in support of his defense.

The patient's response under the aroused instructions to manual stimulation of an adult female's genitals was 29% of his full erection, as compared to a 51% of his full erection for similar child interaction. Under these conditions, he experienced a Pedophile Index of 1.78. When comparing his response to engaging in penile-vaginal intercourse with an adult female, he experienced 40% of his full erection as compared to 99% of his full erection when listening to tape descriptions of engaging in vaginal intercourse with a child. The index for this comparison was 2.47. Combining the data under all aroused conditions we came up with a final mean index of 2.18.

Under suppressed instructions as outlined previously, the patient's responses in one condition to adult interaction was 49% compared to interaction with a child of 39%, giving a mean index of only .79. However, in the other condition, his arousal response to adult interaction was 29% of an erection compared to 51% erection leading to an index of 1.58, with an overall mean index for both suppressed conditions of 1.05. This data indicated definite arousal response to child cues even though the patient *verbally reported* little arousal to most of the tapes.

Based on the results of the arousal measurement, the patient was then shown the data, and after some preliminary attempts at deception he finally confessed to a long-standing pattern of behavior with children throughout his career. Based on the data gathered by us, the defense changed its plea, and we testified to our findings at his trial. The person is now receiving treatment along the outlines provided by the assessment done by us.

Both of us have had experiences where clients have been able to deceive us and to continue their behaviors without change. As a result, both of us will now no longer work with referred "volunteers" unless they are willing to also undergo arousal assessment. On the other hand, of course, there are questions about the generalization of responses assessed on the arousal measurement cues and just what can be predicted, but, at the present time that is the state of the art. It certainly does provide leads that can then be more systematically followed for further elaboration.

Of course, at this time we can also not predict which therapeutic technique will work best for which person with what particular behavior of concern. For example, we have used a *covert conditioning* procedure with one person that had no effect whatsoever (see following case study), whereas with many others the procedure has been highly effective. In another case *satiation therapy* was found to be highly effective, whereas it failed completely on another. At best, we select procedures that appear to offer the most promise based on a careful integrated treatment program as outlined previously. Although we have had considerable overall success when following the procedures, we have also had our failures. It is hoped that by reporting our procedures in detail in this chapter that researchers and other clinicians might experimentally approach the many variables that we struggle with in our daily clinical practices. To this end we next turn to a case study.

Case Study

In 1975, Joe was arrested and charged with sexually related attacks against several women. After his arrest, a court-appointed panel of three psychiatrists recommended that Joe be conditionally released, concluding that he was suffering from a "compulsive neurosis." Because he would receive treatment, he was considered unlikely to be a danger to himself or to others. Two years later in 1977, while continuing outpatient psychotherapy because of the past rape incidents, Joe raped and stabbed a 13-year-old girl. The attempted murder occurred while the girl was trying to resist the rape. By 1979, Joe had been acquitted of attempted murder and rape by reason of insanity and committed to the state hospital. Interestingly, a second commission involving three different psychiatrists seemed in basic agreement with the original commission, diagnostically; however, they now found him to be extremely dangerous to other persons.

After he was committed to the hospital for the criminally insane, we were asked to assess and treat Joe if possible. The assessment period and various treatment strategies employed in this case are perhaps more than might typically be required. However, the methods described here may at least provide the reader with an idea of some of the options available in working with deviant sexual behavior.

The assessment alone in this case took slightly over 6 months and involved a wide range of materials and procedures. There were numerous clinical interviews, forms, inventories, and tests as well as discussions with staff personnel at the state hospital, studies of past records and test results, films, audiotapes, objective arousal measurement, and Joe's own self-monitoring of certain feelings and behaviors. The assessment covered such broad categories as his knowledge, feelings, and skills regarding the social and interpersonal areas, the sexual area, and the educational/vocational areas. We were particularly concerned regarding Joe's repertoire of heterosocial skills (i.e., assertiveness, voice, affect, content of talk, eye contact). Regarding heterosexual skills, concentration centerd on his knowledge, his verbal and behavioral repertoire, and his physiological responses of arousal to consenting, coercive, and aggressive sexual contact. Space limitations here obviously preclude a detailed developmental history of the many complex and intricate dynamics that probably set the stage for Joe's criminal behavior. However, some of the issues from his sexual history that were considered important in helping to formulate a treatment strategy are noted in the sample of excerpts presented later.

During the first interview with Joe, the focus of attention was on establishing rapport and outlining groundrules on such issues as confidentiality, fees, scheduling, and so forth. The major focus next centered on obtaining historical information from him. This part of the evaluation occurred over a 2-week period and involved approximately 6 hours. The first strategy was to have him describe pretty much in his own words the history of his presenting problem (i.e., his sexual aggressiveness). After obtaining these data, we spent time taking a detailed sexual history that involved information as to his early sexual thoughts, feelings, and behaviors, many of which did not necessarily have any apparent direct relationship to the behavior for which he was being treated.

Joe was a very bright, articulate individual whose memory for long- and short-term events seemed excellent. His creditability was considered to be very high, especially because checks were made on some of what he related through other sources such as police records, family, other reports, and the like. It is also worthy to note that because he had already been acquitted and committed "indefinitely," he had no particular reason to think that portraying himself in a positive manner could have any effect on his current situation.

The following samples of transcripts from sessions with him cannot possibly convey many of the important cues that influenced us (and other therapists). For example, the therapists were both repeatedly struck by the very subtle cues Joe put out to suggest "lack of affect." Although he would say the "correct words" regarding how sorry he was and the tragedy it posed for the victims, one never quite got the sense that this was very sincere, though the therapists were continually hard-pressed to identify any specific behaviors that contributed to these feelings or impressions. His apparent lack of affect and the implications this had to treatment strategy will be discussed.

During our first session, the following exchange occurred:

T: Well, Joe, at this point it certainly appears that if we're going to have any chance of helping you move toward your goal, we're going to have to get a lot of very detailed information about many aspects of your life, especially those that relate to the kind of behavior that's gotten you into this kind of trouble.

J: Well, I'm certainly willing to tell you anything you want to know; I sure don't have anything to lose at this point.

T: Since we're going to have several opportunities to get together, today I'd just like to have you take me through the history of your rape activities. Joe, when I talk about rape, I'm referring to any of the things you've done sexually without your partner's consent. Whether it's someone that you knew or a prostitute that you picked up on the street.

J: Are you also talking about what happened when I was overseas in the military?

T: Yes, all incidents. Joe, what I really hope to get from you is information that would tell me about the kind of pattern you learned over a long period of time.

J: Do you want to know the very first time it happened?

T: Fine, Joe, let's start with that, and I'll just periodically ask questions if I want further details or I am unclear.

J: Okay—about 10 years ago while I was stationed overseas, it was towards the end of my tour. I'd been taking Dexedrine for quite some time, you know stuff I could get downtown. I was lonely and would every now and then have vague thoughts about grabbing a woman on the base. Then I started looking around the base for a good place. I started hanging around the airmen's club, kind of planning what I'd do and then I got a small pocket knife.

T: Joe, do you recall the kinds of sexual fantasies or daydreams you were having around this period of time?

J: Not particularly. I mean like I never had thoughts about wanting to hurt anyone. One night outside the enlisted men's club this WAVE came out—I'd been kind of loitering around and then I started walking ahead of her. I slowed down as I got to this drainage ditch; I suddenly turned around and punched her in the stomach. She dropped to her knees and started to yell so I grabbed her behind, dragged her ass, and then she whispered she couldn't breathe; I moved her down to the drainage ditch, turned her around and told her to take her clothes off. She just stood there and said nothing. I then told her to "do what I tell you or I'm going to hit you again." Then I hit her in the stomach and started yanking her dress down. I remember being "supercharged" though at this point not really sexually aroused. She was wearing a bra, panty hose, shoes, and as I pulled her clothes off she was just silent; then I pulled her to her feet and told her to kneel down and tied her hands with the panty hose. That's when I took my pants down, took off my shirt and rolled her on her back and spread her legs.

T: How aroused, sexually, were you at this point?

J: I had a hard on and was very excited. I tried to French kiss her but she refused, and then I tried to enter her but it was really difficult because of movements she was making. And then in about 5 seconds I came on her belly, never did make entry. There was some relief of tension but I was still very high. I tried to kiss her and she turned away, then I grabbed her head and said, "Do what I tell you"; she refused again. Then I was really mad and I banged her head on the cement several times. I rolled off of her. I was still breathing like I had run 2 miles and weak all over. She was unconscious but breathing. So, I put my clothes on. It's funny, it was raining when I went back to the barracks but it felt very refreshing. I just felt kind of exhilarated. It wasn't until I changed my clothes and laid down at the bed that I started to have some fears about the consequences, which is the first time that even entered my mind. The next day I overheard a discussion about this girl being found wandering around near the ditch suffering from concussion and amnesia, and the theory was that she'd been involved in black market activities and they figured someone just got to her. This is the first time anything like this had ever occurred and when I look back on it, it was the one that I was most excited by as compared to all the others later on.

T: Joe, please try to recall as much as you can about the kinds of sexual fantasies or daydreams you'd have following this incident. I mean like any thoughts or fantasies you'd have when you masturbated or to sexual-type daydreams, or night dreams.

J: It was about 3 months before I was discharged from the military and I didn't have any sex during that time; however, I masturbated a lot of times to thoughts about that incident. In fact, the most arousing part of the whole fantasy was seeing myself looking at the girl's breasts when she was on her back with her hands tied.

Later incidents were described by Joe in clear detail with a very similar behavioral pattern. Sometimes he would be very aggressive toward his victims, unpredictably punching them, and other times he would show unexplained "kindness" like driving the woman back to where he originally abducted her. The onset of an episode was typically perceived by some feelings that he could best describe as restless or a slight agitation, and he would go to his van for the purpose of cruising. He kept a knife beneath the seat, and a piece of rope was readily available. He seldom paid very close attention to the victim's physical characteristics and was much more alert to the person's availability. After he would get someone in the car, as soon as he was away from heavy traffic, he would pull the knife and order the victim down on the floor and tie her hands. He would then drive to some secluded spot and rape her. Some suggestions or hints as to Joe's earlier memories and experiences that contributed to some extent to his sexual aggressive pattern were evidenced through the following dialogue, which occurred during the second interview period.

T: Joe, you've brought me up to date on all of the rape incidents, however, at this point I'd like to spend some time trying to get some idea of your sexual history. Here, I'm talking about things like early sexual dreams and fantasies, when you started masturbating, where you learned about sex, and so on. First of all, what are some of your earliest memories about yourself as a sexual person?

J: No one ever talked about sex in our house, and I was always very bashful and shy. I think I first learned about masturbation through friends at school when I was maybe around 12. I started masturbating maybe around three times a week when I was an early teenager, though when I got to be older it increased to about four to six times weekly.

T: Joe, what would you find yourself thinking about when you'd masturbate?

J: Well, in the beginning I'd look at women in magazine advertisements, I'd imagine touching or kissing their breasts or legs or hips. I think around 14 or 15 I started having fantasies regarding my mother; these were really kind of sadistic. I'd imagine her bound by her hands to the front door, nude, and gagged.

Joe was never able to clarify why these particular fantasies were so stimulating; however, he does recall that the aggressive fantasy of his mother was the most frequent one he had with masturbation. By the time he was undergoing assessment, he was fantasizing aggressive- or sadistic-type themes about 70% of all the times he would masturbate, and the fact that he had been committed indefinitely because of this kind of behavior seemed to have had no apparent affect on the frequency with which he would masturbate to the fantasy of such behavior. We would like to especially emphasize here that continuing to masturbate to the fantasy of the kinds of activities that may have led to the person's incarceration is very typical and appears to be a heavy contributor to the high recidivism rates seen with sexual offenders following their release.

After the first rape and 3 months prior to his discharge from the military, Joe continued to masturbate to the fantasy of the rape incident, with the most arousing part still being his looking at the girl's breasts while she was on her back with her hands tied and helpless. Following discharge, he rejoined his wife. Later when she became pregnant and he was having difficulties with an employer at work, he started to think much more about picking up women, and he began to specifically plot how he would do this. He still had a supply of Dexedrine left from his military days and in retrospect admits this probably contributed much to his feelings of excitation, anticipation, and other physiological responses. His second rape, and most of the others, involved his picking up females who were either hitchhiking or at bus stops, and his coercive and aggressive pattern of behavior with them was quite consistent from one incident to the next. The only exception was when he would occasionally punch his victim for no apparent reason, and he never could give any idea as to what might have elicited this form of assaultiveness. Whether he physically assaulted or not, the terror and helplessness of his victims were always present.

During one session, futile attempts to get some sense of Joe's affect are described by the following excerpt:

J: It just really turned me on when I would see how helpless they were.
T: Joe, did you find yourself having any particular concerns or worries about the impact on your victim, or after the rape did you have any thoughts about how bad they might be hurt?
J: No, I never really intended to hurt anyone anyway, and as soon as I would take off I would put it out of my mind except when I might masturbate to the thought of one of the victims being helpless, laying nude, and seeing her breasts.
T: Joe, what kinds of thoughts and feelings do you have nowadays about what you did?
J: Now that I've turned to God, I ask for forgiveness of anything I've done bad. That's a big turning point for me.
T: That sounds real good, Joe. What about any thoughts or feelings you might have about the various women you raped?
J: Well, I'm sorry about Joanne and for her family [*this is the victim whom he almost murdered*]. However, I don't think I really ever intended to hurt anybody anyway and that was really an accident.

This sort of dialogue was one of many where it simply seemed that Joe was devoid of any real feelings whatsoever about the impact of what he had done on the lives of others. By the time this initial history taking was complete, Joe was masturbating once or twice a day and estimated that around 70% of his fantasies involved "inappropriate aggressive behavior." These fantasies would typically involve a woman in some form of bondage and regardless of the form of sexual activity that he was engaging in with her, she would "not be enjoying it," and she would be displaying some sounds of discomfort. It should be stressed here that on no occasion did Joe seem to delude himself, like many rapists, that his victim was indeed enjoying his aggressive actions. Of all sexual fantasies, he reported that only 20 to 30% involved a cooperative partner who was enjoying the activity.

From the information the therapists acquired during these evaluation sessions as well as the data generated by some of the assessment forms such as the Sexual Fear Inventory, Sexual Behavior Inventory, and the like, a three-phase treatment program was formulated. Conceptually, each phase of treatment was largely based on a psychological learning model that seemed quite adequate when looking at Joe's learning history and the subsequent behavior that led to his trouble. A multitude of treatment decisions were made over a lengthy period of time that sequentially covered the cognitive, affective, and the overt repertoire areas. The following is an overview of the treatment procedures.

Cognitive Aspects of Treatment

This first treatment phase acquainted Joe with the principles of learning and provided possible explanations as to how he might have acquired the kinds of feelings and behaviors that led to his problems. His above average intellect facilitated communication on a variety of cognitive methods such as *thought stopping, impulse control, chain breaking,* and the like. Additionally, he was provided with books (for example, on assertiveness) and films regarding sexual information and behavior.

During this phase and throughout the other two, he continued to provide data regarding his masturbation fantasies, with special attention being paid to the percentage of his fantasies that involved coercion and aggression.

Affective Phase of Treatment

The initial assessment indicated that Joe had much difficulty in expressing himself in a direct and honest way. He was certainly aware of the "correct" words to say, though one could not help but sense a continual "detachment" from him. During this phase he was first helped in becoming aware of the distinction between *thinking* and *feeling,* to be more precisely aware of his own emotions, and to be able to express these to others in an appropriate way.

However, the most important part of this phase was the assessment of his sexual arousal to various stimuli that had been eliciting and reinforcing his inappropriate and illegal sexual behavior. The penile tumescence monitor (penile plethysmograph) was extensively used throughout this phase. During initial assessment, details regarding his behavior and feelings to each of the numerous rapes that he could recall were obtained from Joe. From these data a series of 12 audiotapes was created that covered (a) four depictions of mutually consenting sexual relationships; (b) four sexual encounters where verbal coercion was used by him; and (c) four sexual encounters where he used physical aggression or force. Of the four tapes from each category, two involved actual experiences he had, and two involved fantasies he had about such an experience. These tapes relied exclusively on the information Joe had given regarding what he felt were the most erotic cues in the various situations. However, because the plethysmograph often yields indications of arousal to cues of which the person may not be aware, an additional data base was generated following his listening to all 12 tapes presented in random order while being measured by the plethysmograph. Then, six new tapes were created that placed even greater emphasis on the cues that he most strongly responded to on the first tape series. Conversely, content that seemed to have no association with increasing levels of sexual arousal was eliminated.

The "second generation" of tapes did, indeed, produce an even greater level of arousal response than the original set and thus became the tool for pretreatment assessment, probes during treatment, and posttreatment assessment. At this point, an index of Joe's response to rape cues was derived by dividing the mean level of arousal to the coercion tapes by the mean level of arousal to the mutually consenting tapes. Joe's index of arousal on the coercion tapes was 1.36 and 2.7 for the aggression series.

After this evaluation, the first therapeutic intervention involved suggesting to Joe that he change the content of his masturbatory fantasies. Prior to intervention, only 20 to 30% of his fantasies involved "cooperative or positive imagery," though after 3 months he reported 56% of an "appropriate" fantasy. This attempt to build his responses to positive sexual imagery was then accompanied by *aversion therapy* to reduce his arousal response to inappropriate cues. Valeric acid was selected as the noxious stimulus. (n.b., covert conditioning procedures were not selected because of his pattern of responses to the Composite Fear Inventory.) After 36 aversion therapy sessions, assessment revealed that his overall sexual response, expressed as percentage of erection, was reduced with all three themes (i.e., mutually consenting, 10%; coercion, 26.5%; and aggression, 36%). However, because his response to the mutually consenting tapes was also significantly reduced, his rape index was as high, or even higher, than when first calculated (2.6 and 3.6).

The fact that he had not responded nearly as negatively as expected to the Valeric acid was indeed perplexing to the therapists until a careful review of earlier discussions with Joe was made. In going over notes and transcripts from the session when the smell of Valeric acid was introduced to him, it suddenly became clear that the therapists' personal negative reaction to Valeric acid contributed to their assumption that Joe would respond likewise. However, note what he actually said:

J: Well, I have been looking forward to your coming today, to get started with whatever we're going to do. Did you bring any of the stuff you were talking about?

T: Yeah, Joe, Valeric acid is specifically what I meant and I have some in a vial here. In fact, when I let you take a brief smell of it, try to cap it as quickly as possible in that the smell permeates the room very rapidly. When we actually begin using the stuff, we will be able to control the odor such that we can let you smell it very directly, intensely, and not have to worry about the smell escaping. Here, why don't you take a whiff and tell us your reactions?

At this point, he took a smell, did not pull his head back in any sudden way, but proceeded to take a second smell before recapping the vial. His comment:

J: Well, it sure doesn't smell very good, though it's not really as bad as I thought it was going to be.

In retrospect, it turned out to be a big mistake for the therapists not to have paid more attention to Joe's evaluation. This was largely because they were too busy holding their own breath so as not to smell the noxious substance. At this point, consultation with Dr. Gene Abel and Dr. William Marshall from Canada led to a relatively new procedure then, called *satiation therapy.*

This procedure was first described by Marshall in 1979. Noting that uninterrupted performance of certain behaviors may lead to a reduction in the future probability of these behaviors, Marshall extended this to the treatment of males with deviant sexual interests. This procedure was selected particularly where more traditional aversive therapy or covert sensitization strategies had not been effective in reducing deviant arousal. To briefly summarize, the procedure involves having the patient experience periods of excessive, prolonged masturbation while fantasizing the deviant sexual activity. In order to control the fantasizing, the individual must verbalize into a tape recorder throughout the entire period. The notion here is that the preferred sexual activity will soon lose its attractiveness, although theoretically, the loss could be explained in a variety of ways.

This procedure was carried out over a 4-month period. The results showed a significant drop in arousal to a mean of 7% erection response to the mutually consenting tapes, 7% to the coercion tapes (Rape Index of 1.1), and 8% to the aggressive tape (Rape Index of 1.2). However, as Abel points out, anything below a 10% erection response could likely be caused by artifact, and therefore it was concluded that there had been a significant reduction in his arousal response to the unwanted cues. Because his arousal to the mutually consenting tapes was also still low, at this time he was started on a *positive reconditioning* procedure for 2 months. This mainly involved having him fantasize socially and sexually appropriate stimuli while masturbating in a comfortable nonthreatening private atmosphere. The last assessment of arousal responses in 1981 indicated his low overall response to coercion and rape cues was still being maintained, and he reported that almost 100% of his sexual fantasies with masturbation involved mutually consenting situations. The therapists might also note here that assessment was made on how well he could consciously suppress arousal cues by periodically instructing him to do so, thus giving some indication of his ability to distort data if he chose to. Repeated checks indicated that he appeared to be responding in a way consistent with what he reported.

Overt-Behavior Phase of Treatment

In the final phase of treatment, close attention was particularly given to Joe's repertoire of social skills. His social assets and deficits were evaluated in several different ways. He first completed the Social Performance Survey Schedule (Lowe & Cautela, 1978). This 100-item self-report inventory attempts to assess two classes of behavior: the frequency with which certain positive social behaviors are performed (example, initiating conversation with others), and the frequency with which negative social behaviors are performed (example, interrupting others). The data here indicated that Joe generally knew what "not to do" socially; however, he did *not* engage in the positive social behaviors nearly as much as would be expected from males his age. This assessment certainly was consistent with the type of heterosocial history he had given us.

To further pinpoint possible social assets and deficits, the Heterosocial Skills

Behavior Checklist for Males (Barlow *et al.*, 1977) was used. Next, one of the therapists' female employees, whom Joe had never met, roleplayed a social situation with him while he was evaluated by three impartial assessors. His responses were compared to a norm group described as "white socially adequate males" (WSAM), and the results indicated that Joe scored significantly lower than the norm group in two of the categories as well as in his overall performance.

At this point, two female social workers from the state's Sex Abuse Treatment Center and one female crisis worker who was working as a volunteer in the People against Rape organization were asked to assist in the treatment program. All assessment data in the social skills area were given to the volunteers, and they began a series of training sessions with Joe that extended over a 2-month period. In addition to social skills training, the volunteers worked with Joe, assisting him in expressing his feelings more comfortably and directly as well as involving him in a variety of role-playing situations that he might encounter if, and when, he was released from the state hospital. To keep Joe as "unprepared and off guard" as possible, he was never told when the female volunteers would show up for a session, nor was he briefed in advance on any of the scenarios he would be required to roleplay. One example of a fairly stressful role-playing activity required him to appropriately deal with the situation where he was released from the hospital and recognized in a social setting by someone who knew of his criminal background.

At the end of this training program, he was evaluated on the Social Performance Survey Schedule and again overt behavior was assessed via the Heterosocial Skills Checklist. On the survey schedule, his overall score significantly shifted to compare favorably with the norm group score, and on the Checklist he scored 100% in all three categories. At this point, it was apparent that Joe was much more in touch with his feelings, and on occasion he would cry when talking with the volunteer workers about what he had done to his victims. By this time, it was mutually agreed to terminate treatment until such time as he became eligible for conditional release.

The preceding overview of the treatment program unfortunately must be condensed because of space limitations. However, the amount of time, effort, and money spent to adequately treat a case such as this can be phenomenal. For example, in this case we personally were involved in over 250 hours (at half our usual fee) of evaluation and treatment. An additional 200 free hours were provided by psychology interns whom we were supervising, and another 40 hours were devoted by the volunteer social workers.

Assessment and Treatment Problems Encountered

Case studies in the literature often seem to proceed with an orderly series of assessment and treatment interventions with the resulting data usually clearly suggesting the efficacy of the methods employed. We would like to emphasize that this was certainly not the situation in this case nor for that matter in many others in which we have been involved. All of the problems with assessment noted earlier in our general discussion of the subject indeed occurred with this case. For example, how reliable is self-report from an incarcerated rapist? How much can one generalize from the apparent social skills he has acquired via role playing to the world outside the institution? And these questions should not obscure the more practical problems such as transporting bulky equipment from the office to the hospital, using seclusion rooms where there are many outside distracting noises, no electrical outlets, and a variety of other obstacles. However, it goes without saying that the need for ongoing assessment of one sort or another is very critical if one is to have any confidence whatsoever in the effect of treatment interventions. The most glaring example of this is what happened during the phase of aversion therapy with Valeric acid. Had we relied on self-report, we would have assumed that Joe was getting more and more turned off to inappropriate sexual stimuli. However, physiological measurement showed this not to be the case and because of these data, an entirely new treatment intervention was employed.

There were numerous treatment problems that would be analogous to those noted previously under assessment difficulties. The most unexpected and uncontrollable factors frequently posed problems for treatment. For example, because this particular case was a rather notorious one in the community, each time the press covered a particularly lengthy rape trial, this case would usually be mentioned. These stories caused much anxiety and some degree of depression for Joe to the extent that this had to be dealt with therapeutically before proceeding with the treatment strategy described earlier. Another unexpected development was during the phase when we attempted to recruit and train female volunteers to assist us with the social skills training portion of treatment. It was noted on the front page of a leading newspaper that Joe would possibly be considered by the courts for eventual release into the community. The outcry against this possibility led to the withdrawal of two of our initial volunteers from the treatment program and made it almost impossible for the recruitment of other appropriate volunteers. Also, anybody who even remotely appeared to be providing assistance to an individual like Joe (maintaining confidentiality under these circumstances is virtually impossible) is subject to a variety of negative social pressures. Finally, there is the futility of ever trying to determine exactly which procedure had which effect when any number of procedures are being simultaneously employed. To further complicate the issue regarding the assessment of treatment efficacy is the fact that Joe still has not been released. If he is eventually released long after treatment has been officially terminated, and does not repeat his behavior, what if anything one can really say about the treatment's being effective?

Follow-up is crucial in cases such as this, and possible post-formal-therapy booster sessions or even further interventions may be necessary. We usually set up agreements with patients to have continuing ongoing contact and follow-up visits with objective measures for at least 5 years, if not for the rest of their lives (along the lines of a "behavioral checkup" once or twice a year, as a person would visit a dentist).

Assuming eventual objective measures of success and appropriate court action for the institutionalized person, the last area of consideration is possible rehabilitation into the community. This would mean gradual reintroduction into society; possibly speaking about such persons and their treatment to special groups; making meaningful contributions of time and effort to socially approved public and private community associations; and other appropriate activities. If the institutionalized person is to be released on some form of probation or parole in another area of the country, it is important that he or she also makes arrangements for continued ongoing contact and follow-up visits with a therapist familiar with, and experienced in, this type of approach to treatment, one who would be available for continuing follow-up and perhaps occasional booster sessions, or further interventions, as might be called for.

The final results of the patient's physiological arousal measurement, although no absolute guarantee of future behavior, are now the best scientific data that we have so far in this area on predicting such behaviors in the future. As was mentioned earlier, there are no guarantees of "success" with this approach, or any others; however, with continued objective measurements and the use of coordinated selected interventions as described, it is our strong belief that the prognosis for a lasting behavior change has a much higher probability of being achieved than with no treatment, incarceration alone, standardized indirect treatment approaches, or any combination of the foregoing.

Summary

This chapter began with the point that there are very few, if any, areas of human behavior in American culture that can generate as much concern, controversy, and confusion as that of sexual deviation. The cultural context is an extremely important factor in determining what is considered "deviant," as well as whether such behavior is viewed from a statistical, legal, psychiatric, or psychological viewpoint. The ROBI descriptive classification scheme for assumed or possible sexual disorders was briefly described.

An overview of assessment approaches was then discussed with emphasis on the contrasting approaches of an *indirect* or *dynamic viewpoint* with that of a *psychological learning model*. An individualized assessment approach from within the later viewpoint was then described along with the various assessment materials and procedures utilized by such an approach. The data thus collected are then used in order to carefully formulate an individualized treatment program that focuses on interventions in three major areas of functioning: the cognitive-thinking area, the affective-emotional area, and the overt-behavioral area. Various treatment procedures and techniques were then described for intervention in these three areas of concern.

It was pointed out that there are inherent difficulties with some of the assessment materials that then contribute toward the ineffectiveness of the treatment procedures. Stress was placed on the importance of the use of a penile transducer for (a) determining what are the most erotic cues that elicit arousal responses so as to not rely entirely on what the person may report verbally as most arousing; (b) uncovering or discovering unacknowledged or unknown arousal responses to other unwanted or illegal behaviors not initially presented; (c) assessment probes during treatment to see the effect of various interventions; and (d) to obtain pre- and post-treatment indexes of the person for possible prediction purposes.

A case study was then presented to illustrate the use of assessment materials and treatment techniques within the psychological learning model proposed by the authors. Finally, this was followed by a discussion of some of the assessment and treatment problems that are encountered by clinical treatment in nonideal settings, with difficult long-term behaviors that have a lasting negative impact on society, as contrasted with straightforward research in an academic setting where most variables can be controlled. When it comes to treatment for the sexual offender, it is our strong, though not popular, position that even if the person is institutionalized in some manner, eventually most such persons will be released, and, therefore, it is extremely important to society, as well as the individual, to do whatever is possible with the therapeutic assessment and effective treatment techniques that currently exist within the state of the art to reduce the probability that such behaviors occur again in the future.

References

Abel, G. G., & Annon, J. S. (1982, April). *Reducing deviant sexual arousal through satiation.* Workshop presented at the Fourth National Conference and Workshops on Sexual Aggression, Prevention of Child Molestation and Rape, Prevention Strategies and Plans for Action, Denver.

Abel, G. G., & Blanchard, E. B. (1976). The measurement and generation of sexual arousal in male sexual deviates. In M. Hersen, R. M. Eisler, & P. M. Miller (Eds.), *Progress in behavior modification* (Vol. 2). New York: Academic Press.

Abel, G. G., Barlow, D. H., Blanchard, E. G., & Mavissakalian, M. (1974, September). *The relationship of aggressive cues to the sexual arousal of rapists.* Paper presented at the American Psychological Association, New Orleans.

Abel, G. G., Barlow, D. H., Blanchard, E. B., & Guild, D. (1975, May). *The components of rapists' sexual arousal.* Paper presented at the Annual Meeting of the American Psychiatric Association, Anaheim, California.

Annon, J. S. (1971a). *The extension of learning principles to the analysis and treatment of sexual problems. Dissertation Abstracts International, 32* (6-B), 3627. (University Microfilms N. 72-290, 570)

Annon, J. S. (1971b, September). *The therapeutic use of masturbation in the treatment of sexual disorders.* Paper presented at the Annual Meeting of the Association for the Advancement of Behavior Therapy, Washington, DC.

Annon, J. S. (1972, May). *The extension of learning principles to the analysis and treatment of a pedophilic problem.* Paper presented at the Annual Meeting of the Hawaii Psychological Association, Honolulu.

Annon, J. S. (1973a). The Behavior Assessment Form. In A. L. Comrey, T. E. Becker, & E. M. Glaser (Eds.), *A sourcebook for mental health measures.* Los Angeles: Human Interaction Research Institute.

Annon, J. S. (1973b). The Composite Fear Inventory. In A. L. Comrey, T. E. Becker, & E. M. Glaser (Eds.), *A sourcebook for mental health measures.* Los Angeles: Human Interaction Research Institute.

Annon, J. S. (1973c). The Life History Questionnaire. In A. L. Comrey, T. E. Becker, & E. M. Glaser (Eds.), *A sourcebook for mental health measures.* Los Angeles: Human Interaction Research Institute.

Annon, J. S. (1973d). The therapeutic use of masturbation in the treatment of sexual disorders. In R. D. Rubin, J. P. Brady, & J. D. Henderson (Eds.), *Advances in behavior therapy* (Vol. 4). New York: Academic Press.

Annon, J. S. (1975a). *The behavioral treatment of sexual problems: Intensive therapy.* Honolulu: Enabling Systems.

Annon, J. S. (1975b). *The Sexual Fear Inventory (Male Form and Female Form)*. Honolulu: Enabling Systems.

Annon, J. S. (1975c). *The Sexual History Form*. Princeton, NJ: Educational Testing Service.

Annon, J. S. (1975d). *The Sexual Pleasure Inventory (Male Form and Female Form)*. Honolulu: Enabling Systems.

Annon, J. S. (1976a). *The behavioral treatment of sexual problems: Brief therapy*. New York: Harper & Row.

Annon, J. S. (1976b). The PLISSIT model: A proposed conceptual scheme for the behavioral treatment of sexual problems. *Journal of Sex Education and Therapy, 2,* 1–15.

Annon, J. S. (1981). PLISSIT therapy. In R. J. Corsini (Ed.), *Handbook of innovative psychotherapies*. New York: Wiley Interscience.

Annon, J. S., & Robinson, C. H. (1978). The use of vicarious learning in the treatment of sexual concerns. In J. LoPiccolo & L. LoPiccolo (Eds.), *Handbook of sex therapy*. New York: Plenum Press.

Annon, J. S., & Robinson, C. H. (1980a). Sexual disorders. In A. E. Kazdin, A. S. Bellack, & M. Hersen (Eds.), *New perspectives in abnormal psychology*. New York: Oxford University Press.

Annon, J. S., & Robinson, C. H. (1980b). Treatment of common male and female sexual concerns. In J. M. Ferguson & C. Barr Taylor (Eds.), *The comprehensive handbook of behavioral medicine (Vol. 1). Systems intervention.* Jamaica, NY: SP Medical and Scientific Books.

Annon, J. S., & Robinson, C. H. (1981a). The behavioral treatment of sexual dysfunctions. In A. Sha'Ked (Ed.), *Human sexuality in rehabilitation medicine*. Baltimore: Waverly Press.

Annon, J. S., & Robinson, C. H. (1981b). Contributor's comments. In R. S. Daniel (Ed.), *Human sexuality methods and material for the education, family life and health professions (Vol. A). An annotated guide to the audiovisuals.* Brea, CA: Heuristicus.

Annon, J. S., & Robinson, C. H. (1981c). A practical approach to day to day sexual problems. In D. A. Shore & H. L. Gochros (Eds.), *Sexual problems of adolescents in institutions.* Springfield, IL: C C Thomas.

Annon, J. S., & Robinson, C. H. (1981d). Video in sex therapy. In J. L. Fryrear & R. Fleshman (Eds.), *Videotherapy in mental health.* Springfield, IL: C C Thomas.

Barlow, D. H. Abel, G. G., Blanchard, E. B., Bristow, A. R., & Young, L. D. (1977). A heterosocial skills behavior checklist for males. *Behavior Therapy, 8,* 229–239.

Cautela, J. R., & Kastenbaum, R. (1967). A reinforcement survey schedule for use in therapy, training, and research. *Psychological Reports, 10,* 1115–1130.

Eysenck, H. J., & Rachman, S. (1965). *The causes and cures of neurosis*. San Diego: Robert A. Knapp.

Hartung, J. (1983, November). *A guide for therapists who treat sex offenders*. Paper presented at the Annual Convention of the American Society of Criminology, Denver.

Lester, D. (1975). *Unusual sexual behavior: The standard deviations*. Springfield, IL: C C Thomas.

Lowe, M. R., & Cautela, J. R. (1978). A self-report measure of social skill. *Behavior Therapy, 9,* 535–544.

Marshall, W. L. (1973). The modification of sexual fantasies: A combined treatment approach to the reduction of deviant sexual behavior. *Behaviour Research and Therapy, 2,* 557–564.

Marshall, W. L. (1979). Satiation therapy: A procedure for reducing deviant sexual arousal. *Journal of Applied Behavior Analysis, 12,* 377–389.

McHugh, G. (1976). *Sex Knowledge Inventory: Form Y: Vocabulary and Anatomy*. Saluda, NC: Family Life Publications.

McHugh, G. (1979). *Sex Knowledge Inventory: Form X*. Saluda, NC: Family Life Publications.

Quinsey, V. L., Chaplin, T. C., & Carrigan, W. F. (1980). Biofeedback and signaled punishment in the modification of inappropriate sexual age preferences. *Behavior Therapy, 11,* 567–576.

Robinson, C. H. (1974, November). *The effects of observational learning on the masturbation patterns of preorgasmic females*. Paper presented at the Annual Meeting of the Society for the Scientific Study of Sex, Las Vegas.

Robinson, C. H. (1975a). The effects of observational learning on sexual behaviors and attitudes in orgasmically dysfunctional women. *Dissertation Abstracts International,* Vol. XXXV, 9. (University Microfilms No. 75-5040, 221)

Robinson, C. H. (1976b, December). Sexual problems and vicarious learning. In R. J. Pion (Chair), *Human sexuality.* Symposium conducted at the annual clinical convention of the American Medical Association, Honolulu.

Robinson, C. H. (1976, May). The use of observational learning in the treatment of sexual concerns. In R. J. Pion (Chair), *A brief therapy approach to the office management of sexual problems.* Postgraduate course presented at the annual meeting of the American College of Obstetricians and Gynecologists, Dallas.

Robinson, C. H. (1977, May). The treatment of sexual problems through vicarious learning. In R. J. Pion (Chair), *Management of sexual problems*. Postgraduate course presented at the annual meeting of the American College of Obstetricians and Gynecologists, Chicago.

Robinson, C. H., & Annon, J. S. (1975a). *The Heterosexual Attitude Scale (Male Form and Female Form)*. Honolulu: Enabling Systems.

Robinson, C. H., & Annon, J. S. (1975b). *The Heterosexual Behavior Inventory (Male Form and Female Form)*. Honolulu: Enabling Systems.

Staats, A. W., & Staats, C. K. (1963). *Complex human behavior: A systematic extension of learning principles*. New York: Holt, Rinehart & Winston.

Ullmann, L. P., & Krasner, L. (1975). *A psychological approach to abnormal behavior* (2nd ed.). Englewood Cliffs, NJ: Prentice-Hall.

Psychosexual Dysfunction

Nathaniel McConaghy

Introduction

A considerable research literature exists evaluating the assessment and treatment of psychosexual dysfunctions from a behavioral perspective (Friedman, Weiler, LoPiccolo, & Hogan, 1982; McConaghy, 1984). However, this literature focuses mainly on specific behavioral techniques and provides little additional assistance to the therapist who believes the patient's personality has an important bearing on his or her response to treatment. Of course, the learning theory the therapist adopts influences the degree to which he or she believes the patient has a personality: that is, a tendency to show consistent behavioral patterns over a wide variety of situations, including, of course, the therapeutic situation (McConaghy, 1985). Therapists adopting a cognitive approach tend to accept the existence of such consistent behavioral patterns based on irreversible cognitive categorizations established by learning especially in early childhood. Therapists adopting a strict classical conditioning approach also consider such patterns important and to be based on constitutional differences in psychological characteristics as well as learning. Those adopting a behaviorist or social learning position award them little significance:

> Social-learning theory makes no assumptions about the generality or consistency of behavior patterns across stimulus situations . . . there is no reason to expect behaviors such as aggression and dependency to be stable across situations unless the situations and contingencies are similar. (Mischel, 1967, pp. 66–67)

NATHANIEL McCONAGHY • Psychiatry Unit, Prince of Wales Hospital, Randwick, New South Wales 2031, Australia.

A related issue that has an important influence on the therapist's approach is the extent to which he or she believes patients can be unconscious of aspects of their behaviors.

There has so far been little effort directed toward comparing the efficacy of behavioral approaches based on different attitudes to the existence of personality traits and unconscious factors. The author believes them to be of considerable importance not only in determining the outcome of those patients who are admitted to and remain in research studies evaluating treatment of behavioral dysfunctions, but also in influencing the type of patient who decides not to be admitted to or to drop out of such studies. If this belief is correct, these factors, whether appreciated by the therapist or not, have influenced the reported outcome of the studies already published, even though this outcome has usually been interpreted as reflecting the influence only of specific aspects of behavioral therapies. The author believes he is markedly influenced in his clinical assessment and treatment of patients with sexual dysfunctions by the general theory of behavior he has adopted as being most useful in understanding the behavior of people in general and patients in particular, though aware that this general theory has not been empirically validated.

It is surely a truism that many aspects of voluntary behavior are unconscious. When we speak, drive a car, or hit a tennis ball we are not aware of many of the processes that select the order of the words we employ or determine the strength and direction of our motor responses. However, presumably students of behavior still exist who question that we can be unconscious of the nature of our motives when we express emotional behaviors. My view concerning unconscious emotions tends to approximate that of the 19th-century observers of human behavior as expressed in their novels and writings, rather than the view advanced subsequently by Freud. The 19th-century concept was that it is not abnormal to be unconscious of many of one's motives and that such unconsciousness is not motivated solely by defense mechanisms that protect the ego from anxiety concerning sex or aggression. Rather, we all are at times partly or completely unconscious of many of our motives, often but not invariably, in order to feel better about ourselves:

> with that subtle, selfish, ambiguous sophistry to which the minds of all men are so subject, he taught himself to think that in doing much for the promotion of his own interests he was doing much also for the promotion of religion. (Trollope, 1967, pp. 115–116)

> Mrs. Norris had not the least intention of being at any expense whatever in her [niece's] maintenance . . . though perhaps she might so little know herself, as to walk home to the Parsonage after this conversation, in the happy belief of being the most liberal-minded sister and aunt in the world. (Austen, 1945, pp. 6–7)

However, the motivation for unconscious behaviors might be no more than to strengthen an argument by quoting an authority:

> Mr. Woodhouse was rather agitated by such harsh reflections on his friend Perry [the local apothecary] to whom he had, in fact, though unconsciously, been attributing many of his own feelings and expressions. (Austen, 1946, p. 94)

Certainly, most 19th-century writers were more likely to observe unattractive unconscious motives underlying attractive conscious ones rather than the reverse: "In modesty I can always find a repressed urge towards pride" (Tolstoy, 1970, p. 138). This was possibly not true of Dickens, whose heroines (though never the reader) were often unaware of their excellent qualities:

> The people even praise Me as the doctor's wife. The people even like Me as I
> go about, and make so much of me that I am quite abashed. I owe it all to him,
> my love, my pride! They like me for his sake . . . (Dickens, 1963, p. 796)

What then should be the response of the therapist who believes a patient is showing motives of which he or she is unconscious? The patient might, for example, report difficulties in carrying out the treatment program, which suggests an unconscious unwillingness to comply with it, or show a strong tendency to reject the possibility that his or her symptoms are psychologically caused, for example, appearing to regard such a suggestion as questioning his or her masculinity or femininity.

Trainee therapists may be taught that the appropriate response to such patients is to confront them with the suggestion that they are acting under the influence of such unconscious motives, though I am unaware of any empirical evidence comparing the outcome of this technique with that of other possible approaches. Certainly, confrontation appears in the short term to have the desired effect in some patients of causing them to change their behavior so as to become more compliant with the therapist's wishes. However, in others it appears to produce negative feelings, manifest by strong denial and at times signs of resentment and anger. If the interpretation is correct and the patient has unconscious motives that lead him or her to resist treatment and that the patient is not prepared to acknowledge, it might be expected that he or she would prove difficult to treat. Certainly, this is the author's experience. If the therapist persists in confronting such patients, their resultant hostility could lead them to terminate contact with the therapist.

The therapist's method of dealing with unconscious behavior may therefore give him or her the power to cause some patients who are difficult to treat to decide not to accept treatment after initial assessment, or to cease treatment prematurely. It is unlikely that many therapists use this power consciously to avoid treating difficult patients. However motivated by such factors as increasing the effectiveness of treatment, some therapists, for example, make contractual agreements with patients that continuation of therapy is contingent on the patient's meeting certain requirements, such as carrying out a specified number of homework sexual activities between interviews. This can have the effect of excluding from treatment some patients with unconscious resistances.

The nature of the therapists' practice is likely to influence this aspect of their assessment and treatment of patients. Understandably and indeed possibly desirably, the therapeutic zeal of many therapists at the commencement of their careers in unrealistically high, as it has not yet been tempered by the experience of difficulties and failures. Such therapists are less likely to notice the presence of unconscious motives in their patients and may respond to these motives in a way that will certainly retain the patient in treatment but may retard his or her progress.

The patient who subtly conveys the information that he or she has been treated unsuccessfully by a number of practitioners but was never really understood until he or she met the present therapist often has surprising success with the young and inevitably somewhat insecure therapist who is likely to respond to such a pleasing comment with overinvolvement. The patient, after initial progress, may relapse into chronicity and require to be seen more and more frequently, perhaps at times for crisis interventions outside office hours. Only then may the therapist realize he or she cannot maintain the degree of therapeutic involvement he or she has initiated, yet feel unsure as to how to reduce it without harming the patient. A danger is that the therapist may react with denial and hostility and reject the patient, using such labels as *demanding* and *manipulative,* not to objectively describe the patient's behavior, but to excuse his or her own. Such patient's numerous unsuccessful therapeutic experiences may have all been of this nature, each sufficiently rewarding initially to encourage the patient to seek further such destructive encounters. Until the therapist has learned to recognize the unconscious flattery, seductiveness, or other manipulations to which he or she may be particularly susceptible, a principle that can help obviate such overinvolvement is never to set up a therapeutic relationship of an intensity or frequency that cannot be maintained indefinitely.

Another aspect of therapy of which the therapist may only be partly conscious is the degree to which his or her behavior changes in response to differences in the degree of psychological and intellectual sophistication of the patient. Such sophistication can, of course, in part reflect differences in the level of education, social class, and intelligence. I find myself at times adopting a more direct, matter-of-fact manner with some patients, presumably believing this will improve the therapeutic relationship. Also, I have come to believe that certain difficulties in communication can be due to biological differences in patients. One such difference is allusive thinking (Armstrong & McConaghy, 1977; McConaghy, 1960), which is shown in marked form by a percentage of normal people who, when talking about abstract issues including their feelings, express themselves in a vague, "woolly," and usually verbose fashion, which may be so imprecise as to make it impossible to determine their meaning. Another is a reduced ability to conceptualize about personal relationships shown by some subjects, usually men, who demonstrate no other evidence of intellectual impairment. Though such beliefs concerning biologically determined individual differences in communication skills are unacceptable to many students of human behavior, some would appear to agree with the observation on which the latter belief is based, though they may attribute the deficiency to childhood experiences that "get set in concrete":

> Another example is of men who don't express their feelings . . . the problem seems to go way back and change is difficult. . . . Whether the man has had years of psychoanalysis, courses of assertiveness training and communication work, or whatever, he remains somewhat reluctant to express himself and when he does you can almost hear the tumblers turning. (Zilbergeld, 1983, pp. 235–236)

The therapist who accepts that such limitations to communication in a patient may be intrinsic or at least largely unmodifiable is likely to be less challenging or confronting to that patient than the therapist who regards them as evidence of unconscious resistance.

Another decision that the behaviorally orientated clinician must make with little empirical data to guide him or her concerns the procedure to adopt with the patient who requests treatment for sexual dysfunction but presents obvious evidence of being in a difficult relationship with the sexual partner. To some extent, it could be considered exploitive to persuade patients to accept treatment for problems the therapist decides they have, in addition to the ones for which they sought treatment. A considerable percentage of the population who come to the attention of the therapeutically oriented, for example in surveys, has been considered to have emotional problems that could require treatment. Dohrenwend and Dohrenwend (1963) in reviewing such surveys pointed out that the prevalence of psychological disorder reported has at times reached 60%. Frank, Anderson, and Rubinstein (1978) reported a prevalence in this range of sexual dysfunctions alone. One of the advantages of a behavioral, as opposed to a psychodynamic, approach to psychological problems is that a behavioral approach is problem oriented and does not seek to establish in the patient some ideal state of mental health in order to successfully treat his or her complaint. Accepting that the patient can be unconscious of important aspects of his or her emotional behavior could encourage the therapist to search for such behaviors that warrant treatment. The results of the surveys quoted suggest that few persons subject to such a therapist's scrutiny would escape showing indications for treatment, whether they be sexual difficulties, communication problems, lack of assertiveness, or difficulty in controlling aggression.

However, to adopt a strict problem-oriented approach can be as unreasonable as to enthusiastically search for additional problems. A behavioral approach to sexual dysfunctions usually requires that the patient's partner cooperate in the treatment program. Adequate cooperation is unlikely if the relationship with the partner is in part hostile or otherwise unsatisfactory. Indeed, it is frequently reported that patients with sexual dysfunctions whose marital relationships are unsatisfactory respond poorly to behavioral approaches (McGovern, Stewart, & LoPiccolo, 1975; Munjack, Cristol, Goldstein, Phillips, Goldberg, Whipple, Staples, & Kanno, 1976). The therapist who detects evidence of a poor relationship with the sexual partner therefore needs to decide to what extent emphasis should be put on treating this relationship in addition, or even prior to, focusing on the patient's sexual dysfunction.

Assessment and Treatment of Sexual Dysfunctions in Women

The DSM-III classification of mental disorders separates psychosexual dysfunctions in women into inhibited sexual desire, inhibited sexual excitement, inhibited orgasm, functional dyspareunia (painful intercourse), and functional vaginismus (involuntary spasm of the outer vaginal musculature). Though failure to experience orgasm in the intercouse situation appears to be the commonest dysfunction for which women seek treatment, it is commonly associated with complaints of inadequate interest in and ability to be aroused by sexual activities, and not uncommonly with some degree of pain with intercouse. Vaginismus sufficient to prevent penetration has virtually disappeared in the author's practice in the last few years, perhaps reflecting reduced anxiety concerning sexual activity in the community.

Case Study 1

Couple A. was referred by their medical practitioner because, as he wrote in the letter of referral, Mrs. A. "had been anorgasmic all her life and feels she has been made to feel all the blame for this and this has made it difficult for them to make progress with another therapist."

Mr. Brian A. was 30 and Mrs. Wilma A. 28 years of age, and they had a 4-year-old daughter, Marilyn. They had been married 9 years.

AUTHOR: What do you see as the problem that brought you to see me?

MRS. A.: Well, our sexual relationship has never been successful. I've never had an orgasm. I'm getting to the stage I'm just not interested in sex. . . . I realize this is hard for Brian.

AUTHOR: Do you have any physical discomfort with sex?

MRS. A.: With intercourse at times it's painful.

AUTHOR: Does it prevent your husband's penis from entering you.

MRS. A.: It can make it difficult and then the pain is worse afterwards.

AUTHOR: Where do you experience the pain?

MRS. A.: Mainly on the surface.

AUTHOR: Are there times when you find intercourse pleasurable?

MRS. A.: Hardly ever. At most about 10 times since our marriage.

AUTHOR: Do you enjoy any aspects of your sexual relationships—like the foreplay before intercourse?

MRS. A.: Yes, if I'm properly aroused. Brian often doesn't do this. He can be very heavy handed.

AUTHOR: Are you able to tell him how to stimulate you?

MRS. A.: I've told him. He never seems to understand.

AUTHOR [*to Mr. A.*]: How do you see that?

MR. A.: I try to do what Wilma wants. At times however I do it, it seems to be wrong.

AUTHOR [*to Mrs. A.*]: Can you tell him then what he's doing wrong.

MRS. A.: Sometimes I just can't get aroused.

AUTHOR: Couldn't you decide on those occasions to leave it till another time?

MRS. A.: I don't always know. Sometimes if Brain persists then I will get aroused. Then I'll enjoy it.

AUTHOR: Do you ever feel you get near to a climax—say with your husband stimulating your clitoris?

MRS. A.: At times I feel I get very close. But I have to tell him to stop. I can't stand it anymore.

AUTHOR: Why?

MRS. A.: The feeling becomes unbearable.

AUTHOR: How do you get along together in your general relationship?

MRS. A.: Oh, we get along well. Perhaps too well.

AUTHOR: Why do you say that?

MRS. A.: Well, we agree on most things.

AUTHOR: Why perhaps too well, though?

MRS. A.: Well, we never shout at each other. People say you should at times, but I don't like arguments.

AUTHOR: Do you feel like shouting at times?

MRS. A.: I have to control my emotions. Our daughter is very sensitive. She couldn't stand us shouting.

AUTHOR: How do you know that?

MRS. A.: When my brother visits, we used to have mock fights, just for fun, but she was terribly upset, she would cry and say "Mummy, don't, don't . . . "

AUTHOR [to Mr. A.]: How do you see the situation?

MR. A.: Yes, it's like that.

AUTHOR: Do you ever feel like shouting, or arguing.

MR. A.: No, not really.

AUTHOR: Was your family against fighting or getting angry?

MRS. A.: Brian's family wasn't close, not like mine. He didn't get on with his two brothers.

AUTHOR: Did you fight with them?

MR. A.: As kids we fought a lot . . . not later.

AUTHOR [to Mrs. A.]: How did your family feel about arguing?

MRS. A.: Oh, there was very little fighting in our family. My father would apologize if he'd been wrongly angry.

AUTHOR: What would make him angry?

MRS. A.: Hardly anything, even if I'd done something wrong. He was my step-father. Our natural father died when I was 3½ and my mother married again when I was 8.

AUTHOR: Did you have problems getting on with your step-father at first?

MRS. A.: Oh, no. We accepted him as our father straight away.

AUTHOR: In regard to your present problem, what has led to your seeking treatment now?

MR. A.: Dr. G. [their medical practitioner] did suggest we have treatment about 3 years after we were married and Wilma still wasn't having a climax.

MRS. A.: In the last 9 months, my health hasn't been good and I've thought perhaps it was due to sex.

AUTHOR: In what way?

MRS. A.: I've had a lot of trouble from adhesions since I had my appendix out 3 years ago. Our doctor thought sexual frustration might be the cause.

AUTHOR: What was your physical health like before the operation?

MRS. A.: I've never had much energy. I've always tired easily. Our doctor put it down to my low blood pressure; and I'm bordering on anemia.

AUTHOR: What was your health like at school?

MRS. A.: I was never robust. I did run around a lot and would be up till all hours and tire myself out. Then I'd be too tired to do anything.

AUTHOR: How about after you left school?

MRS. A.: I was sick for about 4 years after I left school.

AUTHOR: Were you able to work?

MRS. A.: Yes. I was generally sick at weekends. After we married I worked part-time till Marilyn was born.

AUTHOR: How was your health after you married.

MRS. A.: It was alright. I never had much energy.

AUTHOR [to Mr. A.]: How has your health been since childhood?

MR. A.: Pretty good. I never needed much time off from school or work.

AUTHOR: With your wife often not enjoying sex, I suppose at times she doesn't want it when you do. How do you feel about that?

MR. A.: I accept that.

MRS. A.: Not really. Brian can go really quiet and sulky if we haven't had sex for some weeks, or if I tell him I can't. Sometimes I have it because I know it will put him in a good mood.

AUTHOR [*to couple*]: You've seen another therapist recently about your problem. How did he try to help you?

MRS. A.: He said it was all my problem.

AUTHOR: What did he suggest?

MRS. A.: He gave me books to read—*How to Become Orgasmic, My Secret Garden* and told me I was to masturbate 3 hours a week for 9 weeks on my own.

AUTHOR: How did you feel about that?

MRS. A.: Pretty horrified. I've never masturbated . . . Nor have any of my friends.

AUTHOR: How do you feel about your husband masturbating you?

MRS. A.: That can be alright.

AUTHOR: Well, the approach I suggest will be based on the same theory the other therapist was using. This is that sexual feelings are blocked by anxiety, perhaps say fear of losing emotional control, though you might not be aware of this anxiety.

MRS. A.: No, I certainly don't feel that I am anxious about sex.

AUTHOR: No, as I said, often patients don't seem to be aware of being anxious but if we treat them on this basis they often respond. The way we try to reduce this possible anxiety and encourage you to experience feelings is to ask you to experience being in the sexual situation repeatedly without attempting intercourse so that there is no pressure on you to become sexually aroused and you are to concentrate more on just enjoying the physical sensual sensations of being stroked and cuddled.

MRS. A.: O, I do that already. I really enjoy just being cuddled.

AUTHOR: Yes, though I get the feeling that your husband at times doesn't pick up your cues as to how you like to be cuddled and stroked, so these sessions could help that. Also I wonder if he isn't much less communicative than you. In this interview I haven't got much of an impression as to how he feels about the situation. So these sessions might also help him to communicate more. In the sessions I want you to cuddle naked, one to be passive for about half an hour and the other to do the stroking. But the passive one is to say how and where they want to be stroked or kissed, what things feel pleasant, not necessarily sexually arousing. You might like to have your feet, your hands, or your back stroked. In these first sessions you are not to include the sexual organs or the breasts in the stroking. You need to put aside an hour three or four times a week when you aren't under any time pressure to enjoy these sessions in a relaxed state.

MRS. A.: That's going to be hard. Marilyn doesn't like going to bed till late, sometimes after midnight.

AUTHOR: Perhaps you could let her stay in her room looking at books or playing till she goes to sleep.

MRS. A.: She wouldn't do that—she often comes into our room during the night.

AUTHOR: Couldn't you just lock the door and tell her you and your husband were not to be disturbed.

MRS. A.: We couldn't do that. She is a very sensitive child. We couldn't lock her out. She would be terribly upset.

AUTHOR: Well you have to make some decision about your priorities. I would think it is not good for Marilyn to allow her to be so dependent on you and to control your behavior in that way.

MR. A.: We'll try and work something out.

AUTHOR: Well, I would like to see you in a few weeks so you can let me know what is happening and I can decide if you are ready to move onto the next stage.

MRS. A.: That's going to be a problem for us. It's a 4-hour drive from where we live to get here. If you could see us as late as possible, I can arrange for Marilyn to be looked after in the afternoon and evening.

AUTHOR: That does make it hard for you. Perhaps we could try to find a therapist nearer to where you live, as I will need to see you at regular intervals to assess your response and discuss what you are to continue to do.

MRS. A.: Dr. G. said there's no one near us who does this treatment so we have to come to Sydney. He has a lot of faith in you and said you've helped a lot of his patients.

AUTHOR: Well we can see if you can manage. I could see you at 6 P.M. in 3-weeks' time.

Comment

My reply to the referring doctor commenced with "Thanks for referring Mr. and Mrs. A. Mrs. A., in particular, impresses me as a determined woman who believes very firmly her own views and isn't going to have them easily modified." I based this impression on her reluctance to consider any change, for example, in her handling of her daughter and the determined manner in which she demonstrated this reluctance in the interview and indeed in which she presented most of her views and attitudes. There were a number of other aspects of Mrs. A.'s presentation that made me feel pessimistic about my ability to help the couple. There were indications she was unwilling to accept responsibility for her behavior, blaming her husband for not adequately stimulating her, yet not showing interest in adequately instructing him. She was not prepared to tolerate unusual sensations, that is, those of approaching orgasm, and was prone to sickness behavior, lacking energy and in her earlier life being sick most weekends. I considered the most ominous feature in regard to prognosis was her general lack of insight in that she presented the evidence of her negativism and poor health very openly without apparent awareness that it could be revealing of underlying psychological attitudes.

In the interview 3 weeks later, Mrs. A. reported that she had enjoyed and experienced pleasurable feelings in the first few sessions of the treatment in the first week after they saw me, but subsequently she had felt "more tired after her day's work and didn't have any interest to continue" in the subsequent 2 weeks. She said, "I can often go for weeks without any interest in sex." I suggested that they might try in the mornings instead, and when she countered that they did not wake in time, I suggested they use an alarm. The couple could not attend the third interview until a month later. They had only been able to average sessions once a week due to Mrs. A.'s illness and tiredness. They had resumed having intercourse as Mrs. A. said she had not realized I wanted them to continue the treatment sessions. However, though she had no enjoyable feelings with the act of intercourse she had had no pain with it and was continuing to enjoy foreplay more.

AUTHOR: I want you to return to not attempting intercourse in your sessions, but to include your sexual organs in your love play. One is still to be passive for a half hour and the other to do the stimulating, but the passive one to say how they like their sex organs stimulated. It is O.K. for you to try to reach orgasm or ejaculate, but not by intercourse. It's important to realize it can take up to an hour or so for you, Wilma, to reach orgasm with masturbation the first few times, but then as you start to learn how to come you should respond more rapidly.

At the fourth interview after another month, Mrs. A. reported: "I have felt I was getting near to a climax with Brian masturbating me, but he complained his hand was getting tired."

AUTHOR: How would you feel about taking over from him for a while at those times?

MRS. A.: Well I'll try.

AUTHOR: Also, if it is an unconscious fear of losing control that is stopping you from coming, it might help if you act out having an orgasm when you make love—that is, if you move without inhibitions and call out and try to feel free to express high excitement.

MRS. A.: I'm still not interested at all in some of our sessions.

AUTHOR: On those times could you concentrate more on just enjoying the physical feelings and try to find activities that are pleasurable without sexual excitement, say having your back rubbed.

The couple canceled their next few appointments so that the fifth interview was 3 months later. They told me their daughter had been very sick and also there had been extra work pressure for Mr. A. Initially, Mrs. A. said they had been carrying out treatment sessions at least once a week. She felt she was enjoying their relationship more but was not closer to climax.

AUTHOR: Did you try to act out having a climax at times?

MRS. A. No. I'm sure it wouldn't help. I am a very emotional person. I don't feel any blocks about that. Brian has been getting moody at times when I haven't been interested in having sex for a while.

AUTHOR: Though you have been having sessions at least once a week?

MRS. A.: I think so. At times I've just done it to put Brian in a better mood.

AUTHOR [to Mr. A.]: Are you coming by some method—masturbation or oral sex—in the sessions?

MR. A.: Yes, usually I masturbate myself.

AUTHOR: Do you feel you can accept that as a substitute for intercourse for the time being?

MR. A.: Yes.

AUTHOR [to Mrs. A.]: Perhaps in sessions if you feel no negative feelings to intercourse, you could go ahead with it, but in most sessions still not go beyond foreplay.

At the sixth interview a month later, Mrs. A. reported her response was still variable; at times she was aroused, and she enjoyed stimulation of her nipples and clitoris but not intercourse.

AUTHOR: From now on would you try to continue to intercouse in roughly half the sessions; the other half stay at foreplay with emphasis on the nipple and clitoral stimulation. Also I want you to prolong the clitoral stimulation by using a vibrator. The "Pifco" is the best one and most chemists stock it. It has a few attachments, so if you'll just experiment with the one which seems to stimulate you best. Some women require stimulation right on the clitoris; others find that too intense and place it near the clitoris, so you need to work this out. When you do use it, be prepared at first to continue for at least 40 minutes.

The couple could not keep their seventh appointment for 2 months. They then reported Mrs. A. was responding sexually more, so that in most sessions she was sexually aroused. However, she was unable to reach a climax with the vibrator although the sensation was initially pleasurable it became unpleasant after some minutes and they had to stop. Mrs. A. added "Brian tries too hard to get me aroused at times and it only turns me off."

AUTHOR: Could you tell Brian then that it's not going to work and perhaps if he comes himself and tries another time.

MRS. A.: But sometimes when he persists I do finally get aroused and enjoy it.

AUTHOR: Perhaps then if Brian waits about 10 minutes, but if he thinks you're still not responding, but as you are getting to the point that it's unpleasant could you try what I suggested earlier, acting as if you're coming, being really excited, so that your acting in that way could incorporate the increase in clitoral sensation, so it continues to be pleasant, rather than becoming unpleasant.

At the eighth interview, 6 weeks later, Mrs. A. reported: "We haven't made any progress with the vibrator. It's really more frustrating, as I feel I get so close, then I have to stop."

AUTHOR: Did you try to act out coming?

MRS. A.: Not really. I didn't feel it would help. I felt too frustrated to try.

AUTHOR: Perhaps if you have a few drinks of alcohol before your sessions, that might just reduce any inhibitions and get you started.

MRS. A.: Oh, I get so silly even with just one drink; I'd just laugh and not be able to try.

AUTHOR: But perhaps if you had sex in a kind of laughing mood now and then this could make it easier for you to accept these feelings. [Sensing a negative response] Would it be better to try the effect of reducing any possible anxiety with a minor tranquilizer?

MRS. A.: Well we could try, though any drugs have a very powerful effect on me.

AUTHOR: Right. Continue your sessions as you have been doing. I'll give you a prescription for these tablets [Lorazepam 1 mg] and an hour before a session when you are going to use the vibrator take one. If you don't get a definite reaction, try two the next time.

The ninth appointment was 6 weeks later, in late January.

MRS. A.: We've had an additional problem since we saw you. Brian had better tell you about it.

MR. A.: I've been getting very depressed for the last month.

MRS. A.: He stole a light fitting from a shop in our local town and he's on a theft charge. Our solicitor asked if you could give him a report of his psychological state.

In early January, Brian had called Wilma during the day to confirm the type of fitting he intended to buy. After the phone call, he had the idea of taking it rather than paying for it—the value was about $40. He took wrapping paper with him to the shop to put the fitting in, so it would look as if he had not bought it in the store, proving he had planned the crime. Subsequently, I asked about their sexual life in the 4 weeks following the last interview before this incident occurred and if the tranquilizer had helped.

MRS. A.: I didn't get around to trying it. Before Christmas wasn't a sensible time with so much to do. Then we had a lot of visitors after Christmas, before this happened. Also Marilyn had to have her last injection and I didn't want anything that might make me not compos mentis. Since Brian was charged we haven't tried. I was shocked and had no sleep and since then I've been in a state of exhaustion. If the people in the town find out it will be terribly embarrassing. I'm treasurer of the parent's association of the preschool. I'm wondering if I should resign.

AUTHOR: Do you feel you were improving before this happened with Brian?

MRS. A.: I don't know whether improvement is the right word. At times I was, at others not. Of course the problem had been there 9 years. I didn't expect improvement in a few months [*I had first seen them 9 months previously*]. Brian has seemed unhappy for months. He gets very impatient with everybody, especially Marilyn, in spasms. At times it's directly related to how good it's been the night before. At least that's how it appeared to me.

AUTHOR: When you have felt improvement, what have you noticed?

MRS. A.: Brian seems to feel I respond more quickly. If I am slow he can lose interest and if he doesn't get excited it's hard for me to stay excited.

AUTHOR: But the times you feel improvement, what you you notice?

MRS. A.: Well, sex is more enjoyable, maybe not as frustrating.

AUTHOR: As Brian has never shown any tendency to criminal behavior before, I believe that his stealing could be due to stress. You [*to Mr. A.*] haven't said much in these interviews and I really haven't obtained an impression of how you feel. However, asking you to refrain from intercourse for these months could have made you angry—perhaps even unconsciously to want to punish Wilma.

MRS. A.: Yes, I could believe that.

AUTHOR: If you accept that idea I could write a report along those lines. With no previous history, I think at most you should get a fine. What do you feel about continuing the therapy?

MRS. A.: Yes, when I have settled down.

AUTHOR: Then when you are ready would you continue your sessions, only proceeding to intercourse on half the occasions. Continue using the vibrator and trying the effect of the tablet. Also, it would help me to assess your progress if you start to keep a record of every session—what you did, for how long, and your response.

The couple did not keep subsequent appointments. After about 9 months I rang and spoke to Mrs. A. Brian had been found guilty and fined $120.

MRS. A.: I was good till the court case was over. Then I lost weight and was shaking all over. For Brian, once the case was finished, that was that.

AUTHOR: How have you been getting along together?

MRS. A.: A bit strained. I've asked Brian to give me room for a while. I've got to try and get myself back again. Brian is inclined to leave things to me.

AUTHOR: And on the sexual side?

MRS. A.: We haven't had sex since Easter [*6 months ago*]. I haven't felt up to it. Perhaps when I feel O.K. we'll get in touch with you.

Comment

My failure in this case and the possibility that Brian's stealing was a potentially tragic result of this raises very strongly the question of whether I could have used other approaches that would have been successful; whether I should have terminated the treatment earlier as a failure or referred the couple to another therapist. Other approaches I could have used would have included confronting Mrs. A. with her apparent failure to comply with the treatment as evidence of negativism, that was possibly related to hostility to her husband or a need to control their relationship. This might have encouraged the husband to be less passive; alternatively, it could have made her more reluctant to report their behavior accurately. I find I am not so comfortable with a more confronting approach, and perhaps for that reason feel I do not get good results when I attempt it. The couple was unwilling for financial reasons to undertake more intensive treatment. However, I could have threatened termination of treatment unless they accepted admission to a unit for brief intensive therapy. Such techniques could have been instituted as systematic desensitization for unconscious anxiety concerning orgasm in Mrs. A., assertive training for Mr. A., and joint marriage therapy.

In fact, subsequently Mrs. A. wrote to me requesting further help, particularly with communication problems. I referred the couple to a family therapist who I believe tends to be more confronting than I am. After 10 sessions with that therapist I will see the couple for further assessment.

Without research data to guide the therapist he or she must reach his or her decision on these aspects of treatment, including their likely cost-effectiveness on the basis of intuition.

Case Study 2

Couple B. was referred for difficulties in their sexual relationship following a period of separation. Mrs. B. was at times experiencing negative feelings during intercourse. The referring doctor stressed they were both "strict Catholics."

MRS. B.: I feel if I'm more dominant sex is better but I don't like being dominant.

MR. B.: I'm tense all the time, worried I'll do the wrong thing. I feel Betty goes frigid suddenly. At times it can be devastating—leaves us feeling dreadful. We've been reading *Forum Magazine* and *The Art of Love Making* in the last few months but I don't think it's helped much.

AUTHOR: How long have you been having a problem?

MRS. B.: I've never been sure to be aroused with sex since we married 10 years ago. I knew I had polycystic ovaries and I probably wouldn't get pregnant, but I was frightened if I did something might go wrong.

MR. B.: It's only been a real problem since we've been trying to get over our great unhappiness with Karen.

Their daughter, Karen, was born 6 years ago, and at the age of 3½ years developed a cerebral tumor and died after 5 months of distressing treatment. During her illness, Mr. B. expressed homosexual feelings.

MR. B.: I think I was aware of being interested in boys since I was 14. But I had healthy relationships with girls. I always respected them and took them out to behave properly. I was a member of Catholic Youth and had a strict moral code. When our little girl was born it was an overwhelming feeling. I felt that proves I'm a man, I'm not gay, it's the living evidence. Then when she died . . . got sick . . . I felt I was responsible, I'd been punished.

The couple had come under the influence of spiritualists when their daughter was 6 months old. They were told she had a great future, would be "a world's wonder."

MR. B.: I fell for it, got lots of literature on it, I got right into it.

MRS. B.: I was never totally believing. The man was very dominant, interfering in our lives. He was a great orator. We were fruit for the picking.

MR. B.: When Karen became ill we felt terrible guilt—we thought if we were truly following spiritualism she wouldn't be sick. For 3 weeks after she died I thought I'd put that tumor in her head. When Karen was ill, sex was out. We were living with a homosexual friend to be near the hospital. He talked about his homosexuality a lot. Three days after the specialists told us Karen was going to die I made an advance to him. I felt terrible guilt. I told Betty when she came back from visiting Karen. It decimated her.

MRS. B.: I just thought Peter's very vulnerable. We had all different religions praying for Karen and it didn't sink in. Only a year later it came to the surface. I felt dreadful . . . really dirty.

AUTHOR: Had it affected your sex life?

MRS. B.: We were hardly ever having sex. But I wanted another child.

MR. B.: I never wanted to think about it. Once during sex, Betty said, "You're not making love to a man, you're making love to a woman." Then a year later she said, "Why did you approach David?"

MRS. B.: When Karen was ill, Peter started to dress in a more flamboyant way. I put it down to stress and grief. Peter coped by cracking jokes, being humorous. Inside he was devastated. I told him I felt angry and hurt. I felt my womanhood was being threatened.

MR. B.: One night we had a dreadful argument. Pressure had built up through lack of communication and we split up.

MRS. B.: Prior to that I tried to talk about it.

MR. B.: I felt guilty, dirty.

MRS. B.: But Peter didn't say that at the time.

MR. B.: I ran away. I didn't want to talk about it. I denied it.

MRS. B.: Before we separated we became involved in Marriage Encounters. We even gave talks to other couples, but I resented it; I felt we should be going out and enjoying ourselves. All our free time was going in voluntary work. Then I met a naval officer—I opened up to him. I couldn't talk to my parents or friends. I became very involved with him. I ended up having a relationship with him.

MR. B.: I'd cry alone, but I was using the marriage counseling to deny it.

MRS. B.: Peter had this thing that he had to make up for his guilt.

MR. B.: Then after that dreadful night we separated. A friend asked me to go and tell Betty how I felt. I went and told her to her face I didn't love her. After that I felt I was kicking my heart around. It was one of the most horrible things I've ever done. In the 7 months we were apart I got involved in the gay scene—was promiscuous. After I told Betty, I went off with a man, Derek. I said, "I feel we can make it together." He said, "Don't be taken in by the image." All I talked about to him was Karen. He talked about he and I spending the next 50 years together. I felt, "Oh my God, with a man." I took stock of myself. I wanted children. I had a dreadful period of depression. I talked to a close friend at work. He persuaded me on my suggestion, motivation, that we try to resolve the marriage. I approached Betty and we got together with the help of Marriage Guidance Counseling. The barrier was very hard to work through. My mind has homosexual urges, but my body doesn't want it.

AUTHOR: And in your sexual relationship?

MRS. B.: I feel "Is Peter really making love to me?" I can't get aroused. When he takes charge more I feel better.

MR. B.: I think, "Is she enjoying this, does she like it?" She feels my negativity, it puts her off.

AUTHOR: Well there is treatment to reduce the intensity of any homosexual thoughts you might have, Peter. And I think you would both benefit by learning more about how to make love to each other and turn each other on. This should make you, Peter, more confident in your approach and you, Betty, be more comfortable with being more assertive when you feel like it, without thinking you are threatening your femininity or Peter's masculinity. The treatment for Peter we carry out over a week in hospital. You receive three sessions a day in which you are trained to relax and are asked to visualize situations which might have caused you to become homosexually aroused in the past but instead you visualize staying relaxed. If this is successful it has the effect of weakening the intensity of your homosexual feelings and thoughts [*McConaghy, 1982; McConaghy, Armstrong, & Blaszczynski, 1985*]. In the meantime I'd like you both to have sessions at home three or four times a week. The sessions should be about an hour and at a time when you're both relaxed and have the time. You are to cuddle together naked, but not attempt intercourse. One is to be passive for half an hour and the other stimulates them. The passive partner is to say how they'd like to be stimulated. The stimulation is not to include your sexual organs for the first 10 minutes. After half an hour you change roles, the passive one becoming active. You can come anyway you like except by intercourse.

Comment

In addition to the problems reported in this interview, Mr. B. had rather effeminate mannerisms. Yet I felt much more confident that this couple would respond well to treatment, as compared with the previous couple. They showed concern and sensitivity to each other's feelings not only in what they said but in their nonverbal behavior, regarding each other sympathetically and at times supportively touching each other.

When I saw Mr. B. 3 weeks later on his admission to hospital, he reported their sexual relationship had improved. They had initially complied with the instruction to avoid intercourse.

MR. B.: The night before I came into hospital we had two bottles of wine. We made love very beautifully. Betty was very responsive and climaxed just with intercourse. Before that she only reached a climax with masturbation.

AUTHOR: How have you felt about your homosexual feelings?

MR. B.: At times when we were cuddling, flashes of homosexual relationships would come through. I would feel guilty, lose confidence.

When I saw Mr. B. a month later he reported:

MR. B.: Since the treatment I'm not besotted by the thoughts of homosexuality anymore. I feel much more confident and our sexual relationship is really good. Betty is very responsive.

I saw the couple a fortnight later when they had found out that Betty had become pregnant the night before his admission.

MR. B.: I feel as I did when she became pregnant with Karen.

At follow-up 3 months later the couple confirmed they were still very happy in their emotional and sexual relationship. Three months later their referring doctor reported that Mr. B. was sharing in his wife's pregnancy and their improvement in all areas was maintained.

Case Study 3

Miss C., aged 22, was referred because she "did not enjoy sex at all."

AUTHOR: Do you have any response to private masturbation?

MISS C.: No, I don't enjoy it. It does nothing for me. My father used to expose himself to me when I was 3 or 4. He used to handle my sex organs and I used to enjoy it then. My mother found out when I was 4½ and they split up. But he used to come to my school, so my mother had to call for me. The last time I saw him he came up to me at a bus stop when I was 12. I was upset for a week. I feel disgusted with my father—*hate* would be a good word. I distrust any man I meet.

AUTHOR: Do you get pleasure from any kind of physical contact?

MISS C.: Sometimes I enjoy kissing. But I feel scared if it gets more sexual. As a child I enjoyed it, but he was warped and he made me get aggressive to other people. He spoilt me so if anyone crossed me at all I was really violent. He indulged me completely, treated me like a little girlfriend.

AUTHOR: When did you start to date with boys?

MISS C.: When I was 13. I've had lots of boyfriends. They could last a couple of weeks to a few months. I'd tend to get restless before anything could develop. At times I'd enjoy cuddling, if I found the particular man attractive; some I can't stand getting near me— my flesh crawls. Men I find attractive I don't like as people. Those I do, I couldn't think of sleeping with. I find it hard to say no to invitations from men even if I don't want to go out with them. I like men a lot older than me. I've no patience with young men. When I was 15, I was attracted to men in their 30s, if they had good looks and were intelligent and kind. They needed to be physically fit. I can't stand fat bottoms.

Miss C. had not been out with a man or had intercourse for some months. Then she had not enjoyed it though she had got aroused to a certain extent beforehand. She had never experienced a climax. Miss C. said she got depressed at times and often found it difficult to get to sleep. She felt "fat all the time" but "half the time I don't care." She binged when upset and her doctor wanted her to do exercises, but she was "tired and couldn't be bothered." She had a volatile temper and was easily crossed. If she was in a good mood it was O.K. She developed a bust and body hair when 10. She said, "I hate my bust, I feel it's too big. It draws attention to me. I get yelled at in the street by some idiot." She had been living with a step-sister 4 years older for the past 5 years and feels she lets this sister dominate her. She had previous psychiatric treatment—1-year play therapy when aged 5; also for a few months when 15 or 16, as her mother thought there was something wrong with her as they fought a lot (the psychiatrist said, "It's your mother who's neurotic, not you"); when 17, for some months at a clinic, where the first therapist said, "Not everyone's trying to get up you, you know," and the second wanted to watch her masturbate and help her. She said the last therapist continued to ring her after she stopped attending and came to her house once. She continued: "I get so sick of people thinking of me only in sexual terms." She denied awareness of feelings of sexual attraction to women.

Comment

Miss C. was a very attractive girl who dressed sufficiently strikingly to be likely to attract attention of the type of which she complained, that is, being seen as a sex object. I found her manner in the interview somewhat sexually provocative; this possibly explained the responses of the two previous therapists if her report were true, as it was likely she would behave similarly in other relationships both in therapy and in normal life. Readiness to reveal involvement in what are generally regarding as disturbing sexual behaviors, such as incest, is, in my experience, consistent with a somewhat histrionic or attention-seeking personality. And this combined with her report of moodiness suggested that she was likely to set up somewhat neurotic relationships, apart from her sexual difficulties. Without this possible complication, as she was without a partner, one way of treating her sexual difficulties would be referral to a male surrogate therapist. However, most of my women patients have not been prepared to accept the nature or expense of this therapy. I decided to treat her initially with systematic desensitization and directed masturbation. Hierarchy items I used in systematic desensitization included such stimuli as sitting next to a man she finds attractive, his putting his arm around her, her feeling pleasure in response, her expressing her pleasure and excitement by putting her arm around him saying how she felt, and so on through foreplay activity to intercourse and to reaching orgasm both with intercourse and in private masturbation. Items in which she behaved more assertively with her sister were also included. I saw her in weekly sessions between which I asked her to practice relaxation four times a week for 10 minutes, without images in the first 4 weeks, but including images after that.

After a fortnight she reported she had met a male friend and had felt more relaxed in intercourse. He did not continue the relationship, and I encouraged her to cope with her resulting depression by developing new interests she would enjoy, using a pleasant events schedule to help her identify these. She enrolled in drama classes and started singing lessons. After 4 weeks I asked her to masturbate in private, giving up to an hour to the initial sessions. After 8 weeks she commenced a relationship with another man with whom she said she enjoyed intercourse but was not reaching a climax. She felt insufficient response to persist with masturbation either privately or with him. I suggested using a vibrator, but she was not motivated to do so. After two more sessions, she expressed satisfaction with her response and said she felt she would continue to improve without further treatment and was discharged. She answered a letter a year later to say she had maintained her improvement and was involved in a relationship she enjoyed. She was not reaching orgasm in sexual relations but did not see this as a problem.

Assessment of Sexual Dysfunctions

As is evidenced in the case histories reported, I consider that assessment of sexual dysfunctions in women can be carried out almost exclusively by clinical interview. The major aims of the interviewer should be first, to establish the nature of the patient's problem and second, to determine if any aspects of her personality or her relationship with her partner are of importance in maintaining this problem, or whether it can be attributed entirely to faulty learning experiences. Such faulty experiences may be lack of adequate exposure to appropriate sexual stimulation, or experiences that have caused the patient to fear such stimulation or to fear her emotional response to it.

Though the patient presents complaining of lack of sexual responsiveness or failure to achieve orgasm, in the initial interview or occasionally not until she has had a few sessions of treatment it may become obvious that the patient is seeking help for another problem. She may indicate that she is content to achieve orgasm by other means than intercourse, but her partner is insisting that she achieve it by intercourse "as all his other girlfriends did." Though having presented as a patient seeking help for failure to achieve orgasm by the act of intercourse, she may in fact be seeking support from the therapist to resist the pressure from her partner. It may be his need that she reinforce his concept of masculinity by achieving orgasm through his activity alone. The likelihood that many of his previous partners satisfied this need in him by faking orgasm could by explored with him. Women who report lack of sexual interest but resist involving their partner in therapy at times seek treatment because they wish to leave their present relationship but are guilty and require the approval of an authority figure to do so.

In agreement with the conclusions of other workers (Hatch, 1981), I have not found physiological measures of women's sexual arousal of value in assessment of their sexual dysfunctions or of their response to treatment. Nor in such assessment have I found that psychological tests or inventories add significant information to that obtained by clinical interview. I have at times requested patients who are responding poorly to monitor their behavior in home assignments, but have not found it necessary with the majority of patients.

Treatment of Sexual Dysfunctions

In treating sexual dysfunctions in women I have followed the procedure outlined in Figure 1.

Assessment and Treatment of Sexual Dysfunctions in Men

The DSM-III classification of mental disorders separates psychosexual dysfunctions in men into inhibited sexual desire, inhibited sexual excitement (partial or complete failure to attain or maintain erection until completion of the sexual act), inhibited orgasm, premature ejaculation, and functional dyspareunia. The complaints for which men commonly seek treatment are failure to attain or maintain erection, frequently termed impotence, and premature ejaculation. In my experience men who complain of pain in heterosexual intercourse often have a marked personality disorder with hypochondriacal and psychotic features and require treatment for this rather than directly for the sexual problem. In the past, men have presented complaining of pain when penetrated rectally in homosexual relationships. Therapy was equivalent to that used in the treatment of women with vaginismus. Intercourse is temporarily proscribed and graduated manual anal dilation practiced by patients or their partners during sex foreplay sessions. In recent years I have seen very few patients who experience this or other psychosexual dysfunctions in homosexual relationships. Most now attend therapists whose practice is largely limited to subjects who identify themselves as homosexual.

Case Study 1

Mr. A., aged 36, reported he had "severe impotence" for 12 months or more, "I can't get an erection when I want to have intercourse." He had separated from his wife 10 months previously, and when he had subsequently attempted intercourse with other women, he had obtained no or only a partial erection inadequate for intercourse.

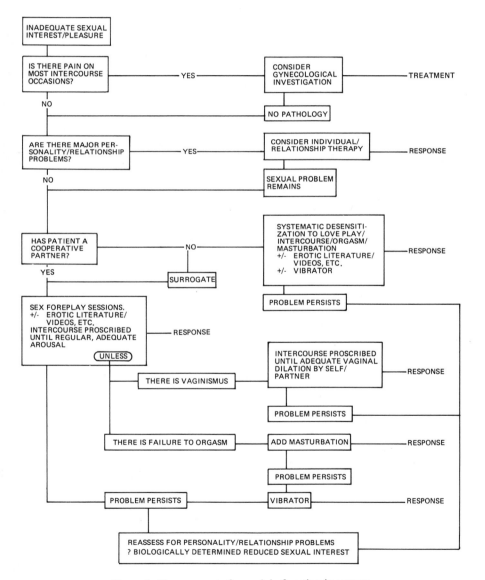

Figure 1. Management of sexual dysfunction in women.

AUTHOR: Do you wake up with an erection during the night or in the morning?

MR. A.: Once or twice a week I wake up with one, but it only lasts a short period.

AUTHOR: Would it be firm enough for penetration?

MR. A.: Perhaps.

AUTHOR: How about with masturbation, do you get a firm erection then?

MR. A.: Yes, if I come in about half a minute. Otherwise I lose about half the erection.

AUTHOR: Do you fantasize during masturbation?

MR. A.: Yes, I tried fantasies of women, but it makes no difference.

AUTHOR: How often are you coming?

MR. A.: Well, under pressure I've been going to masturbation about once a week.

AUTHOR: Do you have any wet dreams?

MR. A.: I haven't noticed any.

AUTHOR: Do you get aroused to sexual stimuli—say seeing an attractive girl, or with erotic pictures?

MR. A.: I haven't seen any pornography in the last year or so. I have gone to the beach to see if I got sexually excited—there was only a small tendency for my penis to get hard.

AUTHOR: Have you always had some problem with getting erections with intercourse?

MR. A.: No, I had a tremendous sex life with my wife. We married 15 years ago. In the first year we had sex five or six times a day. My wife had a lot of health problems. She fell pregnant 10 or 11 times in the first 10 years. We had to marry, but she miscarried then and about five more times before our son was born. After his birth she had several more miscarriages and finally she needed a tubal ligation. After her first miscarriage when she was pregnant she wouldn't have intercourse for some months. After about 5 years, I started to feel uncertain of getting an erection when we had foreplay. She never liked to masturbate me. This got worse 5 years ago. Then she returned to work for up to 14 hours a day. A couple of nights she didn't come home. At times I relieved the pressure by masturbation. Three years ago I could masturbate two or three times a night. The erection would last several minutes. Eighteen months ago I wouldn't keep the erection with masturbation. I was getting suspicious of her, she was popular, attractive. Ten months ago she walked out on me and our son. I lost two stone in the next 2 months— I became a bag of bones. But then I cut myself off, started to enjoy myself.

AUTHOR: Do you have difficulty dating women, asking them out?

MR. A.: No.

AUTHOR: Who are you currently involved with?

MR. A.: I'm seeing two girls regularly, one, there's no sex; the other, we've gone to bed several times; one occasion I got an erection, but it died.

AUTHOR: Are you both able to enjoy sex without actual intercourse?

MR. A.: The message is that she prefers intercourse to oral sex and so on.

AUTHOR: Would she be prepared to work with you on this problem?

MR. A.: I don't think so. We are friends, but not to the extent she would bend over backwards to help me out.

In view of Mr. A.'s emotional response to the termination of his marriage I sought evidence of underlying continued depression. He agreed he was depressed but considered it due to his sexual problem rather than to the loss of his wife. He found it difficult to get to sleep, but though this was worse in the last year, it had always been a problem. His appetite was excellent, and his interest in his work, sporting, and other leisure activities and in his son was strong. He was progressing well in his work and was "still getting promotions." I found nothing of relevance in events of his earlier life. His health had always been good. The referring doctor had carried out hormone investigations on Mr. A. that were normal. Otherwise, in view of the gradual onset of his failure to maintain an erection with masturbation I would have considered referring him for endocrine investigation.

At the end of the interview, I said, "Your referring doctor said you have read *Understanding Human Sexual Inadequacy,* so you will be aware that the current belief is that erection problems like yours are due to anxiety about whether you will get and maintain an erection in order to perform sexually to your and your partner's satisfaction. To reduce this anxiety it is necessary to take the pressure off you to feel you have to perform. This is done by getting you to restrict yourself to foreplay activities with a partner who puts no pressure on you to get an erection. You are not to attempt intercourse in your sexual activity with your partner until you are regularly getting and maintaining erections in the foreplay. As your present partner may not work with you, and you think she puts a lot of emphasis on intercourse, I think you would respond most quickly and best if you worked with a surrogate therapist. Surrogates professionally help people with sexual problems by working with them to reduce their anxiety and improve their ability in actual sexual situations. She will take on the role of your partner initially in nonsexual physical contact and later, in foreplay activities, but not intercourse, until you have lost your anxiety and preoccupation concerning getting an erection. You will probably need about 10 or 12 sessions of treatment with her. If you agree to this approach, I will refer you to her and supervise the treatment by interviewing you after you have had four or five sessions and subsequently a few more times as appropriate. She will also report your progress to me by phone. Present health care insurance does not cover the cost of this treatment, so you will need to pay her for each session. The last time I found this out from her the fee was $50 a session, but if you accept this treatment, you can discuss this with her when she calls you to make the first appointment. She has asked me not to give her phone number to anyone whom she has not interviewed."

The surrogate accepted the referral, and when I saw Mr. A. a few months later he reported he was getting better erections that he considered were not hard enough, but they were sufficient for penetration. The erection would weaken in 2 to 3 minutes if he did not ejaculate by then. He had become involved with another girlfriend who "accepts what I've got." On their last occasional of intercourse he had lost his erection twice but finally was able to ejaculate. He was concerned the girlfriend was getting too involved with him. He considered that his erection with masturbation was firmer and he was getting a better climax. The surrogate considered that in sessions with her his erection was satisfactory and maintained till ejaculation. She felt he had become involved with a woman very like his wife who was chasing him and stressing she wanted a permanent relationship and a baby. She intended to cease treatment in about a month. I saw him 2 months following cessation of treatment. He had broken off the relationship, "the scene was getting too much." He was taking some girls out but not having intercourse currently. He considered he was able to attain an erection more quickly and maintain it for 5 minutes or more and was pleased with his response. He would return if there were future problems.

Comment

When patients do not obtain and maintain an adequate erection with private masturbation, unless one can obtain evidence that the patient is anxious in this situation or is suffering from a depressive illness, the possibility of an organic factor should be excluded. If they are getting an adequate erection at times, for example, when awakening during the night or the morning, impairment of vascular penile flow is unlikely, but investigation for endocrine abnormalities, diabetes, excessive use of alcohol, or intake of other drugs, prescribed or otherwise, should be carried out. If no abnormalities are found, treatment is undertaken on the assumption that anxiety is causing the problem. It is possible that disuse may play a role in impairment of erection, and if the patient is not having regular ejaculations, encouragement to attempt this, either in sexual relationships or by private masturbation, at times appears effective.

The fact that Mr. A.'s partner preferred intercourse as part of the sexual relationship is not unusual in my clinical experience. I have noticed that articles in the lay press commonly state that male sexuality is excessively penis–vagina oriented, and men with impotence need not consider it a problem because many women prefer to reach orgasm by other methods than intercourse. Though this may well be correct, at least in clinical populations most women appear to expect intercourse to be an important part of their sexual relationships.

Case Study 2

Mr. B., aged 38, divorced, complained that in his 9-month relationship with a woman friend he either could not maintain an erection, or if he did, he could not ejaculate.

AUTHOR: How long do you continue in intercourse until you decide you won't ejaculate?
MR. B.: At least 10 minutes, until my girlfriend is bored with it.
AUTHOR: When did you first have sexual difficulties?
MR. B.: In the last 3 years. I had a vasectomy in 1980 and afterwards I found it difficult to maintain an erection and I was slower to come. The surgeon said there was no physical problem.
AUTHOR: What was your sex life like in your marriage?
MR. B.: When I first married at 25, for 3 or 4 years we had sex up to three times a week. I didn't have any difficulty with erections or coming. But before we split up 7 years ago, at times I found erections hard to maintain. Since then it gradually got worse.
AUTHOR: What are your erections like in situations where there is no need for you to feel under pressure to get one—with masturbation on your own, with pornographic photos, or with sexual fantasies.
MR. B.: With masturbation I might think of a woman I met, or I work with and get a good erection which lasts till I come. Pornography used to turn me on once, but in the last few years I haven't had any response.
AUTHOR: Do you wake with erections at night or in the morning?
MR. B.: Before I was divorced I might have but not often. I haven't since.
AUTHOR: Do you feel under pressure to get an erection with your girlfriend or find yourself thinking about whether you're getting one or whether it is lasting?
MR. B.: No, I just have jumbled thoughts.

AUTHOR: Well, the current theory is that anxiety is the major cause of problems with erection and normally we treat these by trying to get you to relax in the sexual situation with your partner. Would your present girlfriend work with you on this problem?

MR. B.: Yes. She's tried a lot of ways already to help me maintain the erection. She thinks I'm too tense, I can't relax enough. I am under a lot of stress.

Mr. B. had considerable work pressures and was continuing to live in the same house as his wife and children, "in a different area," during a prolonged legal settlement. His wife was denying him access to the children, preventing him from taking them away on weekends and holidays: "She wants the house, children, everything." He saw his girlfriend once during the week and at the weekend and was "very relaxed with her."

Clearly, there were psychological factors contributing to Mr. B's sexual dysfunction as he obtained satisfactory erections with masturbation. However, as he reported absence of erections nocturnally or in response to pornography, I thought organic factors might also be contributing and referred him to a physician for an opinion. His endocrine assessment, lipids, blood glucose, liver, and renal functions were normal. I then interviewed Mr. B. with his girlfriend and outlined the homework assignments of presexual foreplay with stimulation of the sexual organs and intercourse proscribed, as with the first couple discussed in the treatment of dysfunctions in women. When I saw the present couple 3 weeks later they had carried out sessions twice a week for 3 weeks. Mr. B. reported he felt relaxed to the extent that at times he fell asleep while being stimulated. Though at times he felt sensually aroused, it was not enough to cause an erection. His girlfriend commented, "Even his touch is more relaxed." I trained Mr. B. in relaxation exercises of alternately contracting and relaxing muscles and asked him to practice these at the start of their sessions for 10 minutes. Also, I instructed the couple to continue not to attempt intercourse in the sessions but to include their sexual organs in the stimulation. Three weeks later the couple reported Mr. B. was maintaining his erection for an adequate period and was able to come reasonably rapidly with masturbation. I instructed them to persist with this approach in half the sessions and to proceed to intercourse in the other half. A month later they reported they were having satisfactory intercourse when they attempted it, and I instructed them to gradually increase the relative number of sessions in which they proceeded to intercourse. At follow-up 3 months later they had maintained the improvement.

Comment

In this patient a general high level of tension may have been more important in maintaining his erectile difficulties than anxiety specifically concerning his ability to perform sexually. I find I tend to be rather arbitrary in making the decision as to whether or not to proscribe stimulation of the sexual organs as well as intercourse in the foreplay homework sessions. If I consider there is likely to be significant anxiety concerning such stimulation, related, say, to past discomfort or pain in women or to a marked need to produce an erection as evidence of masculinity in men, I proscribe it. However, as it is possible that regular achievement of orgasm is a factor in maintaining normal sexual functioning, if the anxiety is mainly related to the act of intercourse it would seem preferable that the couple does reach a climax in these homework sessions, but of course not by intercourse. Whether this procedural difference is of importance in determining the outcome of therapy would of course be easily resolved by research, but to my knowledge such research has not been reported.

Case Study 3

Mr. C., a 49-year-old single man, was referred as having "primary impotence." Recently, he had attempted intercourse for the first time and found he was impotent in that situation. He had lived with his parents, and after his father's death 9 years previously he cared for his mother who was confined to a wheelchair with arthritis and heart disease, till her death 2 years previously. He had felt happy with his life and explained his lack of sexual involvement throughout his earlier life as due to the fact that he "had so many other things to do." Since his mother's death, he "had time on his hands," and 18 months previously developed a relationship with a recently widowed woman. He attempted intercourse but did not obtain an erection on the first two occasions and ejaculated prematurely on the third. He considered his partner "had her own troubles," She was moody, very overbearing, nervous, and rather critical. He said, "It was rubbing off on me, everything was always on her terms." The relationship terminated 6 months previously, and in the last 3 months he had become involved with another woman, whom he felt was much more compatible. He obtained an erection and urethral discharge when he cuddled with her, though he had not attempted intercourse. She was divorced with a 30-year-old daughter and was 8 years older than the patient. He considered his sister was trying to break off this relationship and had been responsible for the termination of the previous one, but he had forgiven her for that.

He had commenced masturbation when about age 15 and subsequently maintained a frequency of a few times a week at most. He had no difficulty obtaining an erection that lasted some minutes. He never had a steady girlfriend in adolescence or early adulthood, as he "did not desire it." Prior to his involvement 18 months previously, he was masturbating once or twice a month with a good erection. Since then, the frequency had reduced, and at times when he attempted masturbation he did not get an erection and he desisted. He had not felt any urge in the last 6 months. He woke in the mornings with erections occasionally, but during the night noticed he had firm, maintained erections regularly. His present partner had not had intercourse for 8 years, and he felt no pressure from her to commence until he felt ready. He considered he would have no problem and had only kept the appointment with me because it was made by his doctor. I suggested that it might help when he later attempted intercourse if he immediately recommenced masturbation about twice a week and persisted for several minutes even if he did not get or maintain an erection initially. In his referring letter the doctor reported that Mr. C.'s hormone levels were normal. Mr. C. did not smoke and only took alcohol occasionally; otherwise, I would have advised him that both these activities are believed to impair erectile ability. I informed him that many men around the age of 50 did not get erections readily with only psychological stimulation and cuddling but needed masturbation by their partner as well. To easily incorporate this into his sexual relationship, I suggested he and his partner commence cuddling together naked in sessions of foreplay and not proceed to intercourse until he was regularly attaining and maintaining an erection without anxiety. If there were any problems, I asked him to return to see me with his partner.

Comment

Mr. C.'s reduced frequency of sexual outlets and poor erection with masturbation suggested an organic component was present. However, as he reported good nocturnal erections I thought a vascular problem was unlikely. His hormone levels were reported as normal, so I merely ensured that his doctor had excluded diabetes and that his general level of health and physical activity was satisfactory.

Five months later Mr. C. returned without his partner to discuss "family problems." His sister was "putting on turns" to break up his relationship with his partner, carrying out "poisonous work," spreading false rumors about them to his friends. He had stopped seeing his sister and felt content about this. When I asked about his sexual life, he said he and his partner were carrying out foreplay regularly. He was only getting an erection briefly and had not attempted intercourse. His parter reached a climax with masturbation, but he did not. He considered she was quite happy with their sexual activity and put no pressure on him to attain an erection. He rarely obtained a full erection with masturbation on his own—"Only half a one, and then I have to squeeze it at the base to keep it." About once a fortnight he was waking with a firm erection, but felt his nocturnal erections were less frequent than when I saw him last, but added that he was now sleeping sounder.

Comment

Mr. C. seemed an uncomplicated, frank, relaxed person. When subjects do not obtain adequate erection on their own with masturbation in the absence of definite evidence of anxiety, I have found that organic factors are usually present. Though his hormone levels were reported to be normal, such measures have proved unreliable in my past experience. I referred him to an endocrinologist to have them repeated.

Mr. C.'s testosterone level was low at 8.8 nmol/1. There was borderline elevation of serum F.S.H., though the L.H. was normal, "suggesting some tubular degeneration." The endocrinologist commenced Mr. C. on Depot Testosterone, 250 mg monthly, but referred him back to me when after 3 months there was no improvement. At my request, he attended with his partner, Joan. He still reported obtaining normal erections lasting several minutes on wakening about once every 1 or 2 weeks. He and his partner were cuddling together naked a couple of times a week, but his erections in this situation remained very brief. His partner showed no evidence of a negative attitude, saying "Sex doesn't matter to me, though I know it's important to Jack. It's really the companionship I value and I want him to be happy." I asked them to continue to refrain from intercourse in their sessions but to continue masturbation of Mr. C. until ejaculation if possible. A month later the couple reported no significant improvement following continued foreplay sessions five nights out of seven. Mr. C.'s erections came "up to half-mast and off again." He reported that the previous night, when alone at his home after a session, he had an erection of the shaft for 10 minutes, "but no head erection."

> AUTHOR: Well, I believe you Jack must still be somewhat anxious in the foreplay sessions about getting an erection as you get better erections when you are alone. However, your report of no "head erection" suggests there may also be a problem with the blood supply to your penis. I think almost all men when they start to have a problem with erections of whatever cause would be somewhat anxious about it. While there is a physical cause operating, it will be difficult to eliminate that anxiety altogether. So I will refer you to a vascular surgeon for his opinion as to whether you have a problem which he can help.

The surgeon reported that infrared photoplethysomography revealed evidence of reduced penile blood flow of a degree, which, in his opinion, would make it impossible for Mr. C. to obtain an erection adequate for intercourse. There was no evidence of large vessel disease or of other conditions for which vascular surgery has yet been shown to produce significant lasting improvement. I had a final discussion with the couple in which I informed them of the surgeon's findings and continued:

> Though there is this evidence that the blood flow to your penis is reduced, there are no actual physical changes in your blood vessels which can be found. So the only operation that could help at present is to have a form of implant put into your penis, Jack. The cheapest procedure, which still costs some hundreds of dollars, is to have an implant which keeps your penis rigid without making it longer, so it is capable of penetration, but doesn't remain in an erect position all the time. More complex procedures costing some thousands of dollars are carried out overseas which produce an implant you can pump up, so that they produce a more complete erection only when you need it. Research is being carried out to develop operations which could improve the blood supply to the penis in cases like yours but so far the results are not good enough. It does seem likely that in the next 4 to 5 years such operations will be developed, and if so they will enable you to attain a more normal erection. If you have an implant now, it will mean some interference with the structure of your penis, making it unlikely that you could have such an operation later, supposing of course one is developed. Despite the reduced blood flow you did get an erection of the penis shaft recently when you were on your own. If your relationship develops to the extent that you feel able to sleep together regularly and you continue your sexual sessions, you should get to the stage where you will get an erection like that at a time when you are together. If you can use that erection to have intercourse it should increase your confidence and reduce your anxiety more. Also, you could try what some couples call "stuffing." You, Jack, lie on your back and you, Joan, sit on him and stuff his nonerect penis into your vagina, using extra lubrication if you need it. Then you should be able to move on Jack so that he gets the kind of erection he is now getting with masturbation in your sessions together and with the extra excitement, possibly a better one. Again,

the main thing is to do these things only for the enjoyment, keeping in mind any pressure you feel, Jack, to get an erection is likely to take your mind off your enjoyable sensations and so reduce your excitement. So these are the possibilities at present. Do you feel you'd like to obtain further information about the operation from a surgeon who carries them out regularly?

The couple decided to do so, and I said I would be happy to see them again if they felt I could help in any way. The surgeon later informed me that they decided against the operation at that time.

Comment

There appeared to be a contradiction between the surgeon's opinion that Mr. C's penile blood flow would not maintain an erection adequate for intercourse and the patient's report of occasional erections that would seem adequate. This has not been unusual in my experience. I believe the procedures used to assess organic contributions to erectile difficulties require further validation. Though it is assumed that erections during or following sleep are equivalent to those obtained in sexual situations, it seems possible that they may not be produced by identical neurophysiological mechanisms. Some patients with older husbands have reported that they only have intercourse when their husband wakes them during the night and that their husband is not prepared to discuss the situation with them. It is possible the husbands are no longer able to obtain erections in sexual situations and are too concerned by what they regard as evidence of failure of masculinity to confront the situation. By making use of noctural erections they can maintain this avoidance.

Case Study 4

Mr. D. was a well-built man of 27. The referring doctor reported that he presented with complaints of reduced enjoyment of orgasm and volume of ejaculate for the past 6 years. The doctor's letter continued:

> Of late he stated that orgasms make him 'feel funny in the head and in the rear.' He seems to have sexual relationships in difficult situations which he calls 'cagey sex.' His lack of enjoyment of these occasions makes me wonder if he is anhedonic.

Bizarre physical symptoms attributed to sexual difficulties or concern with the nature of the ejaculate have been, in my experience, associated with nonsexual psychological problems, commonly a personality disorder with obsessive or psychotic features. The doctor's stress on the patient's use of idiosyncratic verbal expressions suggested he might show a degree of allusive thinking, as discussed in the introduction to this chapter. This proved to be the case. The patient's answers to questions were vague, imprecise, and often hard to follow or irrelevant. He apparently had some awareness of his communication problem as he gave me two notes he had written, one, a list of his good and bad features and one reporting loss of confidence and self-consciousness.

AUTHOR: What is the problem that caused you to come and see me?

MR. D.: It's in the mind. I'm too self-conscious, my mind can't concentrate on one thing. I'm always thinking . . . a hell of a worrier.

AUTHOR: Your doctor's referring letter says you have a sexual problem.

MR. D.: Well, I do have a problem in the ejaculation department.

AUTHOR: In what way?

MR. D.: The ejaculation isn't happening to the fullest.

AUTHOR: How do you mean?

MR. D.: It's frustrating.

AUTHOR: But what do you mean that the ejaculation isn't happening to the fullest?

MR. D.: The volume isn't full either . . . the build up is so quick.

AUTHOR: Do you mean you come too soon?

MR. D.: No it's not that, when I'm ready it happens too quick, I can just feel it's not right.

AUTHOR: Is it different if you come in intercourse or by masturbation?

MR. D.: Half and half.

By persistent questioning aimed at obtaining as clear an idea as possible of Mr. D.'s complaints, it seemed that when he was aged 17 he felt ejaculation had a slower build up and a fuller volume; it felt "proper." Since then, it gradually felt less proper. Asked about his complaint that ejaculation made him feel funny in the head and in the rear, he said that that was how it used to feel when it was right. "It should have a draining effect." He believed the problem affected his life-style, making him less at ease, and that it was not really a sexual problem, but was in his mind because if he tried to exclude thoughts from his mind when he ejaculated, this improved it. It was difficult to determine if he had any definite psychotic symptoms, such as believing people were trying to harm him, or hearing voices of people who were not present, because of the lack of clarity of his replies concerning this.

AUTHOR: Do you feel people talk about you?

MR. D.: People feel uneasy with me. When you speak to them you can see their face drop. When I leave it's a relief. I've released the pressure. They can sign to each other and release the pressure.

Mr. D. showed no evidence of intellectual or social deterioration that would be expected if he had been suffering from schizophrenia for some years. He was living with his parents and two younger siblings—"our family are close together mentally but not physically." He had had steady employment as an automobile electrician. He was currently having a clandestine sexual relationship with a married woman. He had a few long-term relationships in the past and claimed that he had illegitimate children in two of these. "I feel evil telling you this." He had had 9 months' psychotherapy 2 years previously that he considered had not helped him, but having reported this, he said he believed nothing could help him. He aims from treatment were to continue body building and "to settle down," that is, marry. However, his body building currently took up all his spare time, "even running I've got to limit, as it takes up time, makes you slim." He had taken up body building because

I get dead proud. I don't like to think a fellow's better than me. Like a woman watching that fellow and I feel . . . and I don't like to think . . . if you know what

I mean. That's why I took up body building . . . the physical to try and help the mental side of things.

Comment

In my experience, people with these bizarre somatic preoccupations with sexual activity do poorly with any therapy, and particularly with that focused on their sexual complaints. Nevertheless, it would seem desirable to have empirical data with which to evaluate complaints of variations in sensation with orgasm in men. To my knowledge, no data have been collected concerning such variation and the factors that influence it. I considered that low self-esteem was the basis of many of this patient's feelings of discomfort and referred him for communication skills training and cognitive therapy aimed at raising his self-esteem, but he did not continue in therapy. Other therapists may have treated him with direct sexual therapy, for example, training him to concentrate on his physical sensations, initially during sessions of foreplay and later during intercourse and ejaculation.

Case Study 5

Mr. E. was a 30-year-old man who had been married 9 years. He was referred for treatment of premature ejaculation. He reported that he and his wife had intercourse about once a fortnight, but that he ejaculated within a minute of penetration. His wife usually had a climax by masturbation after he ejaculated. He would like intercourse more often, but his wife was tired. "The three kids [aged from 15 months to 5 years] tire her out." He had masturbated about twice a week till a few months ago, but then ceased. When asked why, he thought it could have been because he was uptight about that time as they were three men short in the drawing office of which he was in charge. He felt he was always somewhat uptight, but more so in the last 2 years when he had to cease playing in a band to help more at home. "It was one of my favorite things." However, he was able to continue some leisure activities, including squash twice a week and listening to music with his wife. He had always "come a bit fast" in sexual relations, but this had become much more marked in the last few months.

I arranged to see him with his wife and assessed their relationship in the interview as basically loving and supportive. His wife felt he was a somewhat uptight person. I gave Mr. E. a brief training in relaxation and asked him to continue this at home in 10-minute sessions three times a week. I advised the couple to arrange a period of an hour two or three times a week at home when they were free from pressure. In these periods they were to cuddle together naked in foreplay sessions in which one was to stimulate the other for a half hour, and then change roles. I continued:

AUTHOR: You are not to attempt intercourse but towards the end of these sessions you can come by any other means such as oral sex or masturbation, if you feel like it. However, before you come, Mr. E., you are to get to the point of coming and then stop, three or four times in a session. This will enable you to learn to control your coming, and obtain confidence that you can maintain an erection for some minutes. One way of stopping yourself coming is for you, Mrs. E. to firmly but not painfully squeeze the head of your husband's penis when he tells you he feels it is inevitable that he will come. It is easiest if you sit between his legs and masturbate him. When he is on the point of coming you quickly put your first finger around the head of his penis, your second finger just under the head on the top of the shaft, and the ball of your thumb under the head where it joins the shaft. I'll draw it for you. Do you understand? Then you squeeze firmly, but not hard enough for it to be painful. Probably you'll both need a few attempts before you get the timing right. When you have, it will stop Mr. E. coming and his erection will go down to an extent, but then you masturbate him again to that point and repeat it three or four times. Do you both feel happy about that procedure?

They said they did, and when I saw the couple 3 weeks later, Mr. E. reported he was much less uptight and had stopped smoking. The squeeze technique was working, and he was keeping his erection for several minutes in their sessions.

AUTHOR: Now would you proceed to have intercourse in about half your sessions, with you, Mr. E., lying on your back. You, Mrs. E., are to sit on his penis so that it enters your vagina. Mr. E. is to stay still and you, Mrs. E., are to move and if Mr. E. feels he is about to come, he tells you and you lift yourself off his penis and sit back between his legs and stop him with the squeeze. Then you masturbate him to erection and again sit on his penis and repeat the procedure till you, Mr. E., have kept your erection for 10 minutes or so within your wife's vagina. The other half of your sessions continue the foreplay and practice the squeeze without attempting intercourse.

I saw them again 4 weeks later. They had only been able to have sessions about weekly, but they reported that Mr. E. was maintaining erections in intercourse for up to 15 minutes without needing the squeeze, and they had commenced to adopt other positions. Mrs. E. was reaching a climax during intercourse. I advised them to continue as they had been doing, but to return to sessions of practicing the squeeze without intercourse if there was any sign of relapse, and to return to see me if any problem persisted.

Comment

Some workers use the Seman's (1956) rather than the squeeze technique in treating premature ejaculation. The female partner still repeatedly masturbates the male to the point of orgasm, but merely desists temporarily when he says he is about to ejaculate, rather than using the squeeze to stop him. I am unaware of any research comparing the two techniques.

Assessment of Sexual Dysfunctions

The role of hormonal and penile blood flow disturbances is better understood in relation to male than to female sexual dysfunctions, so that indications for their assessment by physical investigation are easier to determine and are outlined in Figure 2 and were discussed in relation to Case 3.

I have not found the assessment of nocturnal erections by penile plethysmography to add anything of value to the patient's report (McConaghy, 1984).

The main source of information in assessment of sexual dysfunctions in men as in women is the clinical interview. In the interview, in addition to obtaining exact information about the patient's complaint and sexual activities, evidence is sought as to whether anxiety could be playing a significant role in producing the problem and whether other personality or relationship factors could be of importance.

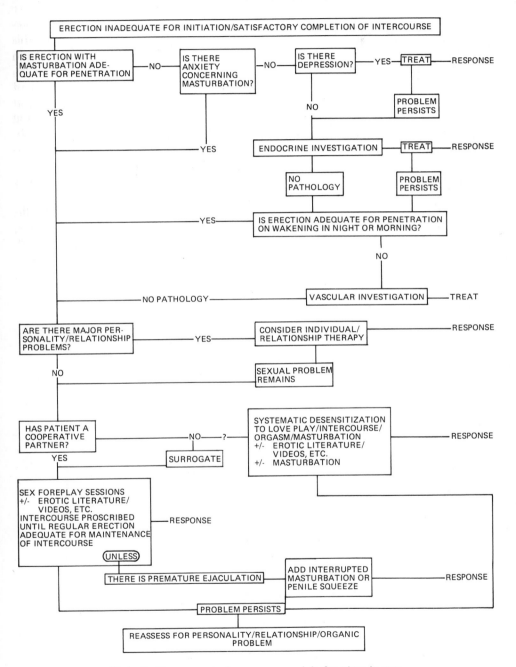

Figure 2. Management of common sexual dysfunctions in men.

In treating the common sexual dysfunctions of erectile impairment and premature ejaculation, I have followed the procedure outlined in Figure 2. As far as possible, I encourage the patient to work with his partner or employ a surrogate. With these conditions I have found systematic desensitization without a partner to be far less effective. When hormonal abnormalities are found, often their correction does not result in recovery, and the patient still needs behavior therapy.

The rather rare patients who report inability to ejaculate within the vagina and who have a cooperative partner I instruct to have sex foreplay sessions similar to those described, with the addition that the man masturbates to the point where ejaculation is inevitable and then penetrates his partner. When this has been successful on a number of occasions, I instruct him to penetrate slightly before this point and if this is successful to gradually lengthen the period between penetration and ejaculation. If this fails or he does not have a cooperative partner at the time, I have found systematic desensitization to be effective, employing a hierarchy of items of love play, intercourse, and ejaculation during intercourse. Emphasis is put on the patient's letting his sexual feelings take over, so that he visualizes expressing his excitement in a completely uninhibited manner. My impression is that such subjects, like many women with anorgasmia, fear loss of emotional control in the presence of their partner.

Patients who report minimal sexual desire without erectile or ejaculatory problems and whose hormonal status is normal, I have treated as if they have erectile problems as outlined in Figure 2. Emphasis is placed on the use of erotic literature and videos and the enjoyment of sensuous experiences such as massages, steam baths, concerts, and art exhibitions as seem appropriate. I insist they work with a partner, which usually necessitates referral to a surrogate therapist.

Summary

Difficulties in dealing with unconscious motives and relationship problems that contribute to sexual dysfunctions are discussed, and the lack of research data to guide the therapists' intuition in their management of these difficulties is pointed out. Sexual dysfunctions in women are classified, and case histories outlined of the assessment and therapy of three women with sexual dysfunctions. The first was a married woman who had never experienced orgasm and showed marked unconscious resistance to therapy that largely consisted of homework sessions of presexual and sexual foreplay with her husband. In the course of treatment, the husband carried out a minor theft that possibly related to his communication difficulties. The second case was a married woman who experienced negative feelings to intercourse following a period of separation from her husband in which he had homosexual involvements. She was also treated with homework sessions of sexual foreplay. The third case was a single woman who reported lack of enjoyment of sexual relationships and who responded to systematic desensitization. The assessment of sexual dysfunctions in women by clinical interview is briefly discussed, and a treatment outline is given.

Sexual dysfunctions in men are classified, and case histories of five men with dysfunctions are outlined. One developed erectile dysfunction after separation from his wife 12 months previously and responded to presexual and sexual foreplay sessions with a therapist surrogate partner. The second complained of erectile dysfunction and retarded ejaculation following a vasectomy. He generally felt tense and responded to relaxation and sessions of presexual and sexual foreplay with his partner. The third had attempted intercourse for the first time in middle age and found he was impotent in that situation. He no longer obtained adequate erections with masturbation. He did not respond to regular masturbation and sexual foreplay sessions with his partner, and on investigation showed hormonal deficiency and reduced penile blood flow. He considered having a penile implant inserted. The fourth patient presented with reduced enjoyment of orgasm but showed marked communication difficulties. It was considered that his problem was primarily due to low self-esteem rather than being specifically sexual. The final patient suffered from premature ejaculation and responded to sexual foreplay sessions involving regular masturbation and inhibition of ejaculation by penile squeeze. Indications for physical investigation of sexual dysfunctions in men are discussed, and the importance of the clinical interview is emphasized. A treatment outline for dysfunctions is given.

References

Armstrong, M. S., & McConaghy, N. (1977). Allusive thinking, the word halo and verbosity. *Psychological Medicine, 7,* 439–445.

Austen, J. (1945). *Mansfield Park.* London: Oxford University Press.

Austen, J. (1946). *Emma.* London: Oxford University Press.

Dickens, C. (1963). *Bleak House.* London: Collins.

Dohrenwend, B. P., & Dohrenwend, B. S. (1965). The problem of validity in field studies of psychological disorder. *Journal of Abnormal Psychology, 70,* 52–69.

Frank, E., Anderson, C., & Rubinstein, D. (1978). Frequency of sexual dysfunction in "normal" couples. *New England Journal of Medicine, 299,* 111–115.

Friedman, J. M., Weiler, S. J., LoPiccolo, J., & Hogan, D. R. (1982). Sexual dysfunctions and their treatment: Current status. In A. S. Bellack, M. Hersen, & A. E. Kazdin (Eds.), *International handbook of behavior modification and therapy* (pp. 653–682). New York: Plenum Press.

Hatch, J. P. (1981). Psychophysiological aspects of sexual dysfunction. *Archives of Sexual Behavior, 10,* 49–64.

McConaghy, N. (1960). Modes of abstract thinking and psychosis. *American Journal of Psychiatry, 117,* 106–110.

McConaghy, N. (1982). Sexual deviation. In A. S. Bellack, M. Hersen, & A. E. Kazdin (Eds.), *International handbook of behavior modification and therapy* (pp. 683–716). New York: Plenum Press.

McConaghy, N. (1984) Psychosexual disorders. In S. M. Turner & M. Hersen (Eds.), *Adult psychopathology and diagnosis* (pp. 370–406). New York: Wiley.

McConaghy, N. (1985). Learning approach. In J. H. Geer & W. T. O'Donohue (Eds.), *Paradigms and approaches to sexuality.* New York: Plenum Press.

McConaghy, N., Armstrong, M. S., & Blaszczynski, A. (1985). Expectancy, covert sensitization and imaginal desensitization in compulsive sexuality. *Acta Psychiatrica Scandinavica.*

McGovern, K. B., Stewart, R. C., & LoPiccolo, J. (1975). Secondary orgasmic dysfunction. I. Analysis and strategies for treatment. *Archives of Sexual Behavior, 4,* 265–275.

Mischel, W. (1967). A social learning view of sex differences in behavior. In E. E. Maccoby (Ed.), *The development of sex differences.* London: Tavistock.

Munjack, D., Cristol, A., Goldstein, A., Phillips, D., Goldberg, A., Whipple, K., Staples, F., & Kanno, P. (1976). Behavioral treatment of orgasmic dysfunction: A controlled study. *British Journal of Psychiatry, 129,* 497–502.

Semans, J. H. (1956). Premature ejaculation: A new approach. *Southern Medical Journal, 49,* 353–357.

Troyat, H. The Caueasus [A quotation by Tolstoy from a draft of Childhood]. In H. Troyat, *Tolstoy* (pp.109–149). Harmondworth: Penguin Books.

Trollope, A. (1967). *Barchester Towers.* London: Zodiac Press.

Zilbergeld, B. (1983). *The shrinking of America.* Boston: Little, Brown.

Marital Dysfunction

GAYLA MARGOLIN AND VIVIAN FERNANDEZ

Introduction

Despite the prevalence of marital dysfunction in our society, it is a difficult phenomenon to define. Spouses themselves do not always reach the same conclusions about whether or not their marriage is in trouble or about the extent of that trouble. They are judging the same relationship but from different perspectives, using different criteria, and having different expectations about whether the problems are temporary or permanent. Outsiders' judgments about a couple's marital adjustment depend, to a large degree, on the extent to which the spouses overtly vocalize their dissatisfaction or demonstrate their conflicts. Even those suffering severe marital distress are able to conceal their discontent in certain circumstances if they so choose. Neither clinically sophisticated observers nor the very close associates of the couple possess X-ray vision that uncovers more than the spouses themselves wish to reveal.

In thinking about marital dysfunction, we must consider a continuum ranging from benign forms of marital dissatisfaction to severe forms of marital dysfunction. Marital dissatisfaction, as opposed to severe dysfunction, permeates all relationships at some time or another. Although often a discomforting process, it is a normal part of adult intimacy. In many instances, marital discord alerts the couple to the fact that there is a problem and thus serves a growth-producing function. Marital dissatisfaction also tends to occur at times of major life transition, such as a child's birth, a child's leave taking from the home, the start of a new job, being fired from a previous job, and so on. Although these events may be temporarily

GAYLA MARGOLIN and VIVIAN FERNANDEZ • Department of Psychology, University of Southern California, Seeley G. Mudd Building, University Park, Los Angeles, California 90089. Preparation of this chapter was supported by Grants MH 32616 and MH 36595.

associated with increased marital tensions, they do not necessarily trigger the long-range decline of a marriage. If anything, the spouses may perceive that there is a logical and nonthreatening explanation for their dissatisfactions at these times and thus may be motivated to cope constructively with the tensions.

Data pertaining to the other end of the continuum—severe marital dysfunction and the dissolution of marriages—leave no doubt that this, too, is a relatively common phenomenon. For every two marriages, there is one divorce (Divorce American Style, 1983). Furthermore, because over a fifth of all marriages are now remarriages involving one previously divorced partner, the ratio between marriages and divorces may be misleading (Harris, 1981). The 1981 divorce figures of 5.3 per 1,000 population is 2% higher than in 1980 (Peterson, 1983). Since 1960, the overall rate has tripled, and the rate for people under 30 has quadrupled (Harris, 1981). It is obvious from these figures that only a small percentage of couples who experience marital discord to the point of dissolution seek therapy during the course of this process. Rather than seek assistance, spouses choose instead to terminate the marriage.

What is less clear is the incidence and prevalence of marital dysfunction among those who do not divorce. We know that, of all persons seeking therapy, a high number complain of relationship problems. Surveys of mental health consumers indicate that between 25% and 50% of all outpatient referrals are for marriage-related problems (Gurin, Veroff, & Feld, 1960; Gurman & Klein, 1980; Overall, Henry, & Woodward, 1974). Unfortunately, data on marital dysfunction among those who do not seek professional services are unavailable. It is also likely, however, that only a small percentage of the general population of distressed couples seeks therapy. Unlike certain problems that demand outside help, marital dysfunction can go untreated. Many couples believe that they can weather a stormy marriage on their own without outside intervention. Furthermore, there is the option for most couples that, if things get too rough, they can remove themselves from the situation.

Models of marital dysfunction often suffer from oversimplification. At the very minimum, a model of marital distress must take into consideration the role of two separate individuals, with their own behavioral, cognitive, and affective elements as well as the relationship between them. Some models of marital functioning focus exclusively on the global characteristics of each individual. Borrowing from the language of individual psychopathology, those models assign separate labels to each spouse and then propose that certain combinations of labels are particularly troublesome. Martin (1976), for example, identifies the *hysterical* wife and the *obsessional* husband as a most difficult therapeutic combination. Such models are limited by a static view that explains relationship problems through personality characteristics that existed prior to the marriage.

Other models of marital distress focus more on process dimensions of the interaction, for example, how the couples communicate and how they solve problems. Although this is an important dimension of relationships, it, too, can be overly narrow, assuming that all couples suffer a similar type of communication deficit. Increased quarreling, for example, often is a sign that the relationship is undergoing stress, and yet the absence of quarreling does not mean that the relationship is going satisfactorily. Spouses also can drift apart by failing to discuss and deal with important issues (Levinger, 1983).

What are the indicators of marital dysfunction? Because marital dysfunction is not a monolithic entity, it is difficult to pinpoint, in DSM-III style, a range of precise signs indicating the presence or absence this clinical phenomenon. Although we can expect a variety of personal problems and dysfunctional relationship patterns, we also can expect that the spouses will function competently in certain realms. Some couples who argue about most everything work together remarkably well as a parenting team. Other highly distressed couples enjoy a rich and satisfying sexual relationship. As Wile (1981) points out, however, individuals in distressed relationships "look and often feel ridiculous. They argue over trifles, exchange barbed endearments, sulk, and rage"(p. 2). Generally, it is the presence of the partner that serves as the stimulus for these unattractive qualities. The spouse's demeanor in an individual session or when alone for a brief moment in the waiting room can be quite different from what is observed when the partner is present. We also may find that, although these individuals generally have rational and understandable perceptions of the world, their perceptions regarding the spouse are distorted. In other words, their negative perceptions of one another (because rarely if ever are they distorted in a positive direction) are quite different from what we as therapists observe about that person. These cognitive distortions may be a function of expectations and assumptions brought to the relationship from previous relationships, of vulnerabilities and personal self-doubts, or of anxiety and emotional turmoil due to the fact that the major relationship of their lives is in jeopardy. Lastly, although the relationship patterns also take many forms, the most common and easily recognized patterns are mutual attacking, mutual withdrawal, or a combination of attack and withdrawal. In examining patterns as signs of marital dysfunction, it is important to understand the consequence of these patterns for the couple. Being either volatile or distancing as a couple is dysfunctional *if* it causes discomfort to the spouses and causes them to evaluate the relationship in a negative way.

What typically occurs with distressed couples is that the individual characteristics and dysfunctional patterns mutually support and fuel each other. The mutually shaped dysfunctional patterns elicit the cognitive distortions and the signs of individual pathology; likewise, the spouses' individual characteristics elicit behavior patterns from the partner that reinforce the cognitive distortions.

Confusion in the identification of marital distress also arises from its overlap with other intrapersonal and interpersonal realms. Marital distress has been shown to be associated with a variety of emotional and health-related concerns, most notably depression and psychosomatic complaints (e.g., Bloom, Asher, & White, 1978; Gove, Huges, & Style, 1983; Weiss & Aved, 1978). Marital disturbance also has been related to disturbances in social networks. Children of maritally disturbed couples show a greater incidence of problems themselves (Christensen & Margolin, 1981; Emery, 1982). Whether the child's problems preceded the marital problems or were an outcome of them, the two sets of problems can be mutually maintaining

(Margolin, 1981b). Marital relationships also can affect or be affected by other changes in a spouse's larger social network: that is, a change in relationships with extended family, friends, or work associates. Spouses who are maritally distressed often suffer from social isolation, having let slide couple-based relationships and not having devoted the energy to developing individual friendships. Thus, the presenting complaints of the maritally distressed client may include any one of these factors in conjunction with or in lieu of an emphasis on marital problems.

Finally, the understanding and treatment of marital dysfunction also must take into account the sequential unfolding of relationship difficulties. Couples who seek marital therapy vary considerably in the extent to which they have progressed toward terminating their relationship. Some seek therapy explicitly to avoid that possibility. These couples request therapy more for preventative than reparative purposes, wanting to nip in the bud what they perceive as early signs of discontent. Others turn to therapy as a last-ditch effort before filing for divorce. Helping to place couples along this continuum, Weiss and Cerreto (1980) offer a stepwise progression of events describing the pathway toward marital dissolution. Their model, which assumes that spouses can be at very different places along this progression, evolved into a 14-step scale, with items ranging from occasional thoughts of divorce, specific plans for divorce, discussing the issue with others, taking financial steps toward independence, discussing the issue seriously with one's spouse, contacting a lawyer, and then finally separation and/or divorce.

Duck (1984) presents another model of the progression of relationship dysfunction that includes five steps:

> (1) *the breakdown period,* when the relationship sustains its existence but becomes less rewarding because of turbulence or disorder in its conduct; (2) *the intrapsychic phase,* where one or both individuals brood and recriminate about their partner and the relationship; (3) *the dyadic phase,* where one or both persons bring their dissatisfactions into the open and adopt a confrontational position; (4) *the social phase,* where the partners consult and involve the network concerning the threat to their relationship; and (5) *the grave-dressing phase,* when the partners and their relevant networks construct publicly negotiable accounts of the course of the dead relationship and create an agreed history for the relationship and its demise. (p. 7)

Contrary to the Weiss and Cerreto model, Duck suggests that the overall progression can be reversed and that the processes that occur are not all that different from what always occurs in relationships. What differentiates satisfied from dissatisfied couples are not the actual processes that spouses engage in but their interpretations, formulations, and evaluations of these processes. At all times in a relationship, including during these five stages, partners assess and evaluate themselves, one another, and the relationship. During unstressful times, the products of these evaluations are positive but, as spouses progress through these five stages, the outcomes are increasingly negative.

These two models illustrate the large degree of variability in how marital dysfunction is exhibited. Spouses enter therapy having progressed to different stages along the continuum toward dissolution. Based on these models we see that, despite the fact that the couple may be suffering from relationship dysfunction, marital therapy may not be the treatment of choice. In some cases the couple has progressed so far toward relationship dissolution that attempts to improve the relationship would be at the expense of the well-being of the individuals involved.

The therapist's task in diagnosing marital dysfunction is, first of all, to determine whether marital problems exist. Although most couples readily acknowledge the presence of marital problems, the determination is sometimes clouded by the presence of other psychological problems that also demand attention. Given the overlap between individual and marital problems, our bias is to inquire into the strength of the marital relationship even if the primary presenting complaint is something quite different. If marital dysfunction is an issue, the second task is to evaluate the scope and intensity of the marital problems. To what degree have the spouses' lives been disrupted by these problems? How have their own personal evaluations of the problems affected their decision to remain in the marriage? By evaluating these dimensions, the therapist and the couple together can decide whether repairing the relationship is the goal that both spouses seek and whether this can be done to the benefit rather than to the expense of each participant. Specific strategies for sorting out and assessing these issues are presented next.

Assessment

In line with the objectives stated previously, this section proposes ways to evaluate marital distress with a focus on both the individual and the relationship. There are quite a few chapters and books that detail the methodologies behind marital assessment (e.g., Filsinger, 1983; Jacobson, Ellwood, & Dallas, 1981; Margolin, 1983c; Margolin & Jacobson, 1981; Weiss & Margolin, in press). Our purpose here is to identify targets for assessment and then to indicate how each target might be assessed. The foremost targets when focusing on the individual are satisfaction, stability, requested changes, and individual skills and resources. The relationship focus examines patterns of interaction that occur between the two partners. Patterns may be found in moment-to-moment interactions, daily or weekly interactions, or interactions that unfold over several months or even years.

Individual Perspectives

Satisfaction

The complexities and confusion in measuring marital satisfaction have led some to conclude "perhaps it is time to discard the global concept of marital happiness altogether" (Hicks & Platt, 1970, p. 569), whereas others conclude that satisfaction may be the most important measure of therapy success versus failure (Baucom, 1983). Marital satisfaction, as strictly a subjective measure, is assessed through interview procedures and through questionnaires. The difficulty with this measure, however, is the lack of comparability across spouses. Does one spouse's rating as "moderately unhappy" differ from the other's rating as "severely unhappy"? Rather than measure discrepancies between spouses, an evaluation of satisfaction actually measures a within-person discrepancy, that is, the difference between what a person anticipated from his or her marriage and what currently is experienced. Spouses with low dissatisfaction simply may have low expectations or may indeed be quite satisfied. As still another confound, satisfaction is influenced by social desirability and demand factors. Some spouses are not yet ready to admit to themselves, let alone to someone else, the nature of their feelings about the relationship. Other spouses, particularly at the beginning of therapy, are quite keen on communicating their dissatisfaction in the hope of getting the attention and assistance of the therapist and/or mate.

Despite these qualifications, because increased satisfaction is generally what we strive for in marital therapy, it should be assessed. Two well-known questionnaires that serve this purpose are the Locke-Wallace Marital Adjustment Scale (MAS) (Locke & Wallace, 1959) and the Dyadic Adjustment Scale (DAS) (Spanier, 1976). These brief, easily administered questionnaires have been shown to be internally consistent and accurate discriminators between satisfied and dissatisfied couples. As such, they are popular choices as screening measurements and as treatment outcome measurements. The overall score on these measurements gives a general index of global satisfaction. Therapists also tend to be interested in specific questions found on these inventories such as, "If you had your life to live over, would you marry the same person?" or "How much do you confide in your spouse?"

A somewhat newer scale is the Marital Satisfaction Inventory (MSI) (Snyder & Regts, 1982; Snyder, Wills, & Keiser, 1981) designed to assess multiple dimensions of marital satisfaction. Rather than give one measure of overall satisfaction, this instrument produces an MMPI-type profile, including 1 validity scale, 1 global affective scale, and 11 additional scales assessing affective communication, problem-solving communication, quality and quantity of leisure time, finances, sexual dissatisfaction, sex role orientation, history of family and marital disruption, dissatisfaction with children, and conflict over child rearing. Although the scales of this instrument overlap with the MAS, it assists the therapist in identifying spouses' relative satisfaction in different areas.

Information about satisfaction also can be gleaned from the interview, although here, less direct questions often prove more productive. Finding out what initially attracted the spouses to each other is one possible direction. Likewise, inquiries can be made into what they currently like about one another. These questions are best avoided, however, if it seems likely that one or both spouses will have nothing positive to say. Spouses' satisfaction also is evidenced by the way they relate to each other in the session. Do they spontaneously reveal good points about the relationship? Are there signs of mutual pleasure, shared enjoyment, or playfulness? Because couples vary considerably in the way they actually exhibit these "soft" signs of marital satisfaction, the therapist should refrain from having too set an idea about how to identify satisfied versus dissatisfied couples.

As indicated previously, stability is the dimension that measures how far along toward separation or divorce a couple has progressed. More often than not, the dissolution of a marriage is determined by the unilateral decision of one spouse rather than a consensus decision. What is more important, then, is assessing how far each spouse has moved toward divorce. Because most every spouse, at some point, entertains notions of separation, therapists' discomfort in assessing this dimension generally is unwarranted. To directly ask "How has your current marital situation affected your thoughts about separation?" or "Where do you stand in terms of staying together versus separating?" no more plants new ideas in a spouse's mind than asking a depressed client whether he or she has considered suicide. It is possible, however, that in a conjoint interview, a spouse will not reveal the full extent of his or her feelings for fear of upsetting the partner. To counter this tendency, the therapist can communicate that it is understandable, and even expected, for spouses in unhappy relationships to consider divorce and even express surprise if this is not the case.

The assessment of stability is essential in the determination of whether or not marital therapy is indeed the appropriate mode of therapy. To work effectively on improving the marriage, both partners must be willing to direct much time and emotional energy toward this goal. This generally is not possible or advisable for a spouse who is seriously contemplating divorce. It likewise is not advisable for a committed spouse who is married to an uncommitted spouse. Increasing the hopes of the committed spouse may set this person up for more disappointment in the long run. Thus, information regarding stability is used to decide whether to focus on marital improvement, on decision making about continuing the marriage, or on helping spouses adjust to a separation.

A standardized assessment of stability is found in the Marital Status Inventory, the 14-item, true-false Guttman scaling referred to previously in the Weiss and Cerreto (1980) model of marital dissolution. This listing of steps toward divorce can be supplemented by interview questions. In addition, some of the most compelling information about a spouse's commitment to the marriage often surfaces in his or her reactions to therapy assignments. Repeated failures to complete a therapy assignment may signal a lack of commitment to the marriage. Finding that changes in the marriage do not produce the anticipated positive effect may be a signal of emotional estrangement from the spouse.

Requests for Change

As a contrast to the global measures of satisfaction and stability, assessment also must be directed to the delineation of specific changes requested by each spouse. These changes, which, of course, are idiosyncratic to each couple, often become the basis of treatment goals. The Areas of Change Questionnaire (AC) (Weiss, Hops, & Patterson, 1973; Weiss & Perry, 1979) assesses which of 34 specific behaviors each spouse wants changed, whether the behaviors are to be accelerated or decelerated, and whether the behaviors are to be changed a little or a lot. The instrument also asks each spouse to predict what types of changes the partner desires. Thus, use of this instrument helps not only to pinpoint major relationship problems but also to determine whether the couple's communication regarding these problems is clear. Through careful examination of each item, the therapist identifies changes desired by both spouses (an optimistic sign for therapy!), changes desired by only one spouse, and changes desired that are in direct opposition to one another (e.g., "I want to spend more time together" is the request of one, whereas "I want to spend less time together" is the request of the other).

Delving into particular problem areas also comprises a major part of the intake procedures. However, for spouses to discuss these requests in a constructive fashion often entails much shaping on the part of the therapist. Spouses typically present their requests in a vague and global manner, stressing their dissatisfactions rather than what would be desirable alternatives. Although the expression of complaints also has its place in therapy, there can be considerable benefit to the requester and listener from hearing instead what the desired action entails. By stating these requests in specific and neutral language, they become much less threatening to hear and thus actually have more impact. It is important, however, that in stating requests, there is no implied pressure that the requests are to be met. Quite to the contrary, the therapist should indicate that this is not the time to respond to these requests. The intention is to create an environment in which the listener simply can hear the request rather than mount a defense as to why the request has not or will not be met.

Individual Skills and Resources

Marital interaction is highly influenced by each spouse's behavioral repertoires, their cognitive styles and abilities, their emotional predispositions, and their physiological makeups. The marital therapist's task, rather than assessing each of these dimensions in full, is to assess how these dimensions influence the relationship. Formalized assessment procedures from individual psychotherapy are available, although informal observations generally suffice. Perhaps it goes without comment, but it is necessary to become acquainted with each spouse as an individual. What comprises his or her life outside the marital relationship? What type of employment does each engage in, and how satisfying is that employment? In addition to obtaining clinically useful information about the skills, demands, and responsibilities required of each spouse in his or her job, the therapist can use this as an opportunity to validate the worth of each individual. Unfortunately, reminders still are needed that equal attention should be paid to the workload of the woman who makes mothering and housekeeping her full-time job; the same questions apply here as well. In addition to work-related questions, it is important to assess other activities that define each spouse as a unique individual and to determine what social support systems are available to each.

Among the behaviors deemed important to relationship functioning are the couple's problem-solving abilities, sexual repertoires, and specific skills in child raising, financial decision making, and so on. Complicating the assessment of behavior competencies is the issue of performance versus skill (Margolin, 1983c). Consider the case of a husband who is not physically affectionate. Is that a skills deficit indicating that he never learned to be affectionate or that his previous attempts at being affectionate resulted in failure? Or, is his lack of affection simply a reflection of how he feels toward his wife? Training for skills deficits offers an easier and more straightforward intervention than coping with performance deficits. Only through adequate assessment, however, can we determine if skills training really is necessary.

The cognitive variables of interest are equally diversified as the behavioral variables. Long-standing "cognitive sets" about relationships, including attitudes, beliefs, and expectations for intimate relationships, comprise one category of cognitive variables. These typically are assessed through the interview or through Sager's (1976) structured writing task. Expectations, for example, can be identified by inquiring into the meaning of a problem area. In a case where the wife is disturbed by the husband's refusal to attend church, it is necessary to determine the meaning each one attaches to that husband's refusal. The wife's view of family life may cause her to interpret the refusal as a lack of caring, whereas the husband's message may simply reflect a disinterest in religion.

Another cognitive variable concerns the way a spouse processes relationship information. Does that spouse amplify the negative side of a message and filter out the positive side? Assessment of this important cognitive process has been obtained by having spouses rate ongoing communications or else rate videotape playbacks of communication (Gottman, Notarius, Markman, Bank, Yoppi, & Rubin, 1976; Margolin, Hattem, John, & Yost, in press; Markman, 1979, 1981; Weiss, 1984a). In each of these procedures, spouses make regular standardized ratings, usually on a 1–5 scale of negative to positive, of what was just said. Alternatively, we can explore cognitive explanations of marital distress by having spouses become commentators on their own moment-to-moment communications. Simply asking a spouse to repeat or paraphrase what the partner has said may identify cognitive distortions and selective attention. Often, we find that it is attributions about the spouse's behavior or conclusions drawn from the partner's behavior, rather than the behavior *per se*, which constitute the primary problem (Doherty, 1981a,b; Epstein, 1982; Weiss, 1980).

Consideration of cognitive variables also must take into account spouses' differences in cognitive abilities and styles. One spouse might take a systematic, methodological approach to problem solving, whereas the other enjoys a more spontaneous, free-wheeling discussion. This is not an issue of one approach's being more or less effective, but it reflects an incongruity of approaches that can potentially result in frustration and miscommunication.

Affective factors constitute the third type of individual variables to be considered. Margolin and Weinstein (1983) suggest that the assessment of affect must consider the related but separate dimensions of affective experience and affective expression. The first dimension considers whether or not partners respond to a wide range of stimuli with the appropriate quality and quantity of feeling. Spouses either can suffer from (a) affective deficits, or a lack of emotional charge in their lives; (b) affective excesses, or the persistence of a particular emotion to the exclusion of other emotional experiences; or (c) a discrepancy between spouses, such that they experience vastly different levels of emotionality. The second dimension—affective expression—concerns how partners transmit to one another the feelings that they experience. Here, too, spouses may have (a) deficits of expression, in which emotional experiences are not acknowledged nor labeled; (b) excesses, in which emotional expressions are ill timed or are overwhelming to the listener; or (c) misinterpretations, in which there is a difference between the emotional statement that is sent and that that is received.

The assessment of affective experience and expression can take several forms. The most common is simply observing how spouses respond to one another in the interview. A husband who explodes with frustration each time the wife begins to speak or a wife who cries throughout the interview would be examples of affective excesses. Some spouses are quite good at making meta-comments regarding their own affective experience: that is, they temporarily can step back from the ongoing process and reflect upon what they were feeling in the midst of an interchange. Other spouses, however, have much difficulty monitoring and reporting upon their own emotional state. These spouses draw a blank at the question, how did you feel when your partner made that last remark?

A second procedure for assessing the range of affective experience is the direct sampling of couples' communication through videotaping or audiotaping conversations in the office or at home. Gottman (1979) was the first to develop a system for coding such samples for affect, based on a hierarchical scanning of facial cues, voice tone, and body posture.

As a third procedure, spouses can be asked to monitor affective experiences through behavioral records or diaries. In one case, for example, a couple was instructed to rate emotional closeness versus distance three times per day along a 5-point rating scale and to indicate what factors contributed to each rating. Monitoring procedures such as these often illustrate to spouses ways in which they are not in touch with the variability or intensity of their own feelings.

Physiological factors, which have received the least attention in marital assessment, can play an important role in the relationship. Variables to consider include, for example, general energy or activity levels, hormonal or chemical inbalances, or the presence or absence of psychoactive drugs (Goldfried, 1977). The marriage between a "night owl" and a "morning lark" can be a source of frustration for each spouse, particularly if they misattribute the source of their problems to a lack of interest in being together rather than their differences in diurnal cycles.

Relationship Perspective

Taking a relationship perspective in marital assessment means focusing on interactional as opposed to individual units. Any one event simultaneously (a) reveals something about the actor's state; (b) serves as a reaction to the other person's previous behavior; (c) is an action directed toward the other person; and (d) commands a response in return (Peterson, 1977). The key factor in understanding interactional units is to examine actions and reactions across time.

Moment-to-Moment Patterns

Moment-to-moment interactions provide the first level for examining sequences of exchange. Even in the simplest exchange, each person experiences a chain of events, including affect, thought, and action. By observing interactions, we can see how one action triggers another action, and a third action, and so on. By interrupting the process, we also can determine how actions trigger cognitions and feelings as well as further actions in the other person.

There are two basic strategies for assessing these interlinking chains. The first is "stop-action" procedures used in the interview. Having identified an exchange of interest, for example, a rapid-fire or a repeating exchange, the therapist inquires into each spouse's interpretations and feelings regarding what just transpired. This procedure not only slows down the interaction, which may be useful therapeutically, but also points out instances in which there was provocation on the part of the speaker or an overreaction on the part of the listener.

The other, more structured, assessment strategy is for spouses to engage in a time-limited discussion in which they attempt to solve a problem that is troublesome to their relationship. These discussions, which typically are audiotaped or videotaped, can then be observed by the therapist and couple together using the same "stop-action" approach just discussed. Another alternative for these discussions, used more in research and treatment outcome studies, is for trained observers to code the interaction samples. The focus here, with outside observers, is strictly on overt transactions. The two predominant systems that have evolved for coding these transactions are the Marital Interaction Coding System (Hops, Wills, Patterson, & Weiss, 1972) and the Couples Interaction Scoring System (Gottman, 1979), both of which can be analyzed for overall frequencies of specific behaviors as well as for sequential patterns.

Daily and Weekly Patterns

The second level of patterns concerns those exchanges that occur on a daily or weekly basis and are assessed by having spouses monitor behavioral, affective, and cognitive events in their home environment. Here, too, the emphasis is on identifying patterns in which one person's reactions affect the other and vice versa. These procedures can be tailor made, as in the previously given example about rating emotional closeness or distance. The procedure takes on an interactional perspective when spouses' separate records are used to determine how each partner's behavior altered the other's feelings.

The most well-known structured procedure for observing daily and weekly patterns is the Spouse Observation Checklist (SOC) (Weiss & Perry, 1979). The 400 items in this inventory, each categorized as a pleasing or displeasing relationship event, span 12 relationship dimensions: companionship, affection, sex, communication, consideration, coupling activities, household management, child rearing, financial decision making, employment education, personal habits, and independent activities. "Spouse called me just to say hello" is an example of a consideration please, whereas "spouse refused to make a decision on a significant issue" is an example of a communication displease. Spouses read through the inventory at the end of each day indicating what specific events occurred during the previous 24 hours. They also rate, on a 1–9 scale, their overall satisfaction with the relationship for that day. These data can be used to generate hypotheses about what one spouse does that affects the other's satisfaction rating. For example, if satisfaction ranged from 2 to 7 across the week for one spouse, the objective would be to identify specific behaviors that occurred on the day rated as highly satisfying versus the day rated as highly unsatisfying. The data also can be examined for congruent patterns across the two spouses. Is there a similarity in the pattern of good or bad days? What accounts for the fact that one spouse recovers more quickly than the other from a bad day? All told, the SOC contains a high amount of information that readily translates into treatment ideas for improving spouses' daily satisfaction.

Peterson's (1979) Interaction Record (IR), another structured procedure for monitoring daily interaction patterns, is based on a critical events format rather than the frequency count format of the SOC. Spouses identify the most important interaction that occurs each day and then write independent accounts describing (a) the conditions under which the exchange took place; (b) how the interaction started; and (c) a detailed description of what occurred, what was thought and felt, and what the outcome was. The records first are coded for frequencies of specific affective states, construals, and expectations. They then are examined for interaction sequences or action–reaction units, for example, mutual enjoyment, aggression, and mutual affection. This instrument, like the SOC, helps identify the repeating cycles that have major impact on spouses' day-to-day relationship reactions.

Long-Range Patterns

There also are patterns that occur at infrequent intervals, maybe once or twice a year or even less than that but that have high impact for the relationship. As suggested by Margolin (in press), problems with jealousy and trust typically fall into this category.

> The repetitive cycles surrounding these issues tend to be self-maintaining. The first blow dealt to trust in the relationship, e.g., discovering that the partner had an affair or gambled away the family savings, often is followed by an overly solic- itous attempt to correct the situation, e.g., showing extra concern, being overly compliant with the jealous spouse's demands. While there often is immediate improvement in the relationship, the long range reaction is increased resent- ment and further disappointment when the demands no longer are met. The low frequency of these events coupled with their tremendous emotional impact and the tendency for immediate self-corrective reactions present a particular challenge in therapy. (p. 4)

Because of their infrequent nature, these long-range patterns also are difficult to assess. Some couples enter therapy in the midst of a crisis that then abates soon after therapy has begun. How this crisis fits into a repeating pattern over time will be clear only if the couple is able to provide a historical accounting of similar crises and their resolution. If not, the therapist may wait until the crisis reemerges to learn about its cyclical patterning. Due to the tendency for crises to reemerge, therapists typically should be wary of rapidly resolving crises.

The SOC, if repeatedly given over a long period of time, also may provide clues into these patterns. One couple, for example, consistently experienced a difficult few days in anticipation of semiweekly visits from the husband's children from a previous marriage. The couple, although very much aware of their roller-coaster pattern, had not made the temporal association to the children's weekend visits. Such patterns seem quite obvious once discovered. Prior to that time, however, they can be the source of considerable mystery and misattribution.

As discussed in the next section on therapy procedures, relationship patterns at one or more of these levels typically are the target of intervention.

Treatment Techniques

Marital therapy is, by and large, a process of hypothesis testing. Because couples generally enter therapy feeling that the relationship either is stuck or deteriorating, one level of testing is to discover strategies that are likely to move the relationship in a more positive direction. This first level of discovery entails setting up conditions so that the couple can break away from their dysfunctional patterns. The second level of discovery concerns the subjective impact of those changes on the couple. If they begin to interact in a different manner, do they then feel differently about each other and also evaluate the relationship differently?

In most cases, intervention occurs simultaneously on the dyadic and the individual levels. Rather than beginning therapy by changing the way spouses think or feel about the relationship, it generally is more efficacious to change thoughts and feelings *within the context of changing interaction patterns*. Modifying interaction patterns provides data for the spouses to evaluate and reconsider their underlying assumptions about the relationship. Alternatively, changes in those background assumptions provide the motivation for taking larger risks in changing patterns.

Later we discuss some strategies for bringing about these changes. For the sake of consistency, we will discuss changes according to the three types of patterns presented in the assessment section. Before beginning, however, we will briefly outline some of the conditions that help to establish a therapeutic atmosphere conducive to this hypothesis testing.

Therapeutic Conditions

First, one of the most obvious, yet most challenging, aspects of marital therapy is creating a balance in one's relationship with each spouse. For such a balance to occur, the therapist must demonstrate that she or he is definitely each partner's advocate. Because the balance is unlikely to exist at every single moment in therapy, there must be an overall balancing so that neither spouse feels that his or her personal welfare is repeatedly sacrificed for the good of the other.

The creation of such a balance comes from the therapist's efforts at understanding each spouse's perspective coupled with clear demonstrations of that understanding. As Wile (1981) eloquently argues, spouses entering marital therapy generally are deprived of ordinary adult needs. Although their actions may appear manipulative or exploitative, they are feeling deprived and isolated. Formation of a strong relationship with each spouse comes from clarifying each partner's position and then validating the lack of relationship gratification that is behind those feelings.

The second therapeutic condition in a couples therapy is the need for an active, directive therapist. For the argumentative couple, there is nothing to be gained by spending the therapy hour engaging in the same types of arguments that occur at home. Although it is important for the therapist to get a sample of the couple's characteristic interaction style, it is more important that the therapy setting become a safe place for trying out new interaction patterns. To meet this objective, the therapist must be able to interrupt typical destructive patterns and then either to slow down and explore those patterns or else to examine what important issues are being ignored by the retreat to a ritualized pattern. It takes hard work to break through couples' well-rehearsed "cassettes" and help the couples to examine their problems in a different fashion.

A related objective is to test the couple's capacity for a wide range of affective interactions. Weiss (1980) recommends that the therapist test the couple's capacity for positive interaction. What is needed for them to laugh and joke with each other? Are there signs of playfulness or tenderness? In some instances, it is equally important to test for the expression of negative affect, for example, with couples who avoid anything controversial for fear that the relationship quickly will disintegrate.

Being directive also entails setting a structure for the therapy session so that goals eventually are met. As suggested by Jacobson (1983c), the structure sometimes is built into the format of a treatment session by the inclusion of rules and guidelines. If a "no-sidetracking" rule has been discussed with a couple, the therapist must consistently respond to rule violations by interrupting sidetracks and redirecting the couple to the original topic.

The therapist also directs aspects of the couple's interaction outside the session through the use of homework assignments. Rather than leave it to chance whether or not in-session progress gets incorporated into a couple's everyday life, the therapist directly facilitates generalization by making structured homework assignments. Assignments are set up carefully so that both spouses have similar expectations about what events will occur and agree to enact those events. The therapist then follows up on these assignments through a detailed debriefing at the start of the next therapy session.

A third consideration for the therapist is to recognize that the couple rarely seeks therapy before they have tried a number of solutions on their own. There is much to be learned by finding out about those efforts. Even if the efforts do not work, the spouses will feel validated by the therapist's interest in those attempts. In addition, it is often the case that the spouses' efforts to improve the situation are actually what make it worse. As Watzlawick, Weakland, and Fisch (1974) point out, an analysis of how couples solve their problems often shows both spouses engaging in behavior which they individually consider the most appropriate reaction to something wrong that the other is doing. That is, in the eyes of each of them the particular corrective behavior of the other is seen as that behavior which needs correction. (p. 35)

In such instances, it is important for the therapist to understand how good intentions can result in negative consequences for the couple. If the therapist simply labels and tries to change negative consequences, the client is likely to resist, thinking: "This therapist doesn't understand that what I am doing is for the best." More cooperation will be elicited if the therapist highlights the good intentions but then points out the incongruities that sometimes exist between intentions and consequences.

Changing Moment-to-Moment Patterns

Much of what goes on in marital therapy is directed toward changing the recurring patterns that are observed in therapy and that also characterize the couple's interaction at home. In general, the types of patterns to be changed are those that quickly escalate into rote, rather meaningless, and often painful exchanges that interfere with what the couple would like to experience or accomplish in their relationship. Instead of eliminating the negative aspect of such exchanges, our recommended goal is for negative behavior to become the stimulus for constructive behavior: that is, for negative interaction to be recognized by the couple as a signal to change their mode of communication rather than as a signal of defeat. *Communication training* is the general rubric for such interventions, but this constitutes a number of different specific strategies, some directed more toward the speaker and others directed more toward the listener.

Good listening often fails to occur in couples' communication because the listener (a) quickly tunes out, having decided that she or he has heard all this information before; (b) focuses on only part of the message; or (c) busily plans his or her rebuttal. Intervention on the behavioral level to elicit accurate listening involves training in paraphrase and reflection skills. Rather than allowing the conversation to go off on a tangent or misperception, the listener frequently checks out his or her perceptions and seeks clarification if the perceptions are inaccurate. Taking a more cognitive focus, the therapist may have the listener go beyond a passive paraphrasing of content and indicate what was the impact of the speaker's statement (e.g., "Her refusal to acknowledge my idea seemed like a rejection of me as a person"). Likewise, emphasis can be placed on identifying the listener's feelings (e.g., "The statement made me feel worthless, but I also wanted to fight back!").

Speaker–listener discrepancies can be a function of either party. Typical speaker faults include (a) being repetitous or long-winded; (b) stating discontent in a blaming fashion; (c) making demands rather than requests; and (d) emphasizing only a superficial component of the topic. At a minimum, the content must be clear in the speaker's statement. Once this condition is met, the next step is for the therapist to help the client explore the meaning of his or her statement. Does the content of the speaker's statement actually express the nature of his or her true concern? When the wife, for example, complains that the husband leaves his dirty clothes scattered around the bedroom, is that the extent of her issue, or is she feeling taken for granted and frustrated over the distribution of household responsibilities? Examining what about the dirty clothes makes them upsetting helps spouses identify their more serious concerns (Wile, 1981) as well as identify unrealistic expectations and unwarranted causal attributions (Jacobson, 1983c).

It is equally important for the speaker to communicate the affective component of his or her message accurately. Correction is needed if the speaker underplays the affect (e.g., acts as though a significant issue is not significant), overstates the affect (particularly if the affect is related to another unstated issue), or miscommunicates the type of affect (showing anger when the feeling really is one of hurt).

Due to the constant interplay between the listener and speaker, changing these behaviors actually is a change in interaction patterns. The hypothesis to be tested at this stage of intervention is whether or not these types of speaker and listener changes affect the response of the next person. What is the response, for example, if the speaker accurately states his or her pressing concern with affect that is congruent to that concern but that avoids putting the listener on the defensive? These skills, if effective, become the building blocks for negotiation and problem solving, which is the more complicated next stage of communication training.

Problem-solving skills, the aspect of communication training that has received the most attention in behavioral marital therapy, is an opportunity for spouses to apply their listener–speaker skills to a specific conflictual topic, with the objective of making long-range change on that topic. Rather than assume that the accurate exchange of information on a topic will lead to a better outcome, this training makes explicit the steps that are necessary for coping more constructively with a conflictual area.

Jacobson and Margolin (1979, chap. 7) offer a manual of guidelines for problem solving training in couples. After reading this manual and discussing the basic concepts with a therapist, couples then are ready to apply the procedures to a specific problem area. Although the procedures seem straightforward, it is a major accomplishment if a couple reaches *one* problem resolution in an hour session.

The Jacobson and Margolin model separates the problem of definition stage from the problem solution stage. *In developing a clear, well-defined problem statement, spouses are to*

1. Always begin with something positive when stating the problem.
2. Use specific behaviors to describe what is bothersome rather than derogatory labels or overgeneralizations.
3. Make connections between those specific behaviors and feelings that arise in response to them.
4. Admit one's own role in the development of the problem.

5. Be brief and maintain a current or future focus: that is, do not list all previous incidents of the problem, analyze cases, or ask "why" questions.

When deciding what action is in order to solve the problem, spouses are to

6. Focus on solutions by brainstorming as many solutions as possible.
7. Focus on mutuality and compromise by considering solutions that involve change by both partners.
8. Offer to change something in one's own behavior.
9. Accept, for a beginning, a change less than the ideal solution.
10. Discuss the advantages and disadvantages of each suggestion before reaching agreement.
11. Prepare a final change agreement that is spelled out in clear, descriptive behavioral terms, that is recorded in writing, and that includes cues reminding each partner of changes she or he has agreed to make.

There are, in addition, the following general guidelines for problem solving:

12. Develop an agenda for each problem-solving discussion.
13. Discuss only one problem at a time: that is, be aware of sidetracking.
14. Do not make inferences; talk about only what you can observe.
15. Paraphrase what the partner has said and check out perceptions to what was said before responding to the statement.

In order to follow the problem-solving rules, the couple must adopt a collaborative attitude in which problems are viewed as mutual. The earlier speaker–listener skills are essential for moving couples from a stance of "that's your problem! I can't help it if you're unhappy about . . . " to "this is our problem because it affects both our lives." If this later position has not yet been reached, it is unlikely that reasonable agreements will evolve, and it is best to postpone problem solving until a later time.

The final stage of problem solving is a written change agreement or contract specifying what exact actions are to follow from this discussion (Weiss *et al.,* 1973). It is urged that agreements be put in writing so that (a) there is no need to rely on memory to recall the conditions of the agreement; (b) the contract can act as a cue, reminding spouses to carry out the agreement; and (c) the written format, requiring signatures and perhaps a witness, underscores the significance of the agreement (Jacobson & Margolin, 1979).

As will be illustrated in the case example, an important aspect of changing moment-to-moment patterns is to have a systematic approach for teaching specific skills. Jacobson (1977, 1981) divides the teaching procedures into three components: instruction, feedback, and behavioral rehearsal. *Instruction* refers to the way that the therapist actually imparts information about what is necessary for effective communication. This might be accomplished through written materials (e.g., the Jacobson and Margolin problem-solving manual) or through roleplayed demonstrations in which the therapist takes the place of one of the spouses. *Behavioral rehearsal* refers to the actual practicing of specific skills: for example, repeated trials that get closer and closer to expressing exactly what is on one's mind. *Feedback* is, of course, a crucial component of that behavioral rehearsal with the spouses as well as the therapist all participating in that process. Although reinforcement from the therapist is quite powerful in refining the spouse's interaction (e.g., "That was a great brainstorming idea"), constructive suggestions and prompts also are necessary (e.g., "I was confused by the fact that you agreed to go along with her idea but at the same time looked furious"). An equally powerful type of feedback comes from the spouses themselves. Watching themselves on videotape, for example, increases spouses' awareness of themselves as communicators and of their impact on one another. It is this repeated process of trying out and observing new transactions rather than abstract discussion of transactions that ultimately leads to change.

Changing Daily Patterns

The second major type of intervention, directed toward the home setting, involves both reducing undesirable patterns and also introducing new desirable transactions. Although we present several predominant strategies that have evolved to meet these objectives, the actual range of options is limitless.

Behavior Exchange

In the early days of behavioral marital therapy, behavioral exchange simply meant that each spouse made a request of the other, which was then met through a quid pro quo type of exchange (Rappaport & Harrell, 1972; Stuart, 1969). In other words, each spouse would agree to the other's request contingent upon having his or her own request met in return. Although the exchanges generally would be implemented, there did prove to be some problems with this approach. First, spouses often made external rather than internal attributions (e.g., "She or he did it just because I asked . . . or just because it was agreed upon on therapy . . . or just to receive his or her own request in return"). "Wanting to please the spouse" was rarely the attribution that was made. Second, the research data began to indicate that distressed, compared to nondistressed, couples already relied more heavily on contingency control. As Jacobson and Moore (1981) point out, it may be self-defeating to have distressed couples use contingency exchanges more extensively.

In view of these problems, a new format for behavior exchange procedures evolved whereby spouses were given considerably more latitude in choosing how they wanted to please the partner. In other words, the exchange is determined by the giver rather than by the recipient. Givers, however, often are caught in the bind of doing something that they think is pleasing only to have it unappreciated by the spouse. To avoid this unfortunate outcome, spouses must carefully analyze what, in their own behavior, has an impact of the partner. Jacobson (1981) described how the SOC may be adopted for this purpose. Discussion of the SOC in the session can be directed to determining what each spouse does that makes the partner satisfied or dissatisfied with the relationship. Spouses also can examine each other's

SOC forms to generate their own hypotheses about what they can do to increase the partner's satisfaction.

The agreement made in the therapy session is that, during the upcoming week, each spouse will devote energy toward increasing the partner's overall satisfaction. According to Jacobson (1983):

> As task directives become less specific and client options become broader, the likelihood that subsequent changes will be well-received is maximized. Consider a husband who chooses to fulfill the assignment by being more affectionate. The wife leaves the previous therapy session without knowing what to expect from him during the coming week. He has not been asked to be more affectionate, nor has he committed himself in advance to increased affection. Rather, both from the perspective of the wife and in reality, he is choosing to be affectionate. An external attribution which would neutralize the reinforcing impact of his behavior is unlikely. (p. 9)

Weiss *et al.* (1973), Stuart (1980), and Margolin and Weinstein (1983) instigate similar interventions with their respective "love days," "caring days," and "consideration" interventions, which are prespecified times for spouses to increase the number of pleasing actions that they emit. Stuart has couples contract to provide a certain number of desired behaviors each day. The giver is to choose these requests from a larger list of what would be pleasing. Weiss's procedure calls for dramatic increases of pleasing actions: that is, doubling one's usual rate on a certain day of the week. Margolin and Weinstein's procedure asks spouses to show more consideration at least once a day and to keep a record of these actions. In debriefing this task, the giver rather than the receiver reports on what has been done.

Shared Pleasures

Sometimes, rather than have spouses doing activities for one another, the intervention of choice is to have spouses engage in mutually rewarding experiences. These strategies are designed to increase intimacy and to put the couple in touch with good things that can occur in marriage. Stuart (1975), for example, has couples reevoke core symbols, which are events, places, rituals, or objects that have special meaning in terms of the couple's relationship. These symbols, such as special celebrations, going to favorite places, and resurrecting long-time private jokes, help the spouses experience one another in ways that may have been buried under layers of hostility and discouragement (Liberman, Wheeler, de Visser, Kuehnel, & Kuehnel, 1980). For couples with devitalized relationships, therapy can be directed toward developing mutually enjoyable shared activities that may serve as new core symbols. One such strategy is to have couples engage in an activity that sounds like fun but is something they never quite imagined themselves doing. The more novel and even risky the situation, the more likely that the couple will be jarred out of their typically dreary or conflictual interactions (Margolin, 1983a).

Thus far we have presented a number of action-oriented interventions designed to change daily patterns. With each intervention, the couple is challenged to experiment with interactions that are more positive than what currently is occurring. The therapeutic question being asked is whether doing more positive activities creates more positive feelings in the spouses. The feelings generated by these interventions do not replace the hostility and pain but tend to make positive feelings more salient as well as to minimize distorted perceptions about how the relationship is overwhelmingly negative.

Positive Tracking

Although some couples respond well to the actions-speak-louder-than words approach, others benefit more from positive attention paid to what already is happening. *Positive tracking* exercises are designed to undo the taken-for-granted attitude that characterizes many long-term relationships. The SOC, once again, offers one possibility. Analyzing data collected through this instrument increases spouses' awareness about what pleasing activities go on in the relationship. A second strategy that appears quite simple but that we have found to be very useful is the use of "appreciation notes." Through the daily exchange of written messages, spouses inform each other what they have welcomed and enjoyed in each other during that day. Writing rather than verbalizing the messages proves to be very important. Spouses tend to be more thoughtful and careful about what they put in writing. A written note also provides the concrete evidence that, in fact, the appreciation has been expressed. Spouses occasionally get quite creative with how and where they write these notes. One woman surprised both her husband and the therapist by writing one of her notes on her thigh and revealing the message to him while they were out for dinner.

Decreasing Ritualistic Negative Exchanges

Although there has been considerable attention paid to increasing positive exchanges, the restructuring of daily interaction also can be directed to negative patterns. The first step is the identification of repeating negative cycles, of which, in most instances, couples are painfully aware. Detailed observation and exploration are needed, however, when couples are not aware what exact stimuli trigger those cycles. At what point did you start to feel irritated? What did you observe and what were you thinking at that time? To change the overall pattern, spouses need to be aware of exactly what expectations each one brings to the situation. Rather than discounting the expectations, they must be dealt with in a realistic way.

Escalating negative interaction patterns can be changed if very early stimuli that set the sequences into motion become cues for a more positive interaction. For example, it is very common for negative patterns to occur when partners get together at the end of the day. In Wile's (1981, p. 6) portrayal of this meeting, each partner may have had a difficult day and may be "looking forward to this meeting with the fantasy that the partner will compensate for these difficulties." The reality that typically awaits these spouses, however, is a hectic household with multiple demands placed on each spouse and little time to attend to or comfort the other. Changing this pattern means developing a new series of events to follow from the initial greeting. If the couple decides that what they really need is a few minutes just by themselves, they then must orchestrate what happens with the rest of the household (e.g., "What are the children doing?" "Can dinner preparations wait?"). Alternatively, they may decide to postpone their few private moments until the children are in bed. Having that as a goal eliminates the repeated disappointment of not being cared for earlier. With this solution, they still might experience a perfunctory initial greeting, but at least the attribution will be different (e.g., "Things sure are hectic now, but we'll make time for each other later"). Couples who have conflicting needs for closeness versus distance at the end of a long day must plan accordingly with a clear demarcation between time that is private and time that is shared.

Changes in Long-Term Patterns

Changing long-term patterns follows a strategy very similar to changing the negative daily interactions. However, the infrequency with which the patterns repeat makes it more difficult to identify the point at which the negative escalation actually begins. By *long-term patterns* we mean situations that periodically escalate to crisis proportions. Couples' attempts to avoid dealing with these issues altogether often account for both the long periods of quiescence as well as the high-amplitude escalations. Issues of trust, for example, either over extramarital affairs or gambling away the family's savings, tend to fit this pattern: the initial action or perceived action that shakes the foundation of trust in the relationship may be followed by an overly solicitous action to repair some of the damage done to the relationship. However, if the issue is not fully resolved, a background of tension, resentment, and possibly deceit lingers on, providing an atmosphere that is ripe for another escalation (Margolin, 1981a). The perpetuation of these cycles involves both partners. One spouse may transgress a relationship rule but the other partner's response, which typically includes either guilt, withdrawal, or excessive demands, only compounds the problem.

Disruption of these patterns first involves learning what spouses currently are doing to cope and then evaluating whether, in some fashion, they inadvertently exacerbate the problem. A couple who believed that the only way to avoid conflict was to see very little of each other had scheduled their work shifts so that days went by with no contact. What resulted was that, without an opportunity for consultation, each spouse was forced to make independent decisions regarding the children and the household. More often than not, the other objected to the decision. Thus, the strategy of limited contact, rather than being a benefit, was a disadvantage. The same couple also believed that they were happiest on days when they were apart and, thus, rarely gave themselves the luxury of a relaxed day together. As it turned out, the days they did spend together during the course of therapy proved to be quite pleasant and contradicted their mutually accepted assumption.

Challenging spouses to give up what they believe to be the best solution to the problem is not easily accomplished and takes very careful direction on the part of the therapist. Interventions tend to work best when they include both a cognitive and behavioral change on the part of both spouses. Thus, the spouse who works hard to control his or her anger but periodically explodes anyway can be encouraged to express rather than conceal low-intensity anger. Permission, or in fact, instruction to express the anger will lessen the likelihood of major blowups. The other spouse also may conceal important feelings, thinking this is the way to avoid provoking the first partner. More direct expressions of feeling, rather than this protective, condescending stance would be an improvement for this partner. For this intervention to be instigated, the couple first would have to entertain the idea that withdrawal is not necessarily the best solution. Then, for the couple actually to experiment with a new pattern would require specific training in the constructive expression of feelings.

Changes in long-range patterns are difficult to evaluate because it takes some time to determine whether or not the intervention has been effective. Effectiveness would be demonstrated, however, if dealing with the problem area in a more immediate and straightforward fashion avoids the larger, more damaging negative escalation.

Limitations of Treatment Procedures

The procedures just described partially reflect the traditional behavioral marital approach, but they also reflect attempts of the authors and others to expand upon and to correct some of the limitations of that model (e.g., Jacobson, 1983b,c; Jacobson, Berley, Newport, Elwood, & Phelps, in press; Margolin, 1981a, 1983b, in press; Margolin & Weinstein, 1983; Revenstorf, 1984; Weiss, 1984b). The predominant differences between what is presented here from the more standardized behavioral model are (a) the emphasis on affect alone as well as affective cognitive behavioral linkages; (b) flexibility in ordering and sequencing of therapy steps; and (c) attention to patterns as opposed to discrete behaviors. The approach attempts to integrate the behavioral approach with nonbehavioral approaches, such as systems, ego analytic, and psychoanalytic models (e.g. Segraves, 1982; Watzlawick *et al.*, 1974; Wile, 1981).

Relationship of Assessment to Treatment

As argued elsewhere (e.g., Margolin & Jacobson, 1981), the primary reason for doing a careful assessment is to obtain information that directs our treatment efforts. Answers to assessment questions should be associated with the decision to implement certain procedures as well as to rule out other procedures. These types of decisions, however, presume a basis for predicting what type of treatment strategies are effective with what types of couples. This matching, unfortunately, has not been addressed.

The way marital therapy actually has been carried out reflects the therapist's theoretical orientation more than the particulars of a given case. Therapists tend to assess only what fits with their particular treatment model and then to treat only what they assess. What evolves from this undifferentiated approach to treatment is that a given therapist does very similar types of interventions with widely divergent types of couples. Behavior marital therapy, in particular, has had a tradition of attempting to develop a programmatic approach to therapy: that is, a standard set of procedures and a consistent ordering of those procedures. Implementing a programmatic treatment means that assessment plays only a minimum role in the treatment planning for a given couple. Other theoretical models, although less oriented toward a programmatic approach, in reality, are just as likely to advocate one particular type of intervention to the exclusion of others. As Becvar, Becvar, and Bender (1982) point out:

> Any theory is circular in that its assumptions and concepts guide feelings and actions which logically follow from its basic premises. Such actions tend to confirm the fundamental assumptions and concepts of the theory. (p. 388)

The major problem facing marital therapists is the lack of a typology for identifying types of marital dysfunctions. Despite the diversity of couples seen in marital therapy, we do not have a system for categorizing couples nor a common language for describing the differences. The best we have done is to describe couples on the basis of their presenting complaints. This is a start, but it still does not fulfill the need for a typology of interactional styles. An outcome study by Bennum, as reported in Bennum, Margolin, and Christensen (1983), found that the following four presenting complaints did not respond to standard behavioral marital therapy: jealousy, dependence/independence, individual psychopathology, care and nonsexual affection. According to Bennum, problems requiring affective change more than behavioral change were less responsive to behaviorally oriented treatment. The question still to be tested, however, is whether problems of affect are successfully treated with interventions that directly focus on that dimension. The effects of more affectively oriented therapies, either by behaviorally oriented therapists or by others, have yet to be subjected to the same degree of scrutiny as strictly behavioral or even behavioral/cognitive therapies.

Focus on Change

A predominant characteristic of the standardized behavioral models is the emphasis on change. This still is true, although to a lesser degree, of the model just presented. In some respects, this represents an optimistic approach because it suggests that relationships can and do change (Bennum *et al.*, 1983). It is important to point out, however, that change is not the goal in all marital therapy cases. Some couples request therapy strictly for decision-making purposes (e.g., Should they stay together? Is this a good time to have children?). Others enter therapy with problems that are not amenable to an action-oriented approach. A direct clash in values, for example, over whether or not to have children or whether or not to have a monogamous marriage, does not lend itself to a hypothesis-testing approach in which one or more solutions are implemented and then examined for their varying impact.

Clashes on core issues as well as on some less significant issues illustrate the limitations of a model built on negotiation and compromise. The outcome of compromise, in some instances, is that neither partner is satisfied with the solution (Wile, 1981). One could argue that dissatisfaction with a compromise means that the optimal negotiation has not yet been reached. Alternatively, we argue that, in certain cases, the optimal solution simply is acceptance of the spouse as she or he is. Some of the predominant characteristics that a spouse brings to a relationship, such as the need for distance, can be slightly modified but probably never to the point that satisfies his or her partner. The important intervention in this case is an understanding and acceptance of this characteristic coupled with a reinterpretation of its meaning (i.e., it is not a sign of rejection).

Couples also may present long-term despair over an incident that is long finished but that cannot be undone, for example, an affair or a decision that resulted in the loss of a significant amount of money. Although never able to accept such an incident, spouses need to decide whether they want to accept the current relationship and not do it further damage. The primary agenda for therapy is addressing, understanding, and possibly coming to terms with the core issue. After that, a change strategy, such as reevoking positive events, might be in order.

Last, it should be noted that the action-oriented approach of behavioral marital therapy may reflect subtle but nonetheless powerful sex role biases (Jacobson, 1983a; Margolin, Talovic, Fernandez, & Onorato, 1983). The skills training that is done, particularly in problem solving, relies more on rational than emotional processes. This, of course, reflects a stereotypically masculine rather than feminine approach. In doing skills training, we also may overlook the fact that, due to sex role conditioning, spouses may not give themselves permission to emit certain types of behaviors. Rather than a skills deficit, what may be lacking is self-permission on the part of women to express their desires assertively and, on the part of men, to acknowledge and express their feelings. Gurman and Klein (1983) further point out that the tendency in behavioral marital therapy to accept requests at face value, to make them highly specific, and to deal with them on a one-by-one basis may result in our overlooking an underlying theme of the requests, such as sex role conflict. This is one of the reasons that the approach presented here recommends exploring the *meaning and impact* of spouses' complaints.

Increasing Intimacy

In a previous article (Margolin, 1983b), one of us argued that there are important aspects of intimacy that have been neglected in behavioral marital therapy: namely playfulness and passion. Our discussion here of daily interaction patterns focused to a large extent on increasing couples' positive exchanges with the goal being for couples to become involved in mutually enjoyable, recreational activities. These strategies, although fostering a formalized type of positive interaction, do not fulfill couples' hopes for spontaneous intimate play. Spontaneous play, which, according to Betcher (1981), is the aspect spouses would most miss if their relationship ended, consists of "idiosyncratic forms of playfulness that evolve over time in an intimate dyad, such as private nicknames, shared jokes and fantasies, and mock fighting" (p. 13). It is a contradiction of terms to plan for this type of interaction. However, it is possible that the predominantly instructional approach of behavioral marital therapy would be enhanced "by bringing spontaneity, humor, and exaggeration into the therapy session and by challenging the couples' own creativity through subtle suggestions or paradoxical directions" (Margolin, 1983b, p. 67). Most likely, this dimension already is incorporated into the style of some behavioral marital therapists and may even account for some of the variance in outcome across therapists and couples.

The intense emotion of passion, as distinct from the more bland feeling of liking, is another dimension often desired by spouses but overlooked in therapy (Margolin, 1983b). Based on an informal survey by Jacobson (1983b), most marital therapists do not anticipate increased passion to be an outcome of therapy. If anything, therapists espouse a pragmatic stance, maintaining that passion is a transient phenomenon associated with the beginning phases of marriage. The problem, however, is that therapists may too readily dismiss such desires on the part of spouses and thereby overlook the possibility of a realistic expression of those desires (Wile, 1981). Some spouses are quite aware that their idealized notions of passion cannot be met. Nonetheless, addressing these issues may relieve some of the unspoken pressures and may lead to a better understanding between spouses.

Evaluating Successful Outcome

Estimates of the effectiveness of behavioral marital therapy range considerably from slightly over 50% (Jacobson, Follette, Baucom, Hahlweg, & Margolin, 1984) to 90% (Liberman, Wheeler, & Kuehnel, 1983). Jacobson *et al.* indicate that slightly more than one-third of the couples receiving treatment changed from a "distressed" to a "nondistressed" status. In about 40% of the improved couples, positive changes were confined to one spouse.

These data, which are based on highly standardized models of behavioral marital therapy, reflect some of the issues in measuring change. Is it our goal for distressed couples to become more like nondistressed couples? On the one hand, this constitutes a fairly ambitious goal. Perhaps it is sufficient for couples simply to improve from where they began rather than to change to nondistressed status. On the other hand, change to nondistressed status also may be somewhat of a misguided goal. Using typical relationships as the standard of comparison or as the basis of formulating treatment targets means relying on culturally dominant or traditional conceptualizations of intimate relationships (Gurman & Klein, 1983).

A second issue concerns whether we anticipate change on the part of both spouses. Only recently have recommendations been made that, rather than using average couple scores, it may be better to examine outcome data separately for husbands and wives (Baucom, 1983; Jacobson, Follette, & Ellwood, 1984) or to examine difference scores (Baucom & Mehlman, 1984). As Jacobson *et al.* (1984) suggest, perhaps the most important information comes from improvement data on the more distressed spouse, which is concealed with our current procedures. Considerable discussion and debate on these issues currently is underway. Hopefully, attention to these issues will result in recommendations that help us examine couples' variability in response to therapy and that eventually teach us how to match treatment and client variables.

Case Description

The following case was chosen for presentation for a variety of reasons. First, the presentation of complaints was complicated by the fact that there were child problems as well as marital problems. Second, the case was part of a treatment project so that outcome data were available. Third, the case is a good illustration of how certain procedures work better than others for a given couple.

The case was seen as part of the University Family Studies Project,[1] which provides treatment to multiproblem families, who according to interview impressions and self-report measures, demonstrated distress in both the family and marital domains. All families receive both marital and family therapy but random assignment is used to determine the sequencing of these two types of therapies. This family, the W.'s, first were seen for 12 weeks in family therapy and then for 12 weeks in marital therapy.[2] Assessment data were collected at pretreatment, after family therapy, and after marital therapy. After a brief overview of the family therapy, we will focus in depth on the marital therapy.

David and Doris were referred to the clinic by Doris's brother who was concerned about his sister's impatience with her youngest child, Bob. In the initial telephone call, Doris promptly took responsibility for the family problems, claiming that she was responding uncontrollably to her son's tantrums and noncompliance by occasionally hitting him and frequently yelling and crying. She further reported that she relied heavily on her husband to control the child. Doris keenly portrayed her desperation and motivation for therapy, even lying about her son's age so that the family would qualify for this particular treatment project.

Doris and David had been married 3½ years; this was David's first and Doris's second marriage. David, age 32, not having completed high school, worked for the past 16 years in a factory. Doris, age 29, had 2 years of college and currently was a full-time mother.

For the initial session, David dressed elegantly in a three-piece suit and smoked a pipe. Doris, on the other hand, came across somewhat disheveled, in baggy jeans and a smocked blouse, and wearing dark glasses that she never removed. Doris also appeared to be "high" on drugs, which later was verified. The oldest child, Betty, age 6, was Doris's daughter from a previous marriage. She presented as a quiet child but actively responded to her mother's crying by touching and caressing her in apparent gestures of comfort. Bob, age 2½, was quite active, frequently distracting the family and making himself the focus of attention. Doris's attempts at repri-

[1]The University Family Studies Project (Grant MH 32616) was codirected by A. Christensen at the University of California, Los Angeles, and G. Margolin at the University of Southern California.
[2]The second author served as therapist under the supervision of the first author. Names and identifying information on this family have been altered to protect their anonymity.

manding Bob were unsuccessful, whereas David could elicit compliance with merely a stare.

The couple presented Doris as the "identified patient," agreeing that she suffered from drug and alcohol overuse, depression, hyperirritability with the children, and difficulty communicating in the marriage. Despite her full load of responsibilities at home, Doris spent approximately 10 hours per day lying on the couch, either watching television or sleeping, and she averaged four marijuana joints per day. Doris's MMPI profile further supported this picture of someone "crying for help." Her elevations on eight of the nine clinical scales portrayed her as depressed, anxious, rebellious, and with a high number of somatic complaints. David's MMPI profile also was suggestive of depression and of a tendency to be rebellious.

Indices of marital adjustment showed more dissatisfaction on the part of Doris than David. DAS measurements of marital satisfaction revealed scores of 73 for Doris and 88 for David; both of these are considerably below cutoffs indicative of marital distress. A total couple AC score of 41 was similarly well into the distressed range. Areas identified by both spouses as needing change included more interesting conversations, more appreciation, more expression of emotion, less arguing, and more discipline for the children. Doris revealed more dissatisfaction with David on these questionnaires than she did in the interview session. In addition to wanting more assistance around the house, she was angry with David for having to work nights.

Family Therapy

The primary treatment goal for family therapy was to improve Doris's and David's parenting skills. This was accomplished by instructing them to monitor target behaviors, to use time-out to extinguish undesired behaviors such as tantrums, and to use behavioral charting and reinforcement to increase desired behaviors. The secondary goal, also accomplished through these procedures, was for both parents (but primarily Doris) to feel that they had more control over the children's behavior. The structure of these procedures coupled with tremendous support and encouragement on the part of the therapist helped Doris function contingently and effectively. Relevant to the marital intervention that was to follow, Doris began to exhibit a sense of competence and initiative as she gained control of the children. She stopped spending time during the day lying on the sofa. Her marijuana use also decreased although it was not eliminated, and even her physical appearance improved. By the end of this phase of treatment, she was developing treatment programs on her own with little advice from the therapist. David cooperated with the treatment strategies, particularly in implementing time-out, but his impact was felt most strongly in supporting Doris's efforts.

Results from the family intervention indicated that the children's tantrums decreased and their compliance with chores increased. The children seemed pleased with the charting and reinforcement system and particularly with the positive attention they were receiving from their mother.

The family intervention did not have much impact on the W.'s marital relationship, however. Their overall AC score (39) remained unchanged, indicating that there was an equivalent number of marital complaints before and after the child treatment. David's DAS score (78) indicated decreased marital satisfaction, whereas Doris's (71) remained approximately the same from pretreatment. As contrasted with the questionnaire data, the couple reported somewhat more energy in their marriage, as exhibited in increased sexual activity. Although the family intervention certainly did not resolve their marital problems, it may have created an atmosphere that was more conducive for working on these problems.

Marital Therapy

Based on their formal assessment data and their work in family therapy, several general goals had been set for marital therapy. First, communication skills were needed to improve both their affective expression and their problem-solving skills. Second, there was a need for more structure and routine in this couple's lives to help them avoid miscommunications about what was expected of one another. Third, more positive interaction was desired because this had waned in the face of repeated frustrations and difficulties in coping. Fourth, there was an unspoken need for a greater sense of security in the relationship. Both spouses desperately wanted the relationship to continue but doubted their own abilities to keep it intact.

Unfortunately, there was an unforeseen month-and-a-half lapse between the end of family therapy and the beginning of marital therapy. The primary reason for this delay was a crisis surrounding David's work. Despite his seniority at his job, David was part of a large-scale layoff. His initial response to this devastating situation was a thorough job search, which resulted in an offer as a traveling salesman. David was shattered, however, when Doris vehemently objected to this job on the grounds that it would take him away from the family. During a several week "cooling-off" period, David withdrew from Doris and from therapy. Thus, when this couple returned to therapy to begin working on the marriage, they were in crisis. Both appeared for that session looking depressed, unkempt, and having gained weight.

The therapeutic dilemma at the first marital session was whether to focus on the job crisis or whether to begin interventions toward more long-range goals for this couple. Focusing on the crisis was what they had done for the past month and, to some degree, they were comfortable with this. However, because there were no easy answers to that situation, the decision was to engage them in something that would have a more immediate impact. The first session followed the Jacobson and Margolin (1979) format for a relationship history, with the objective being to improve the tone of the couple's interaction. As hoped, this exercise elicited laughter and warmth and reminded this couple of the tremendous sexual and emotional attraction that they experienced at the beginning of their relationship.

This theme of altering their current pattern of interaction was followed up in the second marital session, which again began with the W.'s being depressed and anxious about the employment issue. From an emphasis on how each could be supportive of the other, the concern that emerged was their desire for more appreciation. "Appreciation notes," as described earlier, were introduced at this time. For practice, each one wrote an appreciation note in the session, to which they giggled and blushed, and they obviously were pleased. To avoid the possibility of forgetting to write these notes during the week, each spouse was to take responsibility to remind the partner if, by 8:00 P.M., she or he had not yet received a note. Such prompting proved unnecessary, however, because the couple enthusiastically embraced this procedure. They expressed appreciation for help with the children and with household maintenance as well as for something that they laughingly said: "Not even our therapist can know about!"

The next step was the introduction of "considerations." Based on SOC data that had been collected, each spouse met with the therapist to plan a special consideration during the week. Doris decided to prepare David's favorite meal one day when the children were not around, whereas David chose to take Doris out to lunch, complete with corsage. This couple continued, and in fact, improvised on these interventions over the next several weeks with minimal prompting from the therapist.

Simultaneous to working at home on the overall emotional tone of the relationship, the in-session work moved toward communication training. Their current strategy for coping with their communication was that Doris would withdraw "to avoid David's blowups," and David then would nag her to talk to him. Both readily acknowledged that they felt stuck in this pattern but also took some pride in what a "challenge" they would be for the therapist.

Communication training began by having the couple read the Jacobson and Margolin (1979) problem-solving manual at home and by viewing demonstration videotapes in the session, both of which were discussed in detail in the therapy session. Having observed but not directly practiced these skills, the couple were assigned a reflection exercise for homework. Spouses were to alternate, in 5-minute blocks, between listener and speaker roles with the speaker's choosing a relatively neutral topic (i.e., the contents of her or his day). The speaker was to go no longer than two sentences before pausing to allow the listener to reflect back what was said. Although both spouses agreed to the assignment, making this assignment without direct practice, coaching, and feedback was a mistake. This couple's familiar pattern interfered with homework completion. Doris withdrew from opportunities to do the assignment, and David nagged. Recognizing that the exercise had been assigned prematurely, the therapist decided to work on the skills in the therapy session. The couple agreed a second time to practice this exercise at home but again failed to complete the assignment. Moreover, they missed the next three therapy sessions.

At this point, the therapeutic question was whether to pursue an emotionally oriented approach to communication training or to focus on making more behaviorally oriented changes. Because this couple had responded well to action-oriented approaches, the decision was to introduce behavioral contracting.

David and Doris were asked to identify a specific, but not major, problem they currently were facing. Quickly, they identified a project they had been avoiding for quite some time—rearranging the children's bedroom. Through problem identification and brainstorming, the couple identified the steps needed to complete the project as well as ways they could incorporate fun and playfulness into the task. A detailed contract titled *Project Bunkbed* was drawn up which specified (a) the date and time of the project; (b) the duties of each; (c) permission for working topless and for "free grabs"; and (d) reinforcement for themselves contingent on completion of the job. This contract was successful and motivated them for subsequent contracts, the most important of which was the Sunday Night Planning Contract, in which they agreed to sit down and plan for the upcoming week. In addition to introducing a systematic weekly discussion, this contract provided the couple with a much needed structure and routine in their daily interactions.

Verbal communication, however, continued to be a source of disgruntlement and discouragement. David complained of Doris's tendency to withdraw whenever they argued or discussed anything emotional, and Doris complained of David's tendency to nag her to talk. Clearly, the couple's lack of skills in this area interfered with their being able to resolve long-range problems. It seemed, however, that both were invested in maintaining the appearance of Doris's being inadequate relative to David in communication abilities. In examining the couple's resistance to improving their communication, the issue of power emerged as a possible key.

From what was known from the relationship history and from impressions gathered during the course of therapy, both David and Doris held very traditional values. They considered men to be the heads of households and the providers and protectors of women. In fact, the roles they played in their own relationship from its onset were in accordance with these views. At this time, however, David was unemployed and experienced himself as inadequate in his masculine role. Meanwhile, Doris was becoming increasingly competent in her management of household tasks and of the children. Their established system seemed to be experiencing transition and consequent stress. Competence in communication was the most salient skill that David continued to hold over Doris, and, on overt level, this may have symbolized that David maintained control in the relationship. However, on a covert level, what was occurring was that neither spouse experienced much power. David's attempts to bring out Doris appeared forceful and directive, yet they were ineffective as evidenced by Doris's nonreinforcing response of withdrawal. Doris's withdrawal managed to get David to attend to her, yet the eventual consequence of this pattern was fighting, which she found aversive.

This conceptualization of the couple's dilemma led to the intervention goal of making it safe for both spouses to increase their power and effectiveness while not disrupting the traditional role structure with which they were comfortable. Each spouse was challenged to temporarily give up some of their current, albeit ineffective, power in the hope of gaining increased power in the long run. The therapist met individually with each spouse to explain their separate roles. For David, the specific challenge was to give up his current power of being *the only* competent communicator. He was to stop initiating conversations with Doris and to wait for her to come to him. This strategy was in line with his ultimate goal of promoting more effective communication overall. For Doris, the specific challenge was to get David to stop nagging her by taking the initiative and approaching David herself. Both were somewhat perplexed by the challenge but agreed to try it out for 1 week as an experiment.

In response to this therapeutic task, Doris actually did initiate discussion on more than one occasion, whereas David restrained himself from bringing up major issues. Both spouses were intrigued with this "experiment" and agreed to repeat it the following week.

From then on, the W.'s were more receptive to trying out a variety of communication exercises. The predominant format was for the spouses to take turns initiating and discussing issues while the other paraphrased what she or he had heard. Through videotape playback, each spouse critiqued his or her own performance, identifying desirable behaviors as well as behaviors to change. This time, the spouses did follow through at home practicing what they learned in the session. Eventually, these general communication skills were combined with the contracting format to negotiate several more difficult topics. As they approached their final treatment session in this time-limited therapy, the W.'s negotiated an End of Therapy contract in which they specified that, on their own, they would continue (a) keeping up the children's charts regarding chores; (b) using time-out for tantrums; (c) expressing appreciation verbally or in writing; (d) giving "considerations"; (e) planning weekly activities and dates; and (f) working on communication through Doris's initiating discussions, David's listening and not dominating, and both using their new listening skills.

Case Critique

The time-limited 12-week marital therapy ended with both spouses verbalizing increased satisfaction with their relationship. They had recaptured some of their original enjoyment of one another and exercised more control over the direction that the marriage was heading toward as well as the management of their children. No longer were they locked into the rigid communication pattern in which (a) David overwhelmed and actually drove Doris away, thinking that was the only way to get anything accomplished; and (b) Doris automatically retreated from David, thinking that was her only protection. The change in this pattern did not result from an intellectual understanding of this interaction but from their willingness to follow the therapist's injunction simply to try something new.

Certain characteristics of this couple made their treatment go more smoothly. Probably their most important strength was their basic attraction for one another, which was revived with relative ease. Likewise, their basic desire for the relationship to continue facilitated treatment. Third, these spouses did, in fact, exhibit skills deficits, which are easier to treat than certain other problems, such as a lack of motivation.

On the other hand, what complicated treatment was the individual problems experienced by each spouse. Although Doris showed much improvement, she continued to suffer from drug dependency and depression. David's disappointment over his unemployment was exacerbated by the personal standards he held for achievement coupled with his reluctance to reveal his vulnerabilities to Doris. Had therapy not been time limited, it would have been helpful for this couple to work on accepting their own and one another's strengths and vulnerabilities. One step in this regard would be to examine how this couple's traditional sex role values affected their personal self-esteem as well as the relationship.

As it turned out, concerns over David's continued unemployment prompted an additional therapy session 2 months after the formal termination of therapy. With little help from the therapist, the couple verbalized some of their insecurities and doubts to each other. David considered whether leaving the household would help the family by enabling them to be eligible for welfare assistance. Doris wondered whether David's desperate concerns over money would lead him to abandon the family. Through a remarkably clear expression of feelings by this couple, it became apparent that neither spouse wanted to leave the relationship and that they truly cared for one another. In essence, they used this opportunity to renew their commitment to each other.

The data on this case portray a couple that has made substantial relationship changes. As seen in the overview in Table 1, marital satisfaction measures, which remained unchanged during the child intervention, show improvement concurrent with the marital intervention. Postmarital treatment DAS scores are borderline between the distressed and nondistressed range, whereas the AC score is now well within the nondistressed range. In other words, there was a substantial reduction in their number of specific complaints. The child measures, which improved during the child treatment, either maintained or showed more improvement during marital treatment.

Table 1. Questionnaire Data for Case Example

Measurements	Pretreatment	Postfamily treatment	Postmarital treatment
Marital			
DAS	80.5	74.5	96.5
AC	41.0	39.0	9.0
Child			
CBC—Bob	71.0	64.0	62.0
BAC—Bob	42.0	28.5	28.5
CBC—Betty	64.0	62.5	56.2
BAC—Betty	−14.5	−11.0	−16.0

Note. DAS = Dyadic Adjustment Scale; AC = Areas of Change Questionnaire; CBC = Child Behavior Checklist (Externalizing Scale); BAC = Becker Adjective Checklist. All scores are the average for husband and wife except for the AC, which is the husband–wife total. Higher scores indicate greater distress, except on the DAS for which a higher score indicates higher marital satisfaction. Cutoff scores for distress are as follows: <97 on the DAS; >14 on the AC; >60 on the CBC; and >20 on the BAC.

Summary

This chapter has been written to illustrate the complexities involved in carrying out marital therapy. First, there are a variety of definitional issues surrounding the identification of marital problems and the decision about whether marital therapy is the treatment of choice. Second, assessment is complicated by the multiple dimensions of marital relationships, with individual as well as relationship variables to be considered. Third, treatment procedures were described for three levels of interaction—moment-to-moment, daily, and long-term exchanges. Decisions about the implementation and continuation of any particular intervention with any one couple can be made on the basis of a hypothesis-testing approach. As seen in the case example, considerable flexibility is exercised in using these procedures, with feedback from one intervention being the basis for making the next decision. To progress from case-by-case decision making to more general recommendations, we need to collect systematic information on what couples respond to what treatment. The match between types of interventions and client characteristics is the issue to which we must direct future attention.

References

Baucom, D. H. (1983). Conceptual and psychometric issues in evaluating the effectiveness in behavioral marital therapy. In J. P. Vincent (Ed.), *Advances in family intervention, assessment and theory: An annual compilation of research* (Vol. 3). Greenwich, CT: JAI Press.

Baucom, D. H., & Mehlman, S. K. (1984). Predicting marital states following behavioral marital therapy: A comparison of models of marital relationships. In K. Hahlweg & N. S. Jacobson (Eds.), *Marital interaction: Analysis and modification.* New York: Guilford Press.

Becvar, R. J., Becvar, D. S., & Bender, A. E. (1982). Let us do no harm. *Journal of Marital and Family Therapy, 8,* 385–392.

Bennum, I., Margolin, G., & Christensen, A. (1983, December). *The treatment targets of behavioral marital therapy: Application to specific populations.* Paper presented at the 17th Annual Convention of the Association for the Advancement of Behavior Therapy, Washington, DC.

Betcher, R. W. (1981). Intimate play and marital adaptation. *Psychiatry, 44,* 13–33.

Bloom, B. L., Asher, S. J., & White, S. W. (1978). Marital disruption as a stressor: A review and analysis. *Psychological Bulletin, 85,* 867–894.

Christensen, A., & Margolin, G. (1981, August). *Correlational and sequential analysis of marital and child problems.* Paper presented at the American Psychological Association Convention, Los Angeles.

Divorce American Style. (1983, January 10). *Newsweek,* pp. 42–48.

Doherty, W. T. (1981a). Cognitive processes in intimate conflict: I. Extending attribution theory. *American Journal of Family Therapy, 9*(1), 3–12.

Doherty, W. J. (1981b). Cognitive processes in intimate conflict: II. Efficacy and learned helplessness. *American Journal of Family Therapy, 9*(2), 35–44.

Duck, S. (1984). A perspective on the repair of personal relationships. In S. Duck (Ed.), *Personal relationships 5: Repairing personal relationships.* New York: Academic Press.

Emery, R. E. (1982). Interparental conflict and the children of discord and divorce. *Psychological Bulletin, 92,* 310–330.

Epstein, N. (1982). Cognitive therapy with couples. *American Journal of Family Therapy, 10,* 5–16.

Filsinger, E. E. (Ed.). (1983). *Marriage and family assessment.* Beverly Hills: Sage.

Goldfried, M. R. (1977). Behavioral assessment in perspective. In J. D. Cone & R. P. Hawkins (Eds.), *Behavioral assessment: New directions in clinical psychology.* New York: Brunner/Mazel.

Gottman, J. M. (1979). *Marital interaction: Experimental investigations.* New York: Academic Press.

Gottman, J., Notarius, C., Markman, H., Banks, S., Yoppi, B., & Rubin, M. E. (1976). Behavior exchange theory and marital decision making. *Journal of Personality and Social Psychology, 34,* 14–23.

Gove, W. R., Hughes, M., & Style, C. B. (1983). Does marriage have positive effects on the psychological well-being of the individual? *Journal of Health and Social Behavior, 27,* 122–131.

Gurin, E., Veroff, J., & Feld, S. (1960). *Americans view their mental health.* New York: Basic Books.

Gurman, A. S., & Klein, M. H. (1980). Marital and family conflicts. In A. M. Brodsky & R. T. Hare-Mustin (Eds.), *Women and psychotherapy: An assessment of research and practice.* New York: Guilford Press.

Gurman, A. S., & Klein, M. H. (1983). Marriage and the family: An unconscious bias in behavioral treatment? In E. A. Blechman (Ed.), *Behavior modification with women.* New York: Guilford Press.

Harris, M. (1981, December 23). Growing conservatism? Not in family patterns. *Los Angeles Times,* part II, p. 5.

Hicks, M. W., & Platt, M. (1970). Marital happiness and stability: a review of the research in the sixties. *Journal of Marriage and the Family, 32,* 553–574.

Hops, H., Wills, T. A., Patterson, G. R., & Weiss, R. L. (1972). *Marital Interaction Coding System.* Unpublished manuscript, University of Oregon and Oregon Research Institute.

Jacobson, N. S. (1977). Training couples to solve their marital problems: A behavioral approach to relationship discord. Part II: Intervention strategies. *International Journal of Family Counseling, 5*(2), 20–28.

Jacobson, N. S. (1981). Behavioral marital therapy. In A. S. Gurman & D. P. Kniskern (Eds.), *Handbook of family therapy.* New York: Brunner/Mazel.

Jacobson, N. S. (1983a). Beyond empiricism: The politics of marital therapy. *American Journal of Family Therapy, 11,* 11–24.

Jacobson, N. S. (1983b). Expanding the range and applicability of behavioral marital therapy. *Behavior Therapist, 6,* 189–191.

Jacobson, N. S. (1983c). Clinical innovations in behavioral marital therapy. In K. Craig & D. McMahon (Eds.), *Advances in clinical behavior therapy.* New York: Brunner/Mazel.

Jacobson, N. S., & Margolin, G. (1979). *Marital therapy: Strategies based on social learning and behavior exchange principles.* New York: Brunner/Mazel.

Jacobson, N. S., & Moore, D. (1981). Behavior exchange theory of marriage: Reconnaisance and reconsideration. In J. P. Vincent (Ed.), *Advances in family intervention, assessment and theory: A research annual* (II). Greenwich, CT: JAI Press.

Jacobson, N. S., Elwood, R., & Dallas, M. (1981). The behavioral assessment of marital dysfunction. In D. H. Barlow (Ed.), *Behavioral assessment of adult disorders.* New York: Guilford Press.

Jacobson, N. S., Follette, W. C., & Elwood, R. W. (1984). Outcome research on behavioral marital therapy: A methodological and conceptual reappraisal. In K. Hahlweg & N. S. Jacobson (Eds.), *Marital interaction: Analysis and modification.* New York: Guilford Press.

Jacobson, N. S., Berley, R., Newport, K., Elwood, R., & Phelps, C. (in press). Failure in behavioral marital therapy. In S. Colemen (Ed.), *Failure in family therapy.* New York: Guilford Press.

Jacobson, N. S., Follette, W. C., Baucom, D. H., Hahlweg, K., & Margolin, G. (1984). Variability in outcome and clinical significance of behavioral marital therapy: A reanalysis of outcome data. *Journal of Consulting and Clinical Psychology, 52,* 497–509.

Levinger, G. (1983). Development and change. In H. H. Kelley, E. Berscheid, A. Christensen, J. H. Harvey, T. L. Huston, G. Levinger, E. McClintock, L. A. Peplou, & D. R. Peterson (Eds.), *Close relationships.* San Francisco: W. H. Freeman.

Libermann, R. P., Wheeler, E. G., de Visser, L. A., Kuehnel, J., & Kuehnel, T. (1980). *Handbook of marital therapy.* New York: Plenum Press.

Liberman, R. P., Wheeler, E. G., & Kuehnel, J. M. (1983). Failures in behavioral marital therapy. In E. B. Foa & P. M. G. Emmelkamp (Eds.), *Failures in behavior therapy* (pp. 378–391). New York: Wiley.

Locke, H. J., & Wallace, K. M. (1959). Short-term marital adjustment and prediction tests: Their reliability and validity. *Journal of Marriage and Family Living, 21,* 251–255.

Margolin, G. (1981a). A behavioral-systems approach to the treatment of marital jealousy. *Clinical Psychology Review, 1,* 469–487.

Margolin, G. (1981b). The reciprocal relationship between marital and child problems. In J. P. Vincent (Ed.), *Advances in family intervention, assessment and theory: An annual compilation of research* (Vol. 2). Greenwich, CT: JAI Press.

Margolin, G. (1983a). Behavioral marital therapy. In B. B. Wolman & G. Stricker (Eds.), *Handbook of family and marital therapy*. New York: Plenum Press.

Margolin G. (1983b). Behavioral marital therapy: Is there a place for passion, play, and other non-negotiable dimensions? *Behavior Therapist, 6,* 65–68.

Margolin, G. (1983c). An interactional model for the assessment of marital relationships. *Behavioral Assessment, 5,* 103–127.

Margolin, G. (in press). Building marital trust and treating sexual problems. In A. S. Gurman (Ed.), *Casebook of marital therapy*. New York: Guilford Press.

Margolin, G., & Jacobson, N. S. (1981). The assessment of marital dysfunction. In M. Hersen & A. S. Bellack (Eds.), *Behavioral assessment: A practical handbook*. New York: Pergamon Press.

Margolin, G., & Weinstein, C. D. (1983). The role of affect in behavioral marital therapy. In M. L. Aronson & L. R. Wolberg (Eds.), *Group and family therapy 1982: An overview*. New York: Brunner/Mazel.

Margolin, G., Talovic, S., Fernandez, V., & Onorato, R. (1983). Sex role considerations and behavioral marital therapy: Equal does not mean identical. *Journal of Marital and Family Therapy, 9,* 131–146.

Margolin, G., Hattem, D. John, R. S., & Yost, K. (in press). Perceptual agreement between spouses and outside observers when coding themselves and a stranger dyad. *Behavioral Assessment.*

Markman, H. J. (1979). Application of a behavioral model of marriage in predicting relationship satisfaction of couples planning marriage. *Journal of Consulting and Clinical Psychology, 47,* 743–749.

Markman, H. J. (1981). Prediction of marital distress: A 5-year follow-up. *Journal of Consulting and Clinical Psychology, 49,* 760–762.

Martin, P. A. (1976). *A marital therapy manual*. New York: Brunner/Mazel.

Overall, J. E., Henry, B. W., & Woodward, A. (1974). Dependence of marital problems on parental family history. *Journal of Abnormal Psychology, 83,* 446–450.

Peterson, D. R. (1977). A plan for studying interpersonal behavior. In D. Magnusson & N. Endler (Eds.), *Personality at the crossroads: Current issues in interactional psychology*. New York: Wiley.

Peterson, D. R. (1979). Assessing interpersonal relationships by means of interaction records. *Behavioral Assessment, 1,* 221–236.

Peterson, L. (1983, May–June). Marriage and divorce rates continue increase. *Family Therapy News*, p. 16.

Rappaport, A. F., & Harrell, J. (1972). A behavioral exchange model for marital counseling. *Family Coordinator, 22,* 203–212.

Revenstorf, D. (1984). The role of attribution of marital distress in therapy. In K. Hahlweg & N. S. Jacobson (Eds.), *Marital interaction: Analysis and modification*. New York: Guilford Press.

Sager, C. (1976). *Marriage contracts and couple therapy: Hidden forces in intimate relationships*. New York: Brunner/Mazel.

Segraves, R. T. (1982). *Marital therapy: A combined psychodynamic-behavioral approach*. New York: Plenum Press.

Snyder, D. K., & Regts, J. M. (1982). Factor scales for assessing marital disharmony and disaffection. *Journal of Consulting and Clinical Psychology, 50,* 615–623.

Snyder, D. K., Wills, R. M., & Keiser, T. W. (1981). Empirical validation of the Marital Satisfaction Inventory: An actuarial approach. *Journal of Consulting and Clinical Psychology, 49,* 262–268.

Spanier, G. B. (1976). Measuring dyadic adjustment: New scales for assessing the quality of marriage and similar dyads. *Journal of Marriage and the Family, 38,* 15–28.

Stuart, R. B. (1969). Operant interpersonal treatment of marital discord. *Journal of Consulting and Clinical Psychology, 33,* 675–682.

Stuart, R. B. (1975). Behavioral remedies for marital ills: A guide to the use of operant-interpersonal techniques. In A. S. Gurman & D. G. Rice (Eds.), *Couples in conflict: New directions in marital therapy*. New York: Aronson.

Stuart, R. B. (1980). *Helping couples change: A social learning approach to marital therapy*. New York: Guilford Press.

Watzlawick, P., Weakland, J., & Fisch, R. (1974). *Change: Principles of problem formation and problem resolution*. New York: W. W. Norton.

Weiss, R. L. (1980). Strategic behavioral marital therapy: Toward a model for assessment and intervention. In J. P. Vincent (Ed.), *Advances in family intervention, assessment, and theory: An annual compilation of research* (Vol. 1). Greenwich, CT: JAI Press.

Weiss, R. L. (1984a). Cognitive and behavioral measures of marital interaction. In N. S. Jacobson & K. Hahlweg (Eds.), *Marital interaction: Analysis and modification*. New York: Guilford Press.

Weiss, R. L. (1984b). Cognitive and strategic interventions in behavioral marital therapy. In K. Hahlweg & N. S. Jacobson (Eds.), *Marital interaction: Analysis and modification.* New York: Guilford Press.

Weiss, R. L., & Aved, B. M. (1978). Marital satisfaction and depression as predictors of physical health status. *Journal of Consulting and Clinical Psychology, 46,* 1370–1384.

Weiss, R. L., & Cerreto, M. C. (1980). The Marital Status Inventory: Development of a measure of dissolution potential. *American Journal of Family Therapy, 8,* 80–85.

Weiss, R. L., & Margolin, G. (in press). Assessment of conflict and accord: A second look. In A. Ciminero (Ed.), *Handbook of behavioral assessment* (Vol. 2). New York: Wiley.

Weiss, R. L., & Perry, B. A. (1979). *Assessment and treatment of marital dysfunction.* Eugene: University of Oregon and Oregon Marital Studies Program.

Weiss, R. L., Hops, H., & Patterson, G. R. (1973). A framework for conceptualizing marital conflict, a technology for altering it, some data for evaluating it. In L. A. Hamerlynck, L. C. Handy, & E. J. Mash (Eds.), *Behavior change: Methodology, concepts, and practice.* Champaign, IL: Research Press.

Wile, D. B. (1981). *Couples therapy: A nontraditional approach.* New York: Wiley.

Index